# Tumors of the Heart and Great Vessels

## AFIP Atlas
## of
## Tumor Pathology

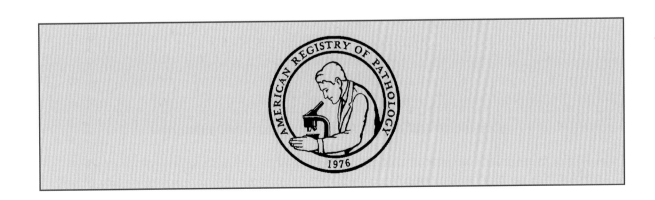

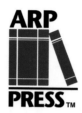

# *ARP PRESS*

*Silver Spring, Maryland*

Editorial Director:  Mirlinda Q. Caton
Production Editor:  Dian S. Thomas
Editorial Assistant:  Magdalena C. Silva
Editorial Assistant:  Alana N. Black
Copyeditor:  Audrey Kahn

Available from the American Registry of Pathology
Silver Spring, Maryland 20910
www.arppress.org
ISBN 1-933477-33-4
978-1-933477-33-6

# AFIP ATLAS OF TUMOR PATHOLOGY

Fourth Series
Fascicle 22

# TUMORS OF THE HEART AND GREAT VESSELS

by

**Allen Burke, MD**

Professor of Pathology
University of Maryland School of Medicine
Baltimore, Maryland


**Fabio R. Tavora, MD, PhD**

Associate Medical Director, Argos Laboratory
Head, Surgical Pathology
Messejana Heart and Lung Hospital
Fortaleza, CE, Brazil

**Joseph J. Maleszewski, MD**
Associate Professor of Laboratory Medicine and Pathology
Associate Professor of Medicine
Mayo Clinic
Rochester, Minnesota


**Aletta Ann Frazier, MD**
Chief, Cardiovascular Imaging
American Institute for Radiologic Pathology
Clinical Associate Professor of Diagnostic Radiology
University of Maryland School of Medicine
Baltimore, Maryland

Published by the
*American Registry of Pathology*
Silver Spring, Maryland
2015

# AFIP ATLAS OF TUMOR PATHOLOGY

**EDITOR**
**Steven G. Silverberg, MD**
Department of Pathology
University of Maryland School of Medicine
Baltimore, Maryland

**ASSOCIATE EDITOR**
**Ronald A. DeLellis, MD**
Warren Alpert Medical School
of Brown University
Providence, Rhode Island

**ASSOCIATE EDITOR**
**Leslie H. Sobin, MD**
Armed Forces Institute of Pathology
Washington, DC

## EDITORIAL ADVISORY BOARD

*Manuscript reviewed by:*
Ronald A. DeLellis, MD
E. Rene Rodriguez, MD
Anonymous Reviewer

# EDITORS' NOTE

The Atlas of Tumor Pathology has a long and distinguished history. It was first conceived at a cancer research meeting held in St. Louis in September 1947, as an attempt to standardize the nomenclature of neoplastic diseases. The first series was sponsored by the National Academy of Sciences-National Research Council. The organization of this formidable effort was entrusted to the Subcommittee on Oncology of the Committee on Pathology, and Dr. Arthur Purdy Stout was the first editor-in-chief. Many of the illustrations were provided by the Medical Illustration Service of the Armed Forces Institute of Pathology (AFIP), the type was set by the Government Printing Office, and the final printing was done at the Armed Forces Institute of Pathology. The American Registry of Pathology (ARP) purchased the Fascicles from the Government Printing Office and sold them virtually at cost. Over a period of 20 years, approximately 15,000 copies each of nearly 40 Fascicles were produced. The worldwide impact of these publications over the years has largely surpassed the original goal. They quickly became among the most influential publications on tumor pathology, primarily because of their overall high quality, but also because their low cost made them easily accessible the world over to pathologists and other students of oncology.

Upon completion of the first series, the National Academy of Sciences-National Research Council handed further pursuit of the project over to the newly created Universities Associated for Research and Education in Pathology (UAREP). A second series was started, generously supported by grants from the AFIP, the National Cancer Institute, and the American Cancer Society. Dr. Harlan I. Firminger became the editor-in-chief and was succeeded by Dr. William H. Hartmann. The second series' Fascicles were produced as bound volumes instead of loose leaflets. They featured a more comprehensive coverage of the subjects, to the extent that the Fascicles could no longer be regarded as "atlases" but rather as monographs describing and illustrating in detail the tumors and tumor-like conditions of the various organs and systems.

Once the second series was completed, with a success that matched that of the first, ARP, UAREP, and AFIP decided to embark on a third series. Dr. Juan Rosai was appointed as editor-in-chief, and Dr. Leslie Sobin became associate editor. A distinguished Editorial Advisory Board was also convened, and these outstanding pathologists and educators played a major role in the success of this series, the first publication of which appeared in 1991 and the last (number 32) in 2003.

The same organizational framework applies to the current fourth series, but with UAREP and AFIP no longer functioning, ARP is now the responsible organization. New features include a hardbound cover and illustrations almost exclusively in color. There is also an increased emphasis on the cytopathologic (intraoperative, exfoliative, or fine needle aspiration) and molecular features that are important in diagnosis and prognosis. What does not change from the three previous series, however, is the goal of providing the practicing pathologist with thorough, concise, and up-to-date information on the nomenclature and classification; epidemiologic, clinical, and pathogenetic features; and, most importantly, guidance in the diagnosis of the tumors and tumorlike lesions of all major organ systems and body sites.

As in the third series, a continuous attempt is made to correlate, whenever possible, the nomenclature used in the Fascicles with that proposed by the World Health Organization's Classification of Tumors, as well as to ensure a consistency of style. Close cooperation between the various authors and their respective liaisons from the Editorial Board will continue to be emphasized in order to minimize unnecessary repetition and discrepancies in the text and illustrations.

Particular thanks are due to the members of the Editorial Advisory Board, the reviewers, the editorial and production staff, and the individual Fascicle authors for their ongoing efforts to ensure that this series is a worthy successor to the previous three.

Steven G. Silverberg, MD
Ronald A. DeLellis, MD
Leslie H. Sobin, MD

# PREFACE

Since the publication of the Third Series atlas on heart tumors over a decade ago, there have been several changes in the pathology and classification of these lesions. The current edition updates the status of heart tumors, with emphasis on newer findings, especially molecular advances. Because heart tumors are rare, most data are derived from single case reports, short series, or larger institutional series with emphasis on clinical data. There is a persistent need to standardize terminology for both benign and malignant lesions, as we interpret newer molecular data in light of morphology. In most cases, we have followed the classification of the World Health Organization, whose updated volume on tumors of the lung, heart, and mediastinum is forthcoming. Because newer imaging modalities, especially cardiac magnetic resonance imaging and 3-D echocardiography, are increasingly utilized in preoperative evaluation of heart tumors, we have introduced a chapter devoted exclusively to radiologic diagnosis.

Most heart tumors can be broadly grouped into congenital and acquired forms. Congenital tumors, such as cardiac rhabdomyoma, histiocytoid cardiomyopathy and cardiac fibroma, are unique to the heart and often are associated with specific genetic causes. Little has changed regarding the histologic diagnosis of these lesions. Contemporary research has therefore focused on earlier detection, especially prenatal diagnosis, and molecular characterization. In the case of cardiac rhabdomyoma, mutations in *TSC1* and *TSC2* have been firmly established, whereas the molecular basis for histiocytoid cardiomyopathy (which is much rarer) is far from clear.

Acquired heart tumors encompass a diverse group of neoplastic and non-neoplastic lesions. Like their congenital counterparts, little has changed with respect to histomorphologic diagnosis. However, isolated diagnostically useful reports have been put forth, such as curious collision tumors or associated conditions (e.g., cardiac myxoma and lymphoma). Molecular aspects of acquired tumors such as cardiac myxoma are also increasingly explored, specifically the role that *PRKAR1A* plays in syndromic and non-syndromic types.

Tumors of valves are generally benign, and the more routine use of echocardiography and valve surgery has led to the emergence of papillary fibroelastoma as the most commonly excised heart tumor. A less common tumor of heart valves, inflammatory myofibroblastic tumor, is covered quite differently from the previous volume, since several reports and series of this childhood tumor have emerged.

This atlas has carried over a discussion of lesions that are neither neoplastic nor hamartomatous, such as thrombi and some infections that can mimic tumors. We have decided to keep this section because some of these lesions, especially thrombi, are among the more commonly excised heart masses, and may present diagnostic challenge.

Rare processes that overlap, and are still of unclear classification, include hamartomas of mature cardiac myocytes, hamartomas of valves, some unencapsulated lipomatous tumors, hemangioma-like tumors, and miscellaneous unclassified benign lesions of various tissue types. In this volume we update the classification of these lesions, which are often published as case reports with little pathologic description.

The chapters on cardiac sarcomas presented the authors with the most difficult task. There is ongoing debate among soft tissue pathologists regarding new labels for those tumors that were previously diagnosed as malignant fibrous histiocytoma (MFH), leading to difficulties in classification of these tumors in the heart. Furthermore, if and how pleomorphic spindle cell sarcomas are related to intimal sarcomas of the great arteries (namely pulmonary arteries), remains controversial.

We believe that this work would be a useful source for physicians who wish to find a reference to classify a tumor, or update their knowledge of these lesions.

**Allen Burke, MD**
**Fabio R. Tavora, MD, PhD**
**Joseph J. Maleszewski, MD**
**Aletta Ann Frazier, MD**

# ACKNOWLEDGMENTS

Among the numerous individuals who have contributed to this latest volume, we would like to thank our families for their unrelenting support, and the editorial efforts of Katie Warfield, Mirlinda Caton, and the staff at the American Registry of Pathology. We would also like to thank Dr. William D. Edwards for his critical review of work as well as images and material that he has painstakingly collected over his career. Finally, we would like to thank Dr. Adina Paulk, whose detailed and critical review of the manuscript was indispensable in the final hectic days of the revisions and corrections.

**Allen Burke, MD**
**Fabio R. Tavora, MD, PhD**
**Joseph J. Maleszewski, MD**
**Aletta Ann Frazier, MD**

# CONTENTS

# 1 ANATOMY OF THE HEART AND BLOOD VESSELS

A fundamental knowledge of cardiac anatomy provides a concrete foundation for diagnostic cardiovascular pathology and is requisite for understanding the clinical manifestations of cardiac disease. In this introductory chapter, the anatomy of the heart and blood vessels is presented, with special emphasis on development, gross structure, and histology to allow for a complete understanding of the tumors and tumor-like conditions described in this Fascicle.

## CARDIAC EMBRYOLOGY

### Formation of the Heart Tube

Approximately 2 weeks after fertilization, a crescentic zone of thickened mesoderm, the precursor of the heart and pericardium, appears adjacent to the margin of the embryonic disc (1). A day or two later, this thickened zone of mesoderm splits into somatic and splanchnic layers, which surround the pericardial portion of the coelomic cavity, or pericardial coelom. Endothelial tubes (cardiac primordial) form as paired, lateral structures from the splanchnic mesodermal layer of the primitive pericardial cavity where it lies close against the developing foregut. By the third week, the endocardial tubes have fused in the midline, forming the primitive heart tube, consisting of three basic layers: the endocardial layer, intervening cardiac "jelly," and a mesothelial layer lining the pericardial coelom. The heart tube has arterial and venous poles at the cranial and caudal aspects, respectively, and begins to beat.

### Looping of the Heart Tube and Septation

Rapid bulboventricular growth of the tube, which is tethered to the dorsal aspect of the embryo and contained within the pericardial cavity, causes an anterior and rightward displacement of the primitive ventricular portion and a posterior displacement of its primitive atrial and venous portions. During this time, endocardial cushion tissue, or primitive connective tissue, begins to invade the cardiac jelly lying between the endodermal and mesothelial layers (2).

Over the ensuing weeks, this heart tube will form, through active and passive mechanisms, seven distinct septa. These divide it into a four-chamber structure with two pairs of valves, two large arteries, and typically six distinct venous connections.

It follows from this brief overview that the heart and pericardium are derived entirely from mesodermal structures. All primary tumors of the heart and pericardium are also of mesodermal origin. Cardiac tumors can also primarily consist of mesodermal elements, such as fat, that become entrapped during the process of septation.

The exceptions consist of tumors of misplaced endodermal rests, and neural tumors, which are of ectodermal origin. Cardiac tumors with endodermal elements, such as glandular structures present in bronchogenic cysts, tumors of the atrioventricular (AV) node, are presumed to arise from embryologically misplaced tissues (3). Theoretically, endodermal structures could be incorporated into cardiac tissue early in embryogenesis when the foregut is adjacent to the laterally placed cardiogenic plates (4). Neural tumors of the heart are rare and are virtually limited to paragangliomas and granular cell tumors of the epicardial surfaces and atria.

The histogenesis of some cardiac tumors, such as cardiac myxoma, remains somewhat controversial. The cardiac jelly, which supports the epimyocardial layer and endothelial layer, is present from before 2 weeks of gestation (four-somite embryo), and becomes infiltrated from the endothelial surface by endocardial cushion cells (2). These cells are the putative cells of origin of cardiac myxoma, and are believed to persist in some adults near the fossa ovalis (5). The rare occurrence of glandular structures within cardiac myxoma is an incidental curiosity for the surgical pathologist, who should not

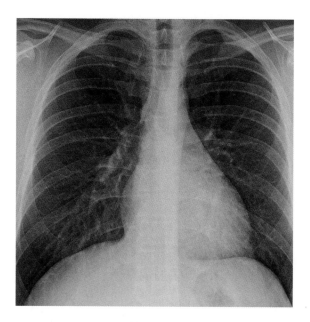

**Figure 1-1**

**CARDIAC SILHOUETTE**

The size of the heart, in relation to the thorax, is demonstrated here on chest radiograph. The heart occupies less than 60 percent of the thorax in this view.

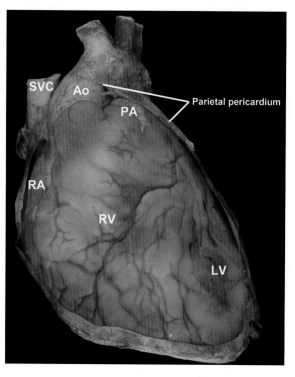

**Figure 1-2**

**PARIETAL PERICARDIUM**

With the anterior aspect of the parietal pericardium removed, the intrapericardial portions of the superior vena cava, aorta, and pulmonary artery are apparent.

mistake them for adenocarcinoma. It is difficult, however, to satisfactorily explain their presence from an embryologic view. In some cases, glandular cells appear to evolve from myxoma cells, casting doubt on the theory that they arise from entrapped endodermal rests (6). It is also possible that cardiac myxoma is a true neoplasm of pluripotent mesodermal cells (endocardial cushion cells) and that the neoplastic alteration is capable of inciting these cells, which are of mesodermal origin, to form mucin-producing glands.

## ANATOMY OF THE HEART AND GREAT VESSELS

### Cardiac Position

Consistent with their embryonic origins as midline structures, the heart and great vessels are situated in the mid-thorax, within the mediastinum. The heart, aortic arch, and descending thoracic aorta are located in the middle, superior, and posterior regions, respectively. Radiologically, the heart occupies less than 60 percent of the thorax when viewed on a posteroanterior chest radiograph (fig. 1-1). The heart is a four-chambered, roughly conical structure, with the atria forming the base and the ventricles forming the apex, which is typically directed leftward, anterior, and inferior.

### External Cardiac Anatomy

The heart is covered and surrounded by the fluid-containing pericardial sac, which consists of both visceral and parietal portions. The visceral pericardium, or epicardium, covers the heart and intrapericardial portions of the great vessels, while the parietal pericardium surrounds the heart, attaching along the great vessels at the reflection of the visceral layer (fig.1-2). The space between these two layers contains serous pericardial fluid (25 mL or less in adults) providing for friction-free movement within the chest.

The AV groove is found at the plane of the base of the heart and contains the circumflex and right coronary arteries, which travel in the left and right AV grooves, respectively. The anterior and inferior interventricular grooves are found at the plane of the ventricular septum and contain the anterior and posterior descending coronary arteries, respectively.

The anterior and inferior free walls of the right ventricle intersect to form the acute margin. The rounded lateral wall of the left ventricle forms a more ill-defined obtuse margin. Vessels supplying these regions are named accordingly; obtuse marginal branches have the circumflex coronary artery and acute marginal branches of the right coronary artery. The intersection of the major lines of division (atrioventricular, interventricular, and interatrial) is along the diaphragmatic surface of the heart and is referred to as the crux of the heart.

Tumor location within the heart is relevant to not only its potential hemodynamic consequences, but also often provides insights into the type of tumor (since certain cardiac tumors tend to have predilections for various locations within the heart). Thus, an understanding of not only the normal size and shape of the cardiac chambers and great vessels, but also their relative positions three dimensionally, is required (fig. 1-3). The right atrium forms the right lateral border of the heart while the right ventricle is situated so that it forms the anterior surface of the heart. The left ventricle is a largely posterior structure, also forming the left lateral heart border. The left atrium lies in a midline-posterior position and is really not a left-sided structure at all.

The pulmonary artery arises anterior, superior, and to the left of the aorta. The superior and inferior vena cavae are continuous with the right lateral heart border formed by the right atrium. The coronary sinus is the major venous drainage conduit for the heart and travels in the left AV groove (in parallel with the circumflex coronary artery), emptying into the right atrium near the atrial septum. The left and right pulmonary veins join the left atrium along its posterolateral aspect and typically consist of a superior and an inferior vessel on each side, totaling four pulmonary veins.

### Internal Cardiac Anatomy

**Atria.** The right and left atria receive blood draining from the systemic and pulmonary venous systems, respectively, and pass the blood into their corresponding ventricles. In addition to their pumping functions, the atria

have an endocrine role by releasing natriuretic hormones in response to atrial stretch, helping to maintain fluid homeostasis (7).

The atria consist of both septal and free wall portions. The free wall of the right atrium is smooth posteriorly and trabeculated anteriorly. The smooth portion, derived from the embryonic sinus venosus, receives the vena cavae and is bordered anteriorly by the crista terminalis. The trabeculated portion contains prominent muscular bands, the pectinate muscles, that arise perpendicular to the crista terminalis and extend anteriorly to involve the pyramidal right atrial appendage (fig. 1-4, left). The free wall of the left atrium includes a dome-shaped body, which receives the pulmonary veins, and a worm-like atrial appendage (fig. 1-4, right). Like the right atrium, the left atrial appendage contains pectinate muscles, although they are not prominent and are isolated to the periphery of the appendage where they are radially arranged. The left atrium contains no crista terminalis.

The atrial septum, when viewed from the right aspect, contains both an interatrial component (between the right and left atria) and an atrioventricular component (between the right atrium and the left ventricle). This is because the tricuspid valve annulus is situated more apically than the mitral valve annulus at the septum (fig. 1-5). The interatrial portion contains the fossa ovalis, with its two major components: a central sheet-like region (the valve of the fossa ovalis) surrounded by a horseshoe-shaped muscular ridge referred to as the limbus of the fossa ovalis (fig. 1-6) (8). In some individuals, the valve and limbus do not fuse after birth and a potential passageway between the two atria persists and is referred to as a patent foramen ovale (9). The atrioventricular portion consists of a muscular and membranous portion and contains the AV node and penetrating bundle of His. When viewed from the left aspect, the atrial septum is entirely interatrial and may be somewhat fenestrated in the region of the valve of the fossa ovalis, corresponding to the embryologic ostium secundum.

**Ventricles.** The ventricles receive blood through their atrioventricular valves from their respective atria and pump it across the semilunar valves into their great arteries. During ventricular systole, the ventricles decrease

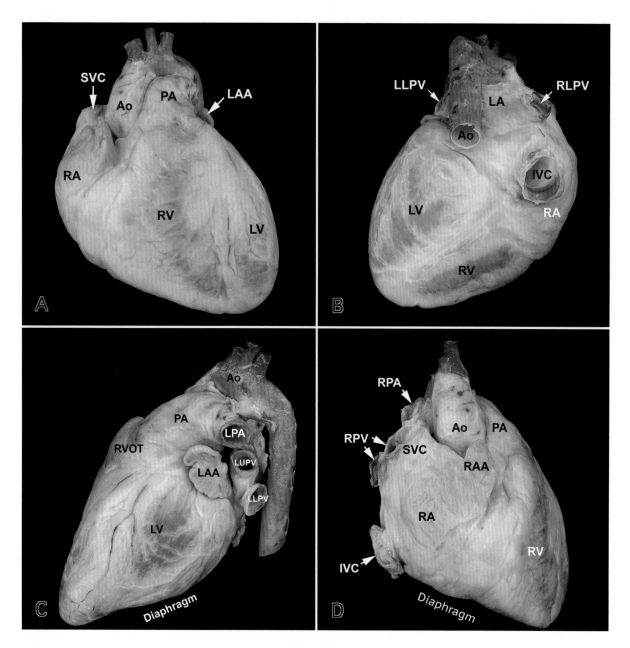

**Figure 1-3**

**EXTERNAL CARDIAC ANATOMY**

The heart and great vessels are exhibited from the anterior (A), inferior (B), left lateral (C), and right anterior oblique (D) anatomic perspectives. (SVC = superior vena cava; RA = right atrium; Ao = aorta; PA = pulmonary artery; LAA = left atrial appendage; RV = right ventricle; LV = left ventricle; LA = left atrium; LLPV = left lower pulmonary vein; RLPV = right lower pulmonary vein; IVC = inferior vena cava; LPA = left pulmonary artery; LUPV = left upper pulmonary vein; RPV = right-sided pulmonary veins; RAA = right atrial appendage.)

their short axis diameters and also their base-apex lengths to expel blood into the arteries and concomitantly close the atrioventricular valves. They are divided into inlet, trabecular, and outlet regions.

The right ventricle is a crescent-shaped chamber when viewed in the short axis plane. The inlet portion is associated with the tricuspid valve with its septal cordal insertions. Antero-apically, trabeculations of muscle extend from

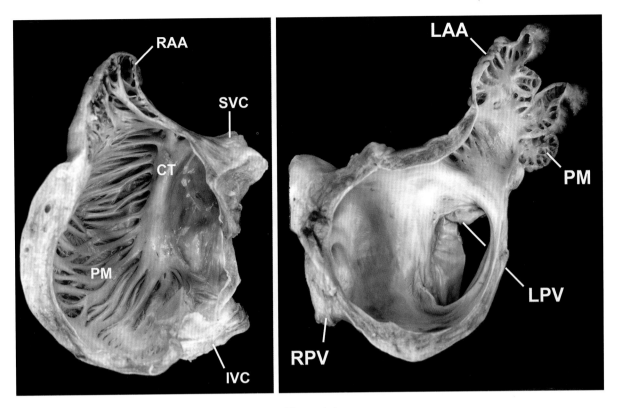

**Figure 1-4**

### COMPARISON OF THE RIGHT AND LEFT ATRIA

Left: The right atrial free wall viewed from the left lateral perspective exhibits the crista terminalis (CT), with the perpendicularly oriented pectinate muscles (PM) extending from the CT, anteriorly. The superior vena cava (SVC) and inferior vena cava (IVC) empty into the smooth-walled portion of the atrium. The pyramidal appendage (RAA) is also evident.

Right: The left atrial free wall viewed from the right lateral perspective exhibits the dome-shaped portion into which the left- and right-sided pulmonary veins (LPV and RPV, respectively) drain. Small radially oriented pectinate muscles are present only in the appendage (LAA).

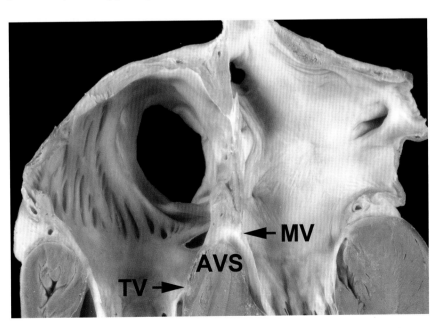

**Figure 1-5**

### CARDIAC SEPTA

The interatrial, interventricular, and atrioventricular (AVS) septa are exhibited in this four-chamber anatomic plane. The more apically positioned tricuspid valve annulus (TV) can be compared to the position of the mitral valve annulus (MV).

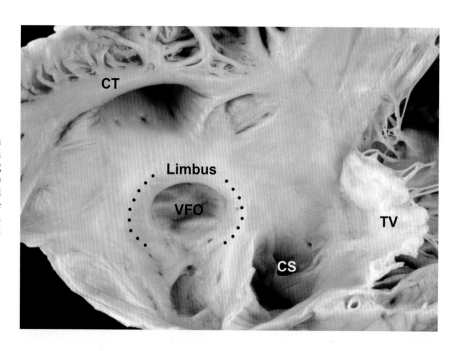

**Figure 1-6**

**ATRIAL SEPTUM**

The opened right atrium exhibits the fossa ovalis portion of the atrial septum, consisting of the valvular component (VFO) as well as the horseshoe-shaped limbus. The opening of the coronary sinus (CS) is seen anteriorly, as well as the septal tricuspid valve leaflet (TV).

the septum to the free wall and serve as a convenient region in which to lodge pacemaker/cardioverter-defibrillator leads or from which to obtain endomyocardial biopsies (fig. 1-7). The remaining smooth-walled outlet region is often referred to as the infundibulum (meaning funnel) or right ventricular outflow tract.

The left ventricle is a circular chamber when viewed in the short axis plane and is composed of muscular myocyte bundles arranged in a complex meshwork, with populations of myocytes aligned both tangential to the epicardial and endocardial surfaces and traversing the thickness of the wall (10). This arrangement results in a twisting motion of the ventricle during systole, wringing the blood into the outflow tract. The inflow region of the valve is bordered by the mitral valve cords, which extend downward onto papillary muscles with no direct septal cordal attachments (as opposed to the right ventricle). The apical region is characterized by trabeculations that are much shallower than those seen in the right ventricle (fig. 1-7). The outflow region of the left ventricle is musculomembranous, consisting of not only the ventricular septum and anterobasal free wall anteriorly, but also the anterior mitral leaflet posteriorly.

**Cardiac Valves.** The AV valves allow for unidirectional blood flow between the atria and the ventricles. They have two basic structural elements: a valvular apparatus (consisting of saddle-shaped annulus, commissures, and leaflets) and a tensor apparatus (consisting of tendinous cords and papillary muscles) (fig. 1-8) (11,12). The leaflets consist of fibrous connective tissue and have an annular edge, free edge, and closing surface. This closing surface is the surface of the leaflet that comes into contact with the apposing leaflet during ventricular systole. Tendinous cords extend from papillary muscles, branching multiple times, to insert along the ventricular aspect and free edge of the leaflet; upwards of 150 cords insert onto each valve, distributing the force along the undersurface of the leaflet (13,14). The cords are anchored to the ventricular walls, either by attaching directly to the ventricular septum (a feature seen only in morphologic tricuspid valves) or to papillary muscles located beneath the commissures. Contraction of the papillary muscles during ventricular systole helps facilitate AV valve closure by bringing the leaflets into apposition.

The AV valves differ in their morphologic appearance. The tricuspid valve has three distinct leaflets, commissures, and papillary muscles whereas the mitral has only two of each. As previously noted, the annulus of the tricuspid valve is situated more apically on the septum. The mitral valve has an anterior leaflet (that forms part of the left ventricular outflow tract) as well as a more shallow, scalloped, posterior leaflet that has three segments (P1, P2, and P3)

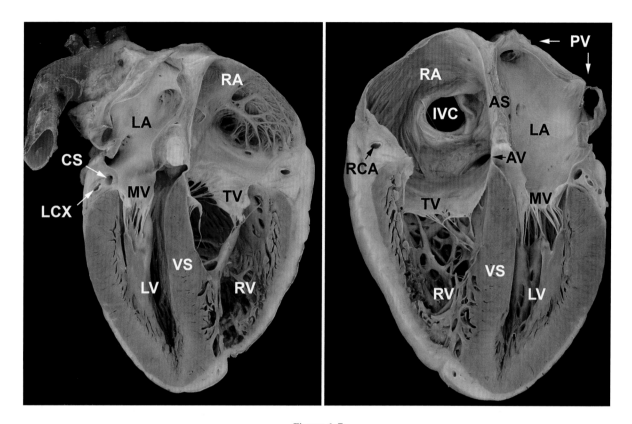

**Figure 1-7**

**INTERNAL CARDIAC ANATOMY**

Four-chamber views shown from the inferior (left) and superior (right) perspectives with the apex directed downward. (CS = coronary sinus; LCX = left circumflex coronary artery; LA = left atrium; MV = mitral valve; LV = left ventricle; VS = ventricular septum; RV = right ventricle; TV = tricuspid valve; RA = right atrium; RCA = right coronary artery; IVC = inferior vena cava; AV = atrioventricular septum; AS = atrial septum; PV = lower pulmonary veins.)

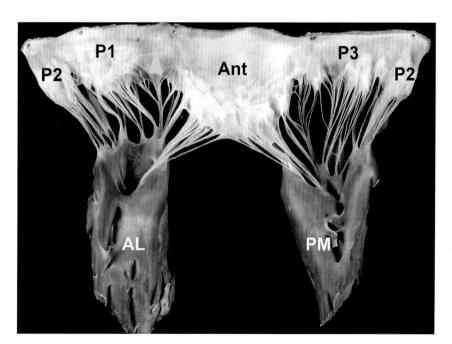

**Figure 1-8**

**MITRAL APPARATUS**

The sail-like anterior mitral leaflet (Ant) is situated between a shallow, tri-scalloped (P1, P2, and P3) posterior leaflet. The posteromedial (PM) and anterolateral (AL) papillary muscles are located directly beneath the commissures (yellow arrowheads).

(fig. 1-8) (15). A morphologic tricuspid valve always empties into a morphologic right ventricle, whereas a morphologic mitral valve always empties into a morphologic left ventricle.

The semilunar valves allow for unidirectional blood flow between the ventricles and great ar-

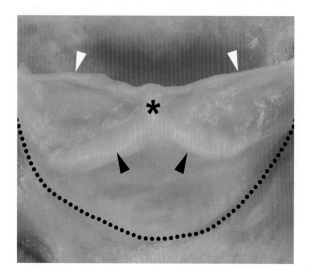

**Figure 1-9**

**AORTIC VALVE CUSP**

Each semilunar valve cusp has a free edge (white arrowhead), a closing edge (black arrowhead), a nodule of Arantius (asterisk), and an annulus (dotted line). The moon-shaped region between the free and closing edges is referred to as the lunula.

teries. Anatomically, they are simpler than their AV counterparts, consisting of an annulus and cusps devoid of a tensor apparatus (papillary muscles and tendinous cords). The annulus is a complex three-dimensional structure, shaped like a triradiate crown, with the three points at the level of the sinotubular junction demarcating the commissures. These commissures are the points where two cusps meet. The cusps themselves are half-moon–shaped (semilunar) structures with various anatomic features (fig. 1-9). The nonannular edge is the free edge, beneath which is situated a biscalloped ridge referred to as the closing edge. The region between the free edge and the closing edge is often referred to as the closing surface, or lunula, and serves as the point of contact with the neighboring cusps (fig. 1-10) (16). The nodule of Arantius is a small fibrous mound situated at the free edge at the center of each cusp. The aortic and pulmonary semilunar valves are anatomically similar, with the aortic valve being slightly thicker.

The relationship of the four major cardiac valves is best understood by an examination of the cardiac base with the atria removed (so-called surgeon's view) (fig. 1-11). The aortic valve is situated in the middle and its annulus is in continuity with the other three major valves: left-posterior commissure to mitral valve, right-posterior commissure to tricuspid valve, and

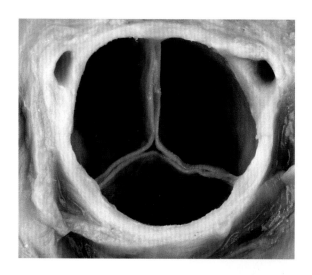
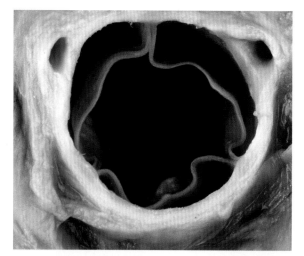

**Figure 1-10**

**AORTIC VALVE**

The aortic valve is in closed position (ventricular diastole) (left), and open position (ventricular systole) (right). The left and right coronary ostia are located slightly above the free edges of the open cusps.

right-left commissure to pulmonary valve. The valves do not reside in the same plane or even parallel planes. Because of the intertwining of the great arteries, the aortic and pulmonary valves are skewed 60 to 90 degrees as the valvular orifices are directed toward opposite shoulders. The tricuspid and mitral valves are skewed 10 to 15 degrees with respect to one another, changing somewhat throughout the cardiac cycle.

**Vascular Supply and Drainage.** The blood supply of the heart is derived primarily from the left and right epicardial coronary arteries, which arise from the left and right aortic sinuses (of Valsalva), respectively, typically just below the sinotubular junction. The left main coronary artery branches to become the left anterior descending (LAD) and left circumflex (LCX) coronary arteries (fig. 1-11).

The LAD courses from the base to apex in the anterior interventricular sulcus and wraps posteriorly at the apex to a variable extent. Consequently, the LAD supplies the anterolateral and anteroseptal left ventricle, the basal- and mid-ventricular levels, and the entire left ventricle at the apical level. Branches arising from the LAD over the surface of the heart are referred to as diagonal branches. The LAD also gives rise to an extensive network of vessels branching into the anterior portion of the ventricular septum (fig. 1-12). The LCX wraps around the left lateral aspect of the heart within the left AV groove, supplying the lateral left ventricle at the basal- and mid-ventricular levels.

After arising from the right aortic sinus, the right coronary artery (RCA) wraps around the right lateral aspect of the heart within the right AV groove to give rise to the posterior descending coronary artery about 70 percent of the time, making it the dominant coronary

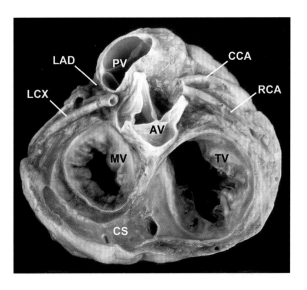

Figure 1-11

**BASE OF THE HEART**

The centrally located aortic valve (AV) is adjacent to the three other major cardiac valves (mitral [MV], tricuspid [TV], and pulmonary [PV] valves). The distribution of the epicardial coronary arteries (LAD = left anterior descending coronary artery; LCX = left circumflex coronary artery; RCA = right coronary artery; CCA = conus coronary artery) and the coronary sinus (CS) is also demonstrated in this view.

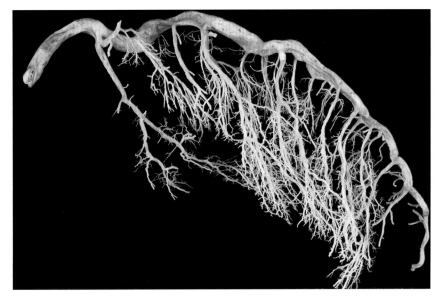

Figure 1-12

**LEFT ANTERIOR DESCENDING CORONARY ARTERY**

The numerous branches, including the downwardly directed septal perforating branches that extend into the anterior ventricular septum, are seen.

artery. Approximately 10 percent of the time, the posterior descending coronary artery arises from the LCX (so-called, left-dominant hearts). The remaining 20 percent of hearts are said to be co-dominant, with both RCA and LCX contributing to the supply of the posterior descending coronary artery.

The sinus node is supplied by the RCA in 60 percent of hearts and from the left circumflex in the remaining 40 percent. The AV node, however, derives its blood supply from the dominant coronary artery.

The venous circulation of the heart is composed of the coronary sinus, anterior cardiac venous system, and thebesian venous system. The great cardiac vein is situated adjacent to the LAD and LCX and receives blood from the territory supplied by both before draining into the coronary sinus. The coronary sinus is located adjacent to the posterior LCX and also receives blood from various small cardiac veins and tributaries; it drains directly into the right atrium (17). Numerous small thebesian veins drain directly into the cardiac chambers, usually the right atrium and ventricle.

**Conduction System.** The cardiac conduction system typically refers to the specialized cardiac myocytes responsible for initiating the cardiac impulse and propagating it from the atria to the ventricles. Normally, the impulse begins in the heart's pacemaker, the sinoatrial (or sinus) node, located subepicardially at the junction of the sinus venosus and the right atrium, just anterior to the superior vena cava. From the sinus node, conduction propagates to the AV node, located subendocardially in the AV septum, by way of several internodal tracts. From the AV node, the impulse is conducted through the cardiac skeleton by the penetrating bundle of His, where it is transmitted to the left and right bundle branches, and ultimately, the Purkinje fibers and the ventricular myocardium.

In addition to being influenced by the sympathetic and parasympathetic nervous systems, as well as circulating catecholamines and electrolytes, the function of the conduction system can be influenced by tumors. Mass effect from histologically benign tumors can have devastating arrhythmic consequences within the heart muscle. Despite the fact that the conduction system tissue itself consists of myocytes, rather than neural tissue, the heart and blood vessels receive rich autonomic innervation from the cervical sympathetic ganglia and parasympathetic vagus nerves, from which neural neoplasms occasionally arise.

Examination of the cardiac conduction system is important when assessing for involvement by various tumors. The sinus node is evaluated by procuring a rectangular portion of tissue at the superior portion of the sulcus terminalis, just anterior to the junction of the superior vena cava and the right atrium (fig. 1-13) (18). Often, a grossly visible artery, the sinus node artery, is seen running through the center of the rectangle, helping to confirm the correct anatomic area. The AV node is evaluated by procuring a rectangular portion of heart that includes the so-called triangle of Koch, which is bordered by the tricuspid valve annulus, the opening of the coronary sinus, and the tendon of Todaro (fig. 1-14). At the apex of this triangle, the AV node is reliably found. Both of these rectangles can then be serially sectioned and submitted in a systematic way to allow for evaluation of the conducting tissue contained within them.

## CARDIAC HISTOLOGY AND ULTRASTRUCTURE

Histologically, the myocardium contains a number of cell types in addition to cardiac myocytes, which comprise the majority of the heart's mass. The myocardium also contains fibroblasts (present in greater numbers than even cardiac myocytes), endothelial cells, and smooth muscle myocytes (19). Cardiac myocytes are 20 to 30 μm in diameter and generally about four times this in length (fig. 1-15). They are characterized by dense cross-bands, called intercalated discs, which represent highly specialized intercellular attachment points that create a branching network of muscle fibers, which are connected physically and electrically. This allows for an electromechanical syncytium that allows the heart to contract and relax in an orderly fashion. Cardiac myocytes contain one or two centrally placed nuclei, helping to differentiate cardiac-type striated muscle from the skeletal variety. The perinuclear region is rich in glycogen, mitochondria, and often lipofuscin pigment granules. Atrial myocytes also typically contain perinuclear granules (0.3 to 0.4 μm in

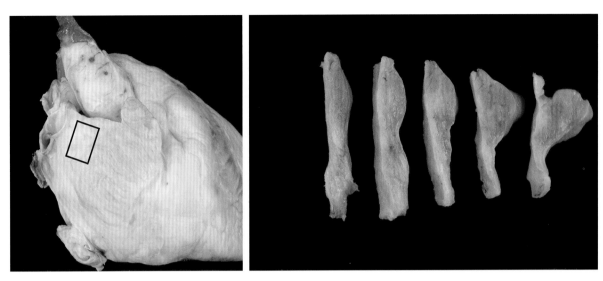

**Figure 1-13**

**SINOATRIAL (SINUS) NODE**

Left: The location of the epicardial sinus node is within the rectangular box. The sinus node artery is faintly seen running through the central portion of this area.

Right: Serial sectioning of the rectangular box allows for histologic evaluation of the sinoatrial (SA) node.

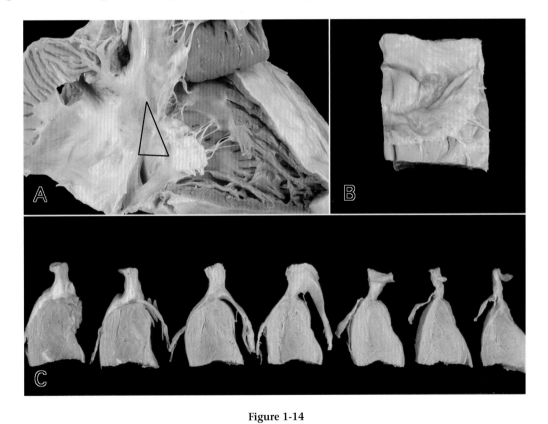

**Figure 1-14**

**ATRIOVENTRICULAR NODE**

The atrioventricular (AV) node is a subendocardial structure that lies within the triangle of Koch (A). Removal of this area (B), followed by serial sectioning (C), allows for histologic evaluation of the AV node.

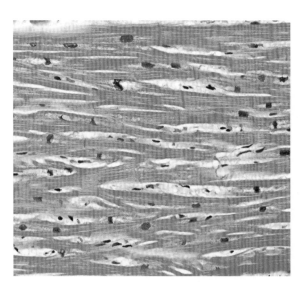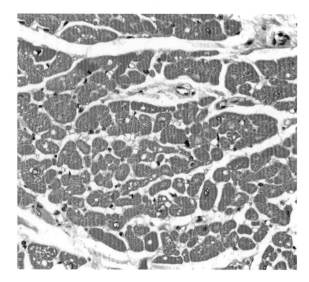

**Figure 1-15**

**MYOCARDIUM**

Normal, branching cardiac myocytes (left, longitudinally oriented; right, oriented in cross section) are 20 to 30 μm in diameter and have one or two centrally placed nuclei.

**Figure 1-16**

**ATRIAL NATRIURETIC PEPTIDE GRANULES**

Perinuclear granules are seen on ultrastructural analysis of the atrial myocardium.

size) that contain atrial natriuretic factor; they are best demonstrated on ultrastructural examination (fig. 1-16).

As alluded to above, a specialized population of myocytes comprises the cardiac conduction system. Although all myocytes are capable of impulse conduction, this population of cells is responsible for generating the impulse and rapidly conducting it along anatomic pathways, allowing for an organized pattern of contraction and relaxation which results in optimal emptying and filling of the chambers. Nodal tissue contains four morphologic types of myocytes in varying proportions: small, pale staining nodal or P cells; contractile-type myocardial cells; transitional cells with a hybrid morphology of nodal- and contractile-type cells; and Purkinje cells (fig. 1-17) (20,21). The Purkinje cells tend to be larger (up to 2 times) than contractile-type myocytes and are paler staining, owing to their glycogen content. While seen in variable quantities in the nodes, particularly the AV node, Purkinje cells are usually identified in the subendocardium, where they form an extensive network by which impulses are conducted to the ventricular myocardium.

Understanding the histomorphologic features of the various cell types, as well as their usual arrangement, is important in diagnosing certain types of cardiac tumors, particularly hamartomas. Hamartoma of mature cardiac myocytes, for example, is a grossly evident white mass that histologically is composed of enlarged myocytes in a haphazard distribution. A poorly understood entity, histiocytoid cardiomyopathy, is thought to represent a hamartomatous lesion composed of Purkinje-type cells.

## ANATOMY AND HISTOLOGY OF BLOOD VESSELS

### Elastic Arteries

The major elastic arteries include the aorta and the pulmonary arteries. While the overall diameters of these two vessels are similar throughout life, the wall of the pulmonary artery is typically less than half the thickness of the aortic wall.

The main pulmonary artery arises from the right ventricle to the left of the ascending aorta, directed toward the left shoulder. As it bifurcates, the left pulmonary artery continues as a smooth arch and courses over the left bronchus, while the right pulmonary artery arises at a right angle and travels beneath the aortic arch, posterior to the superior vena cava.

The aorta arises at the level of the aortic valve annulus and terminates at its bifurcation into the common iliac arteries. The aorta is divided into four primary regions: the ascending aorta (including the aortic root), aortic arch, descending thoracic aorta, and abdominal aorta. The ascending aorta and aortic arch are of neural crest derivation, while the remaining portions are derived from the primitive vascular mesenchyme (22). The ascending aorta is divided into the aortic root (or sinus) and the tubular portion, and arises to the right and posterior of the

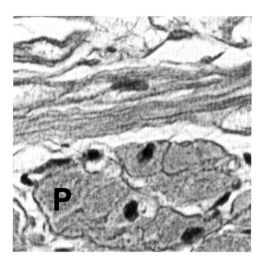

**Figure 1-17**

**PURKINJE CELLS**

Pale Purkinje cells (P) comprise part of the conduction system. These cells contain abundant glycogen and are larger than the contractile cells of the heart (located in the upper segment of this figure).

main pulmonary artery. The tubular ascending aorta transitions to the aortic arch at the takeoff of the brachiocephalic artery, just beyond the pericardial reflection. Consequently, the ascending aorta is almost entirely intrapericardial. The aortic arch normally travels over the left bronchus as well as the right pulmonary artery. The descending thoracic aorta is situated posterior to the left atrium, adjacent to the esophagus. After extending inferiorly to the diaphragm, the aorta is referred to as the abdominal aorta before its iliac bifurcation at the level of the umbilicus.

Histologically, elastic arteries are composed of lamellar units, typically arranged in parallel from the intimal surface to the adventitia (fig. 1-18). The elastic tissue in the pulmonary artery is somewhat discontinuous, imparting a slightly more disorganized-appearing architecture (23). A lamellar unit consists of smooth muscle, collagen, and ground substance sandwiched between elastic fiber plates. The orientation of the elastic fibers, as well as the relative amounts of muscle, collagen, and ground substance, vary between elastic arteries as well as regionally within the same elastic vessel (24). The composition and structure of elastic arteries provide them with an amazing ability to stretch and accommodate the pressures generated by the ventricles.

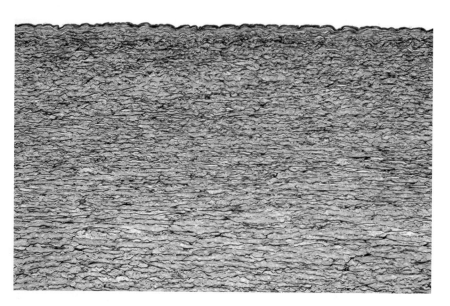

**Figure 1-18**

**ELASTIC ARTERY**

Parallel elastic membranes are located from the adventitial surface to the intimal surface. Juxtaposed between the elastic membranes are smooth muscle myocytes, collagen, and ground substance (aorta, Verhoeff-van Giesson stain).

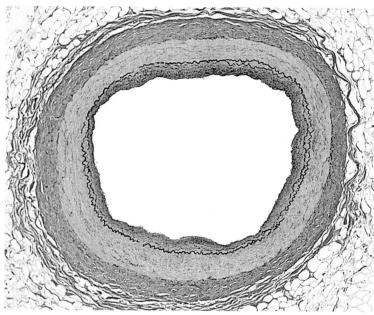

**Figure 1-19**

**MUSCULAR ARTERY**

Muscular arteries contain two prominent elastic membranes: one at the intimal-medial junction and one at the medial-adventitial junction. The internal elastic lamina is typically more prominent, as in this example. Between these membranes are abundant smooth muscle fibers arranged both concentrically and obliquely, maintaining vascular tone and modulating resistance (left anterior descending coronary artery, Verhoeff-van Giesson stain).

## Muscular Arteries

The epicardial coronary arteries, described above, are the prototypical muscular arteries of the heart. While muscular arteries contain the same basic components as elastic arteries, their relative quantities and the arrangement are strikingly different. Instead of parallel lamellar units, a well-developed muscular media with little collagen or elastin characterizes muscular arteries (fig. 1-19). Two distinct elastic layers are usually present: an inner internal elastic membrane at the junction of the media and intima, and an external elastic layer between the media and adventitia.

### Veins

The epicardial cardiac veins, running antiparallel to their arterial counterpart, are relatively thin-walled. In contrast to the muscular arteries, the media is thin, consisting of bundles of smooth muscle and collagen with a haphazard arrangement of elastic fibers in the outer media and adventitia. Cardiac veins do not have distinct elastic membranes.

**REFERENCES**

1. Gittenberger-de Groot AC, Bartelings MM, Deruiter MC, Poelmann RE. Basics of cardiac development for the understanding of congenital heart malformations. Pediatr Res 2005;57:169-176.
2. Wessels A, Sedmera D. Developmental anatomy of the heart: a tale of mice and man. Physiol Genomics 2003;5:165-176.
3. Linder J, Shelburne JD, Sorge JP, Whalen RE, Hackel DB. Congenital endodermal heterotopia of the atrioventricular node: evidence for the endodermal origin of so-called mesotheliomas of the atrioventricular node. Hum Pathol 1984;15:1093-1098.
4. Ariza S, Rafel E, Castillo JA, Garcia-Canton JA. Intracardiac heterotopia—mesenchymal and endodermal. Br Heart J 1978;40:325-327.
5. Orlandi A, Ciucci A, Ferlosio A, Genta R, Spagnoli LG, Gabbiani G. Cardiac myxoma cells exhibit embryonic endocardial stem cell features. J Pathol 2006;209:231-239.
6. Pucci A, Bartoloni G, Tessitore E, Carney JA, Papotti M. Cytokeratin profile and neuroendocrine cells in the glandular component of cardiac myxoma. Virchows Arch 2003;443:618-624.
7. Thibault G, Garcia R, Cantia M, Genest J. Atrial natriuretic factor. Characterization and partial purification. Hypertension 1983;5(Pt 2):I75-180.
8. Sweeney LJ, Rosenquist GC. The normal anatomy of the atrial septum in the human heart. Am Heart J 1979;98:194-199.
9. Hagen PT, Scholz DG, Edwards WD. Incidence and size of patent foramen ovale during the first 10 decades of life: an autopsy study of 965 normal hearts. Mayo Clin Proc 1984;59:17-20.
10. Anderson RH, Smerup M, Sanchez-Quintana D, Loukas M, Lunkenheimer PP. The three-dimensional arrangement of the myocytes in the ventricular walls. Clin Anat 2009;22:64-76.
11. Sonne C, Sugeng L, Watanabe N, et al. Age and body surface area dependency of mitral valve and papillary apparatus parameters: assessment by real-time three-dimensional echocardiography. Eur J Echocardiogr 2009;10:287-294.
12. Badano LP, Agricola E, Perez de Isla L, Gianfagna P, Zamorano JL. Evaluation of the tricuspid valve morphology and function by transthoracic real-time three-dimensional echocardiography. Eur J Echocardiogr 2009;10:477-484.
13. Seccombe JF, Cahill DR, Edwards WD. Quantitative morphology of normal human tricuspid valve: autopsy study of 24 cases. Clin Anat 1993;6:203-212.
14. Roberts WC. Morphologic features of the normal and abnormal mitral valve. Am J Cardiol 1983;51:1005-1028.
15. Morris MF, Maleszewski JJ, Suri RM, et al. CT and MR imaging of the mitral valve: radiologic-pathologic correlation. Radiographics 2010;30:1603-1620.
16. Bennett CJ, Maleszewski JJ, Araoz PA. CT and MR imaging of the aortic valve: radiologic-pathologic correlation. Radiographics 2012;32:1399-1420.
17. Noheria A, Desimone CV, Lachman N, et al. Anatomy of the coronary sinus and epicardial coronary venous system in 620 hearts: an electrophysiology perspective. J Cardiovasc Electrophysiol 2013;24:1-6.
18. Anderson RH, Yanni J, Boyett MR, Chandler NJ, Dobrzynski H. The anatomy of the cardiac conduction system. Clin Anat 2009;22:99-113.
19. Sarantitis I, Papanastasopoulos P, Manousi M, Baikoussis NG, Apostolakis E. The cytoskeleton of the cardiac muscle cell. Hellenic J Cardiol 2012;53:367-379.
20. Waller BF, Gering LE, Branyas NA, Slack JD. Anatomy, histology, and pathology of the cardiac conduction system: Part I. Clin Cardiol 1993;16:249-252.
21. Waller BF, Gering LE, Branyas NA, Slack JD. Anatomy, histology, and pathology of the cardiac conduction system: Part II. Clin Cardiol 1993;16:347-352.
22. Jiang X, Rowitch DH, Soriano P, McMahon AP, Sucov HM. Fate of the mammalian cardiac neural crest. Development 2000;127:1607-1616.
23. de Sa M, Moshkovitz Y, Butany J, David TE. Histologic abnormalities of the ascending aorta and pulmonary trunk in patients with bicuspid aortic valve disease: clinical relevance to the Ross procedure. J Thorac Cardiovasc Surg 1999;118:588-594.
24. O'Connell MK, Murthy S, Phan S, et al. The three-dimensional micro- and nanostructure of the aortic medial lamellar unit measured using 3D confocal and electron microscopy imaging. Matrix Biol 2008;27:171-181.

15

# 2 HEART TUMORS: CLASSIFICATION AND OVERVIEW

## CLASSIFICATION

Lesions that cause masses or tumors in the heart span a wide range of non-neoplastic and neoplastic conditions. Pseudotumors and organized thrombi may clinically and pathologically mimic neoplasms; metastatic lesions also pose difficulties in the differential diagnosis. As in other organs, heart tumors are classified either by the type of proliferation (Table 2-1) or cellular differentiation (Table 2-2). Several lesions are considered congenital (rhabdomyomas, histiocytoid cardiomyopathy, fibromas, and sometimes, hemangiomas). The most common

tumors are myxomas in adults (Table 2-3) and rhabdomyomas in children (Table 2-4). Tumors of the serosal layer of the heart (pericardium) are not covered in this Fascicle.

There are several lesions that are difficult to classify, some of which are variably included in series of heart tumors. The exact nature of cardiac myxoma, the most common heart mass, is still not certain, although the overwhelming consensus is that it is a true neoplasm. Less certain is the nature of papillary fibroelastoma, which shares some features of a reactive process and some of a benign hamartoma. Purkinje cell

Table 2-1

### PATHOGENETIC CLASSIFICATION OF HEART TUMORS

| Broad Classification | Specific Classification | Growth Pattern |
|---|---|---|
| Pseudotumors | Mural thrombi (including CAT[a]) | Intracavitary |
| | Inflammatory masses | Intramural |
| | Vegetations | Intracavitary |
| | Anomalous cords/false tendons | Intracavitary |
| Reactive versus hamartoma | Papillary fibroelastoma[b] | Intracavitary |
| Hamartoma | Rhabdomyoma | Intramural |
| | Purkinje cell hamartoma/histiocytoid cardiomyopathy | Intramural |
| | Fibroma | Intramural |
| | Hamartoma of mature cardiac myocytes | Intramural |
| | Lipomatous hypertrophy, atrial septum | Intramural |
| Ectopic tissues/choristomas | AV nodal tumor | Intramural |
| | Bronchogenic/duplication/developmental cysts | Intramural |
| | Ectopic thyroid, thymus | Intramural |
| Benign neoplasms | Myxoma | Intracavitary |
| | Hemangioma | Intramural |
| | Inflammatory myofibroblastic tumor[c] | Intracavitary |
| | Solitary fibrous tumor | Intramural, pericardial |
| | Lipoma | Intramural, intracavitary |
| | Paraganglioma | Intramural |
| Sarcoma | Angiosarcoma | Intramural, pericardial |
| | Intimal/pleomorphic spindled sarcoma | Intracavitary, intramural |
| | Synovial sarcoma | Intracavitary, intramural |
| | Rhabdomyosarcoma | Intramural |
| Lymphomas | Lymphoma, B cell | Intramural, intracavitary |
| | Other lymphomas, including Hodgkin lymphoma | |
| Germ cell tumors | Teratomas, yolk sac tumors | Intramural, intracavitary |

[a]CAT = calcified amphorous tumor; AV = atrioventricular.
[b]Incidence is increasing; the most common excised tumor in the authors' practice.
[c]Sometimes considered a low-grade sarcoma.

Table 2-2

CLASSIFICATION OF HEART TUMORS
BY CELL DIFFERENTIATION

| Differentiation | Tumor |
|---|---|
| Mesenchymal | |
| Fibrous/myo-fibroblastic tumor | Fibroma |
| | Inflammatory myofibroblastic |
| | Solitary fibrous tumor |
| | Sarcomas of intimal origin |
| Endothelial | Hemangioma |
| | Epithelioid hemangioendothelioma |
| | Angiosarcoma |
| Smooth muscle | Leiomyoma |
| | Leiomyosarcoma |
| Striated muscle | Histiocytoid cardiomyopathy |
| | Rhabdomyoma |
| | Adult cellular rhabdomyoma |
| | Hamartoma of mature cardiac myocytes |
| | Rhabdomyosarcoma |
| Lipomatous | Lipoma |
| | Lipomatous hypertrophy of the atrial septum |
| | Liposarcoma |
| | Hibernoma |
| Matrix-forming | Osteosarcoma, chondrosarcoma (usually a component of intimal sarcomas) |
| Other/unknown | Myxoma |
| | Papillary fibroelastoma |
| | Synovial sarcoma |
| Neuroectodermal | Paraganglioma |
| | Peripheral nerve sheath tumor |
| | Granular cell tumor |
| Epithelial | Bronchogenic cysts |
| | AV nodal tumor |
| Hematopoietic | Lymphoma |
| | Castleman disease |
| | Rosai-Dorfman disease |
| | Other histiocytic tumors (e.g., Erdheim-Chester disease) |
| Germ cell | Teratoma |
| | Yolk sac tumor |

Note: Mesotheliomas will not be discussed in this volume, but this subject is covered in Fascicle 3 of the AFIP Fourth Series of the Atlas of Tumor Pathology: Tumors of the Serosal Membranes.

Table 2-3

CARDIAC TUMORS IN ADULTS:
HISTOLOGIC TYPES AND FREQUENCY[a]

| Tumor Type | Number | % Overall | Range of % by Series |
|---|---|---|---|
| Myxoma | 567 | 69 | 55-83 |
| Papillary fibroelastoma | 117 | 14 | 2-28 |
| Sarcoma (other than angiosarcoma) | 57 | 7 | 0-13 |
| Angiosarcoma | 25 | 3 | 0-7 |
| Lipoma/lipomatous hypertrophy | 24 | 3 | 0-4 |
| Hemangioma | 12 | 1.5 | 0-2 |
| Fibroma | 11 | 1.3 | 0-3 |
| Lymphoma | 2 | 0.2 | 0-1 |
| Inflammatory myo-fibroblastic tumor[b] | 2 | 0.2 | 0-1 |
| Leiomyoma | 1 | 0.1 | 0-1 |
| Hibernoma | 1 | 0.1 | 0-1 |
| Paraganglioma | 1 | 0.1 | 0-1 |
| Solitary fibrous tumor | 1 | 0.1 | 0-1 |
| Teratoma | 1 | 0.1 | 0-1 |
| Total | 822 | 100 | |

[a]822 surgically resected tumors compiled from references 2, 3, 9, 10, 11, 12, and 17–20.
[b]Various designations.

Table 2-4

CARDIAC TUMORS IN CHILDREN:
HISTOLOGIC TYPES AND FREQUENCY[a]

| Tumor Type | Number | % Overall |
|---|---|---|
| Rhabdomyoma[b] | 61 | 39 |
| Fibroma | 35 | 22 |
| Teratoma | 20 | 13 |
| Myxoma | 18 | 11 |
| Hemangioma | 12 | 8 |
| Sarcoma | 6 | 4 |
| Inflammatory myofibroblastic tumor | 5 | 3 |
| Papillary fibroelastoma | 1 | <1 |
| Total | 158 | 100 |

[a]158 surgically resected tumors compiled from references 2, 3, 9, 10, 11, 12, 17, and 20–22.
[b]Frequently multiple.

tumor, or cardiac hamartoma, forms innumerable oncocytic lesions in infants with ventricular tachycardia, and is currently considered a cardiomyopathy with mitochondrial genetic defects. Organized thrombi are very common atrial lesions, but only uncommonly result in diagnostic uncertainty requiring surgical resection; when these calcify, they have been designated as true "tumors" (calcifying amorphous tumor) that are included in tumor series.

The heart, as a midline structure, is prone to developmental rests and germ cell tumors. As a result, there are scattered reports of intrapericardial developmental cysts and germ cell tumors, most of which are within the pericardial space, but some of which are within the heart muscle.

The classification of cardiac sarcomas generally follows that of soft tissue lesions; because many series do not include pathologic documentation, there is likely an over-representation of rhabdomyosarcoma, based on the mistaken notion that tumors within striated muscle will likely demonstrate muscular differentiation. Benign tumors with striated muscle differentiation include rhabdomyoma, a well-defined hamartoma associated with *TSC* mutations, and less common entities that include non-neoplastic hamartoma of mature cardiac myocytes, as well as neoplasms that have been termed adult cellular rhabdomyoma. Lastly, bland spindle-cell myofibroblastic tumors with an inflammatory reaction form a spectrum of lesions ranging from neoplasms (inflammatory myofibroblastic tumors) to reactive inflammatory processes with fibrosis, and occur in the heart as well as other organs in children and young adults.

## CLINICAL FEATURES

Cardiac neoplasms result in widely varied signs and symptoms (1,2–4). The presentation depends on the size, anatomic location, growth rate, and invasiveness of the lesion, and to a lesser degree, the tissue type. Tumor friability affects the rate of embolism for intracavitary tumors such as myxoma and sarcomas (5). Large tumors may be clinically silent, whereas small tumors in a critical location may give rise to devastating clinical consequences. Local extension of the tumor may cause conduction or coronary artery compromise, with chest pain, myocardial infarction, arrhythmia, heart block, and sudden death (6).

The left atrium is the most common location for primary cardiac neoplasms. Left atrial tumors, especially those that are mobile or pedunculated and especially myxomas and papillary fibroelastomas, lead to systemic embolism involving the coronary, cerebral, and peripheral circulations. Left atrial tumors may also interfere with mitral valve function, resulting in mitral stenosis or regurgitation. Cardiac murmurs and a characteristic tumor "plop" may be auscultated. Valve dysfunction manifests as left-sided heart failure with shortness of breath, orthopnea, paroxysmal nocturnal dyspnea, pulmonary edema, fatigue, cough, and chest pain. Intramural left ventricular tumors may be asymptomatic or present with a mass effect. With protrusion into the cavity, hemodynamic compromise may result (7). The most common symptoms relate to mitral valve dysfunction, especially mitral stenosis. Tumors of the valves (generally either papillary fibroelastoma or inflammatory pseudotumor) may prolapse directly into the coronary ostia causing myocardial ischemia.

Right atrial or right ventricular tumors may result in right heart failure from atrioventricular or pulmonary outflow obstruction, resulting in peripheral edema, hepatomegaly, ascites, shortness of breath, syncope, and sometimes, sudden death. If the tumors interfere with valve function, they may result in regurgitation or stenosis (6). Right-sided cardiac tumors may embolize to the lungs and present as pulmonary emboli with chest pain, pulmonary infarction, and hemoptysis (8). Chronic embolization may also mimic chronic thromboembolic disease with signs and symptoms of pulmonary hypertension.

Pericardial tumor involvement may result in the chest pain typical of pericarditis. The tumors may be hemorrhagic and cause pericardial effusion and tamponade. Constrictive pericarditis may also result from tumor infiltration.

Rarely, tumors such as myxoma, considered a "great mimicker," cause constitutional symptoms such as anorexia, weight loss, fatigue, and malaise, which may mimic a variety of systemic disorders. Interestingly, they may also cause hematologic abnormalities, including anemia, polycythemia, leukocytosis, thrombocytosis, and elevated sedimentation rate (7). Tumor production of mediators, including interleukins, has been reported (12).

In large series of heart tumors, between 10 and 20 percent are found incidentally upon investigation for other conditions or in asymptomatic individuals (9). When present, the symptoms include congestive heart failure, embolism, chest pain (9), palpitations, syncope, atrioventricular block (10), and tachyarrhythmias. Elbardissi et al. (11) compared the frequency of the following symptoms caused by heart tumors: dyspnea, chest pain, palpitations, syncope, constitutional symptoms, embolic symptoms, lack of symptoms, atrial fibrillation, and ventricular tachycardia. They found in general no correlation with tumor type. The only exceptions were an increased risk for constitutional symptoms with malignant tumors (p<.0001) and ventricular tachycardia with fibromas and lipomas, which have a frequent intramural ventricular location.

The clinical diagnosis of heart tumors is made by transthoracic echocardiography in over 90 percent of cases (2,13). Angiography is frequently performed preoperatively in patients over 40 years to exclude coexistent coronary disease, and helps identify the feeder vessels characteristic of vascular tumors such as hemangioma. Coronary computerized tomography (CT) was the diagnostic method in 8 percent of tumors in studies by Endo et al. (2). Cardiac magnetic resonance imaging (MRI) is useful for delineating tumor borders and identifying tissue type, for example, fat and vascular lesions.

## PATHOLOGIC FINDINGS

The pathologic features of heart tumors are generally similar to those of their extracardiac counterparts, as in the case of sarcomas, lymphomas, and benign lesions such as fibromas, paragangliomas, teratomas, and hemangiomas. In contrast, there are lesions that are histologically unique to the heart, such as cardiac myxoma, lipomatous hypertrophy of the atrial septum, papillary fibroelastoma, rhabdomyoma, and histiocytoid cardiomyopathy.

The growth pattern of a heart tumor has important implications for tumor resectability. In general, benign lesions are circumscribed and amenable to excision, whereas sarcomas infiltrate the wall of the involved chamber. Some benign tumors are exclusively intracavitary (Table 2-1), including myxoma, papillary fibroelastoma, and many hemangiomas. These tumors are typically attached to the endocardium via a broad-based pedicle or narrow stalk. Benign lesions such as fibromas and rhabdomyomas are typically intramural, and even though they are circumscribed, may be difficult to resect.

Cardiac tumors generally have a propensity for a specific cardiac chamber (Table 2-5). For example, cardiac myxomas and spindle cell sarcomas are usually located in the left atrium, angiosarcomas in the right atrium, and papillary fibroelastomas on the valves. Many tumors, however, especially benign lesions, have little predilection for one chamber or another.

There are several entities other than primary cardiac tumors that occur in similar locations and are often in the clinical and pathologic differential diagnosis. These include metastatic lesions, thrombi, and cysts (Table 2-6). Thrombi are frequently excised from the right atrium, and cysts, although frequent in the pericardial space, are rare within the myocardium.

The surface of the tumor may affect the embolic potential. A minority of myxomas and most papillary fibroelastomas result in embolism, which then causes stroke or even death. A review of cardiac tumors that resulted in these phenomena demonstrates that most were myxomas and papillary fibroelastomas (Table 2-7). Most embolic events related to cardiac tumors are caused by myxomas and papillary fibroelastomas. Embolizing myxomas are typically in the left atrium, and embolizing papillary fibroblastomas on the aortic and mitral valves. Similarly, although left atrial tumors are most likely to result in embolization, aortic and pulmonary valve tumors have the highest frequency of such events.

## STAGING

There is no accepted staging system for cardiac tumors. The College of American Pathologists (CAP) has adopted a checklist for heart tumors without guidance for staging, as none has been adopted by the AJCC/UICC (American Joint Cancer Committee/Union Internationale Contre le Cancer). The protocol applies only to sarcomas, and includes tumor histology, size, site, extension, margins, and lymph-vascular invasion. The histologic grading of sarcomas recommended by the CAP follows that of the Fédération Nationale des Centres de Lutte Contre le Cancer (see chapter 16).

## TREATMENT

The treatment of benign cardiac tumors is surgery. More than 95 percent of tumors that are diagnosed echocardiographically undergo excision (11). For some childhood tumors, treatment is conservative, especially for rhabdomyoma and hemangioma, which have a propensity for regression. Approximately 25 percent of malignant tumors are unresectable at the time of diagnosis, and are biopsied for tissue diagnosis or debulked (13). For some unresectable malignancies, autotransplantation is performed

Table 2-5

**CARDIAC TUMORS IN CHILDREN AND ADULTS: FREQUENCY BY ANATOMIC SITE[a]**

| Chamber | Overall % | Most Frequent Tumor (Percentage in Chamber/Site) |
|---------|-----------|--------------------------------------------------|
| Left atrium | 58 | Myxoma (92)<br>Sarcoma (other than angiosarcoma) (4)<br>Metastasis (1)<br>Angiosarcoma, hemangioma, thrombus, papillary fibroelastoma, lipoma, rhabdomyoma (each <1) |
| Right atrium | 15 | Myxoma (45)<br>Angiosarcoma (12)<br>Other sarcoma (8)<br>Thrombus (8)<br>Lipoma (8)[b]<br>Metastasis (6)[c]<br>Lymphoma (3)<br>Hemangioma (3)<br>Papillary fibroelastoma (2)<br>Rhabdomyoma (2)<br>Fibroma (<1)<br>Paraganglioma (<1)<br>Teratoma (<1) |
| Cardiac valve | 13 | Papillary fibroelastoma (96)<br>Myxoma (2)<br>Lipoma, sarcoma, hemangioma (2) |
| Left ventricle | 8 | Fibroma (38)<br>Rhabdomyoma (19)<br>Myxoma (14)<br>Papillary fibroelastoma (10)<br>Thrombus (5)<br>Metastasis (5)<br>Hemangioma (3)<br>Lipoma (5) |
| Right ventricle | 5 | Rhabdomyoma (28)<br>Myxoma (14)<br>Fibroma (17)<br>Sarcoma (11)<br>Lipoma (11)<br>Papillary fibroelastoma (11)<br>Hemangioma (3)<br>Teratoma (3)<br>Metastasis (3) |
| Biatrial | 1 | Myxoma (80)<br>Thrombus (10)<br>Hemangioma (10) |

[a]Data from 725 surgically resected tumors reported in references 2, 3, 9–12, and 17–23.
[b]Many atrial tumors reported as lipoma are likely more accurately classified as lipomatous hypertrophy (of the atrial septum).
[c]Metastases are under-reported, as not all series included them.

(3,9,11,13). Infiltrative tumors, both benign and malignant, often require patching of the atrial or ventricular wall with autologous pericardium or synthetic material (9,11,13). Tumors that involve the valve leaflet or annulus require repair of the valve (valvuloplasty) or valve replacement. In a series of papillary fibroelastomas, which frequently involve the valve surface, most tumors were excised without damaging the underlying leaflet, although in a minority, concomitant valve repair was necessary (14).

## PROGNOSIS

The prognosis of patients with cardiac tumors depends on the tumor type. In general, patients with benign tumors have an excellent prognosis, whereas those with primary sarcomas have a dismal prognosis.

Operative mortality is between 1 and 5 percent for patients with resected cardiac tumors (10,11,13). The recurrence rate for benign tumors is rare, with occasional recurrences (1 percent)

Table 2-6

FREQUENCY OF METASTASES AND NONTUMOR MASSES IN SERIES OF EXCISED CARDIAC MASSES[a]

|  | n | Total | % |
|---|---|---|---|
| Metastases | 39 | 261 | 15 |
| Thrombi | 14 | 147 | 9.5 |
| Calcified thrombi (CAT) | 10 | 442 | 2.3 |
| Cysts | 6 | 339 | 1.8 |

[a]Data from references 2, 3, and 18–20.

Table 2-7

EMBOLIC SYMPTOMS RESULTING FROM CARDIAC TUMORS[a]

|  | % of Total Embolic Events | % of Tumors that Resulted in Embolic Symptoms |
|---|---|---|
| **Tumor Type** | | |
| Myxoma | 48 | 24 |
| Papillary fibroelastoma | 34 | 34 |
| Sarcoma | 15 | 27 |
| Fibroma | 2 | 11 |
| Lipoma | 1 | 9 |
| **Tumor Location** | | |
| Left atrium | 46 | 26 |
| Aortic valve | 25 | 42 |
| Right atrium | 10 | 19 |
| Left ventricle | 7 | 13 |
| Mitral valve | 7 | 35 |
| Right ventricle | 2 | 12 |
| Pulmonary valve | 1 | 50 |
| Tricuspid valve | 1 | 14 |

[a]Data is modified from reference 11 and includes various types of embolic phenomena.

for myxomas and papillary fibroelastomas (13). Postoperatively, there may be atrioventricular (AV) block in tumors near the membranous septum.

The median survival period for patients with benign tumors is measured in decades compared to months for those with sarcomas (13). Elbardissi et al. (15) compared postoperative survival by cardiac tumor type, and found no difference in survival between myxoma patients and controls. Other benign tumors, however, including lipoma and papillary fibroelastoma, are associated with decreased survival.

The median survival period for patients with primary sarcomas is 17 months if complete excision is possible, versus 6 months if there is persistent disease postoperatively. In general, angiosarcomas impart the worst prognosis (16).

## REFERENCES

1. Veinot JP, Burns BF, Commons AS, Thomas J. Cardiac neoplasms at the Canadian Reference Centre for Cancer Pathology. Can J Cardiol 1999; 15:311-319.
2. Endo A, Ohtahara A, Kinugawa T, et al. Characteristics of 161 patients with cardiac tumors diagnosed during 1993 and 1994 in Japan. Am J Cardiol 1997;79:1708-1711.
3. Grande AM, Ragni T, Vigano M. Primary cardiac tumors. A clinical experience of 12 years. Tex Heart Inst J 1993;20:223-230.
4. Tazelaar HD, Locke TJ, McGregor CG. Pathology of surgically excised primary cardiac tumors. Mayo Clin Proc 1992;67:957-965.
5. Grebenc ML, Rosado de Christenson ML, Burke AP, Green CE, Galvin JR. Primary cardiac and pericardial neoplasms: radiologic-pathologic correlation. Radiographics 2000;20:1073-1103.
6. Shapiro LM. Cardiac tumours: diagnosis and management. Heart. 2001;85:218-222.
7. Majano-Lainez RA. Cardiac tumors: a current clinical and pathological perspective. Crit Rev Oncog 1997;8:293-303.
8. Raaf HN, Raaf JH. Sarcomas related to the heart and vasculature. Semin Surg Oncol 1994;10:374-382.
9. Odim J, Reehal V, Laks H, Mehta U, Fishbein MC. Surgical pathology of cardiac tumors. Two decades at an urban institution. Cardiovasc Pathol 2003;12:267-270.
10. Bossert T, Gummert JF, Battellini R, et al. Surgical experience with 77 primary cardiac tumors. Interact Cardiovasc Thorac Surg 2005;4:311-315.
11. Elbardissi AW, Dearani JA, Daly RC, et al. Embolic potential of cardiac tumors and outcome after resection: a case-control study. Stroke 2009; 40:156-162.
12. Seguin JR, Beigbeder JY, Hvass U, et al. Interleukin 6 production by cardiac myxomas may explain constitutional symptoms. J Thorac Cardiovasc Surg 1992;103:599-600.
13. Bakaeen FG, Reardon MJ, Coselli JS, et al. Surgical outcome in 85 patients with primary cardiac tumors. Am J Surg 2003;186:641-647; discussion 647.
14. Anastacio MM, Moon MR, Damiano RJ Jr, Pasque MK, Maniar HS, Lawton JS. Surgical experience with cardiac papillary fibroelastoma over a 15-year period. Ann Thorac Surg 2012;94:537-541.
15. Elbardissi AW, Dearani JA, Daly RC, et al. Survival after resection of primary cardiac tumors: a 48-year experience. Circulation 2008;118:S7-15.
16. Simpson L, Kumar SK, Okuno SH, et al. Malignant primary cardiac tumors: review of a single institution experience. Cancer 2008;112:2440-2446.
17. Kamiya H, Yasuda T, Nagamine H, et al. Surgical treatment of primary cardiac tumors: 28 years' experience in Kanazawa University Hospital. Jpn Circ J 2001;65:315-319.
18. Matebele MP, Peters P, Mundy J, Shah P. Cardiac tumors in adults: surgical management and follow-up of 19 patients in an Australian tertiary hospital. Interact Cardiovasc Thorac Surg 2010; 10:892-895.
19. Strecker T, Rosch J, Weyand M, Agaimy A. Primary and metastatic cardiac tumors: imaging characteristics, surgical treatment, and histopathological spectrum: a 10-year-experience at a German heart center. Cardiovasc Pathol 2012; 21:436-443.
20. Thomas-de-Montpreville V, Nottin R, Dulmet E, Serraf A. Heart tumors in children and adults: clinicopathological study of 59 patients from a surgical center. Cardiovasc Pathol 2007;16:22-28.
21. Padalino MA, Vida VL, Boccuzzo G, et al. Surgery for primary cardiac tumors in children: Early and late results in a multicenter European Congenital Heart Surgeons Association study. Circulation 2012;126:22-30.
22. Stiller B, Hetzer R, Meyer R, et al. Primary cardiac tumours: when is surgery necessary? Eur J Cardiothorac Surg 2001;20:1002-1006.
23. Kosuga T, Fukunaga S, Kawara T, et al. Surgery for primary cardiac tumors. Clinical experience and surgical results in 60 patients. J Cardiovasc Surg (Torino) 2002;43:581-587.

# 3 IMAGING OF CARDIAC MASSES

The radiologic investigation of a cardiac mass potentially utilizes the modalities of chest radiography, echocardiography (ECG), ECG-gated cardiac computerized tomography (CT) angiography, magnetic resonance imaging (MRI), and even coronary angiography. Plain film chest radiography is only of limited value, and may be normal or show nonspecific cardiac silhouette enlargement.

With multiplanar anatomic as well as functional information, images are analyzed to discern lesion characteristics, including number, location, morphology, margins, tissue character, vascularity, mobility, and evidence of local invasion or metastatic spread. Imaging findings that strongly suggest benignity include well-defined lesion margins, intracavitary location with narrow mural attachment, left-sided location, and the absence of associated pulmonary nodules, pericardial nodularity, or thickening. The imaging features more compatible with malignancy are right-sided location, ill-defined tumor margins, intramural location, wide-based mural attachment (if intracavitary), heterogeneity, and most importantly, the invasion of regional structures including valves, pericardium, regional vessels, or mediastinum. Multifocal intracardiac or pericardial lesions or pulmonary metastases also support an underlying malignant etiology.

If aggressive imaging features are present, the differential diagnosis always begins with metastatic disease; it is 20 to 40 times more frequent than all primary cardiac tumors. Only 25 percent of primary cardiac tumors are malignant, and almost all are sarcomas. Angiosarcoma is the most common cardiac sarcoma with a definable histologic subtype, followed by smaller (and variably reported) numbers of osteosarcoma, malignant fibrous histiocytoma, leiomyosarcoma, rhabdomyosarcoma, fibrosarcoma, myxosarcoma, synovial sarcoma, and liposarcoma. Primary cardiac lymphoma is rarer than the cardiac sarcoma, and characteristically found in immunocompromised individuals.

Although primary malignant cardiac tumors often cannot be distinguished on the basis of their radiologic appearance, benign cardiac neoplasms tend to demonstrate imaging features that reflect their underlying pathology. Cardiac myxomas, for example, are usually left atrial masses and have a narrow base of attachment to the fossa ovalis. Rhabdomyomas are found in the pediatric population, often ventricular in location and commonly multiple. Cardiac fibromas are generally ventricular in location and often calcified. Papillary fibroelastomas are subcentimeter, pedunculated, valvular masses usually discovered incidentally on an aortic valve leaflet. Lipomas and lipomatous hypertrophy of the interatrial septum are distinguished by their homogeneous fat content and location.

Radiologic detection, localization, morphologic contour, and tissue characterization are essential for the differential diagnosis and treatment planning of a cardiac mass. The spectrum of cardiac masses considered during radiologic interpretation includes benign, malignant, and secondary metastatic tumors to the heart. The formulation of a differential diagnosis acknowledges that metastatic disease and thrombus are far more common than primary cardiac tumors, and that most primary tumors are benign histologically.

Cardiac CT angiography performed after intravenous contrast administration uses ECG-synchronized data acquisition to eliminate cardiac motion artifact. This technique provides remarkable visualization of the cardiac anatomy and valvular configuration at any selected moment during the cardiac cycle. Serial axial images, coronal and sagittal multiplanar reconstructions, and three-dimensional renderings are provided for visual analysis. The key features of a cardiac mass evident with this technique include location, morphology, tissue attenuation (soft tissue, fat, calcium, fluid), heterogeneity, contrast enhancement, and occasionally mobility during the cardiac cycle. With postprocessing of the CT image data, curved planar reconstructions are created to display an entire coronary vessel or vascular segment in a single plane. The relationship of a cardiac mass to adjacent coronary arterial anatomy may be delineated prior to surgical intervention.

Cardiac MRI both confirms and complements cardiac CT angiography. MRI acquires data over several cardiac cycles and provides additional dynamic information pertaining to myocardial perfusion, cardiac wall motion, and valvular function. Function is assessed with "cine" imaging, a movie loop of the cardiac cycle showing left ventricular contractile motion, valvular function, and the mobility of certain cardiac masses. Perfusion of the myocardium and the cardiac mass is demonstrated by sequential images obtained immediately following intravenous administration of contrast (the "first pass" series of images) and on delayed sequences (images obtained 10 minutes later). With the application of various sequences, MRI may enhance the soft tissue differentiation of a cardiac mass from adjacent myocardium (especially intramural lesions) as well as delineate characteristic patterns of contrast enhancement (absent, early, or delayed).

The key imaging findings for evaluating cardiac and pericardial masses are location, morphology, tissue character, solitary versus multiple lesions, vascular involvement, and extracardiac findings. Additional important clues to the nature of the lesion include patient age, known extracardiac malignancy, underlying genetic predisposition, human immunodeficiency virus (HIV) positivity, or prior organ transplantation. Unfortunately, any cardiac mass, benign or malignant, may produce rhythm disturbances, valvular entrapment, pulmonary or systemic embolization, heart failure, or sudden death. Therefore, with rare exception, surgical intervention is the cornerstone of therapy, whether palliative or curative.

## IMAGING CHARACTERISTICS AND DIFFERENTIAL DIAGNOSIS OF CARDIAC MASSES

The essential characteristics that refine the radiologic differential diagnosis of a cardiac or pericardial mass include: site, age of patient, and presence of fat or calcifications (Tables 3-1, 3-2).

**Table 3-1**

### SIMPLIFIED APPROACH TO THE DIFFERENTIAL DIAGNOSIS OF CARDIAC TUMORS BY SITE

**Multiple Cardiac Masses**
  Metastases
  Rhabdomyoma (infants)[a]
  Rhabdomyosarcoma (children, young adults)
  Leiomyosarcoma (30% of leiomyosarcoma cases)
  Primary cardiac lymphoma (immunocompromised patients)

**Right Atrial Mass**
  Thrombus
  Metastasis
  Endovascular tumor extension via IVC[b] (hepatic, renal, adrenal, uterine malignancies)
  Angiosarcoma (vascular pooling; +/- hemorrhagic pericardial effusion)
  Liposarcoma (may contain fat)
  Primary cardiac lymphoma (may be multifocal; necrosis unusual)
  Myxoma (may contain calcification)

**Left Atrial Mass**
  Thrombus (left atrial appendage location; +/- mitral valve disease)
  Myxoma (narrow septal attachment near fossa ovalis)
  Metastasis
  Pulmonary venous extension of tumor from the lung
  Leiomyosarcoma
  Osteosarcoma (variably calcified)
  Malignant fibrous histiocytoma
  Paraganglioma (50% produce symptoms due to elevated catecholamines)

**Ventricular Mass (Left > Right)**
  Thrombus
  Metastasis
  Fibroma
  Rhabdomyoma (infants)

**Valvular Mass**
  Vegetation
  Thrombus
  Metastasis (right-sided)
  Papillary fibroelastoma (aortic or mitral)
  Hamartoma
  Myxoma (unusual site)

**Pericardial Mass**
  Metastases (multiple)
  Lymphoma (single or multiple)
  Hemopericardium (blood products may mimic soft tissue)
  Tuberculous pericarditis (loculations, adhesions, +/- calcification)
  Lipoma
  Hemangioma
  Lymphangioma
  Benign teratoma
  Paraganglioma
  Mesothelioma
  Sarcoma

[a]Differentiating features are in parentheses.
[b]IVC = inferior vena cava.

**Table 3-2**

**SIMPLIFIED APPROACH TO THE DIFFERENTIAL DIAGNOSIS OF CARDIAC TUMORS BY PARAMETERS OTHER THAN SITE**

**Cardiac Mass in an Infant or Child**
Rhabdomyoma (multifocal, homogeneous, noncalcified, +/- tuberous sclerosis)[a]
Fibroma (marked T2 hypointensity to myocardium; often calcified)
Teratoma (heterogeneity)
Rhadomyosarcoma (single or multiple, heterogeneity, valvular involvement)

**Fat-Containing Cardiac Mass**
Lipoma
Lipomatous hypertrophy of the interatrial septum (hourglass shaped)
Liposarcoma (mixed with soft tissue components, aggressive features)

**Calcifications in a Cardiac Mass**
Calcified thrombus
Fibroma
Myxoma (if right atrial)
Osteosarcoma (variable)
Carcinoid
Calcified amorphous tumor of the heart (rare)
Tumoral calcinosis
Mitral annular calcification (may mimic a mass)

[a]Differentiating radiologic features are in parentheses.

The radiologic images generated from a cardiac CT angiogram and/or MRI examination are evaluated by the features listed below and the discerning questions associated with them.

**Location.** Which cardiac chamber is affected: right atrium or ventricle, left atrium or ventricle? Is the mass centered in the wall of the heart ("intramural"), filling a cardiac chamber ("intracavitary"), attached to a cardiac valve, or arising within the pericardial sac?

The differential diagnosis of an intracavitary lesion of the right atrium begins with thrombus and metastatic disease, which are far more common entities than primary cardiac neoplasia. Thrombus formation is associated with hypercoagulable states, underlying malignancy, prolonged immobilization, and mural hypokinesis. Thrombi most likely form within an atrial appendage (fig. 3-1) and are not usually adjacent to the interatrial septum. Distant malignancies may metastasize via systemic venous return to the right atrial (or ventricular) chamber, adhere to endothelium and grow into large lesions (fig. 3-2). Direct, contiguous endovascular tumor

extension into the right heart may be traced to a noncardiac primary such as a caval, renal, adrenal, uterine, or hepatic malignancy (fig. 3-3). Uncommonly, an atrial myxoma arises in the right atrium rather than the left.

If a right atrial mass is intramural rather than intracavitary, the differential diagnosis more strongly favors malignancy and comprises metastatic disease (via hematologic or lymphatic pathways) and primary cardiac malignancies including angiosarcoma (fig. 3-4), lymphoma (fig. 3-5), or liposarcoma. The presence of an associated pericardial effusion suggests angiosarcoma or lymphoma. When the lesion is centered in the wall of the right ventricle, a fibroma or rhabdomyoma (in younger patients) should be considered.

If an intracavitary mass is located in the left atrium, it may represent thrombus (particularly in the setting of mitral valve disease, atrial fibrillation, or cardiac transplant), metastatic disease, or contiguous pulmonary venous tumor extension from a lung malignancy. The most important additional diagnostic consideration is myxoma, a benign primary tumor typically attached to the interatrial septum with preferential growth into the left atrial chamber (fig. 3-6). A mass chiefly centered within the left atrial wall (intramural, with or without intracavitary extension) is more likely malignant and may be a leiomyosarcoma, osteosarcoma, malignant fibrous histiocytoma, or rarely, paraganglioma. A mass in the left ventricle may represent thrombus (especially if intracavitary and associated with global or segmental hypokinesis), metastasis, fibroma (fig. 3-7), or rhabdomyoma.

A valvular mass may be discovered on imaging incidentally or in the context of embolic events or valve dysfunction. The differential diagnosis includes thrombus, vegetation from endocarditis, metastasis, papillary fibroelastoma, and valvular myxoma. A valvular bland thrombus lacks enhancement. Leaflet destruction and valvular incompetence are usually seen in endocarditis, but normal valve function is preserved in the presence of a papillary fibroelastoma. Valvular myxomas are usually larger than papillary fibroelastomas, and are differentiated by their heterogeneous or high T2-weighted signal intensity on MRI. Valvular entrapment may occur as a complication of a

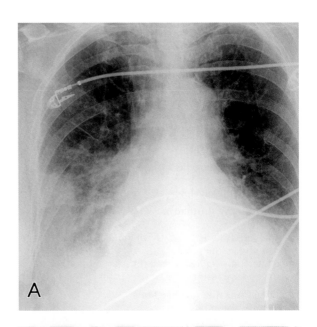

**Figure 3-1**

**LEFT ATRIAL APPENDAGE THROMBUS**

Chest radiograph of a 77-year-old female (A) with congestive heart failure demonstrates cardiac enlargement, pulmonary edema, and bilateral pleural effusions. Contrast-enhanced axial (B) and coronal reformat (C) computerized tomography (CT) images show a filling defect (asterisk) within the left atrial appendage compatible with thrombus.

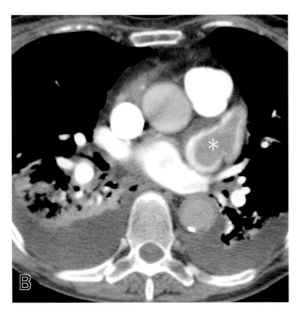

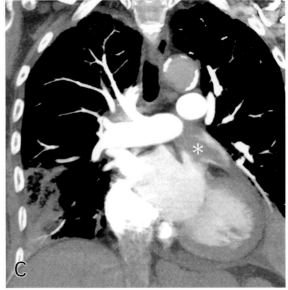

benign but mobile cardiac tumor such as myxoma. When a valve appears invaded or engulfed by an adjacent cardiac mass, a more aggressive histology should be considered.

A mass centered in the pericardial sac is analyzed carefully to discern whether the abnormality is related to a primary cardiac, mediastinal, or pulmonary abnormality. It may represent metastasis (including lymphoma), organizing hemopericardium, or inflammatory exudate. Rarely, the mass is a primary pericardial malignancy such as lymphangioma (fig. 3-8),

hemangioma, benign mature teratoma, paraganglioma, mesothelioma, or sarcoma.

**Morphology.** Is the lesion wide-based or pedunculated with respect to the myocardium? Are the margins of the mass smooth and sharp, or poorly defined and infiltrative?

A wide-based, sharply marginated intracavitary mass may be benign (thrombus, myxoma) or malignant. When a cardiac mass is intracavitary and pedunculated (i.e., connected to the endocardial surface by a narrow stalk such as a typical atrial myxoma), it is most likely histologically

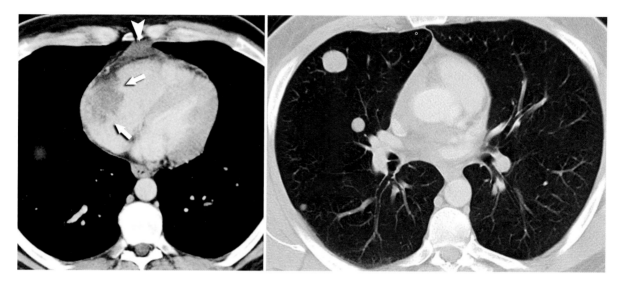

**Figure 3-2**

**METASTATIC SEMINOMA**

Left: The contrast-enhanced axial CT image soft tissue window, in a 43-year-old male demonstrates a poorly marginated, broad-based right atrial filling defect (arrows) representing metastatic deposition of seminoma along with a small pericardial effusion (arrowhead).

Right: Axial CT image lung window shows multiple well-circumscribed nodules compatible with pulmonary metastases.

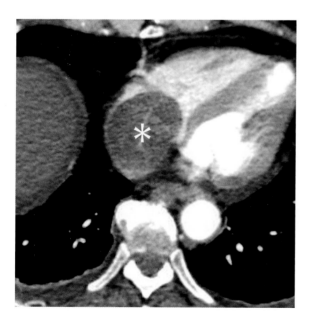
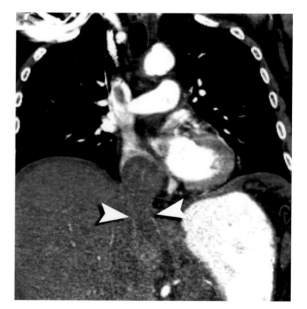

**Figure 3-3**

**RIGHT ATRIAL MASS ARISING FROM A PREVIOUSLY UNRECOGNIZED HEPATOCELLULAR CARCINOMA**

Left: Contrast-enhanced axial CT soft tissue window in a middle-aged adult male shows an intracavitary mass (asterisk) almost completely filling the right atrium.

Right: Coronal CT reconstruction reveals a contiguous soft tissue mass distending the inferior vena cava (arrowheads) and originating from an intrahepatic lesion.

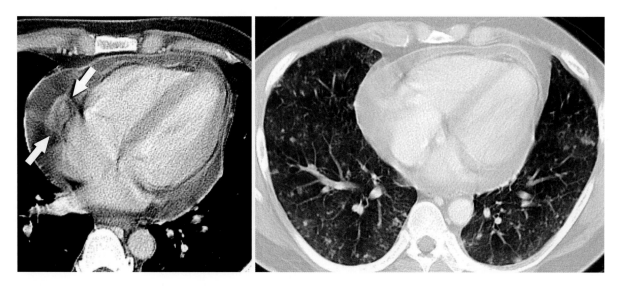

**Figure 3-4**

**ANGIOSARCOMA**

Left: Contrast-enhanced axial CT image in a 33-year-old male (soft tissue window) shows an enhancing, oblong mass within the right atrial wall (arrows). There is diffuse enhancement of the pericardium with a moderate pericardial effusion, compatible with secondary tumor infiltration.

Right: Axial CT image (lung window) reveals widespread pulmonary nodules with halos of ground glass density, compatible with hemorrhagic metastases.

**Figure 3-5**

**PRIMARY CARDIAC LYMPHOMA (NON-HODGKIN)**

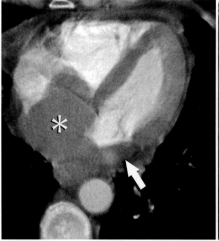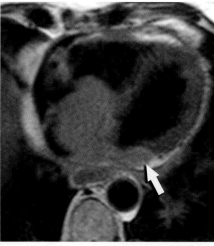

Left: Contrast-enhanced axial CT image in a 74-year-old male with pericardial effusion shows a wide-based right atrial mass (asterisk) extending into the posterior left atrial wall (arrow).

Right: T2-weighted axial magnetic resonance image (MRI) delineates a hyperintense intramural tumor extending within the left atrial wall (arrow).

benign. Nevertheless, a mobile lesion has the capacity for valvular entrapment and embolization (fig. 3-6). An intramural location is highly suggestive of malignant histology, particularly when the margins are ill-defined and suggest adjacent myocardial infiltration (fig. 3-9).

**Tissue Character.** Does the lesion appear homogeneous or heterogeneous? Are there discernable components of soft tissue, fat, calcification, or fluid (of simple or increased attenuation)?

Following administration of intravenous contrast material, does the lesion enhance? If so, is the enhancement immediate or delayed?

The evaluation of a cardiac mass for tissue character and internal features is aided by measuring its radiodensity in Hounsfield units (HU) on CT imaging. Homogeneous soft tissue attenuation (20 to 40 HU) suggests a solid mass. Cystic, necrotic, or myxoid components measure between -20 and 20 HU. Areas of acute

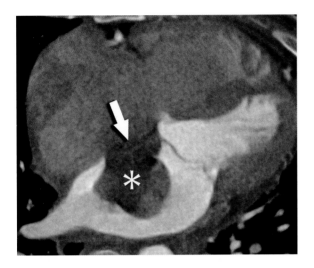
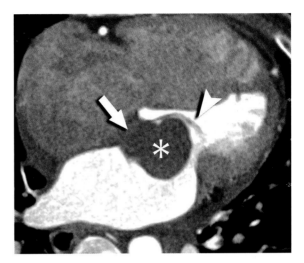

**Figure 3-6**

**ATRIAL MYXOMA**

Contrast-enhanced echocardiogram (ECG)-gated cardiac CT images in a 46-year-old female reconstructed at 20 percent (left) and 60 percent (right) of the R-R interval demonstrate a mobile, intracavitary mass (asterisk) attached to the interatrial septum (arrow) and directly impacting the mitral valve (arrowhead).

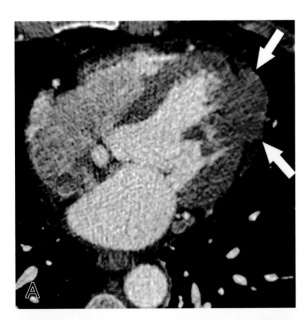

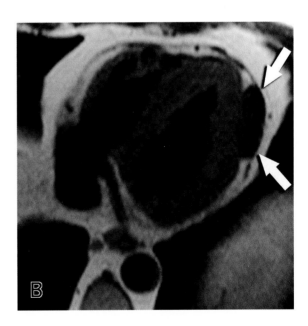

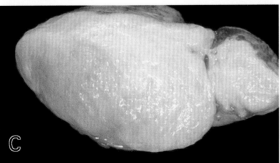

**Figure 3-7**

**LEFT VENTRICULAR FIBROMA**

A: Contrast-enhanced ECG-gated cardiac CT image in an asymptomatic 45-year-old male demonstrates an oblong, homogeneous soft tissue mass (arrows) in the lateral left ventricle, partly surrounded by epicardial fat.

B: Axial MRI (double inversion recovery) confirms an oblong, hypointense mass (arrows) associated with the left ventricular wall, partly outlined by epicardial fat.

C: The ventricular fibroma (on cut section) reveals firm, whorled white tissue.

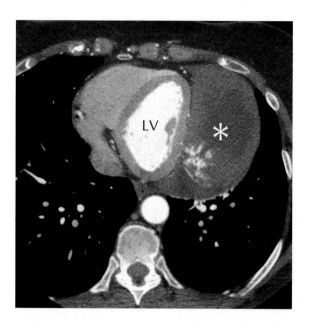
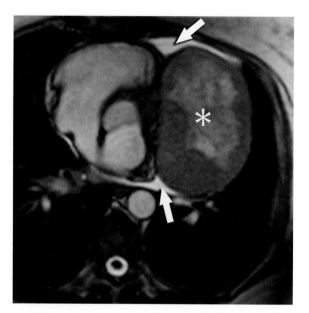

**Figure 3-8**

**PRIMARY PERICARDIAL LYMPHANGIOMA**

Left: Contrast-enhanced axial CT image in a 58-year-old female. The soft tissue window shows a well-defined, heterogeneously enhancing intrapericardial mass (asterisk) exerting extrinsic mass effect upon the left ventricle (LV).

Right: Short axis cine MRI shows the pericardial mass (asterisk) centered in the pericardial sac and framed by a small pericardial effusion (arrows).

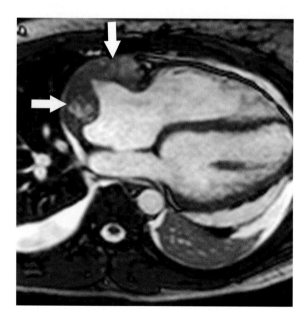
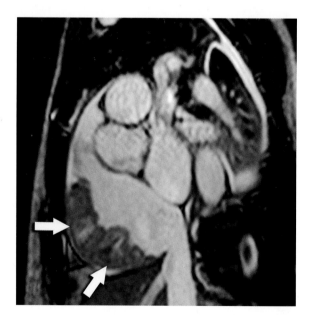

**Figure 3-9**

**ANGIOSARCOMA**

Four-chamber axial (left) and sagittal (right) cardiac MRI steady state free precession (SSFP) images in a 30-year-old male show a multilobulated, heterogeneous intramural mass (arrows) centered within the anterolateral right atrial wall, accompanied by pericardial and bilateral pleural effusions.

hemorrhage tend to measure 50 to 100 HU. Hemorrhagic components are notably found in angiosarcomas and their characteristic tumor extensions into the pericardial sac. Very high attenuation material compatible with calcifications (130 HU or greater) are found within chronic thrombus, fibroma, myxoma (when right-sided), osteosarcoma, carcinoid tumor (fig. 3-10), treated metastases, and calcified amorphous tumor of the heart. Lipomas, lipomatous hypertrophy of the interatrial septum, and liposarcomas are low attenuation lesions of measurable fat density (-100 to -10 HU). A simple lipoma is entirely composed of fat, occasionally with thin internal septations, whereas a liposarcoma typically contains variable fat and soft tissue components (fig. 3-11).

The vascularity of a cardiac mass is demonstrated by the patterns of enhancement observed following the administration of intravenous contrast material. The absence of postcontrast lesion enhancement on CT and MRI (including both immediate and delayed sequences) classically distinguishes a thrombus from other cardiac masses. One exception is organized thrombus, which may demonstrate minimal peripheral enhancement.

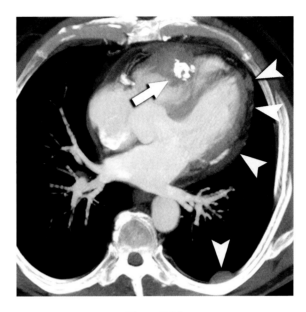

Figure 3-10

**RIGHT VENTRICULAR PRIMARY CARCINOID TUMOR METASTATIC TO PLEURA AND PERICARDIUM**

Postcontrast maximum intensity projection (MIP) axial CT image in a 56-year-old male (soft tissue window) shows an intramural 4 x 5-cm mass centered in the anterior right ventricle wall (arrow) with central calcification. The pericardium and left pleura contain metastatic nodules (arrowheads).

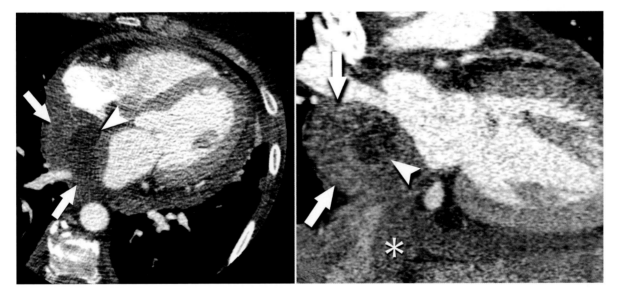

Figure 3-11

**PRIMARY CARDIAC LIPOSARCOMA**

Contrast-enhanced ECG-gated cardiac CT, axial (left) and coronal reformat (right), in a 53-year-old female, show an infiltrative soft tissue mass (arrows) centered within right and left atrial myocardium which contains a component of low attenuation fat density (arrowhead). There is invasion of the inferior vena cava (asterisk) and a pericardial effusion, further supportive of an aggressive rather than benign histology.

Most cardiac tumors enhance only mildly on postcontrast imaging. However, primary cardiac tumors that are characteristically hypervascular and demonstrate avid contrast enhancement include rhabdomyoma, paraganglioma, and angiosarcoma. Fibromas may also demonstrate marked hyperenhancement on delayed MRI, an observation currently attributed to significant extracellular accumulation of the gadolinium. Metastatic disease in the heart demonstrates variable postcontrast enhancement, depending upon the underlying histologic character.

**Solitary Versus Multiple Lesions.** Is the mass unifocal or multifocal within the heart or pericardium?

Multiple cardiac masses are most likely metastases (fig. 3-12) or thrombi. Primary cardiac tumors that may present as multifocal lesions in the heart are rhabdomyoma (in infants), rhabdomyosarcoma (in children and young adults), leiomyosarcoma (in 30 percent of leiomyosarcoma cases), and lymphoma (primary or secondary) (fig. 3-5).

**Vascular Involvement.** Is there contiguous vascular involvement or obstruction? Does the vascular component possibly originate from a primary pulmonary or extrathoracic mass with secondary cardiac invasion?

An intracardiac mass may represent the contiguous extension of tumor or tumor thrombus from an extracardiac malignancy. If the lesion is located in the right heart, the superior and inferior vena cavae are assessed for an endovascular component connected to the intracardiac lesion. For example, a right atrial intracavitary mass may represent direct extension of a subdiaphragmatic primary malignancy via the inferior vena cava (fig. 3-3). If the lesion is identified in the left heart, the pulmonary veins are examined for identifiable extension from a lung malignancy (fig. 3-13), either primary or metastatic. Rarely, a coronary artery contains a related thrombus or a directly invading tumor.

**Associated Findings.** Are there secondary pericardial, pleural, mediastinal, or pulmonary findings?

Effusions, thickened mesothelial linings, nodules (pericardial, pulmonary, pleural), thoracic lymphadenopathy, and contiguous invasion of regional structures by the cardiac mass are important observations and strongly suggest an aggressive malignant process (fig. 3-10). Pericardial or pleural nodularity is characteristic of metastatic disease and often associated with effusion. Multiple pericardial nodules with a hemorrhagic-appearing pericardial effusion in the presence of a right atrial intramural mass is typical of a primary angiosarcoma (fig. 3-4, left). Larger pericardial effusions are associated with cardiac lymphoma. Mediastinal lymphadenopathy in the presence of multiple cardiac or pericardial masses suggests the diagnosis of secondary cardiac lymphoma or metastatic disease. When a right-sided intracavitary or valvular cardiac mass is accompanied by lung nodules or wedge-shaped lung densities, pulmonary embolization is a primary consideration and the origin may be septic or neoplastic (figs. 3-2, right; 3-4, right).

## RADIOLOGIC FEATURES OF PRIMARY CARDIAC NEOPLASMS

### Myxoma

With an incidence of 0.03 percent, cardiac *myxoma* is the most common primary cardiac tumor (almost 50 percent of all benign cardiac tumors). Myxomas often present between the third and sixth decades, with a higher prevalence in women (1–3). A rare autosomal dominant form of cardiac myxoma is the *Carney complex*, which presents, at an average, 26 years earlier than the sporadic form. Associated features of the Carney complex include pigmented skin lesions, cutaneous myxomas, primary pigmented nodular adrenocortical disease, mammary myxoid fibroadenomas, large cell calcifying Sertoli cell tumors, pituitary adenomas, thyroid tumors, and melanotic schwannomas (4,5).

Cardiac myxomas arise from the endothelial surface by either a narrow or broad-based pedicle and extend into the cardiac chamber (intracavitary growth). They vary in size from 1 to 15 cm in diameter (average, 5 to 6 cm) (2). Approximately 75 percent originate in the left atrium, 15 to 20 percent in the right atrium, and 5 percent are biatrial. Myxomas may rarely arise within a ventricular chamber or along an atrioventricular valve. Most are smoothly marginated and firm, but up to half are friable, with a villous or frond-like surface, and thus predispose to embolization (1,6).

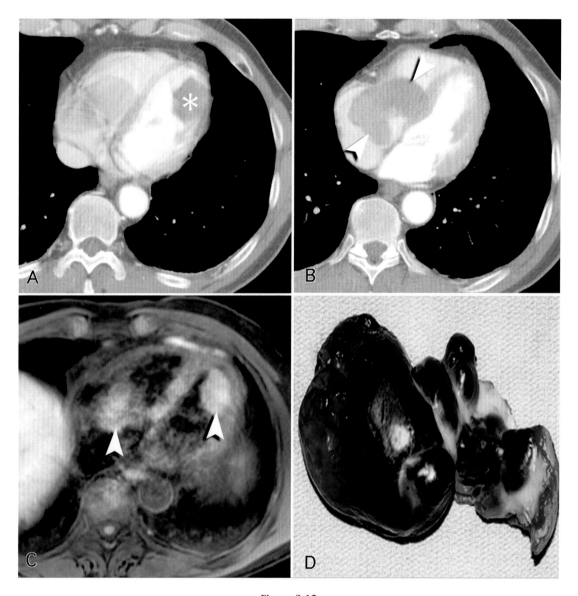

**Figure 3-12**

**METASTATIC MELANOMA**

A,B: Contrast-enhanced axial CT images, soft tissue window in a 68-year-old male show two cardiac masses: one intracavitary rounded lesion adherent to the left ventricle apex (asterisk) and one lesion engulfing the tricuspid valve (arrowheads).

C: Axial T1-weighted MRI image reveals that the masses (arrowheads) have high signal intensity, classic for a paramagnetic substance such as melanin.

D: Resected left ventricular specimen shows a multilobulated, bluish black lesion with a narrow base of attachment to the left ventricular wall.

The clinical presentation depends upon the location, morphology, and size of the lesion. The classic clinical triad is intracardiac obstruction, embolization, and constitutional symptoms but up to 20 percent of patients are asymptomatic (2,5). Obstructive left atrial myxomas mimic mitral valve stenosis, causing dyspnea and orthopnea from pulmonary edema. Obstructive right atrial myxomas produce peripheral edema and syncope. Pedunculated tumors are dynamic lesions prone to intermittent and positional obstruction, occasionally with incomplete closure of, or damage to, the atrioventricular valve apparatus (2,3). Sudden death due to a myxoma is rare

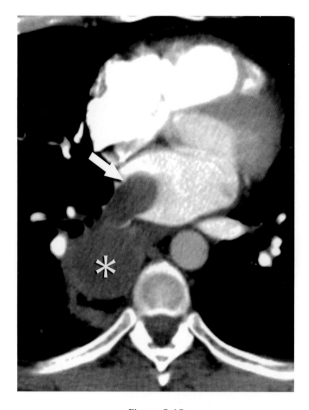

**Figure 3-13**

**LEFT ATRIAL MASS DETECTED IN A PATIENT WITH PRIMARY LUNG CANCER**

Contrast-enhanced axial CT image (soft tissue window) shows a right lower lobe lung mass (asterisk) invading the left atrium (arrow) via the right inferior pulmonary vein.

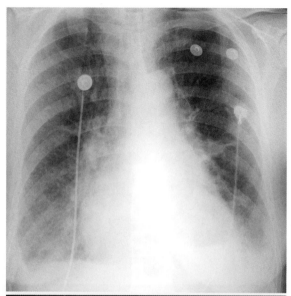

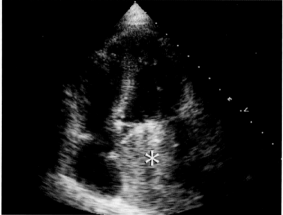

**Figure 3-14**

**LEFT ATRIAL MYXOMA**

This elderly female presented with pulmonary edema.
Top: The chest radiograph shows vascular congestion, small bilateral pleural effusions, and mild cardiomegaly.
Bottom: Two-dimensional transthoracic ECG image (four-chamber view) shows an echogenic mass (asterisk) filling the left atrium.

and caused by temporary complete obstruction of the mitral or tricuspid valve (2). Emboli have been reported in 35 percent of left-sided and 10 percent of right-sided cardiac myxomas. Cerebral, visceral, renal, peripheral, or coronary arteries may be involved by embolic burden (2,3).

On chest radiography, approximately 50 percent of left atrial myxomas have findings suggestive of mitral valve obstruction, such as left atrial enlargement, prominence of the left atrial appendage, and pulmonary edema (fig. 3-14, top) (3). Cardiomegaly and pleural effusions are less frequent findings but may occur with right- or left-sided myxomas (fig. 3-14, top). Radiographic calcifications are reported in 50 percent of right atrial myxomas but are not seen in left atrial myxomas. Approximately one third of chest radiographs are normal (3).

On ECG, myxomas are pedunculated mobile masses, often attached to the interatrial septum by a narrow stalk. The lesion may be homogeneous (fig. 3-14, bottom) or heterogeneous, with echogenic foci due to calcification as well as hypoechoic areas produced by hemorrhage, necrosis, or cysts. Dynamic prolapse of the mass across an atrioventricular valve in concordance with the cardiac cycle is often appreciated (7).

On contrast-enhanced CT, myxomas appear as intracavitary round or ovoid filling defects with smooth, lobulated, or frond-like contours and a

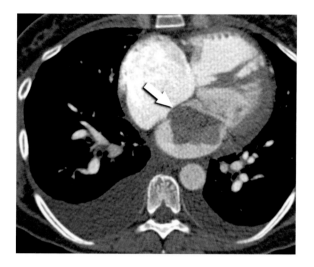
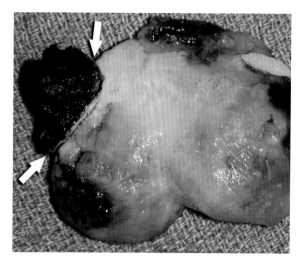

**Figure 3-15**

### LEFT ATRIAL MYXOMA

Left: Contrast-enhanced axial CT image (soft tissue window) in a 42-year-old female demonstrates a lobulated, hypodense mass with a narrow base of attachment (arrow) to the interatrial septum.

Right: The gross specimen is a fleshy white, partly hemorrhagic, 4.5-cm myxoma attached by a narrow stalk (arrows) to the interatrial septum.

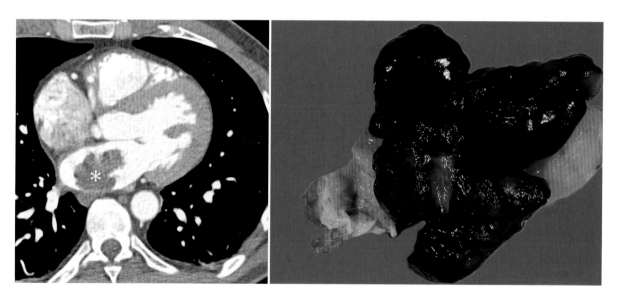

**Figure 3-16**

### LEFT ATRIAL MYXOMA PRESENTING AS CEREBRAL INFARCT

Left: Contrast-enhanced ECG-gated cardiac CT image reconstructed at 78 percent of the R-R interval shows a faintly enhancing intracavitary mass (asterisk) with a frond-like contour and unusual adherence to the left atrial posterior wall.

Right: The myxoma demonstrates a similar frond-like morphology, predisposing to systemic embolization.

connection to the interatrial septum (figs. 3-15, 3-16) (3,5). Most myxomas are hypodense compared to myocardium, but in some cases, they enhance heterogeneously following contrast administration (fig. 3-17) (3). CT delineates either a broad or narrow attachment to the interatrial septum; a pedunculated form of attachment predisposes to mobility and valve prolapse (see fig. 3-6) (7). Calcification may be evident, but for unknown reasons, only in right-sided myxomas

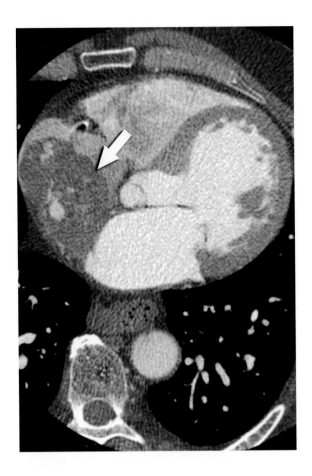

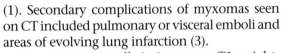

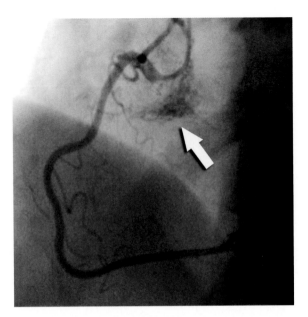

**Figure 3-17**

**RIGHT ATRIAL MYXOMA**

Left: Contrast-enhanced ECG-gated cardiac CT image shows a heterogeneously enhancing myxoma in an uncommon location.

Above: Coronary angiogram performed preoperatively shows tumor arising from the right main coronary artery (arrow).

(1). Secondary complications of myxomas seen on CT included pulmonary or visceral emboli and areas of evolving lung infarction (3).

Myxomas are usually isointense on T1-weighted MRI sequences and high in signal intensity on T2-weighted sequences, likely due to the composition of the myxoid stroma (fig. 3-18) (8). Myxomas are typically heterogeneous, likely reflective of varying components of hemorrhage, calcification, cysts, and myxoid or fibrous tissue (3). Loss of signal intensity occurs with gradient recalled echo (GRE) imaging, perhaps due to magnetic susceptibility from high iron content (3). Myxomas enhance with gadolinium, usually with a heterogeneous pattern on perfusion and delayed enhancement phases (9,10). Cine MRI may demonstrate the point of lesion attachment as well as prolapse of the tumor across a cardiac valve more clearly than CT (fig. 3-19) (3,10).

## Rhabdomyoma

A congenital hamartoma of altered cardiac myocytes, *rhabdomyoma* is the most common cardiac neoplasm in infants and children. It accounts for 50 to 75 percent of pediatric cardiac tumors and occurs equally in males and females (10). Approximately half of all patients with rhabdomyomas have *tuberous sclerosis*; conversely, virtually all infants with tuberous sclerosis have cardiac rhabdomyomas, although this incidence decreases with age due to spontaneous regression (8,11). Rarely, a rhabdomyoma is identified in the setting of a congenital heart disease such as *Ebstein* anomaly, tetralogy of Fallot, and hypoplastic left heart (12).

Rhabdomyomas typically consist of circumscribed mural-based nodules 1 to 3 cm in diameter; multiple nodules are present in up to 90 percent of cases (1). The most common location is the left ventricle or interventricular septum, followed by the right ventricle and atria (13). In up to 50 percent of cases, rhabdomyomas extend into the cardiac chambers; this is less commonly observed in patients with tuberous sclerosis (6,14).

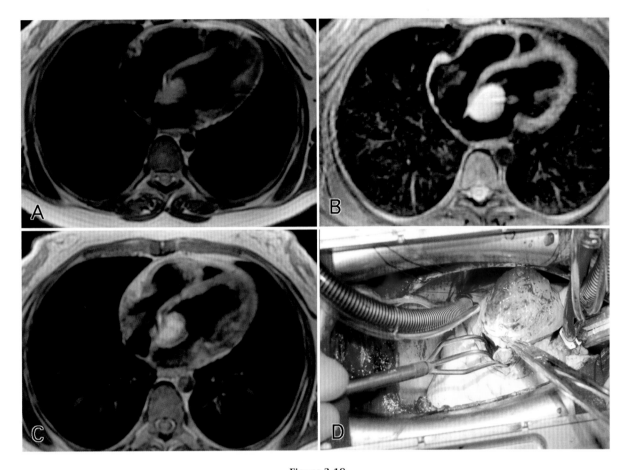

**Figure 3-18**

**LEFT ATRIAL MYXOMA**

A,B: The axial T1-weighted MRI (A) of a 17-year-old male shows an isointense to slightly hyperintense lesion, while the axial T2-weighted MRI (B) shows marked homogeneous high signal intensity.

C: The postgadolinium axial T1-weighted MRI demonstrates heterogeneous enhancement.

D: Intraoperative view of the pedunculated left atrial myxoma. (Courtesy of Dr. G. Boswell, San Diego, CA.)

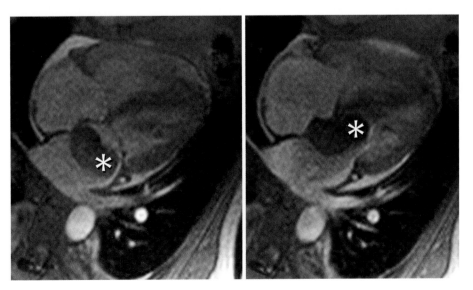

**Figure 3-19**

**LEFT ATRIAL MYXOMA**

Horizontal long axis cine images in both systole and diastole show partial prolapse of the lesion (asterisk) across the mitral valve plane during diastole.

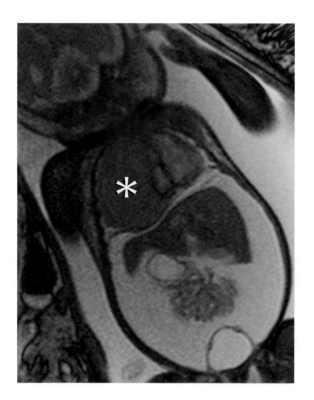 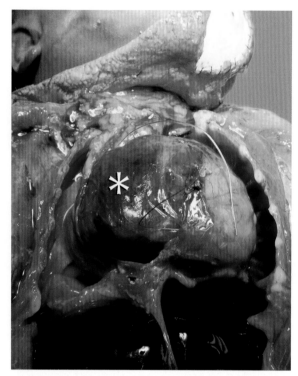

**Figure 3-20**

**CARDIAC RHABDOMYOMA**

A thoracic mass was found in a 33-week-old fetus on obstetric ultrasound.

Left: MRI SSFP oriented to the coronal plane of the fetus shows a large mass-occupying lesion (asterisk) inseparable from the right heart. Abdominal ascites, polyhydramnios, and small bilateral pleural effusions are present.

Right: The autopsy shows a 7 x 5 x 5-cm left ventricular rhabdomyoma (asterisk) that has rotated the heart in an abnormal orientation and produced pulmonary hypoplasia. Residual pacemaker wires are present.

Rhabdomyomas are usually an incidental finding on routine second trimester fetal ultrasounds, but in some cases, critical fetal manifestations include dysrhythmia, hydrops, heart failure, left ventricular outflow obstruction, and death (13,14). Approximately 80 percent of cardiac rhabdomyomas regress spontaneously during childhood. Resection is performed if life-threatening symptoms are present (14). In patients who do not have tuberous sclerosis, rhabdomyomas regress less frequently (8).

The typical imaging appearance of rhabdomyoma is a ventricular, mural-based mass that is usually multiple. Chest radiographs may demonstrate cardiomegaly (12). ECG, both prenatal and postnatal, may reveal intramural, hyperechoic masses often centered in the ventricular myocardium. CT shows multiple intramural nodules that appear either hypodense or hyperdense to normal myocardium (15). On MRI, the intramural masses are isointense on T1-weighted sequences and hyperintense on T2-weighted sequences (fig. 3-20) (8). Rhabdomyomas tend to enhance homogeneously and intensely with gadolinium (8,10). Multiple rhabdomyomas measuring less than 1 mm in size, so-called *rhabdomyomatosis*, may produce the appearance of diffuse myocardial thickening without a perceptible discrete mass (5). Rhabdomyomas may produce focal abnormalities of contractility on MRI (8).

### Fibroma

Cardiac *fibromas* are the second most common tumor in childhood after rhabdomyoma, but unlike rhabdomyomas, they are uniformly solitary (5). One third of patients present before 1 year of age, although 15 percent of cardiac fibromas are discovered in adolescence and adulthood (5). There is no sex predilection (16). Fibromas are associated with *Gorlin syndrome* (also known as *basal cell nevus syndrome*), an autosomal dominant syndrome of multiple basal cell carcinomas, odontogenic keratocysts, skeletal anomalies, and other neoplasms such as medulloblastoma (8).

Fibromas are mural-based masses of homogeneous white tissue with a mean size of 5 cm (range, 2 to 10 cm) (5–7). They are nonencapsulated and have either circumscribed or infiltrating margins. Fibromas are typically located in the interventricular septum or left ventricular free wall (1,6). Patients are asymptomatic in one third to half of cases. Manifestations include heart failure, arrhythmia, chest pain, syncope, and sudden death (1,17,18). Unlike soft tissue fibromatosis, there is little evidence that cardiac fibromas enlarge, and spontaneous regression has been reported (1). Postsurgical recurrence is rare (5).

The most common chest radiograph abnormality is cardiomegaly (fig. 3-21A) (12). A focal bulge of the cardiac contour is also seen (19). In approximately 25 percent of cases, calcification is visualized within the cardiac silhouette and may appear dense or ill-defined (fig. 3-21B) (5,17). On ECG, an echogenic mass (fig. 3-21C) or a focal area of wall thickening mimicking focal hypertrophic cardiomyopathy is seen (5). On CT, cardiac fibromas are circumscribed or infiltrative intramural masses of soft tissue attenuation, often with calcification (figs. 3-7A; 3-21D–E; 3-22A) (8). Enhancement may be either homogeneous or heterogeneous (5,19).

A cardiac fibroma appears as an intramural mass or focal myocardial thickening on T1-weighted MRI sequences, isointense or hypointense to myocardium (fig. 3-7B) (8,20). Unlike other cardiac tumors, fibromas are typically hypointense on T2-weighted and steady state free precession (SSFP) sequences because of their fibrous tissue composition of low water content (figs. 3-21F; 3-22B,C) (8,20,21). Fibrous tissue is also hypovascular, producing little or no evidence of enhancement on perfusion imaging (fig. 3-7C) (20). On the delayed enhancement phase, however, there is marked hyperintensity, a finding currently attributed to the significant

extracellular space for gadolinium accumulation (figs. 3-7C, 3-22D) (20).

## Papillary Fibroelastoma

Cardiac *papillary fibroelastoma* is an endocardial-based mass most commonly found on the aortic valve. Up to 10 percent of benign cardiac tumors that are surgically excised are papillary fibroelastomas (7). Papillary fibroelastomas are most frequently found in the fourth to eighth decades of life, with a mean patient age of 60 years and a slight male predominance. This lesion is the most common tumor of the cardiac valves and is usually solitary (22).

Papillary fibroelastomas consist of multiple fronds attached to the endocardium by a short pedicle (1). Most lesions measure approximately 1 cm in diameter, although lesions up to 7 cm have been reported (22). Over 75 percent of papillary fibroelastomas are found on the cardiac valves, involving, in decreasing order, the aortic, mitral, tricuspid, and pulmonary valves (22). Papillary fibroelastomas on the aortic and pulmonary valves typically protrude into the vascular lumen, whereas those on the atrioventricular valves usually project into the atrial chamber (22). Uncommonly, this lesion arises on the endocardial surfaces of the atria and ventricles or on the Eustachian valve.

Most papillary fibroelastomas do not produce symptoms and are discovered incidentally during imaging, cardiac surgery, or autopsy (22). The tumor itself or an associated thrombus may embolize into the cerebral, visceral, renal, peripheral, coronary, or pulmonary arteries (22). Heart failure, arrhythmia, syncope, and sudden death are less common manifestations.

On ECG, papillary fibroelastomas typically appear as small, homogeneous, valvular masses that are sessile or pedunculated (5). A stippled pattern may be evident along the edges of the lesion, compatible with the papillary projections. Almost half of papillary fibroelastomas are mobile and demonstrate dynamic flutter or prolapse (22,23).

CT detection of papillary fibroelastomas is most often achieved with the ECG-gating technique. A well-defined spherical nodular lesion may be demonstrated attached to a valve leaflet (figs. 3-23, 3-24) (24,25). On MRI, a fibroelastoma is a mobile, nodular mass with

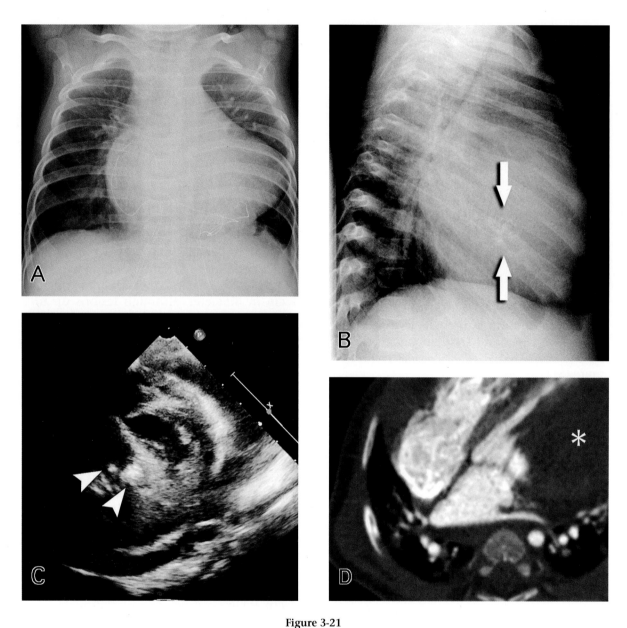

**Figure 3-21**

**LEFT VENTRICULAR FIBROMA**

A: A chest X ray in a 9-month-old male with episodic ventricular tachycardia shows an enlarged cardiac silhouette.

B: A narrow window in a lateral chest radiograph shows a faint group of stippled calcifications (arrows) superimposed over the cardiac silhouette.

C: Two-chamber ECG, long axis view, shows an echogenic mass with central calcifications (arrowheads) filling the left ventricular chamber.

D: Contrast-enhanced axial CT image, soft tissue window, shows a large soft tissue mass (asterisk) indistinguishable from the left ventricle wall.

homogeneous intermediate signal intensity on T1-weighted sequences and intermediate or low signal intensity on T2-weighted sequences (25,26). It may be best appreciated on cine MRI sequences as a small valvular mass with adjacent turbulent blood flow (10). Papillary fibroelastomas are usually hypointense to myocardium on gradient-echo sequences (27). Following the administration of gadolinium, papillary fibroelastomas demonstrate delayed

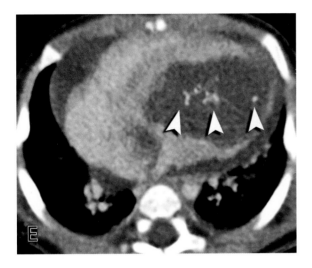
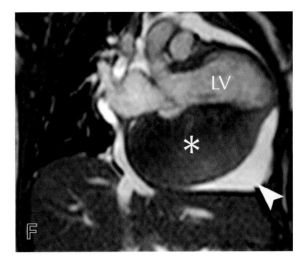

**Figure 3-21, continued**

E: Contrast-enhanced axial CT image obtained at 3-minute delay demonstrates coarse calcifications (arrowheads) within the mass.

F: Coronal T2-weighted MRI shows a large mass slightly hypointense to myocardium (asterisk), centered in the left ventricular wall, compressing left ventricular chamber (LV), and associated with a large pericardial effusion (arrowhead).

hyperenhancement, possibly due to their fibro-elastic composition (24,28).

### Cardiac Sarcomas

Primary *cardiac sarcomas* are rare (less than 25 percent of primary cardiac tumors) and survival is poor, regardless of histologic subtype (1). Although it is often difficult to distinguish a particular subtype of primary cardiac sarcoma radiologically, it is more important to recognize the imaging signs of aggressive biologic behavior. Single or multiple poorly marginated intramural or broad-based intracavitary masses, internal heterogeneity (suggesting necrosis), contiguous invasion of regional vessels or cardiac valves, pulmonary nodules, and pericardial thickening, nodularity, or effusion are findings supportive of malignancy. Two subtypes of cardiac sarcoma with characteristic radiologic features, angiosarcoma and osteosarcoma, are discussed.

**Angiosarcoma.** *Angiosarcomas* are the most common differentiated histologic subtype of cardiac sarcoma (37 percent), but unclassifiable cardiac sarcomas appear to occur with equal frequency (1,29). The mean age at presentation is approximately 40 years, with a male predilection (2.5 to 1.0) (18). Angiosarcomas are located in the right atrium in over 90 percent of cases, in contrast to most other histologic subtypes of cardiac sarcoma, which typically arise in the left atrium. Angiosarcomas often infiltrate the pericardium, leading to malignant pericardial effusion (1).

The clinical presentation is typically the consequence of a malignant, often hemorrhagic pericardial effusion producing pericardial tamponade, pericardial restriction, or right ventricular outflow obstruction (16). The manifestations include chest pain, dyspnea, syncope, fever, and lower extremity swelling (1). Cardiac arrest may occur if the tumor causes valvular obstruction or conduction disturbance. Cardiac rupture due to loss of myocardial integrity has been reported. Right-sided cardiac tumors such as angiosarcoma also produce pulmonary or coronary emboli (29). Metastatic disease at presentation occurs more often with angiosarcoma than with other cardiac sarcomas: 66 to 89 percent of patients have metastases within lung, bone, liver, adrenal gland, or spleen (18).

Chest radiography at diagnosis demonstrates pulmonary nodules in approximately 30 percent of patients with cardiac angiosarcoma (1). Enlargement of the cardiac silhouette may reflect an underlying malignant pericardial effusion (fig. 3-25A). ECG may detect a chiefly intramural right atrial mass located near the inferior vena cava, as well as pericardial effusion or contiguous tumor

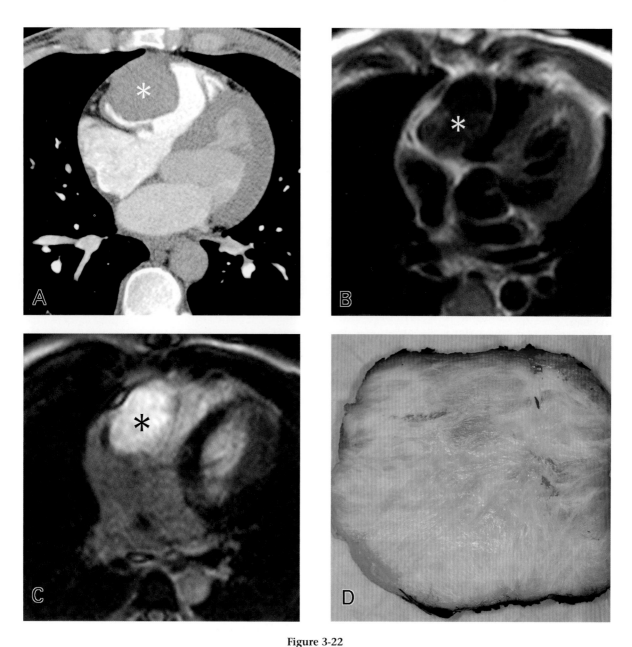

**Figure 3-22**

**RIGHT VENTRICULAR FIBROMA**

A 46-year-old male had right bundle branch block noted on electrocardiogram.

A: Contrast-enhanced axial CT image, soft tissue window, shows a partly intramural, partly intracavitary soft tissue mass (asterisk) centered in the right ventricular wall.

B: Axial T2-weighted MRI reveals that the mass (asterisk) is slightly hypointense to myocardium.

C: Postgadolinium axial T1-weighted MRI demonstrates intense delayed accumulation of contrast material (asterisk).

D: The resected and bivalved specimen is a 4-cm, whitish tan whorled fibroma.

extension into the pericardium, endocardium, and left atrial chamber (14).

CT imaging demonstrates an enhancing right atrial mass centered in the anterolateral myocardium (figs. 3-4; 3-25B; 3-26, left; 3-27A). Peri-cardial thickening, nodularity, and effusion are present in many cases (figs. 3-25B, 3-26B) (29). Pulmonary metastases may be evident, occasion-ally marginated by halos of ground glass due to their hemorrhagic character (fig. 3-4, right).

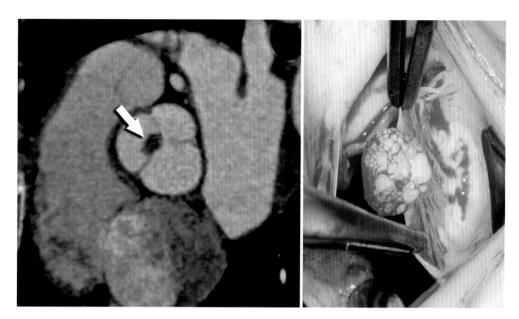

**Figure 3-23**

**PAPILLARY FIBROELASTOMA**

A 59-year-old female with a new cardiac murmur had a lesion identified on the aortic valve by ECG.

Left: Contrast-enhanced ECG-gated cardiac CT image reconstructed through the aortic valve plane demonstrates a 9-mm lesion (arrow) attached to the right aortic valve cusp.

Right: Intraoperative photograph reveals a papillary-appearing lesion at the leading edge of the mid right coronary cusp of the aortic valve.

Angiosarcomas appear as infiltrative masses within the right atrial myocardium on MRI, isointense to the myocardium (with higher signal intensity areas due to focal hemorrhage) on T1-weighted images, isointense on T2-weighted sequences, and heterogeneous areas of high intensity on cine MRI (figs. 3-9, 3-27B). These tumors tend to demonstrate strong, heterogeneous enhancement following contrast administration (reflecting vascularity) (8,10).

**Osteosarcoma.** *Osteosarcomas* account for 3 to 10 percent of cardiac sarcomas (1). Cardiac sarcomas with osteosarcomatous differentiation arise almost exclusively (over 95 percent) in the left atrium and commonly involve the mitral valve (1,8,10). They are typically large tumors (4 to 10 cm), almost uniformly located within the posterior left atrial wall (10).

The clinical presentation includes dyspnea, congestive heart failure, mitral valve obstruction, pulmonary hypertension, and syncope (6). Metastatic disease has been reported in lymph nodes, thyroid gland, skin, lung, and thoracotomy incisions (6). The prognosis is poor (8).

No reports are available concerning specific radiographic manifestations of osteosarcoma, but the most common radiographic abnormality in cardiac sarcomas overall is cardiomegaly (5). In situations of significantly compromised pulmonary venous drainage, features of prominent septal lines and vascular congestion may be seen on chest X ray.

Calcification may be evident on CT images, but interestingly, this is not a consistent feature of cardiac osteosarcoma (figs. 3-28A, 3-29) (8). The features mimic those of myxoma but discerning features include invasion of adjacent structures, a broad base of attachment to the posterior atrial wall, and lack of association with the fossa ovalis (8). This lesion is reported as heterogeneous and isointense compared to myocardium on T1-weighted MRI, heterogeneous and hyperintense on T2-weighted images, and largely hyperintense on cine MRI (figs. 3-28B,C; 3-31). These findings correlate with the variegated gross appearance of the tumor (figs. 3-28D, 3-30).

There is no characteristic postcontrast appearance (8). Although the histologic appearance of

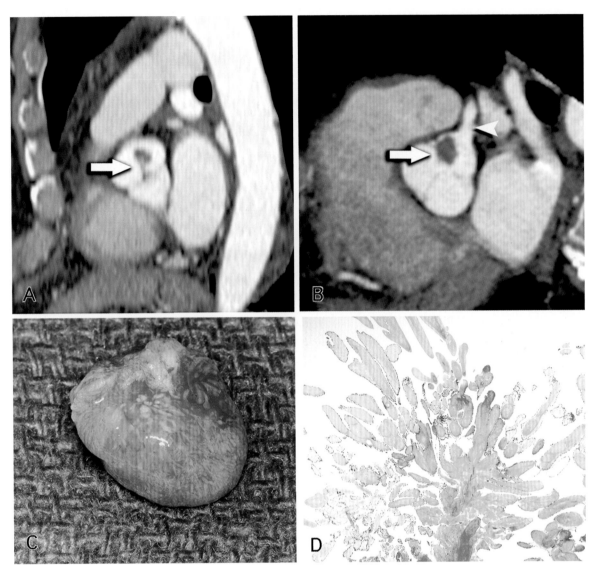

**Figure 3-24**

**PAPILLARY FIBROELASTOMA**

An 83-year-old male with recent cognitive decline showed multiple lacunar infarcts on MRI.

A: Contrast-enhanced ECG-gated cardiac CT image, sagittal plane reconstruction, shows a 1.3-cm papillary lesion (arrow) connected to the left aortic valve by a narrow stalk.

B: Contrast-enhanced ECG-gated cardiac CT image reconstructed through the aortic valve plane shows proximity of the lesion (arrow) to the left main coronary ostium (arrowhead).

C,D: The gross resected specimen (C) and low-power hematoxylin and eosin (H&E)-stained photomicrograph (D) reveal multiple papillary fronds arising from a central stalk.

the tumor is essentially indistinguishable from cardiac metastasis of skeletal osteosarcoma, metastatic osteosarcoma is usually deposited in the right atrium while primary cardiac osteosarcoma arises in the left atrium.

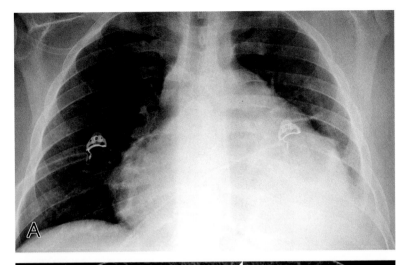

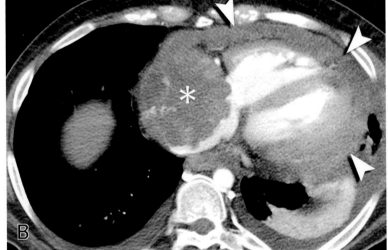

**Figure 3-25**

**ANGIOSARCOMA**

A: The chest radiograph in a 25-year-old female reveals cardiomegaly and left pleural effusion.

B: Contrast-enhanced axial CT image (soft tissue window) shows a heterogeneously enhancing, highly vascular mass (asterisk) arising from the anterolateral right atrial wall. There is associated enhancing pericardial nodularity and thickening (arrowheads) compatible with metastatic involvement.

C: Cardiac autopsy (cut open, four-chamber view) shows a large, spongy, right atrial mass (asterisk) with multiple vacuoles containing hemorrhagic material. There is additional extensive hemorrhagic tumor lining the pericardium (arrowheads).

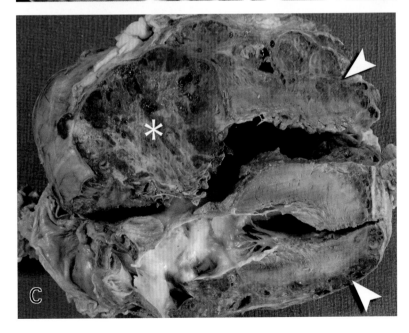

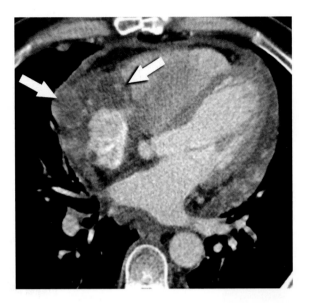
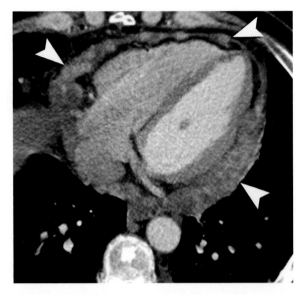

**Figure 3-26**

**RIGHT ATRIAL ANGIOSARCOMA**

Left: Contrast-enhanced ECG-gated cardiac CT image demonstrates a heterogeneous mass centered within the right atrial myocardium (arrows) that contains punctate areas of marked enhancement compatible with highly vascular tumor components.

Right: There is neoplastic involvement of the pericardium, which is studded by multiple enhancing nodules (arrowheads) and contains a pericardial effusion. (Courtesy of Dr. T. L. Mohammed, Seattle, WA.)

**Figure 3-27**

**ANGIOSARCOMA**

A: Contrast-enhanced axial CT scan (soft tissue window) in a 35-year-old female shows a heterogeneously enhancing mass (arrows) filling the right atrial chamber.

B: Coronal T1-weighted MRI (black blood) demonstrates multiple areas of high signal intensity within the mass (arrows), consistent with hemorrhagic foci.

C: Gross specimen of the mass (arrows) in identical orientation to B. There are several areas of purple hemorrhagic material within the tumor and within pericardial metastatic deposits (arrowheads).

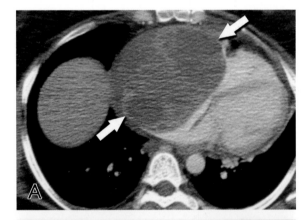

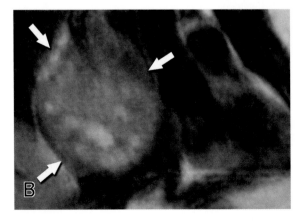
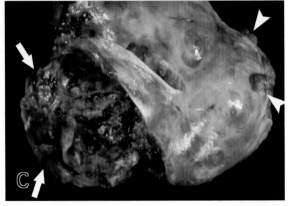

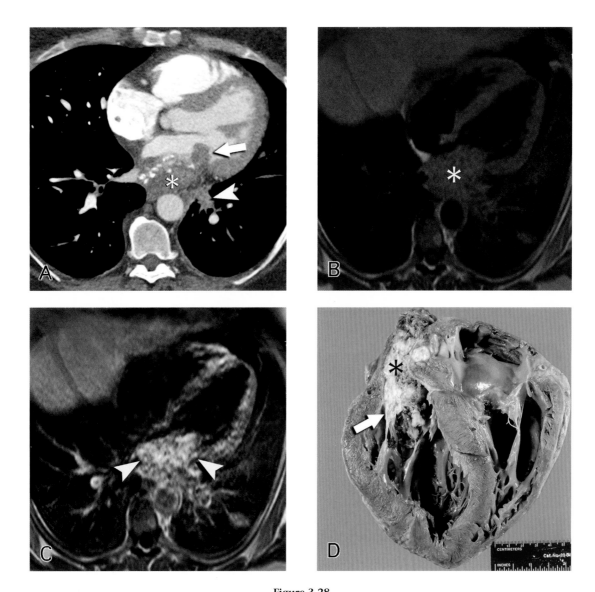

**Figure 3-28**

**LEFT ATRIAL OSTEOSARCOMA**

A: Contrast-enhanced ECG-gated cardiac CT image (75 percent R-R interval) in a 66-year-old female shows a partly calcified, 6 x 5-cm soft tissue mass (asterisk) inseparable from the left atrial posterior wall. The mass engulfs the posterior mitral valve leaflet (arrow) and invades the left inferior pulmonary vein (arrowhead).

B: Axial T1-weighted MRI shows that the mass (asterisk) is isointense to, and contiguous with, normal myocardium.

C: Postgadolinium T1-weighted axial MI (obtained at 10-minute delay) shows intense, diffuse enhancement throughout the mass (arrowheads).

D: Cardiac autopsy specimen (cut open, four-chamber view) shows an infiltrative, pale and gritty mass (asterisk) centered in the left atrium with contiguous mitral valve invasion (arrow).

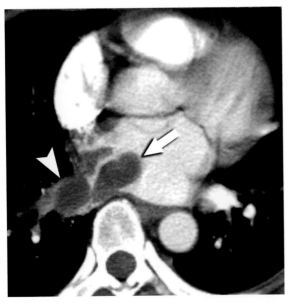

**Figure 3-29**

**LEFT ATRIAL OSTEOSARCOMA**

Contrast-enhanced axial CT scan (soft tissue window) in a 50-year-old female shows a lobulated mass (arrow) in the left atrium that extends into the right inferior pulmonary vein (arrowhead).

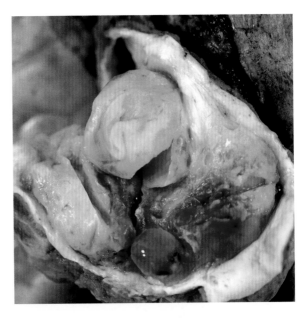

**Figure 3-30**

**LEFT ATRIAL OSTEOSARCOMA**

Surgical specimen of opened left atrium shows a polypoid mass occupying the chamber with features of necrosis, hemorrhage, and cystic change.

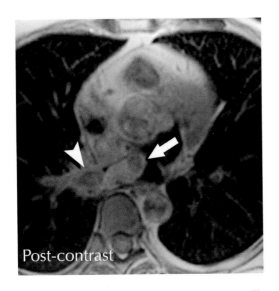

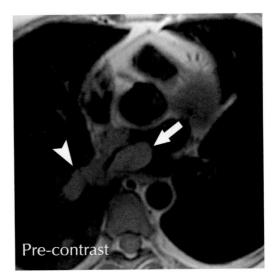

**Figure 3-31**

**LEFT ATRIAL OSTEOSARCOMA**

Axial T1-weighted MRIs, pregadolinium and postgadolinium, show a heterogeneously enhancing, lobulated left atrial mass (arrow) with pulmonary venous extension (arrowhead).

## REFERENCES

1. Virmani R, Farb A, Atkinson JB, eds. Cardiovascular pathology, 2nd ed. Major problems in pathology, Vol. 40. Philadelphia: Saunders; 2001.
2. Reynen K. Cardiac myxomas. N Engl J Med 1995; 333:1610-1617.
3. Grebenc ML, Rosado-de-Christenson ML, Green CE, Burke AP, Galvin JR. Cardiac myxoma: imaging features in 83 patients. Radiographics 2002; 22:673-689.
4. Edwards A, Bermudez C, Piwonka G, et al. Carney's syndrome: complex myxomas. Report of four cases and review of the literature. Cardiovasc Surg 2002;10:264-275.
5. Grebenc ML, Rosado de Christenson ML, Burke AP, Green CE, Galvin JR. Primary cardiac and pericardial neoplasms: radiologic-pathologic correlation. Radiographics 2000;20:1073-1103; quiz 1110-1111, 1112.
6. Virmani R, Burke A, Farb A. Atlas of cardiovascular pathology. Philadelphia: Saunders; 1996.
7. Araoz PA, Mulvagh SL, Tazelaar HD, Julsrud PR, Breen JF. CT and MR imaging of benign primary cardiac neoplasms with echocardiographic correlation. Radiographics 2000;20:1303-1319.
8. Syed IS, Feng D, Harris SR, et al. MR imaging of cardiac masses. Magn Reson Imaging Clin N Am 2008;16:137-164.
9. Sparrow PJ, Kurian JB, Jones TR, Sivananthan MU. MR imaging of cardiac tumors. Radiographics 2005;25:1255-1276.
10. Grizzard JD, Ang GB. Magnetic resonance imaging of pericardial disease and cardiac masses. Magn Reson Imaging Clin N Am 2007;15:579-607, vi.
11. Tworetzky W, McElhinney DB, Margossian R, et al. Association between cardiac tumors and tuberous sclerosis in the fetus and neonate. Am J Cardiol 2003;92:487-489.
12. Isaacs H Jr. Fetal and neonatal cardiac tumors. Pediatr Cardiol 2004;25:252-273.
13. Bader RS, Chitayat D, Kelly E, et al. Fetal rhabdomyoma: prenatal diagnosis, clinical outcome, and incidence of associated tuberous sclerosis complex. J Pediatr 2003;143:620-624.
14. Uzun O, Wilson DG, Vujanic GM, Parsons JM, De Giovanni JV. Cardiac tumours in children. Orphanet J Rare Dis 2007;2:11.
15. Burke A, Jeudy J Jr, Virmani R. Cardiac tumours: an update: Cardiac tumours. Heart 2008;94:117-123.
16. Butany J, Nair V, Naseemuddin A, Nair GM, Catton C, Yau T. Cardiac tumours: diagnosis and management. Lancet Oncol 2005;6:219-228.
17. Iqbal MB, Stavri G, Mittal T, Khaghani A. A calcified cardiac mass. Int J Cardiol 2007;115: e126-128.
18. Cina SJ, Smialek JE, Burke AP, Virmani R, Hutchins GM. Primary cardiac tumors causing sudden death: a review of the literature. Am J Forensic Med Pathol 1996;17:271-281.
19. Burke AP, Rosado-de-Christenson M, Templeton PA, Virmani R. Cardiac fibroma: clinicopathologic correlates and surgical treatment. J Thorac Cardiovasc Surg 1994;108:862-870.
20. De Cobelli F, Esposito A, Mellone R, et al. Images in cardiovascular medicine. Late enhancement of a left ventricular cardiac fibroma assessed with gadolinium-enhanced cardiovascular magnetic resonance. Circulation 2005;112:e242-243.
21. Yan AT, Coffey DM, Li Y, et al. Images in cardiovascular medicine. Myocardial fibroma in gorlin syndrome by cardiac magnetic resonance imaging. Circulation 2006;114:e376-379.
22. Gowda RM, Khan IA, Nair CK, Mehta NJ, Vasavada BC, Sacchi TJ. Cardiac papillary fibroelastoma: a comprehensive analysis of 725 cases. Am Heart J 2003;146:404-410.
23. Sun JP, Asher CR, Yang XS, et al. Clinical and echocardiographic characteristics of papillary fibroelastomas: a retrospective and prospective study in 162 patients. Circulation 2001;103: 2687-2693.
24. Bootsveld A, Puetz J, Grube E. Incidental finding of a papillary fibroelastoma on the aortic valve in 16 slice multi-detector row computed tomography. Heart 2004;90:e35.
25. Lembcke A, Meyer R, Kivelitz D, et al. Images in cardiovascular medicine. Papillary fibroelastoma of the aortic valve: appearance in 64-slice spiral computed tomography, magnetic resonance imaging, and echocardiography. Circulation 2007; 115:e3-6.
26. Luna A, Ribes R, Caro P, Vida J, Erasmus JJ. Evaluation of cardiac tumors with magnetic resonance imaging. Eur Radiol 2005;15:1446-1455.
27. Shiraishi J, Tagawa M, Yamada T, et al. Papillary fibroelastoma of the aortic valve: evaluation with transesophageal echocardiography and magnetic resonance imaging. Jpn Heart J 2003;44:799-803.
28. Kelle S, Chiribiri A, Meyer R, Fleck E, Nagel E. Images in cardiovascular medicine. Papillary fibroelastoma of the tricuspid valve seen on magnetic resonance imaging. Circulation 2008;117:e190-191.
29. Shanmugam G. Primary cardiac sarcoma. Eur J Cardiothorac Surg 2006;29:925-932.

# 4 TUMOR-LIKE LESIONS OF THE HEART

## MURAL THROMBUS

**Definition.** A *mural thrombus* is an admixture of red blood cells, fibrin, and platelets that forms a mass adherent to an endocardium- or endothelium-lined cavity. These are often inappropriately referred to as "blood ," a term that should only be used for extravascular coagulum or nonadherent coagulum formed postmortem within the vasculature.

**General Features.** The factors leading to thrombosis are summarized in the classic description of Virchow's triad: stasis, hypercoagulability, and endothelial injury/dysfunction. From these, it follows that any state that interferes with normal hemodynamic function, coagulability, or endothelial function can result in thrombus formation. Specific examples of diseases or situations affecting these factors are addressed below.

The intricacies of thrombosis are complex and largely beyond the scope of this chapter, but basically are divided into initiation and amplification phases (1). After these phases, the thrombus can organize, sometimes incorporating into the subjacent tissue, or degenerate. The degree of organization or degeneration will affect how a thrombus manifests clinically and pathologically. Thrombotic lesions on the valvular surfaces in the setting of hypercoagulable states (disseminated intravascular coagulation, the antiphospholipid syndrome, or metastatic adenocarcinoma) are referred to as nonbacterial thrombotic endocarditis (NBTE) and are not discussed in this Fascicle.

**Clinical Features.** Mural thrombi form on the endocardial surface of any cardiac chamber with variable protrusion into the cavity. Most mural thrombi are associated with an underlying heart disease that alters hemodynamics by decreasing the contractility of the chamber wall. Left atrial thrombi are frequently associated with mitral valvular disease, especially mitral stenosis, and thrombi form in either atrium in patients with atrial fibrillation or cardiac amyloidosis (2,3). There is an increased risk for their development after cardiac surgery, including mitral valve replacement and the Cox-Maze procedure for atrial fibrillation (4–7). Atrial thrombi also occur after coronary artery bypass graft surgery without valve repair (8).

Right atrial mural thrombi are often asymptomatic. They are frequently incidental findings at autopsy in patients with indwelling catheters or pacemakers (fig. 4-1) (9), and may occur in the setting of right heart failure, tricuspid regurgitation, or underlying coagulopathy. Interestingly, they occur less frequently in atrial fibrillation than left atrial thrombi. Rarely, they are the result of atrial infarctions, either isolated or with ventricular infarctions (10,11). Interventions that predispose to their formation include patch repair of atrial septal defect and radiofrequency ablation (12). Thrombi associated with devices may become infected with bacteria or fungi and result in sepsis; infection of atrial thrombi is otherwise extremely rare (13,14).

Ventricular thrombi are common in dilated cardiomyopathy. They also occur at sites of acute or healed infarctions (fig. 4-2) (15).

While mural thrombi may occur in any chamber in the absence of underlying heart disease, they are most common in the atria. When occurring without underlying heart disease, atrial thrombi may be misdiagnosed as myxomas (16–20). Conversely, atrial neoplasms may be clinically diagnosed as thrombi (4,21). Mural thrombi occurring in the ventricles without underlying heart disease are rare (22–25). Left ventricular thrombi can be found adherent to the mitral annulus when there is severe mitral annular calcification (26). This latter phenomenon may be precipitated by fissuring of the annular calcium or the extrusion of softened material sometimes found at the center of the calcified mass (see below).

In the majority of patients with mural thrombus and no structural heart disease, a

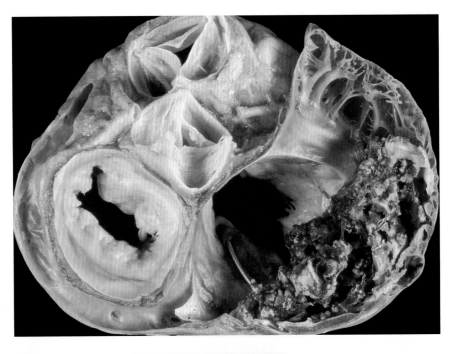

**Figure 4-1**

**DEVICE-ASSOCIATED RIGHT ATRIAL THROMBUS**

A large mural thrombus is present within the posterolateral right atrium. A pacemaker lead can be seen extending through the thrombus, past the tricuspid valve, and into the right ventricle. (Courtesy of Dr. W.D. Edwards, Rochester, MN.)

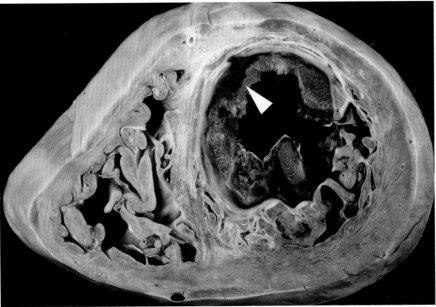

**Figure 4-2**

**POSTINFARCTION VENTRICULAR MURAL THROMBUS**

A large mural thrombus (arrowhead) adheres to the septal, anterior, and anterolateral left ventricle. The abnormal hemodynamics following a left anterior descending coronary artery-territory infarction was the primary inciting factor in this case. (Courtesy of Dr. W.D. Edwards, Rochester, MN.)

coagulation defect is either suspected or documented. Coagulopathies associated with mural thrombi include protein C and S deficiencies (27), heparin-induced thrombocytopenia (28), and disorders of platelet aggregation (29). One of the more common coagulopathies diagnosed in patients with mural thrombi is the antiphospholipid syndrome, with or without other clinical features of systemic lupus erythematosus (19,30,31). Behçet disease may predispose to atrial and ventricular thrombi, particularly on the right side of the heart, by incompletely understood mechanisms that may involve transient proteins C and S deficiency, or endocardial inflammation (32–35). Mural thrombi may occur after erythropoietin administration (24), and can complicate functional paragangliomas or pheochromocytomas because of wall motion abnormalities caused by catecholamine-induced tachycardia (36–38). In some patients, even those with multiple cardiac thrombi, no cardiac disease or coagulopathy is found (22,39).

One complication of mural thrombi is embolization, which causes a variety of symptoms related to pulmonary embolism (9), systemic embolism (e.g., Leriche syndrome) (40), and stroke (36). Rarely, embolism from a ventricular thrombus is triggered by thrombolytic therapy (41).

Mural thrombi are occasionally removed surgically if they are mistaken for a neoplastic process (42), or if there is no response to anticoagulation. In one surgical series of heart tumors, 13 of 84 resected tumors were thrombi that clinically mimicked neoplasms (43). The patients' ages ranged from 29 to 79 years, with no sex predilection. All but 4 thrombi involved the right atrium: 3 were in the left ventricle and the other in the left atrium. Several were multiple, involving also the pulmonary artery or vena cava. Most left atrial thrombi occur at or near the atrial appendage, unlike the typical attachment site near the fossa ovalis for cardiac myxoma.

Compared to atrial thrombi, ventricular thrombi are infrequently removed surgically and rarely come to the attention of the surgical pathologist (22,39). They are, however, sometimes encountered in cardiac explants and apical core specimens procured during the placement of ventricular assist devices. Left ventricular thrombi may also be clinically misdiagnosed as neoplasms (31).

**Radiologic Findings.** The detection of a left atrial thrombus may be difficult by transthoracic echocardiography but is improved with transesophageal echocardiography. Cineangiography, positron emission tomography (PET) (44), and magnetic resonance imaging (MRI) (14) have been used to diagnose mural cardiac thrombus both in patients with underlying heart disease and in those with presumed coagulopathies in the setting of normal cardiac function. If calcified, mural thrombi are seen by chest radiograph (45). In some cases, when the location is intraatrial, the imaging findings are indistinguishable from a primary cardiac tumor, such as myxoma, (46). The distinction is especially difficult if the thrombus is present on a stalk (16,47).

MRI is useful in determining the site of attachment, but tissue characteristics are not specific enough to distinguish myxoma from thrombus. A location in the left atrial append-age, while not entirely specific, is suggestive of thrombus (17). Subacute thrombi likely to embolize have MRI characteristics distinct from organized (older) thrombi or cardiac myxomas, which share similar features and which are less likely to embolize (48). Since no single imaging modality helps differentiate the two entities, a multifactorial assessment (incorporating size, location, shape, and mobility) with multiple imaging techniques is often employed and may still prove indeterminate (fig. 4-3) (49).

**Gross Findings.** Cardiac thrombi are fairly homogeneous, firm, (red to tan-white) masses (figs. 4-4, 4-5), usually without the gelatinous areas characteristic of myxoma. Mural thrombi typically occur in the atrial appendages (figs. 4-6, 4-7) or posterior walls of the atrium, often near the venae cavae, while myxomas tend to occur adjacent to the fossa ovalis in the left atrium. Thrombi may be pedunculated (20,22,47), located on a thin stalk (mimicking a myxoma), or have no attachment site at all (floating ball thrombus) (fig. 4-7) (50–55).

Mural thrombi may be well organized, with little risk for embolization, or friable. The former have been termed *membranous thrombi*, and histologically are smooth muscle cell rich, with a variable proteoglycan matrix and fibroelastic tissue at the base. *Friable thrombi* are frequently polypoid in shape and rich in fibrin and platelets. They may be superimposed on the membranous type. The site of either type is within the left atrial appendage or at the orifice, especially if there is atrial fibrillation.

**Microscopic Findings.** Histologically, organized thrombi are layered, containing degenerated red blood cells with a margin of granulation tissue, and eventually result in fibrosis (fig. 4-8). They also usually contain variable amounts of fibrin and platelets, particularly near the surface.

**Differential Diagnosis.** Ingrowth of endothelium or proliferation of small blood vessels may result in a hemangioma-like appearance (fig. 4-9). Inflammation is variable, and organization at the base has the appearance of neointima. A myxoid matrix is common (fig. 4-10), often mimicking cardiac myxoma, although a thrombus lacks the characteristic myxoma cells and perivascular ring structures of a cardiac myxoma. The endocardium demonstrates

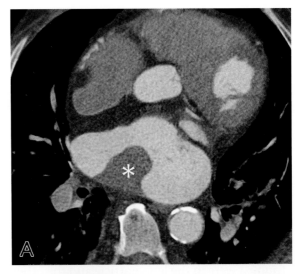

### Figure 4-3

#### LEFT ATRIAL THROMBUS

A: Contrast-enhanced echocardiogram (ECG)-gated axial computerized tomography (CT) image reveals a nonenhancing, well-circumscribed hypodense lesion (asterisk) located in the dependent aspect of the left atrial chamber.

B: Axial magnetic resonance image (MRI), first pass perfusion sequence immediately following administration of gadolinium, demonstrates normal uptake of contrast throughout the myocardium but notable absence of uptake within the thrombus (asterisk).

C: Axial MRI image, phase sensitive inversion recovery sequence (TI=300ms), shows homogeneous low signal intensity in the thrombus (asterisk) compared to all other tissues. This confirms the absence of contrast accumulation within the thrombus on delayed enhancement imaging.

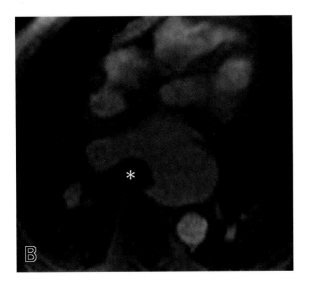

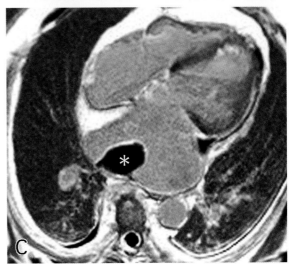

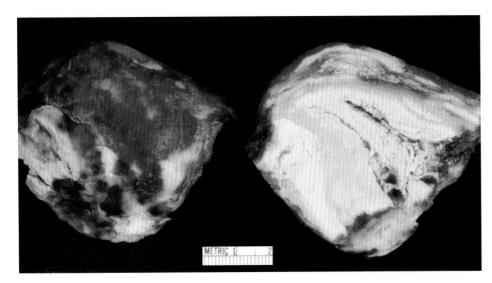

### Figure 4-4

#### ATRIAL THROMBUS

This surgically excised, mobile atrial thrombus (right) exhibits the well-circumscribed gross appearance. A somewhat laminated appearance is seen on cut section (right). (Courtesy of Dr. W.D. Edwards, Rochester, MN.)

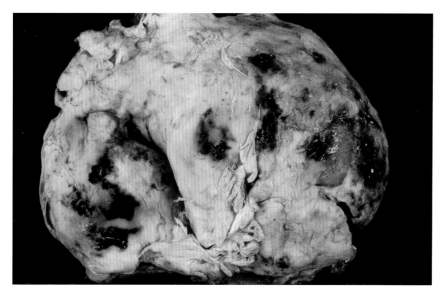

**Figure 4-5**

**ATRIAL THROMBUS**

This surgically excised specimen shows the variegated appearance of these masses as they undergo organization. (Courtesy of Dr. W.D. Edwards, Rochester, MN.)

**Figure 4-6**

**LEFT ATRIAL THROMBUS**

Left-sided atrial thrombi tend to develop within the atrial appendage, as is seen in this example (arrowhead). (Courtesy of Dr. W.D. Edwards, Rochester, MN.)

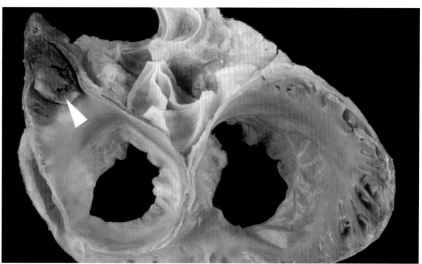

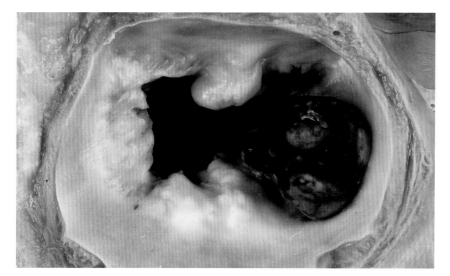

**Figure 4-7**

**MOBILE ATRIAL THROMBUS**

This mobile left atrial thrombus is situated at the mitral valve orifice. It can act like a ball valve during the cardiac cycle. (Courtesy of Dr. W.D. Edwards, Rochester, MN.)

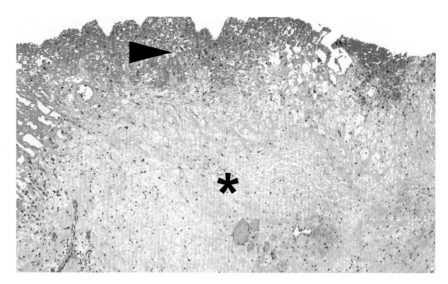

**Figure 4-8**

**ORGANIZING MURAL THROMBUS**

Mural thrombi often exhibit different phases of organization, ranging from fresh (recently formed) thrombus (arrowhead) to more mature fibrotic organization (asterisk). A small amount of granulation tissue is present in the lower left corner.

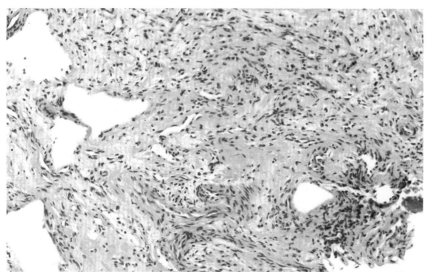

**Figure 4-9**

**ORGANIZING MURAL THROMBUS**

Occasionally, abundant small vessels forming within the organizing thrombi mimic a vascular neoplasm.

thickening and elastosis. Numerous eosinophils and extracellular eosinophilic granules may suggest underlying hypereosinophilic syndrome (eosinophilic endomyocardial disease). Obliteration of intramural arterioles with fibrointimal proliferation suggests a possible essential thrombocytosis or embolic disease resulting in myocardial infarction and mural thrombus. The histologic differential diagnosis of mural thrombi includes cardiac myxoma and metastatic tumor thrombus (56).

Calcification within a mural thrombus often leads to the erroneous clinical diagnosis of cardiac myxoma. Extensively calcified thrombi with areas of amorphous degeneration have been designated *cardiac calcifying amorphous tumor*

(cardiac CAT) (57). These lesions are sometimes considered separately from mural thrombi, and are considered neoplasms (43). Calcified mural thrombi may occur in any cardiac chamber, most commonly the right atrium, and are often associated with antiphospholipid syndrome or renal failure. They may be seen on routine chest radiograph (fig. 4-11) and at surgery as calcified atrial masses (fig. 4-12). The calcification may be diffuse, resulting in a rock-hard mass that must be subjected to days of decalcification before histologic sectioning is possible (fig. 4-13). Histologically, these lesions consist of nodular calcification in a background of amorphous eosinophilic material that likely represents degenerating blood and fibrin (fig. 4-14).

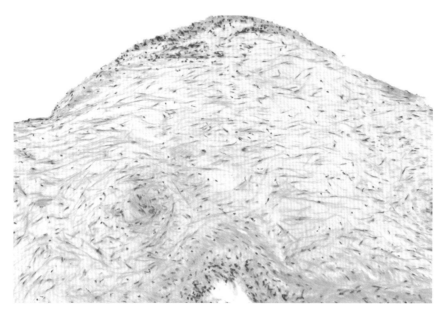

**Figure 4-10**

**ORGANIZING
MURAL THROMBUS**

Thrombi often exhibit focal areas of myxoid change, raising the possibility of a myxoma (particularly when the location of the mass is left atrial). The spindled cells have a tissue culture growth pattern that typical myxoma cells lack. The perivascular ring forms are also absent in these organizing areas of thrombi.

**Figure 4-11**

**CARDIAC CALCIFYING
AMORPHOUS TUMOR**

Frontal (left) and lateral (right) chest views (narrow window) show a mass-like calcified opacity (arrows) centered in the right atrium.

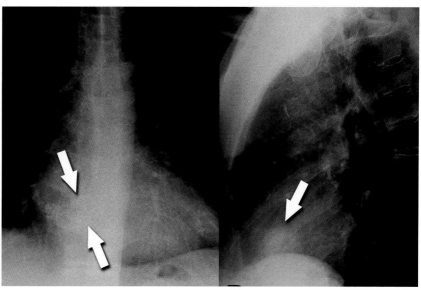

**Treatment and Prognosis.** The treatment for mural thrombus is anticoagulation, and surgery if necessary to prevent embolization (7,8). A pericardial patch repair may be necessary if the thrombus is large (58). If there is no response to anticoagulation, surgery may disclose an unexpected tumor (4). Calcified mural thrombi have been reported to recur and enlarge following surgical excision (59).

## BLOOD CYST

**Definition.** *Blood cysts* are congenital cysts found on the endocardium, particularly along the lines of closure of heart valves. The cysts are lined by flattened endothelium and filled with nonthrombosed blood.

**General Features.** Blood cysts are the result of microscopic invaginations of atrial endothelium into atrioventricular valves and ventricular endothelium into semilunar valves. The cyst lumen is connected to the ventricular cavity or to the aortic or pulmonary arterial lumen, depending on the location. They are, therefore, strictly considered diverticula (60).

**Clinical Features.** Blood cysts are incidental findings on cardiac valves in approximately 50

**Figure 4-12**

**CARDIAC CALCIFYING AMORPHOUS TUMOR**

Intraoperative view into the right atrial chamber shows a glistening, granular, whitish pink mass adherent to the endocardium.

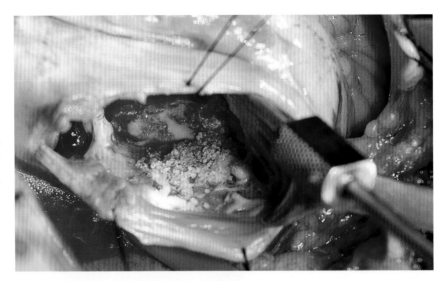

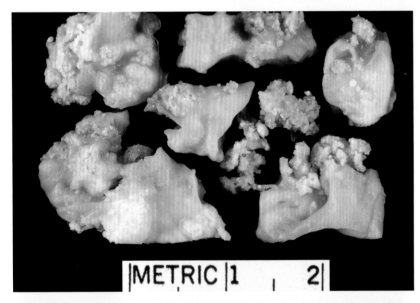

**Figure 4-13**

**CARDIAC CALCIFYING AMORPHOUS TUMOR**

Top: This surgically excised lesion highlights the dense organized nature of these masses and the intimately associated subjacent myocardium.

Bottom: Radiography highlights the calcification within these lesions. (Courtesy of Dr. W.D. Edwards, Rochester, MN.)

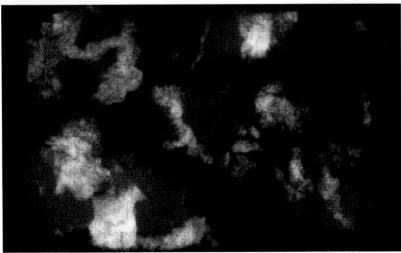

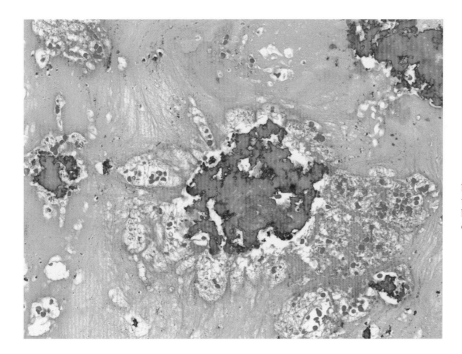

**Figure 4-14**

**CARDIAC CALCIFYING AMORPHOUS TUMOR**

These lesions are characterized by abundant eosinophilic material that contains degenerating blood products and areas of calcification.

percent of children dying under 2 years of age (60). Although they were once believed to be associated with asphyxia, this theory has been refuted (60). Rarely, they achieve a large size and result in obstruction (61,62) or regurgitation (63).

After 2 years of age they are rare; the reason for their disappearance is not clear. It has been suggested that collapse of the cyst with adhesion and fibrosis of opposite surfaces of the endothelium leads to disappearance. Small deposits of hemosiderin, fibrosis, and lymphocytes have been observed adjacent to blood cysts (60), indicating a tissue reaction possibly related to resolution of the cyst. Rare blood cysts are reported in adults, some with devastating embolic consequences (stroke) (64–66).

**Radiologic Findings.** Echocardiography is useful in detecting valvular blood cysts, both because of their location and their cystic character (67). Occasionally, other cystic lesions, such as a parasitic cyst (discussed below), enter into the differential diagnosis. The intensity (hyperintense T1-weighted sequences, hypointense T2-weighted sequences) on MRI distinguishes parasitic cysts from blood cysts, which exhibit an opposite intensity pattern and show no uptake of intravenous contrast media (68).

**Gross and Microscopic Findings.** Blood cysts are multiple in over 50 percent of cases, and up to 20 cysts may coexist. They usually affect the mitral and tricuspid valves, with infrequent pulmonary or aortic valvular involvement (fig. 4-15) (60). They range from microscopic to 3 mm in diameter, although they occasionally grow much larger. Histologically, the cysts are thin walled and lined by cobblestone-shaped endothelial cells.

**Treatment.** Surgical excision is an effective treatment strategy in symptomatic patients (69,70). The role for surgical excision in asymptomatic individuals is less clear.

## CARDIAC VARIX

**Definition.** *Cardiac varices* are endocardial, unilocular, blood-filled cysts lined by endothelial cells and filled with organized thrombus. They are dilated thrombosed veins and are usually found in the right atrium. The term *venous malformation* is preferred by Rose (71), because it implies a congenital, rather than acquired, defect. The term venous malformation, however, may be confused with arteriovenous malformation, which is generally considered a form of hemangioma (see chapter 10). For this reason, the more descriptive term varix is preferred.

**General Features.** The site of virtually all cardiac varices is the inferior rim of the fossa ovalis where the small (thebesian) veins are

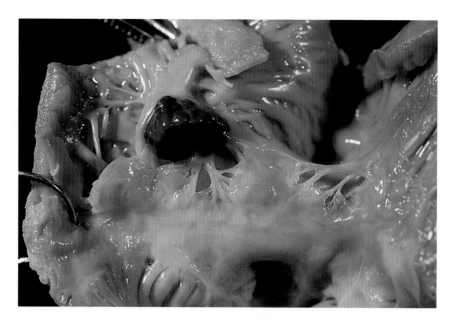

**Figure 4-15**

**BLOOD CYST**

Large blood cyst found incidentally on the tricuspid valve of a 4-month-old infant who died of unrelated causes. This is an unusually large example, since most blood cysts measure less than 2 mm in diameter. Most regress by 2 months of age.

located (fig. 4-15) (71). The cause for their dilatation and formation into varices may be the embryonic incorporation of remnants of the left venous valve into the right side of the interatrial septum (71,72). This explanation, however, does not account for the rare cardiac varices that occur in the ventricles (73).

**Clinical Features.** Atrial varices do not typically cause symptoms. They are usually detected incidentally by imaging or direct surgical inspection (74). The incidence of atrial varices is estimated to be as high as 2.5 percent at autopsy (72), although others estimate a far lower incidence of 0.07 percent (71). In the authors' experience, the latter is closer to reality.

**Radiologic Findings.** Like blood cysts, echocardiography identifies most cases of incidental varices. One example, however, was found by angiography in a patient with atrial myxoma (74).

**Gross and Microscopic Findings.** Grossly, varices are raised, bluish areas inferior to the fossa ovalis (fig. 4-16). Histologically, they are endothelial-lined cysts containing blood with variable organization (fig. 4-17).

**Treatment.** The role for surgical repair/excision is not clear, particularly since asymptomatic presentation is generally the rule. A tumor described as a varix was successfully removed from the right ventricular outflow tract after a loud murmur was detected in an asymptomatic patient (73).

## PARASITIC CYSTS

**Definition.** *Parasitic cysts* that involve the heart derive from tapeworms, and include *echinococcal (hydatid) cysts* and *cysticercosis*. *Echinococcus* is caused by six species of cyclophyllid tapeworms, the most common being *Echinococcus granulosus*, and less commonly, *E. multilocularis*. *Cysticercosis* is caused by larval *Taenia* species, specifically *T. solium*.

**General Features.** These cysts represent a typical phase of the life cycle for parasitic worms. They can achieve a remarkable size. After ingestion, larvae enter the portal or lymphatic circulation, from the gastrointestinal tract where they can deposit and encyst in myocardial tissue. It follows that regional myocardial involvement parallels the relative blood supply (75).

**Clinical Features.** Echinococcal cysts are the only parasitic cysts reported to cause cardiac symptoms. They are in the differential diagnosis of pericardial and intracardiac cysts, generally in developing countries (76). The symptoms, as with other cardiac masses, are largely dependent on size, location, and number of cysts. They can cause heart failure, fatal pulmonary embolism, and anaphylactic reactions (77–80). Cyst rupture may incite embolism or pericardial tamponade (78,79). Pericardial constriction has been reported with hydatid disease (81). Cysts in the tricuspid valve cause heart failure (82–84). Overall, hundreds of echinococcal cysts have been excised from the heart as surgical specimens (85).

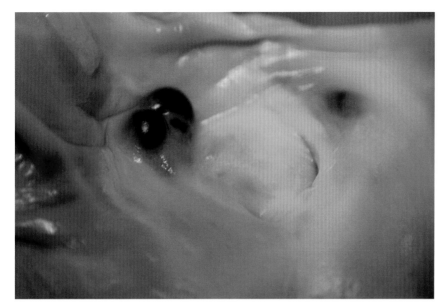

**Figure 4-16**

**CARDIAC VARICES**

Cardiac varices are often found in the region of the limbus of the fossa ovalis. They are well-circumscribed, dark blue lesions that likely represent ectatic thebesian veins.

**Figure 4-17**

**CARDIAC VARICES**

The lesions consist of an attenuated venous wall, complete with an endothelial lining.

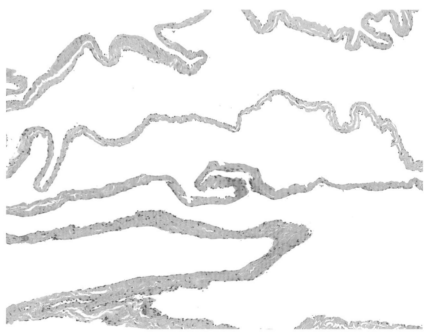

Cardiac echinococcal cysts are found in 0.5 to 2.0 percent of patients infected with *Echinococcus* organisms. In almost half of these cases, the heart is the sole organ involved (77). Overall, only 1 in 80 surgically excised echinococcal cysts involve the heart (85).

Cysticercosis may rarely cause symptomatic cardiac disease, particularly when a mass lesion obstructs normal blood flow (fig. 4-18). The disease has also been described as an incidental finding in the heart at autopsy or at imaging (86,87).

**Radiologic Findings.** Echocardiography is the mainstay for evaluating the heart in the setting of echinococcal disease and is recommended in all cases of systemic disease (75). MRI adds important information regarding the tissue characterization of the cyst and helps to discriminate parasitic cysts from blood cysts or varices. CT and MRI may show a multiloculated cystic lesion with a thin rim of calcific density in a paracardiac location (fig. 4-19). Internal curvilinear structures represent the detached membrane of the daughter

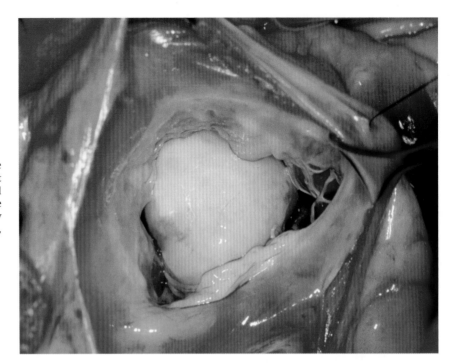

**Figure 4-18**

**CARDIAC CYSTICERCOSIS**

This large cyst arose from the right ventricular outflow tract and interfered with the normal motion of the tricuspid valve leaflets. (Photograph courtesy of Dr. W.D. Edwards, Rochester, MN.)

cysts ("water lily sign"). The lesion may be centered in the paracardiac mediastinum, the pericardium, or the myocardium, and has the potential to rupture into any of these structures.

**Gross and Microscopic Findings.** *Cardiac Cysticercosis.* The metacestode larva of *Taenia solium* is a spherical to oval fluid-filled cyst, measuring up to 1 cm in diameter. A single invaginated protoscolex has four spherical suckers that are 300 μm in diameter. There is a rostellum armed with a double row of 22 to 36 large and small hooklets measuring 100 to 130 μm. These are birefringent, and are sometimes acid-fast. The bladder (cyst) wall is 100 to 200 μm thick, and consists of tegument with microvilli and projections, smooth muscle, tegumental cells, and parenchyma containing calcareous corpuscles 10 to 20 μm in diameter.

*Cardiac Echinococcosis.* In contrast to cysticercosis, echinococcal cysts are several centimeters in diameter (83). The most common sites of these cysts are liver followed by brain and lung, but they may occur in other locations including the spleen, soft tissue, bone, breast, spinal extradural space, and heart. Echinococcal cysts of the left ventricle are usually located in the subepicardium.

Grossly, the cysts appear gelatinous (fig. 4-20). Histologically, the cyst wall has three structural components: 1) an outer acellular laminated membrane; 2) the germinal membrane; and 3) the protoscolices (85). The contents of the cyst are frequently necrotic (fig. 4-21), containing mummified components of the parasite (fig. 4-22). Occasionally, only the isolated hooklets, which can be highlighted with an acid-fast stain, are identified in the abundant necrotic tissue (fig. 4-22, right).

**Treatment and Prognosis.** Early surgical intervention is the optimal treatment for echinococcal cysts. Depending on the location of the cysts, off-bypass surgery may be performed (88). Cross-clamping the downstream artery helps prevent downstream embolization when ventricular cysts are resected (75).

Antiparasitic benzimidazoles, administered preoperatively and postoperatively, are effective in preventing recurrence. In some cases, therapy with these drugs alone has been successful (89).

## INFLAMMATORY MASSES

**Definition.** A number of non-neoplastic *inflammatory masses* have been described in the heart. These include *granulomas* (infectious and noninfectious), *granulomatosis with polyangiitis* (formerly *Wegener granulomatosis*), and *sclerosing mediastinitis*. *Endocarditis* may also manifest as a mass lesion, particularly when associated with fungal infection.

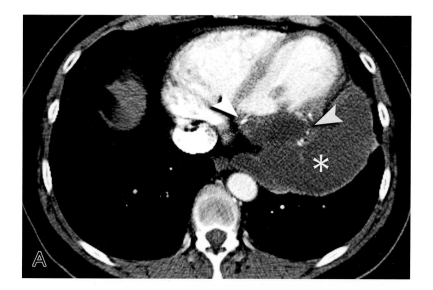

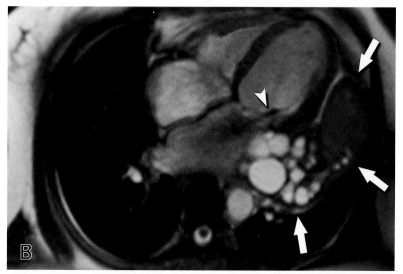

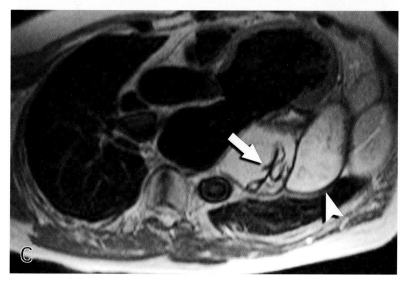

**Figure 4-19**

**CARDIAC CYSTICERCOSIS**

A: Contrast-enhanced axial CT image reveals a multicystic paracardiac mass (asterisk) with scattered marginal calcifications (arrowheads) contiguous with the left ventricular wall.

B: Four-chamber steady-state free precession MRI shows a complex cystic mass (arrows) invading the inferolateral segment of the left ventricle with mitral regurgitation (arrowhead) and left atrial dilatation.

C: Three-chamber inversion recovery black blood T2-weighted MRI shows a hypointense curvilinear lesion (arrow) compatible with a detached daughter cyst membrane. Thin low signal intensity at the periphery (arrowhead) represents the lamellated cyst wall.

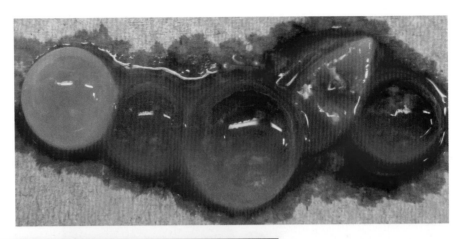

**Figure 4-20**

**CARDIAC ECHINOCOCCAL CYST**

The intrapericardial surgical specimen measured 7 x 3 x 3 cm and consisted of multiple contiguous fluid-filled cysts with fibrous capsules. Microscopic assessment confirmed *Echinococcus granulosus* infection.

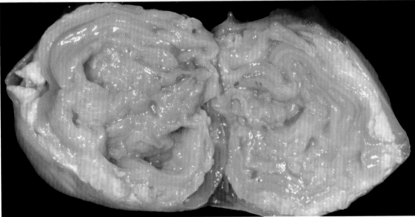

**Figure 4-21**

**CARDIAC ECHINOCOCCAL CYST**

Surgical excised, bisected, echinococcal cyst with necrotic contents. (Courtesy of Dr. W. D. Edwards, Rochester, MN.)

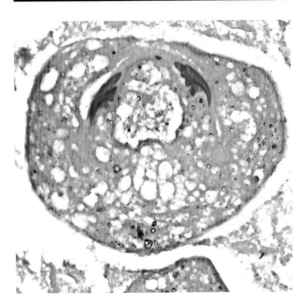
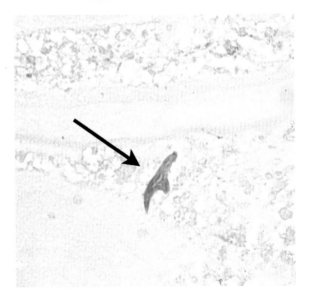

**Figure 4-22**

**CARDIAC ECHINOCOCCOSIS**

Left: An echinococcal scolex with hooklets is present within the necrotic cyst core.

Right: Occasionally, only rare, naked (without associated scolex) hooklets are identified among the necrotic tissue (arrow). (Left and right, acid-fast stains.) (Courtesy of Dr. W.D. Edwards, Rochester, MN.)

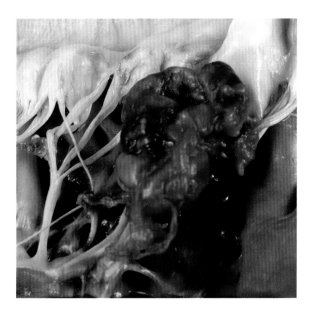

**Figure 4-23**

*ASPERGILLUS* **ENDOCARDITIS**

Above: Fungal endocarditis can present as a mass lesion interfering with valve function.

Right: A silver stain identifies the fungal hyphae. (Courtesy of Dr. W.D. Edwards, Rochester, MN.)

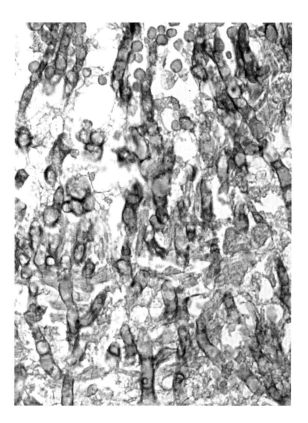

Cardiac inflammatory myofibroblastic tumors (also referred to as *plasma cell granulomas* or *inflammatory pseudotumors*) have often been included in a discussion of non-neoplastic cardiac masses (90,91). It is unclear whether these lesions truly are non-neoplastic, but because at least a subset express ALK-1 immunohistochemically (92) or *ALK-1* rearrangements cytogenetically (93), there is some rationale to include these in the discussion of cardiac neoplasms with primarily benign clinical behavior (see chapter 13).

**General Features.** The etiology of inflammatory masses is primarily either infectious or non-infectious. Endocarditis and infectious granulomas obviously fall into the latter category, while the other entities noted above are primarily in the former category, although some cases of sclerosing mediastinitis have been associated with *Histoplasma capsulatum* infection. Direct fungal infection of the heart itself can also produce mass lesions (fig. 4-23) (94).

**Clinical Features.** The clinical manifestations directly related to inflammatory masses are usually the result of the mechanical-compressive effects of precariously situated lesions.

Most clinical consequences stem from the fact that these lesions are not isolated to the heart, but rather part of a systemic process.

Individuals with infectious masses may exhibit the symptoms of infection (e.g., fever, chills, night sweats), however, occasionally symptoms are related primarily to the hemodynamic consequences of the mass lesion (95). Conduction system disturbances, atrioventricular block in particular, often occur in the setting of myocardial sarcoidosis (96).

**Radiologic Findings.** Inflammatory masses are seen with most imaging modalities. Tissue characterization, as described with CT or MRI, has not been specific for these lesions.

**Gross and Microscopic Findings.** The histopathology of inflammatory masses is varied. A well-formed granuloma associated with fibrosis and a pauci-eosinophilic infiltrate is the usual histologic manifestation of cardiac sarcoidosis (fig. 4-24) (97). The granulomatous inflammation of sarcoidosis can be confluent and extensive, forming large myocardial masses (fig. 4-25). It is not unusual for these granulomas to affect the conduction system, particularly the atrioventricular node and bundle branches (fig. 4-26).

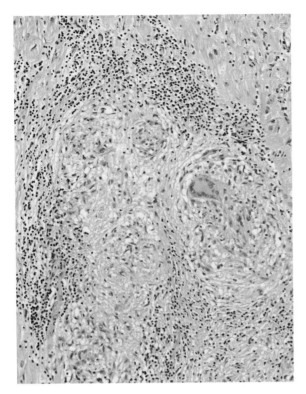

**Figure 4-24**

**CARDIAC SARCOIDOSIS**

The presence of well-formed granulomas containing epithelioid macrophages, giant cells, and a lymphoplasmacytic infiltrate with associated fibrosis is typical of (though not necessarily specific for) sarcoidosis.

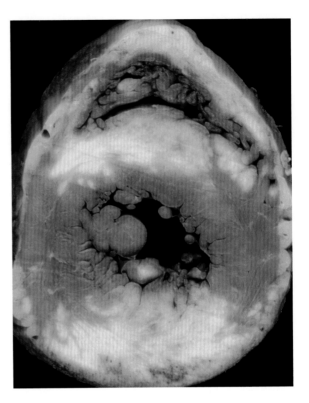

**Figure 4-25**

**CARDIAC SARCOIDOSIS**

Short-axis cut shows a dense, mass-like white infiltrate in the ventricular septum and free walls. Histologically, these areas correspond to coalescing granulomas with associated fibrosis. (Courtesy of Dr. W.D. Edwards, Rochester, MN.)

**Figure 4-26**

**CARDIAC SARCOIDOSIS WITH INVOLVEMENT OF CONDUCTION SYSTEM**

It is not unusual to find granulomatous involvement of the conduction system tissue in the setting of cardiac sarcoidosis. Involvement of the left bundle branch (LBB) is shown here.

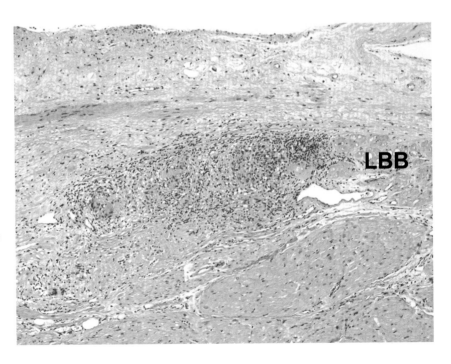

Infectious granulomas in the heart are similar to those identified elsewhere in the body and exhibit collections of epithelioid macrophages with an associated chronic inflammatory infiltrate and variable necrosis. Cardiac tuberculosis is characterized by well-formed necrotizing granulomas containing identifiable acid-fast bacilli (95). Sclerosing mediastinitis manifests as a paucicellular fibrous mass within the atrium (98,99).

**Treatment.** Surgical excision of the mass to alleviate hemodynamic or arrhythmic complications, together with treatment of the underlying disease (e.g., infection) when present, is the treatment of choice (94).

## MITRAL ANNULAR CALCIFICATION RESULTING IN PSEUDOTUMOR (CASEOUS CALCIFICATION)

**Definition.** *Annular calcification* refers to the degenerative deposition of calcium and variable amounts of lipid along the fibrous annulus of the atrioventricular valve. It most often occurs along the posterior mitral valve. It may occasionally protrude into the left atrial or ventricular cavity, producing a mass lesion (100,101). In such cases, the term *caseous necrosis* or *caseous calcification of the mitral valve* is used (102,103).

**General Features.** The etiology of annular calcification is unknown. Some have posited that it is a mechanical stress-induced phenomenon (104), while others maintain it is a manifestation of systemic atherosclerotic disease (105). Rarely, it undergoes central softening or liquefaction, so-called caseous degeneration, although the mechanisms behind this are unclear (106). This gritty material can extrude onto the leaflet surface and incite thrombosis.

Aside from the dystrophic mechanisms of calcification, the annulus can undergo metastatic calcification in the setting of hypercalcemia, such as that seen with hyperparathyroidism (107). Whatever the cause, annular calcification is a common finding that can be seen as a mass lesion either on imaging or at the time of surgery.

**Clinical Features.** Calcification of the mitral annulus is a common finding, seen in 3 to 10 percent of the adult (middle-aged or older) population (108–111). Women are disproportionately affected. It is associated with age over 60 years, obesity, diabetes mellitus, systemic hypertension, atrial fibrillation, and aortic stenosis (110,112).

Mitral valve prolapse is also a well-described association. The association with aortic stenosis and systemic hypertension has been brought into question given that the two diseases have common risk factors (105,110). With that said, the increased strain on the mitral apparatus, imparted by elevated ventricular systolic pressures, is an attractive mechanistic explanation for this degenerative phenomenon.

Annular calcification occasionally leads to left ventricular inflow tract obstruction by restricting leaflet mobility (113). Mitral valve regurgitation has also been reported in the setting of annular calcium (114), but it is likely that valvular regurgitation is more commonly a consequence of underlying valve disease that may also have led to the annular calcification. Conduction system disturbances, such as block (atrioventricular or bundle branch) and bradyarrhythmias, have been observed (115). A report from the Framingham Heart Study (116) has shown the presence of annular calcium to be correlated with adverse outcomes, including a risk of cardiovascular disease (myocardial infarction, heart failure, stroke), cardiovascular disease-related death, and all-cause death (which is increased by 10 percent for each 1 mm increase in thickness of annular calcium). There have been individual reports of annular calcium presenting as a cerebral embolism (100).

Rarely, annular calcification results in a mass that is clinically mistaken for an atrial tumor. (102,103). In such cases, the term caseous necrosis is sometimes used, although the designation is a misnomer.

**Radiologic Findings.** Annular calcification can be visualized on echocardiogram, CT, and MRI. The calcification can be so extensive as to interfere with the proper evaluation of valve function and Doppler-measured flow velocities, particularly on echocardiography (117). The posterior annular distribution is a strong clue suggesting the diagnosis. Occasionally, abscess or cyst is in the differential diagnosis, particularly if central softening is present. A mass lesion may extend into the left atrium, and on imaging appear as a calcified thrombus or neoplasm (100,101).

**Gross and Microscopic Findings.** Annular calcium is distributed primarily along the posterior annulus, with variable encroachment onto the leaflet or into the adjacent myocardium

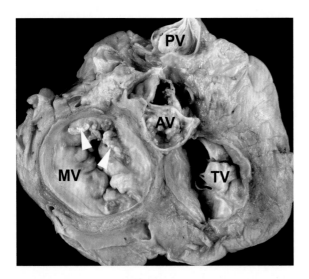

**Figure 4-27**

**ANNULAR CALCIFICATION**

Calcification can protrude from the annulus and extend to involve the leaflet (arrowheads). (Courtesy of Dr. W.D. Edwards, Rochester, MN.)

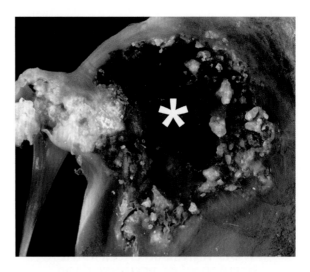

**Figure 4-29**

**ANNULAR CALCIFICATION WITH CENTRAL SOFTENING**

Annular calcification can occasionally undergo central softening (asterisk) which has been termed caseous degeneration. (Courtesy of Dr. W.D. Edwards, Rochester, MN.)

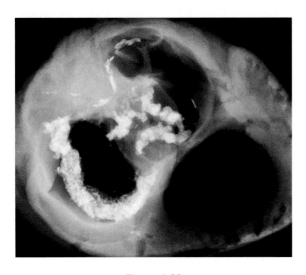

**Figure 4-28**

**ANNULAR CALCIFICATION**

A radiograph highlights the distribution of the annular calcium along the posterior portion of the mitral valve. The dense calcified aortic valve is seen here, a well-known feature associated with annular calcification.

(fig. 4-27). When present, the centrally softened material is typically described as pasty (100). Radiography of the specimen can help assess the extent and distribution of this process (fig. 4-28). Areas of central softening (fig. 4-29) manifest as amorphous eosinophilic material, not unlike that

seen with a cardiac calcifying amorphous tumor. If the calcified shell becomes fractured, this grumous material is extruded out onto the leaflet where it can cause thrombosis or embolize (118,119).

When a mass lesion forms (caseous calcification), it is seen on routine and high resolution imaging (fig. 4-30). Discriminating between cardiac calcifying amorphous tumor and extruded annular calcification can be difficult, although the presence of annular calcification, the position of the mass with respect to the annulus, and the presence of fresh thrombus and giant cells on the surface favor a diagnosis of the latter (fig. 4-31).

Histologically, annular calcification manifests as nodular calcific deposits with admixed and variable amounts of necrotic tissue within a collagenous matrix. Frequently, there is surrounding granulation tissue with a modest lymphoplasmacytic infiltrate. Occasionally, ossification is identified (106). These nodular aggregates may extend to involve the adjacent myocardium, leaflet apparatus, or subvalvular apparatus.

**Treatment.** Treatment of the underlying disorder (e.g., atrial fibrillation or other arrhythmia) is usually recommended, although the impact of such treatment on the annular calcification itself is not clear. Because of the increased operative morbidity and mortality in

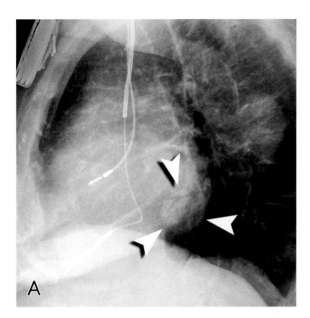

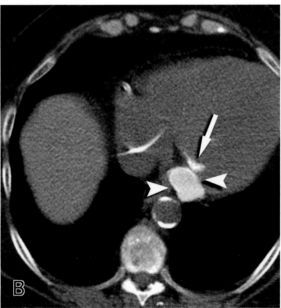

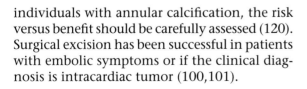

**Figure 4-30**

**ANNULAR CALCIFICATION WITH CASEOUS NECROSIS**

A: Lateral chest radiograph (narrow window) confirms a well-circumscribed, 2-cm calcific density (arrowheads) superimposed over the posterior left atrium.

B: Noncontrast axial CT shows a well-circumscribed, 2-cm lesion of calcium attenuation (arrowheads) closely sited to the posterior left atrial aspect of the mitral valve annulus. There is adjacent mitral annular ring calcification, a common companion finding (arrow).

C: Axial MRI (four-chamber view) immediately following administration of gadolinium (first-pass perfusion) shows total absence of contrast enhancement within the lesion (asterisk). (LA = left atrium, LV = left ventricle.)

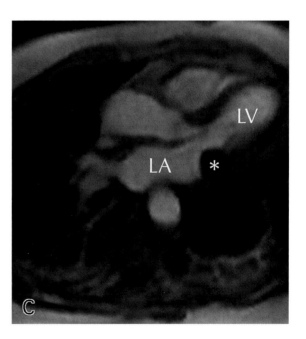

individuals with annular calcification, the risk versus benefit should be carefully assessed (120). Surgical excision has been successful in patients with embolic symptoms or if the clinical diagnosis is intracardiac tumor (100,101).

## MESOTHELIAL INCIDENTAL CARDIAC EXCRESCENCES

**Definition.** *Mesothelial incidental cardiac excrescences* (MICE), sometimes referred to as *mesothelial/macrophage incidental cardiac excrescences*, are fragmented collections of benign mesothelial

cells, fat cells, and macrophages that lack intervening stroma. They are found exclusively within the heart, aorta, or pericardium, generally during cardiac procedures for other causes. They are the cardiac equivalent of so-called lesions of aggregate monocytes and mesothelial cells (LAMM) that are sometimes found in endobronchial biopsy specimens.

**General Features.** Although originally considered a lesion related to histiocytoid hemangioma (121), MICE are now mostly considered artifacts of cardiovascular procedures, having

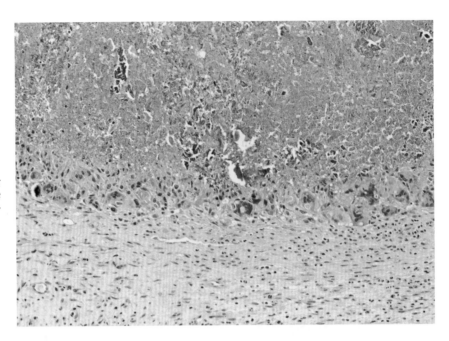

**Figure 4-31**

**EXTRUSION OF ANNULAR CALCIFICATION**

Centrally softened annular calcium extruded through the calcific shell incites a foreign-body giant cell reaction.

been discovered in cardiotomy suction devices (122). This theory does not, however, explain rare similar collections of cells found during transvenous right ventricular biopsy (121). Several cases of MICE have led to the theory that pericardial irritation or trauma may incite their formation, including two cases of metastatic carcinoma without prior cardiac instrumentation (123,124) as well as cases of tuberculous aortitis (125) and rheumatic heart disease (126).

**Clinical Features.** Cardiac MICE are largely considered to be incidental artifacts and therefore usually without clinical relevance. Nevertheless, a single example causing severe acute cardiopulmonary failure has been reported (127). Moreover, a case of metastatic adenocarcinoma found within a MICE highlights the importance of careful histopathologic and immunophenotypic analysis (123). In a series of 14 cases, 7 were in women; 6 were found within atria, 2 on the mitral valve, 1 on the aortic valve, 3 in the pericardium, and 1 in a dissecting aortic aneurysm (121). The fourteenth case was not found at cardiac surgery but at endomyocardial biopsy.

The true incidence of cardiac MICE is unknown. If they are indeed artifacts of instrumentation, they may be common. Less than 40 cases have been reported in the literature. Of 110 cardiac myxomas reviewed at the Armed Forces Institute of Pathology (AFIP), 3 had MICE attachments, indicating that they are probably not rare. Courtice et al. (122)

processed, for light microscopy, the contents of extracorporeal bypass pump filters and material adherent to mediastinal and pericardial drains in cardiac surgery cases. They demonstrated cardiac MICE in 82 percent of pump filters and 13 percent of drains, further suggesting their common occurrence as surgical artifacts.

**Radiologic Findings.** Little is published on the use of imaging modalities to detect MICE. Like most other cardiac masses in this chapter, echocardiography, CT, and MRI may be useful in their identification but are limited in discriminating them from other masses (e.g., thrombus).

**Gross and Microscopic Findings.** Grossly, these lesions are similar to thrombi with a variegated appearance. Histologically, there are compact clusters of histiocytes, fat globules, and mesothelial cells, without intervening stroma (fig. 4-32). The mesothelial components of these lesions stain strongly with antibodies directed against cytokeratin.

**Treatment.** Since these lesions are usually incidental and asymptomatic, simple removal is considered curative. In the single instance of reported clinically consequential MICE, surgical excision was also curative.

### PSEUDOTENDON

**Definition.** *Pseudotendons*, or *false cords*, are fibrotic or fibromuscular bands that attach to two nonvalvular endocardial surfaces within

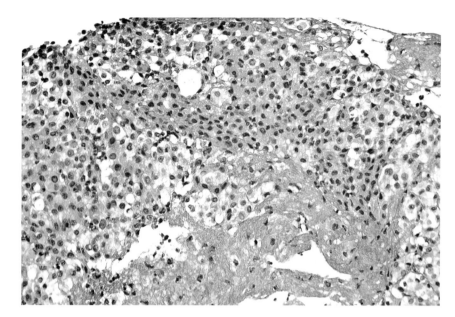

**Figure 4-32**

**MESOTHELIAL INCIDENTAL CARDIAC EXCRESCENCE**

The admixture of fibrin, monocytes, mesothelial cells, and fat is characteristic of these lesions.

**Figure 4-33**

**LEFT VENTRICULAR PSEUDOTENDON**

A membranous band (arrowhead) extends between the septum and the free wall of the left ventricle without attachment to the mitral apparatus. (Courtesy of Dr. W.D. Edwards, Rochester, MN.)

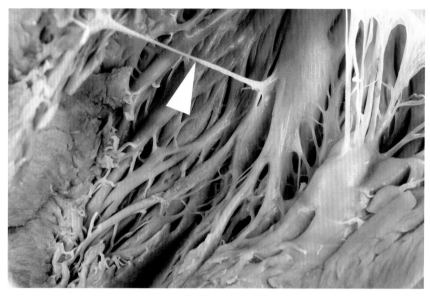

(and occasionally across) a cardiac chamber (fig. 4-33), usually the left ventricle.

**General Features.** The histogenesis of pseudotendons is unknown but is possibly related to localized remnants of noncompacted muscle. Whatever the precise etiology, they are largely believed to represent anatomic variants.

**Clinical Features.** When present in the left ventricle, they are associated with benign murmurs, premature ventricular contractions, and idiopathic ventricular tachycardia; those in the left atrium are associated with patent foramen ovale, Chiari network, and supraventricular arrhythmias. Right atrial false tendons have no known clinical significance.

The prevalence of pseudotendons varies widely, ranging from under 1 percent to over 50 percent (128). This variability is likely a reflection of the method of study.

**Radiologic Findings.** Echocardiography (transesophageal and transthoracic) has identified pseudotendons in both normal and diseased hearts. Several studies that have evaluated the echocardiographic incidence of these lesions have noted an incidence of greater than 50 percent in the general population.

**Gross Findings.** The most common location of pseudotendons is from the left-sided posteromedial papillary muscle to the ventricular septum (66 percent), followed by the cords that connect the anterolateral and posteromedial papillary muscles (12 percent) (129). Least common are cords attached to two points on the left ventricular free wall (less than 1 percent).

**Microscopic Findings.** Histologically, pseudotendons contain fibrous tissue and variable amounts of myocardium, elastic tissue, and blood vessels. Occasionally, they contain conduction tissue, which may serve as the underlying substrate for an associated arrhythmia (130).

**Treatment.** Surgical excision may be warranted in cases of intractable arrhythmia or when the location of the lesion precludes deployment of percutaneous devices (such as septal occluder devices).

## REFERENCES

1. Furie B, Furie BC. Mechanisms of thrombus formation. N Engl J Med 2008;359:938-949.
2. Lee JH, Kang SK, Lee CW, Song JK, Park JS, Choo SJ. Giant left atrial ball thrombus in a patient with chronic nonvalvular atrial fibrillation. Ann Thorac Surg 2008;85:313-315.
3. Feng D, Edwards WD, Oh JK, et al. Intracardiac thrombosis and embolism in patients with cardiac amyloidosis. Circulation 2007;116:2420-2426.
4. de Winkel N, Becker K, Vogt M. Echogenic mass in the right atrium after surgical ventricular septal defect closure: thrombus or tumour? Cardiol Young 2010;20:86-88.
5. Leslie D, Hall TS, Goldstein S, Shindler D. Mural left atrial thrombus: a hidden danger accompanying cardiac surgery. J Cardiovasc Surg (Torino) 1998;39:649-650.
6. Aoyagi S, Tayama E, Fukunaga S, Akaiwa KI, Takagi K, Shojima T. Left atrial thrombosis following mitral valve repair and maze procedure: case report. J Heart Valve Dis 2003;12:714-716.
7. Akalin H, Ozyurda U, Corapçioglu T, Uysalel A, Sonel A. Successful nonsurgical therapy of mural thrombosis of the left atrium after mitral valve replacement. J Thorac Cardiovasc Surg 1988;95:733-734.
8. Darwazah AK. Conservative management of left atrial thrombus after CABG in a patient with normal mitral valve. J Cardiovasc Surg (Torino) 2009;50:821-822.
9. Burns KE, McLaren A. Catheter-related right atrial thrombus and pulmonary embolism: a case report and systematic review of the literature. Can Respir J 2009;16:163-165.
10. Iga K, Konishi T, Kusukawa R. Intracardiac thrombi in both the right atrium and right ventricle after acute inferior-wall myocardial infarction. Int J Cardiol 1994;46:169-171.
11. Datta BN, Khattri HN. Isolated infarction of right atrium and sinu-atrial node. A complication of bleeding diathesis. Case report. Indian Heart J 1981;33:69-72.
12. Ancona R, Comenale Pinto S, Caso P, et al. Right atrial mass following transcatheter radiofrequency ablation for recurrent atrial fibrillation: thrombus, endocarditis or mixoma? Monaldi Arch Chest Dis 2009;72:40-42.
13. Erdem Y, Akpolat T, Oymak O, et al. Magnetic resonance imaging diagnosis of right atrial septic thrombus caused by subclavian catheter in a hemodialysis patient. Nephron 1995;69:174-175.
14. Mathieu P, Marchand R, Tardif J, Perrault LP. Ventriculotomy and resection for left ventricular thrombus infection with Salmonella. Eur J Cardiothorac Surg 2000;18:360-362.
15. Reeder GS, Tajik AJ, Seward JB. Left ventricular mural thrombus: two-dimensional echocardiographic diagnosis. Mayo Clin Proc 1981;56:82-86.
16. Kmetzo J, Peters RW, Plotnick GD, Carliner NH, Baumgartner WA, Fisher ML. Left atrial mass. Thrombus mimicking myxoma. Chest 1985;88:906-907.
17. Kodali S, Yamrozik J, Biederman RW. Left atrial thrombus masquerading as a myxoma in a patient with mitral stenosis. Echocardiography 2011;27:E98-101.

18. Cho HJ, Seol SH, Choi BJ, et al. A case of a right atrial and inferior vena caval thrombus resembling a right atrial myxoma. J Cardiovasc Ultrasound 2010;18:58-61.

19. Gertner E, Leatherman J. Intracardiac mural thrombus mimicking atrial myxoma in the antiphospholipid syndrome. J Rheumatol 1992;19:1293-1298.

20. Lichtenberg J, Tosovský J, Bríza J, Tersíp K, Rohác J, Vondrácková D. Uncommon findings on surgery of benign heart tumours. Czech Med 1991;14:228-235.

21. Cho SF, Lin CJ, Chen YF, Lin SF. Primary cardiac lymphoma mimicking atrial thrombus in a patient who underwent permanent pacemaker implantation. Ann Hematol 2011;90:739-740.

22. Allende NG, Sokn F, Borracci R, et al. Giant pedunculated thrombus with normal left ventricular systolic function mimicking myxoma. Echocardiography 2011;28:E31-33.

23. Alzand BS, Ilhan M. Thrombus in a normal left ventricle. Neth Heart J 2008;16:24-25.

24. Karabinos IK, Koulouris S, Kranidis A, et al. Spontaneous thrombus formation in a normal left ventricle following administration of large doses of epoietin. Hellenic J Cardiol 2007;48:44-46.

25. Paelinck BP, Vrints CJ, Conraads VM. Left ventricular thrombus. Can J Cardiol 2009;25:e390.

26. Sia YT, Dulay D, Burwash IG, Beauchesne LM, Ascah K, Chan KL. Mobile ventricular thrombus arising from the mitral annulus in patients with dense mitral annular calcification. Eur J Echocardiogr 2010;11:198-201.

27. Urgesi R, Zampaletta C, Masini A. Spontaneous right ventricular thrombus in a patient with active ulcerative colitis and protein C deficiency: a review with a case report. Eur Rev Med Pharmacol Sci 2011;14:455-463.

28. Burke AP, Mezzetti T, Farb A, Zech ER, Virmani R. Multiple coronary artery graft occlusion in a fatal case of heparin-induced thrombocytopenia. Chest 1998;114:1492-1495.

29. Schmaier AH, Denenberg B. Left ventricular thrombus with normal left ventricular function and hyperaggregable platelets in a patient with polycystic disease of multiple organs. Am J Med Sci 1984;288:223-237.

30. Acikel S, Akdemir R, Dogan M, Kilic H, Yesilay AB. Antiphospholipid antibody syndrome: coexistence of left ventricular apical thrombus and deep vein thrombosis causing pulmonary thromboembolism in a patient with systemic lupus erythematosus. Echocardiography 2010;27:198-201.

31. Cianciulli TF, Saccheri MC, Lax JA, et al. Left ventricular thrombus mimicking primary cardiac tumor in a patient with primary antiphospholipid syndrome and recurrent systemic embolism. Cardiol J 2009;16:560-563.

32. Gurgun C, Sagcan A, Cinar CS, et al. Right atrial and ventricular thrombi in Behçet's disease: a case report and review of literature. Blood Coagul Fibrinolysis 2000;11:107-110.

33. Amezyane T, Bassou D, Abouzahir A, et al. Unusual right ventricular thrombus in a woman with Hughes-Stovin syndrome. Intern Med 2011;49:207-208.

34. Sayin A, Vural FS, Bozkurt AK, Oz B, Uygun N. Right atrial thrombus mimicking myxoma and bilateral pulmonary artery aneurysms in a patient with Behçet's disease—a case report. Angiology 1993;44:915-918.

35. Mogulkoc N, Burgess MI, Bishop PW. Intracardiac thrombus in Behçet's disease: a systematic review. Chest 2000;118:479-487.

36. Buchbinder NA, Yu R, Rosenbloom BE, Sherman CT, Silberman AW. Left ventricular thrombus and embolic stroke caused by a functional paraganglioma. J Clin Hypertens (Greenwich) 2009;11:734-737.

37. Wiyono SA, Vletter WB, Soliman OI, ten Cate FJ, Geleijnse ML. Thrombus in a normal left ventricle: a cardiac manifestation of pheochromocytoma. Echocardiography 2010;27:195-197.

38. Zhou W, Ding SF. Concurrent pheochromocytoma, ventricular tachycardia, left ventricular thrombus, and systemic embolization. Intern Med 2009;48:1015-1019.

39. Siwach SB, Dua A, Sharma D. Multichamber intracardiac thrombi in a patient without any predisposing cardiac or non-cardiac disease. Int J Cardiol 1992;37:263-265.

40. Berdajs DA, Ruchat P, Tozzi P, von Segesser LK. Acute Leriche syndrome due to the thrombus in the left ventricle. Eur J Cardiothorac Surg 2011;39:423.

41. Bautista RE. Embolic stroke following thrombolytic therapy for myocardial infarction in a patient with preexisting ventricular thrombi. Stroke 1995;26:324-325.

42. Buss SJ, Johanssen C, Katus HA, Mereles D. A trapped thrombus in the right ventricle. Int J Cardiol 2009;133:e60-61.

43. Strecker T, Rösch J, Weyand M, Agaimy A. Primary and metastatic cardiac tumors: imaging characteristics, surgical treatment, and histopathological spectrum: a 10-year-experience at a German heart center. Cardiovasc Pathol 2012;21:436-443.

44. Nonaka A, Stugaard M, Ueda O, Hara H, Shimada T, Shiotani H. Fluorodeoxyglucose-positron emission tomography differentiating thrombus from tumor in the left ventricle. J Am Coll Cardiol 2009;53:894.

45. Lange M, Horstkotte D, Wiemer M. Radiopaque thrombus in right ventricle. Eur Heart J 2008;29:1955.

46. Tehrani F, Eshaghian S. Detection of left ventricular thrombus by coronary computed tomography angiography. Am J Med Sci 2009;338:167-168.

47. Jang KH, Shin DH, Lee C, Jang JK, Cheong S, Yoo SY. Left atrial mass with stalk: thrombus or myxoma? J Cardiovasc Ultrasound 2011;18:154-156.

48. Paydarfar D, Krieger D, Dib N, et al. In vivo magnetic resonance imaging and surgical histopathology of intracardiac masses: distinct features of subacute thrombi. Cardiology 2001;95:40-47.

49. Scheffel H, Baumueller S, Stolzmann P, et al. Atrial myxomas and thrombi: comparison of imaging features on CT. AJR Am J Roentgenol 2009;192:639-645.

50. Kandemir O, Büyükates M, Aktunç E, Turan SA, Aydin M. Coincidentally determined floating right ventricular thrombus in a patient with coronary artery disease. Anadolu Kardiyol Derg 2009;9:E21-22.

51. Karabay CY, Kocabay G, Kalayci A, Zehir R, Mert M, Kirma C. Snake-like thrombus in the right atrium causing pulmonary embolism. Cardiovasc J Afr 2011;22:206-207.

52. Misumi T, Kudo M, Ito T, Matsubara T, Kumamaru H. Floating ball thrombus in the left atrium with mitral stenosis. Jpn J Thorac Cardiovasc Surg 2003;51:387-389.

53. Nurkalem Z, Ergelen M, Özcan S, Uslu N. Case images: free-floating thrombus in the right atrium, ventricle, and outflow tract effectively treated with thrombolysis. Turk Kardiyol Dern Ars 2010;38:380.

54. Sanada A, Fuse K, Ito M, et al. Free-floating ball thrombus in the left ventricle with dilated cardiomyopathy. Int J Cardiol 2007;122:e6-7.

55. Shetty V, Sadiq A, Shani J, Lodha A. Free-floating left ventricular and fixed left atrial thrombus. Am J Med Sci 2009;337:483.

56. Alexandrescu C, Civaia F, Dor V. Tumor thrombus in right atrium from lung adenocarcinoma. Ann Thorac Surg 2009;87:e11-12.

57. Reynolds C, Tazelaar HD, Edwards WD. Calcified amorphous tumor of the heart (cardiac CAT). Hum Pathol 1997;28:601-606.

58. Yoshikai M, Ohnishi H, Fumoto H, Yamamoto T. Surgical technique for massive mural thrombus in the left atrium. J Card Surg 2007;22:443-444.

59. Fealey ME, Edwards WD, Reynolds CA, Pellikka PA, Dearani JA. Recurrent cardiac calcific amorphous tumor: the CAT had a kitten. Cardiovasc Pathol 2007;16:115-118.

60. Zimmerman KG, Paplanus SH, Dong S, Nagle RB. Congenital blood cysts of the heart valves. Hum Pathol 1983;14:699-703.

61. Arnold IR, Hubner PJ, Firmin RK. Blood filled cyst of the papillary muscle of the mitral valve producing severe left ventricular outflow tract obstruction. Br Heart J 1990;63:132-133.

62. Pasaoglu I, Dogan R, Demircin M, Bozer AY. Blood cyst of the pulmonary valve causing pulmonic valve stenosis. Am J Cardiol 1993;72:493-494.

63. Xie SW, Lu OL, Picard MH. Blood cyst of the mitral valve: detection by transthoracic and transesophageal echocardiography. J Am Soc Echocardiogr 1992;5:547-550.

64. Jacob JJ, Jose J, John B. Intracardiac blood-filled cysts of the heart: a rare cause of embolic stroke. Singapore Med J 2007;48:e125-126.

65. Kuvin J, Saha P, Rastegar H, Salomon RN, Pandian N, Denofrio D. Blood cyst of the mitral valve apparatus in a woman with a history of orthotopic liver transplantation. J Am Soc Echocardiogr 2004;17:480-482.

66. Lodha A, Patel J, Haran M, Sadiq A, Shani J. Blood cyst of the mitral valve: a rare cause of stroke. Echocardiography 2009;26:736-738.

67. Pelikan HM, Tsang TS, Seward JB. Giant blood cyst of the mitral valve. J Am Soc Echocardiogr 1999;12:1005-1007.

68. Centella T, Moya JL, Muñoz M, Reguero EM. Images in cardiovascular medicine. Giant endocardial blood cyst in the right atrium: echocardiographic and magnetic resonance imaging features. Circulation 2008;117:3250-3251.

69. Gallucci V, Stritoni P, Fasoli G, Thiene G. Giant blood cyst of tricuspid valve. Successful excision in an infant. Br Heart J 1976;38:990-992.

70. Minneci C, Casolo G, Popoff G, Sulla A, Comin CE, Pedemonti E. A rare case of left ventricular outflow obstruction. Eur J Echocardiogr 2004;5:72-75.

71. Rose AG. Venous malformations of the heart. Arch Pathol Lab Med 1979;103:18-20.

72. Heggtveit HA. Thrombosed varices of the heart. Am J Pathol 1966;48:50a.

73. Murphy MC, Sweeney MS, Putnam JB Jr, et al. Surgical treatment of cardiac tumors: a 25-year experience. Ann Thorac Surg 1990;49:612-7; discussion 617-618.

74. Fueredi GA, Knechtges TE, Czarnecki DJ. Coronary angiography in atrial myxoma: findings in nine cases. AJR Am J Roentgenol 1989;152:737-738.

75. Tuncer E, Tas SG, Mataraci I, et al. Surgical treatment of cardiac hydatid disease in 13 patients. Tex Heart Inst J 2010;37:189-193.

76. Siwach SB, Katyal VK, Jagdish. Intracardiac mass lesions: experience of 14 cases. Indian Heart J 1999;51:414-417.

77. Katewa A, Vaideeswar P, Khandekar JV, et al. Isolated pericardial and intracardiac hydatidosis: presentation as congestive cardiac failure and fatal pulmonary embolism. Cardiovasc Pathol 2009;18:114-118.

78. Charet E, Roudaut R, Lafitte S, Laffort P, Madonna F, de Mascarel A. Echocardiographic demonstration of rupture of intraseptal hydatid cyst. J Am Soc Echocardiogr 2000;13:955-958.

79. Perez-Gomez F, Duran H, Tamames S, Perrote JL, Blanes A. Cardiac echinococcosis: clinical picture and complications. Br Heart J 1973;35:1326-1331.

80. Sinha PR, Jaipuria N, Avasthey P. Intracardiac hydatid cyst and sudden death in a child. Int J Cardiol 1995;51:293-295.

81. DiBello R, Abo JC, Borges UL. Hydatid constrictive pericarditis. A new case and review of the literature. J Thorac Cardiovasc Surg 1970;59:530-532.

82. Geiger AW, Konertz W, Hindricks G, Hachenberg T, Fahrenkamp A, Scheld HH. Echinococcal cyst of the interventricular septum: a rare cause of myocardial ischemia. Thorac Cardiovasc Surg 1992;40:42-44.

83. Rezaian GR, Aslani A. Endocardial hydatid cyst: a rare presentation of echinococcal infection. Eur J Echocardiogr 2008;9:342-343.

84. Shakibi JG, Safavian MH, Azar H, Siassi B. Surgical treatment of echinococcal cyst of the heart. Report of two cases and review of the world literature. J Thorac Cardiovasc Surg 1977;74:941-946.

85. Canda MS, Güray M, Canda T, Astarcioglu H. The pathology of echinococcosis and the current echonicoccosis problem in Western Turkey (A report of patholgic features in 80 cases). Turk J Med Sci 2003;33:369-374.

86. Eberly MD, Soh EK, Bannister SP, Tavaf-Motamen H, Scott JS. Isolated cardiac cysticercosis in an adolescent. Pediatr Infect Dis J 2008;27:369-371.

87. Shogan PJ, Yasmer JF, Monson M. Cardiac cysticercosis. AJR Am J Roentgenol 2009;192:W212-213.

88. Birincioglu CL, Tarcan O, Bardakci H, Saritas A, Tasdemir O. Off-pump technique for the treatment of ventricular myocardial echinococcosis. Ann Thorac Surg 2003;75:1232-1237.

89. Bozbuga N, Erentug V, Akinci E, Yakut C. Is surgical therapy the only treatment of choice for cardiac echinococcosis with multiple organ involvement? Interact Cardiovasc Thorac Surg 2003;2:367-368.

90. Gonzalez-Crussi F, Vanderbilt BL, Miller JK. Unusual intracardiac tumor in a child. Inflammatory pseudotumor or "granulomatous" variant of myxoma? Cancer 1975;36:2214-2226.

91. Rose AG, McCormick S, Cooper K, Titus JL. Inflammatory pseudotumor (plasma cell granuloma) of the heart. Report of two cases and literature review. Arch Pathol Lab Med 1996;120:549-554.

92. Burke A, Li L, Kling E, Kutys R, Virmani R, Miettinen M. Cardiac inflammatory myofibroblastic tumor: a "benign" neoplasm that may result in syncope, myocardial infarction, and sudden death. Am J Surg Pathol 2007;31:1115-1122.

93. Li L, Cerilli LA, Wick MR. Inflammatory pseudotumor (myofibroblastic tumor) of the heart. Ann Diagn Pathol 2002;6:116-121.

94. Rajbanshi BG, Hughes JE, DeSimone DC, Maleszewski JJ, Baddour LM, Dearani JA. Surgical excision of invasive aspergillosis of the right ventricle presenting as intractable ventricular arrhythmia and right ventricular mass. Mayo Clin Proc 2012;87:926-928.

95. Liu PY, Tsai WC, Chen JH, Kan CD, Yan JJ. Coexistence of tuberculous constrictive pericarditis and right atrial tuberculoma: a case report. J Formos Med Assoc 2001;100:336-338.

96. Viles-Gonzalez JF, Pastori L, Fischer A, Wisnivesky JP, Goldman MG, Mehta D. Supraventricular arrhythmias in patients with cardiac sarcoidosis: prevalence, predictors and clinical implications. Chest 2013;143:1085-1090.

97. Okura Y, Dec GW, Hare JM, et al. A clinical and histopathologic comparison of cardiac sarcoidosis and idiopathic giant cell myocarditis. J Am Coll Cardiol 2003;41:322-329.

98. Pereira-da-Silva T, Galrinho A, Ribeiro A, et al. Intracardiac mass due to fibrosing mediastinitis: the first reported case. Can J Cardiol 2013;(12):1475-1474.

99. Kovach TA, Nanda NC, Kim KS, Nath H, Listinksy CM, Chung SM. Transesophageal echocardiographic findings in sclerosing mediastinitis. Echocardiography 1996;13:103-108.

100. Osawa H, Yamaguchi T, Sato H, Ebuoka M. [Surgical removal of left atrial tumor originating from mitral annular calcification in a chronic hemodialysis patient: a case report.] Kyobu Geka 2000;53:1119-1121. [Japanese]

101. Teja K, Gibson RS, Nolan SP. Atrial extension of mitral annular calcification mimicking intracardiac tumor. Clin Cardiol 1987;10:546-548.

102. Blankstein R, Durst R, Picard MH, Cury RC. Progression of mitral annulus calcification to caseous necrosis of the mitral valve: complementary role of multi-modality imaging. Eur Heart J 2009;30:304.

103. Stamou SC, Braverman AC, Kouchoukos NT. Caseous calcification of the anterior mitral valve annulus presenting as intracardiac mass. J Thorac Cardiovasc Surg 2010;140:e9-e10.

104. Silbiger JJ. Anatomy, mechanics, and pathophysiology of the mitral annulus. Am Heart J 2012;164:163-176.

105. Boon A, Cheriex E, Lodder J, Kessels F. Cardiac valve calcification: characteristics of patients with calcification of the mitral annulus or aortic valve. Heart 1997;78:472-474.

106. Warsame TA, Keen OE, Mookadam F, Chaliki HP. Liquefaction necrosis of calcified mitral annulus. Echocardiography 2009;26:1082-1083.

107. Fernandez E, Borràs M, Pais B, Montoliu J. Low-calcium dialysate stimulates parathormone secretion and its long-term use worsens secondary hyperparathyroidism. J Am Soc Nephrol 1995; 6:132-135.

108. Arounlangsy P, Sawabe M, Izumiyama N, Koike M. Histopathogenesis of early-stage mitral annular calcification. J Med Dent Sci 2004;51:35-44.

109. Potpara TS, Vasiljevic ZM, Vujisic-Tesic BD, et al. Mitral annular calcification predicts cardiovascular morbidity and mortality in middle-aged patients with atrial fibrillation: the Belgrade Atrial Fibrillation Study. Chest 2011;140:902-910.

110. Kanjanauthai S, Nasir K, Katz R, et al. Relationships of mitral annular calcification to cardiovascular risk factors: the Multi-Ethnic Study of Atherosclerosis (MESA). Atherosclerosis 2010;213:558-562.

111. Sugiura M, Uchiyama S, Kuwako K, Ohkawa S, Hiraoka K. A clinicopathological study on mitral ring calcification. Jpn Heart J 1977;18:154-163.

112. Savage DD, Garrison RJ, Castelli WP, et al. Prevalence of submitral (anular) calcium and its correlates in a general population-based sample (the Framingham Study). Am J Cardiol 1983;51:1375-1378.

113. Osterberger LE, Goldstein S, Khaja F, Lakier JB. Functional mitral stenosis in patients with massive mitral annular calcification. Circulation 1981;64:472-476.

114. Aronow WS, Kronzon I. Correlation of prevalence and severity of mitral regurgitation and mitral stenosis determined by Doppler echocardiography with physical signs of mitral regurgitation and mitral stenosis in 100 patients aged 62 to 100 years with mitral anular calcium. Am J Cardiol 1987;60:1189-1190.

115. Nair CK, Sketch MH, Desai R, Mohiuddin SM, Runco V. High prevalence of symptomatic bradyarrhythmias due to atrioventricular node-fascicular and sinus node-atrial disease in patients with mitral anular calcification. Am Heart J 1982;103:226-229.

116. Tenenbaum A, Shemesh J, Fisman EZ, Motro M. Advanced mitral annular calcification is associated with severe coronary calcification on fast dual spiral computed tomography. Invest Radiol 2000;35:193-198.

117. Nagueh SF, Appleton CP, Gillebert TC, et al. Recommendations for the evaluation of left ventricular diastolic function by echocardiography. J Am Soc Echocardiogr 2009;22:107-133.

118. Deluca G, Correale M, Ieva R, Del Salvatore B, Gramenzi S, Di Biase M. The incidence and clinical course of caseous calcification of the mitral annulus: a prospective echocardiographic study. J Am Soc Echocardiogr 2008;21:828-833.

119. Davidson MJ, Cohn LH. Surgical treatment of caseous mitral valve annulus calcification. J Thorac Cardiovasc Surg 2006;131:738-739.

120. d'Alessandro C, Vistarini N, Aubert S, et al. Mitral annulus calcification: determinants of repair feasibility, early and late surgical outcome. Eur J Cardiothorac Surg 2007;32:596-603.

121. Luthringer DJ, Virmani R, Weiss SW, Rosai J. A distinctive cardiovascular lesion resembling histiocytoid (epithelioid) hemangioma. Evidence suggesting mesothelial participation. Am J Surg Pathol 1990;14:993-1000.

122. Courtice RW, Stinson WA, Walley VM. Tissue fragments recovered at cardiac surgery masquerading as tumoral proliferations. Evidence suggesting iatrogenic or artefactual origin and common occurrence. Am J Surg Pathol 1994; 18:167-174.

123. Argani P, Sternberg SS, Burt M, Adsay NV, Klimstra DS. Metastatic adenocarcinoma involving a mesothelial/monocytic incidental cardiac excrescence (cardiac MICE). Am J Surg Pathol 1997;21:970-974.

124. Ng MT, Trendell-Smith NJ. A case of mesothelial/monocytic incidental cardiac excrescence (MICE) associated with squamous cell carcinoma of lung. Pathology 2012;44:563-565.

125. Ray R, Kumar N, Gupta R, Mridha AR, Tyagi JS, Kumar AS. Mesothelial/monocytic incidental cardiac excrescences (MICE) with tubercular aortitis: report of the first case with brief review of the literature. J Clin Pathol 2010;63:853-855.

126. Hu ZL, Lü H, Yin HL, Wen JF, Jin O. A case of mesothelial/monocytic incidental cardiac excrescence and literature review. Diagn Pathol 2010;5:40.

127. Pham TT, Antons K, Shishido R, Mullvain J, Salem F, Haghighi P. A case of mesothelial/monocytic cardiac excrescence causing severe acute cardiopulmonary failure. Am J Surg Pathol 2005;29:564-567.

128. Philip S, Cherian KM, Wu MH, Lue HC. Left ventricular false tendons: echocardiographic, morphologic, and histopathologic studies and review of the literature. Pediatr Neonatol 2011;52:279-286.

129. Luetmer PH, Edwards WD, Seward JB, Tajik AJ. Incidence and distribution of left ventricular false tendons: an autopsy study of 483 normal human hearts. J Am Coll Cardiol 1986;8:179-183.

130. Abdulla AK, Frustaci A, Martinez JE, Florio RA, Somerville J, Olsen EG. Echocardiography and pathology of left ventricular "false tendons." Chest 1990;98:129-132.

# 5 CARDIAC MYXOMA

## GENERAL FEATURES

*Cardiac myxoma* is a benign neoplasm of uncertain histogenesis that occurs exclusively on the endocardial surface, usually in the atrium near the fossa ovalis. Cardiac myxoma shares its name and the presence of a mucopolysaccharide matrix with myxomas of soft tissue. The cardiac myxoma cell, however, is histologically and histogenetically distinct from the spindle cells of soft tissue myxomas.

There is a long history of debate concerning the histogenesis of cardiac myxomas. The theory that they are peculiar organizing thrombi or reactive lesions was first put forth over 100 years ago, but there is nearly unanimous agreement today that cardiac myxomas are neoplasms. Myxomas rarely, if ever, occur in regions of the heart that predispose to thrombus formation, namely, the atrial appendages and ventricular apices. There is a subset of histologically typical myxomas that embolize to distant arterial sites, and, unlike thrombi, extend into the arterial wall to form aneurysms. Genetic abnormalities have been found in sporadic cardiac myxomas (1–4). Myxomas occur as an inherited condition in patients with the Carney complex, in whom specific genetic alterations are found with no predisposition to thrombosis. Immunohistochemically, myxomas share little resemblance to the organizing thrombi usually seen in cardiac chambers.

Another issue in the debate regarding cardiac myxoma is the nature of the cell of origin. Immunohistochemically, there is variable expression of epithelial, mesenchymal, endothelial, myofibroblastic, and even neuroendocrine proteins, suggesting activation of primitive pluripotent mesenchymal cells (5–15). In addition, cells of the embryonic endocardial cushion ultrastructurally resemble myxoma cells and may represent myxoma precursors (16). A theory has been advanced that the glandular structures occasionally present in cardiac myxoma (see below) are related to endodermal rests budding from foregut tissues (10). These foregut structures are also thought to represent precursors of cystic tumors of the atrioventricular nodal region. Glandular structures, however, are rare components of myxoma; therefore, this theory is not a comprehensive explanation for its histogenesis. Kodama et al. (17) investigated potential myocyte-specific transcription factors (Nkx2.5/Csx, GATA-4, and eHAND) by immunohistochemistry and mRNA in situ hybridization, and suggested that cardiac myxoma may arise from mesenchymal cardiomyocyte progenitor cells.

Confocal microscopy has shown coexpression of CD34 and alpha-smooth muscle actin in myxoma cells. Upregulation of pathways related to early cardiac differentiation has been shown, by identifying in tumor homogenates, transcripts for Sox9, Notch1, NFATc1, and Smad6. As these molecules are implicated in the endothelial-to-mesenchymal transformation that precedes terminal differentiation of endocardial cushions, it has been suggested that cardiac myxoma cells derive from adult developmental remnants (18). Expression of CD44 and tenascin-c has been detected in a series of cardiac myxomas (19). Tenascin-c was shown in the extracellular matrix and CD44 (hyaluronan receptor) on neoplastic myxoma cells. These markers may have an important role in the angiogenesis related to tumor development and may play a role in the histogenesis of cardiac myxoma.

## CLINICAL FEATURES

Cardiac myxomas account for approximately 70 percent of resected cardiac tumors in adults. The age-standardized incidence rate has been estimated at 0.11 per 100,000 (20). The tumors are extremely uncommon in the pediatric population, occurring occasionally in children and teenagers (21–24). Some reports of valvular cardiac myxomas in infants and children have illustrated myofibroblastic tumors (25,27). More than 90 percent of all cases are solitary and sporadic in nature; the remainder are seen in patients with the Carney complex (myxoma syndrome), an autosomal dominant condition.

Myxomas occur more often in women than men, at a ratio of nearly 2 to 1 (Tables 5-1, 5-2) (26). The average patient age at presentation is 53 years; 90 percent of patients are 30 to 60 years of age. Myxomas, especially sporadic myxomas, rarely occur in children under age 10 years (23–26). There are several reported series of heart tumors in children that include myxomas, not all of which are clearly documented pathologically (21,28–32). In some reports of myxomas occurring in children, the histologic illustrations are more consistent with a myxoid sarcoma than myxoma (29).

Patients with cardiac myxoma have a variety of symptoms, and the tumor is thus termed a "great masquerader." The most common symptoms are those related to heart failure (dyspnea), arrhythmias, and embolization (Table 5-3). Although the diagnosis can be easily made with imaging studies, some patients are symptomatic for long periods before the diagnosis is clinically considered (33). There are three types of symptoms (fever, weight loss, cachexia, fatigue, malaise, arthralgias), sequelae of valvular obstruction, and manifestations of embolic phenomena. Most patients with atrial myxomas present with one or more of these features (33–36). The constitutional symptoms

### Table 5-1

#### CLINICOPATHOLOGIC FEATURES OF CARDIAC MYXOMA[a]

| Feature | Number | % |
|---|---|---|
| Male:Female | 115:196[b] | 37:63 |
| Age (mean years), range | 53.3, 16-81 | – |
| Left atrium, total | 390 | 85 |
| Left atrium, oval fossa | 118 | |
| Left atrium, other sites | 13 | |
| Left atrium, NOS | 259 | |
| Right atrium | 49 | 11 |
| Left ventricle | 8 | 2 |
| Right ventricle | 5 | 1 |
| Biatrial | 4 | 1 |
| Valve | 2 | <1 |
| Size (mean), range | 4.4, 1-11 cm | – |
| Recurrence | 3 | 1 |
| Multiplicity | 3 | 1 |

[a]From published reports of 468 tumors (20,32,37–40,61).
[b]Gender data not available in all series. Specific clinical and pathologic data not available in reference 32.

### Table 5-2

#### MEAN AGE AT PRESENTATION, BY SITE IN HEART[a]

| Site in Heart | Number | Mean Age, Years (Range) | Female:Male |
|---|---|---|---|
| Left atrium, attached to septum | 131 | 54 (7-83) | 69:62 |
| Right atrium, attached to septum | 29 | 56 (15-73) | 17:12 |
| Left atrium other attachment sites | 9 | 51 (32-81) | 7:2 |
| Right atrium, other attachment sites | 8 | 44 (13-77) | 5:3 |
| Biatrial, both sides of septum | 4 | 29 (17-48) | 3:1 |
| Multiple tumors in right atrium | 3 | 39 (24-68) | 2:1 |
| Multiple tumors in left atrium | 2 | 45 (40-50) | 1:1 |
| Left ventricle | 2 | 33 (24-41) | 1:1 |
| Right ventricle | 2 | 46 (28-64) | 2:0 |
| Multiple chambers | 2 | 20 (16-24) | 1:1 |
| Recurrent in right atrium | 1 | 32 | 0:1 |
| Recurrent in left atrium | 1 | 56 | 1:0 |
| Total | 194 | 52 (7-83) | 109:85 |

[a]Data from a series of 194 myxomas seen in consultation by one of the authors. Mean ages of patients with tumors at sites other than atrial septum were significant younger at presentation (p = .007) compared to those with tumors attached to the atrial septum (rows 1 and 2).

**Table 5-3**

**SYMPTOMS AND COMPLICATIONS
OF CARDIAC MYXOMA[a]**

| Symptom | Number | % |
|---|---|---|
| Dyspnea | 126 | 42 |
| Constitutional symptoms | 65 | 22 |
| Embolization | 67 | 22 |
| Chest pain | 52 | 17 |
| Syncope | 47 | 16 |
| No symptoms (asymptomatic) | 36 | 12 |

[a]Data from series presented in Table 5-1, from 302 patients. In patients without symptoms, the mass is inadvertently found on imaging performed for evaluation of conditions unrelated to the tumor.

are associated with laboratory abnormalities such as anemia, increased sedimentation rate, and hypergammaglobulinemia (37–40). Although constitutional symptoms and laboratory abnormalities are not typically the initial problems that lead to the diagnosis, they occur in the majority of patients during the course of illness (41).

The inflammatory features of fever, arthralgias, elevated sedimentation rate, and lupus-like rashes that accompany myxomas have been linked to the production of the proinflammatory cytokine interleukin-6 (IL-6) by the tumor. It has been shown that in sporadic myxoma, tumor size significantly correlates with the preoperative IL-6 level (42). In general, IL-6 levels normalize after the myxoma is excised (43,44). In recurrent myxoma, however, which is characterized by highly myxoid lesions, there is evidence that even small tumors may elaborate high levels of IL-6. Conversely, familial tumors may recur without serologic evidence of IL-6 expression, indicating that screening by imaging is necessary (42). It has been recently demonstrated that circulating monocytes directly contribute to the overproduction of IL-6 in patients with myxoma and constitutional symptoms. Because other inflammatory conditions, such as Castleman disease, are associated with serum elevation of IL-6, cardiac myxoma may be initially diagnosed as a lymphoproliferative disorder (45).

Obstruction of the mitral valve by myxoma leads to a clinical syndrome similar to that seen in chronic rheumatic mitral valve disease.

Right atrial myxomas may obstruct the tricuspid valve and cause the symptoms of right-sided heart failure, peripheral edema, passive hepatic congestion, and syncope. Embolic myxomas lead to ischemia of the extremities, viscera, or brain (30). In most series of cardiac myxomas, symptoms of mitral stenosis are more common than those of embolic phenomena (27,30,46). Myxomas can, however, directly involve the valvular leaflets, and in these cases, the symptoms are usually related to valvular dysfunction. Mitral valve tumors may arise on the annulus, and extend into the left atrium (47), and more rarely arise on the anterior leaflet (3 percent in one series) (37,48).

In right atrial myxomas, computed tomography (CT) scans may demonstrate tricuspid valve obstruction with ascites. Prolapse across the mitral or tricuspid valve, with varying degrees of obstruction, is uncommonly seen with magnetic resonance imaging (MRI) (49).

Left atrial myxomas are commonly incidental findings on imaging, with the increased use of echocardiography and cardiac CT and MRI. Uncommon modes of presentation are cardiac arrhythmias, sudden unexpected death, chest pain or angina, and syncope. Myxoma emboli to the brain cause strokes, transient ischemic attacks, seizures, or hemianopsia. It is currently recommended that patients with cardiac myxoma should undergo surveillance for myxoma-related peripheral embolism, especially to the brain (50). Emboli to iliac arteries and distal vessels cause claudication, gangrene, or Leriche syndrome if located at the iliac bifurcation. Renal emboli result in renal failure, hematuria, or, rarely, rhabdomyolysis.

The typical symptoms of mitral stenosis result from pulmonary hypertension and include dyspnea, orthopnea, and fatigue. Sudden death occurs either because of coronary embolization of tumor fragments, or sudden obstruction of the mitral valve orifice (51); rarely, no evidence of embolism is found in an otherwise normal autopsy (22). Patients with left atrial myxoma may have supraventricular tachycardias and, infrequently, atrial flutter and fibrillation. Tumors found incidentally during life are discovered because of heart murmurs, CT for other causes, or a filling defect during cardiac catheterization for coronary artery disease.

Right atrial myxomas are less frequently symptomatic than left atrial myxomas, and almost half are discovered incidentally. About one quarter of patients have episodes of syncope. Other reported manifestations include peripheral edema, pulmonary embolism, and Budd-Chiari syndrome. Long-term severe pulmonary hypertension has been described in patients with right atrial myxoma (52,53). A report of cardiac myxoma arising in a donor heart after transplant has documented origin in donor tissues (Tables 5-1, 5-2) (54).

Initial auscultatory findings are normal in up to half of patients, even if performed by a cardiologist (33). Abnormal findings include systolic ejection murmur, holosystolic murmur of mitral insufficiency, diastolic murmur of mitral stenosis, loud S1, opening click, loud S2, S4, tumor "plop," and to-and-fro murmurs.

Clinically, left atrial myxoma must be differentiated from mitral stenosis, since the most common symptoms of the latter are of valvular dysfunction, which is usually rheumatic in origin. Unlike myxoma, rheumatic mitral disease commonly results in atrial enlargement, with atrial fibrillation or flutter at later stages. Also in the clinical differential diagnosis of cardiac myxoma is subacute bacterial endocarditis, which, unlike myxoma, is often associated with splenomegaly. Cases of infected myxoma are especially difficult to clinically diagnose and require careful imaging studies to distinguish vegetations from myxoma. The aneurysms of polyarteritis may radiographically resemble those caused by embolic myxoma, and the constitutional symptoms of both entities can overlap. ANCA-related vasculitis may also be in the clinical differential diagnosis, as rarely, cardiac myxoma results in p-ANCA positivity (55).

## CARNEY COMPLEX

Most cases of cardiac myxoma are sporadic; in less than 5 percent of patients, there is a familial history of atrial tumors, multifocal disease, or extracardiac lesions. In 1980, Atherton et al. (56) described a patient with skin pigmentation, neurofibromas, and cardiac myxomas, which was designated NAME syndrome (nevi, atrial myxoma, myxoid neurofibroma, ephelides). The association between cardiac myxoma and adrenal cortical hyperplasia was made in 1982

| Table 5-4 | |
|---|---|
| **CARNEY COMPLEX** | |

| | |
|---|---|
| **Synonyms** | |
| Carney syndrome | |
| LAMB syndrome (lentigines, atrial myxomas, blue nevi) | |
| NAME syndrome (nevi, atrial myxoma, ephelides) | |
| **Genetic Basis** | |
| Mutations in *PRKAR1A* gene, chromosome 17q23-q24 | |
| **Mode of Inheritance** | |
| Autosomal dominant | |

| Features | % Involvement |
|---|---|
| Spotty skin pigmentation | 77 |
| Cardiac myxoma | 53 |
| Cutaneous myxoma | 33 |
| Primary pigmented nodular adreno-cortical disease | 26 |
| Large cell calcifying Sertoli cell tumor of testis | 33 (of male patients) |
| Acromegaly | 10 |
| Psammomatous melanotic schwannoma | 10 |
| Thyroid nodules | 5 |
| Ductal adenoma of breast | 3 (of female patients) |

in Europe (57), at which time the familial nature of the syndrome was noted. In 1984, the acronym was modified to LAMB (lentigines, atrial myxoma, mucocutaneous myxomas, blue nevi), when it was recognized that the myxoid skin lesions were better classified as myxomas than myxoid neurofibromas (58). One year later, Carney et al. (59) defined the myxoma syndrome as the constellation of skin pigmentation, Sertoli cell tumors of the testis, cutaneous myxoma, myxoid fibroadenoma of the breast, primary pigmented nodular adrenocortical disease, and pituitary hyperactivity (gigantism). Several subsequent reports have confirmed these associations (60–62). The previously termed syndromes, LAMB and NAME, now are grouped under a broader category of Carney complex, which accounts for 3 to 7 percent of cardiac myxomas. Carney complex (Table 5-4) should not be confused with Carney syndrome, a triad that is a distinct neoplasia syndrome (63).

Analyses of several large families affected by Carney complex show that the disorder has an autosomal dominant inheritance with variable penetrance (64–66). The linkage to chromosome 17q24, where the *PRKAR1A* gene, encoding the R alpha regulatory subunit of cyclic-AMP-dependent protein kinase A is located, was identified as the cause of Carney complex in most patients

(67,68). In addition, a locus on chromosome 2 (2p15-16) has also been implicated, but the targeted gene not yet identified (64,66,69).

It has been shown by several investigators that familial cardiac myxomas are more often multiple, recurrent at the primary site or distant locations, and right sided than sporadic myxomas. It has been reported that myxomas as part of the Carney complex grow fast, as much as 1.8 cm/year. In the largest series of myxoma syndrome cases, there is a female to male predominance similar to sporadic cases (59), although a male predominance has been reported (70). On average, these patients are 25 years younger than patients with sporadic myxoma, with a mean age of approximately 25 years. Screening two-dimensional echocardiography has been recommended for first-degree relatives of patients with cardiac myxoma, particularly for relatives of younger patients with right-sided or bilateral tumors (71). Germline *PRKAR1A* mutations occur in about two of three patients with Carney complex, allowing for evaluation of family members. In cardiac myxoma tissue mutations are found in a minority of patients with sporadic myxomas, correlating with absent *PRKAR1A* expression by immunohistochemistry (37,37a).

## RADIOLOGIC FINDINGS

The general approach to diagnosing cardiac tumors, including myxoma, is echocardiography, followed by coronary angiography in older patients, and MRI for tissue characterization, location of attachment site, and distinction from mural thrombi (72). In addition to showing typical tumor neovascularization in about 50 percent of myxomas, angiography demonstrates obstructive coronary lesions and the need for revascularization in patients with risk factors for coronary artery disease. Chest radiographs are of little use in the workup of myxoma, but show evidence of mitral valve obstruction in 50 percent of left-sided tumor (signs of pulmonary hypertension), and calcification in about 50 percent of right-sided tumors.

Echocardiography demonstrates tumor size and attachment site, with transesophageal echocardiography providing more precision, especially intraoperatively, to guide tumor excision (73). The typical echocardiographic finding in cardiac myxoma is an atrial lesion attached to the interatrial septum that moves with diastole, usually through the atrioventricular valve. Calcification, which is more often present in right-sided myxomas, is occasionally identified. Mitral or tricuspid insufficiency is uncommon, except for trace degrees noted using color flow Doppler techniques.

CT is capable of precise localization, and can distinguish between fat, thrombus, and tumor, and between benign and infiltrative processes. The typical CT appearance includes a spherical or ovoid lesion with a lobular contour and heterogeneous attenuation (49,74). Myxomas can be hypoattenuated or isoattenuated relative to the myocardium. The site of tumor attachment can be accurately assessed in most cases (49,75). Valvular obstruction and large lesions can cause atrial enlargement.

MRI imaging shows tumor contours similar to those seen on CT; the tumor attachment site is demonstrated in over four fifths of tumors (49). There is typically heterogeneous signal intensity on T1-weighted images, with the myxoid tissue showing low signal intensity (49). In contrast, myxoid tissue has a high signal intensity on T2-weighted images (76). Contrast enhancement is generally moderate, with delayed enhancement in the outer tumor margins (77). Cystic changes, hemorrhage, and calcification are reliably predicted by MRI. MRI with multiplanar imaging is more beneficial than CT for identifying the point of attachment of the tumor, with up to 80 percent accuracy in some series (49).

The radiologic distinction between cardiac myxoma and cardiac sarcoma is not always possible. Many types of cardiac sarcoma are found in the left atrium, and sarcomas can, like myxomas, be attached to the atrial wall by a stalk. Infiltrative growth is much more common in sarcoma than myxoma. When this feature is identified using MRI or CT, the diagnosis of sarcoma should be favored over myxoma.

## GROSS FINDINGS

Most cardiac myxomas are cavitary left atrial masses attached to the atrial septum adjacent to the fossa ovalis (Table 5-1). Right atrial myxomas, which represent most of the remainder, are less likely to be found near the fossa ovalis than left atrial myxomas, although this is still the most common location. In 2 to 5 percent of cases,

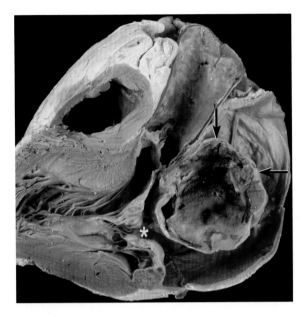

**Figure 5-1**

**CARDIAC MYXOMA**

The tumor (arrows) is attached at the interatrial septum, with close proximity to the mitral orifice (asterisk). The illustration demonstrates the common finding of mitral stenosis or obstruction in patients with left atrial myxoma. There is also significant left atrial dilatation.

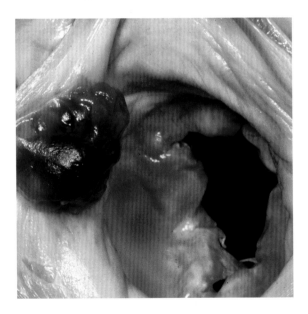

**Figure 5-2**

**CARDIAC MYXOMA**

The left atrium is opened, revealing an unexpected congested tumor attached to the left side of the atrial septum, above the anterior leaflet of the mitral valve. The death was sudden and unexpected, without other findings at autopsy.

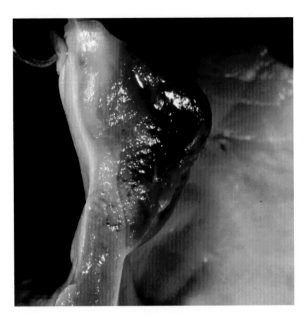

**Figure 5-3**

**CARDIAC MYXOMA**

The heart has been injected with blue dye, indicating vascularity at the base of the tumor. Seen from the anterior perspective, the atrial septum is in the center, with the myxoma at the right, in the left atrium.

cardiac myxomas grow on both sides of the atrial septum and are biatrial tumors that form a single mass. These lesions grow through the interatrial septum or the foramen ovale and are considered a single lesion (78–80). A few cardiac myxomas are truly multiple. These examples, which are typical of the myxoma syndrome, often occur in atrial sites other than the septum, and occasionally, in the ventricles. Single myxomas occurring in the right or left ventricles are rare, as are myxomas attached to the atrioventricular valves or tensor apparatus.

Cardiac myxomas are attached to the atrial septum by either a broad base or a narrow pedicle. Broad-based lesions are more friable and prone to embolism than pedunculated tumors. Cardiac myxomas are typically gelatinous to firm, focally hemorrhagic lesions with a smooth surface (figs. 5-1–5-8). In some cases, they form frond-like excrescences that are likely to embolize (figs. 5-9–5-11). There are often organized thrombi on the surface. On cut section, tumors are variegated in appearance, and may contain gritty calcified areas.

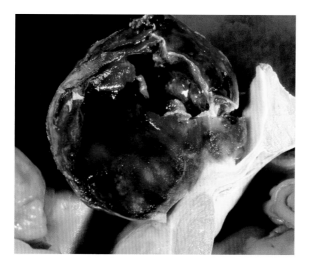

**Figure 5-4**

**CARDIAC MYXOMA**

The left atrium is at the left, with the incidentally found myxoma arising from the endocardial surface. The view is from a posterior perspective.

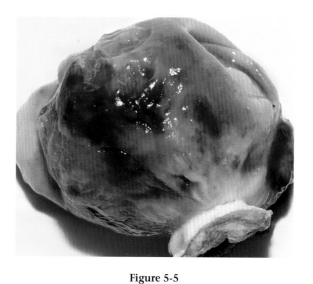

**Figure 5-5**

**CARDIAC MYXOMA**

The atrial attachment site is seen at the bottom.

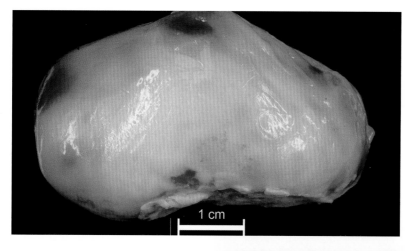

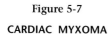

**Figure 5-6**

**CARDIAC MYXOMA**

Most cardiac myxomas have a smooth surface, and do not embolize.

**Figure 5-7**

**CARDIAC MYXOMA**

The bisected cut surface demonstrates a broad-based attachment site, with a 11-mm segment of atrial septum.

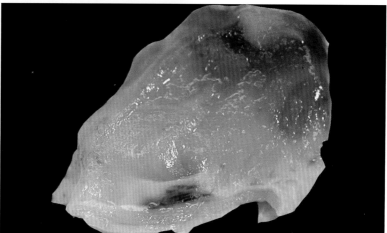

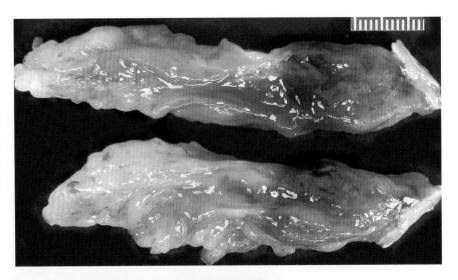

**Figure 5-8**

**CARDIAC MYXOMA**

The tumor is elongated and has a smooth surface. The patient developed symptoms of mitral insufficiency because the lengthening growth prolapsed across the mitral valve and interfered with valve closure.

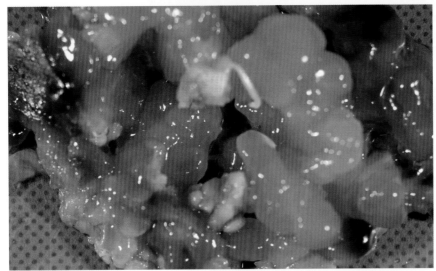

**Figure 5-9**

**CARDIAC MYXOMA**

This tumor has a gelatinous, myxoid appearance, with an irregular surface. This type of myxoma is likely to embolize.

**Figure 5-10**

**CARDIAC MYXOMA**

This tumor has a frond-like surface, similar to that shown in figure 5-9. The tumor was immersed in water for photography. The atrial attachment site is at the bottom right (arrow).

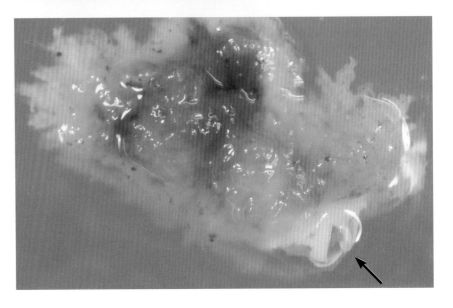

Although small cysts are occasionally noted on gross inspection, myxoma rarely presents as a cystic endocardial mass (52). Cardiac myxomas are usually easily excised with a rim of atrial wall, however, they may invade the atrial wall, requiring reconstructive surgery with patch repair (fig. 5-12).

## MICROSCOPIC FINDINGS

The microscopic diagnosis of cardiac myxoma depends on the identification of the myxoma cell, occasionally called the "lepidic cell." The classic cardiac myxoma cell possesses an oval nucleus with an open chromatin pattern and inconspicuous nucleoli, and is different from the tapered, spindled cell of soft tissue myxomas.

The cardiac myxoma cell has abundant eosinophilic cytoplasm and indistinct cell borders. It may occur singly within a myxoid background, in which case the cytoplasmic outline has a stellate appearance, or, more often, form

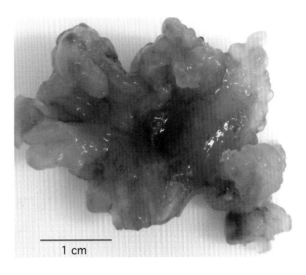

**Figure 5-11**

**CARDIAC MYXOMA**

The tumor is quite myxoid, with an irregular hemorrhagic appearance and mucoid material on the surface. The patient presented with cerebral embolism and stroke.

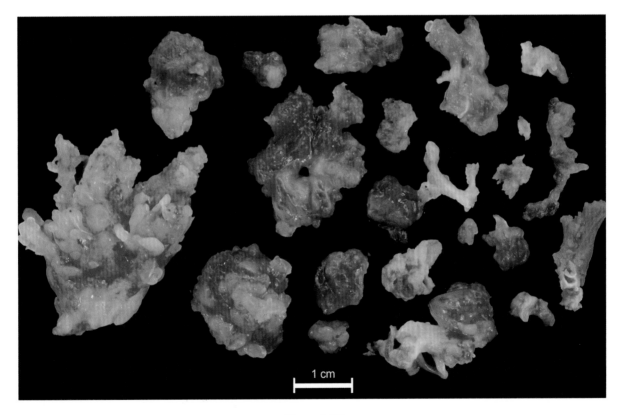

**Figure 5-12**

**CARDIAC MYXOMA: INCOMPLETE EXCISION**

It is rare that a myxoma is not excised in one piece, with a portion of the surrounding endocardium. In this case, the tumor had extensively infiltrated the atrial septum.

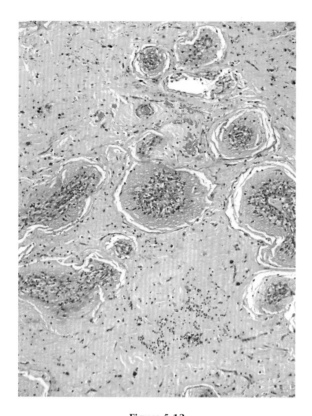

**Figure 5-13**

**CARDIAC MYXOMA:
PERIVASCULAR RING STRUCTURES**

There are often artifactual haloes around the nests of tumor cells. The myxoid stroma is present between the nests, with mild hemorrhage.

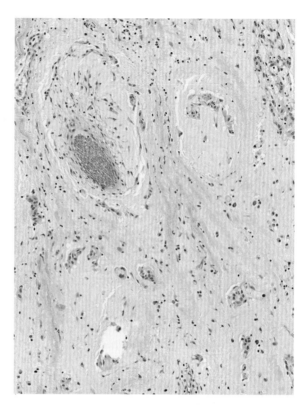

**Figure 5-14**

**CARDIAC MYXOMA:
PERIVASCULAR RING STRUCTURES**

The artifactual peritumoral haloes are prominent.

complex structures (figs. 5-13–5-17). The most common structure is a ring, one or several layers thick, surrounding a blood vessel, and often infiltrated by mononuclear inflammatory cells. The earliest lesions of myxoma are composed of bland ring-like structures without significant inflammation or differentiation into vessels (fig. 5-17). There can occasionally be an epithelioid appearance to the tumor cells (figs. 5-18–5-22). The background matrix may show degenerative changes, hemosiderin macrophages, and intravascular thrombi (fig. 5-23). The demarcation between the endothelium of the vessel and the myxoma cells is sometimes blurred, giving the impression that the myxoma cells are derived from the vessel itself.

Other types of structures present in myxomas are branching cords and tufts that occur on the surface of the tumor. The surface tufts may be quite cellular, and mitotic figures may

occur near the surface of the tumor. Cellularity and mitotic activity, in our experience, are not related to recurrence. The base of the tumor is often infiltrated by inflammatory cells, and prominent, muscularized arteries are typical near the attachment site (figs. 5-24, 5-25).

The presence of a myxoid matrix rich in proteoglycans is variable, and is not diagnostic of myxoma but may be found in any intravascular neoplasm. Secondary changes of fibrosis, thrombosis, and calcification often obscure the underlying nature of the lesion. Calcification is much more common than is appreciated radiographically, and is more prevalent in right-sided tumors. Fibrosis is more extensive in tumors from older patients, and the symptoms in these patients are usually present for long periods. Cardiac myxomas with extensive fibrosis are much less likely to embolize than myxomas with a predominantly myxoid background.

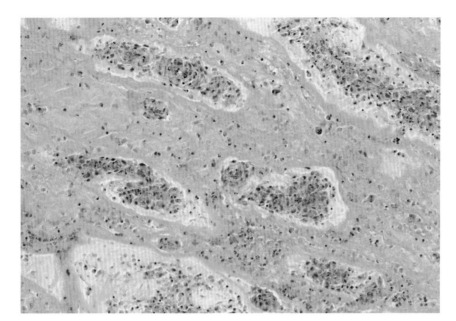

**Figure 5-15**

**CARDIAC MYXOMA:
PERIVASCULAR RING**

The tumor cells cluster around primitive vascular structures, and are infiltrated by inflammatory cells.

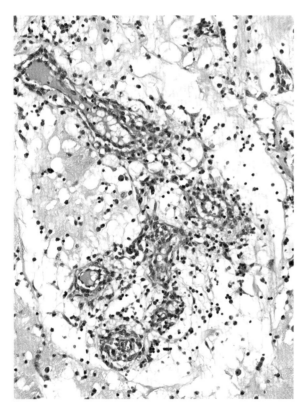

**Figure 5-16**

**CARDIAC MYXOMA:
PERIVASCULAR RING STRUCTURES**

There may be branching of the primitive vascular structures, which show characteristic inflammation and perivascular haloes. The myxoid stroma is prominent at the periphery.

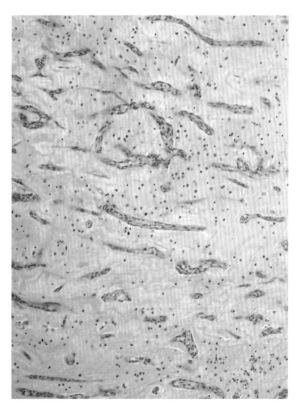

**Figure 5-17**

**CARDIAC MYXOMA: CORD-LIKE STRUCTURES**

The perivascular rings form elongated cords. When cut in a longitudinal section, the myxoid stroma is seen.

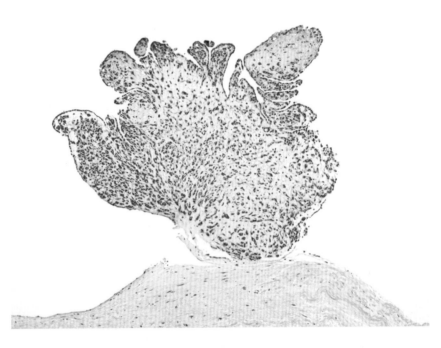

**Figure 5-18**

**CARDIAC MYXOMA**

This incipient incidental tumor shows no features of regression, such as inflammation and hemorrhage. In contrast to papillary fibroelastoma, there are no fibrous papillae, and there is significant cellularity.

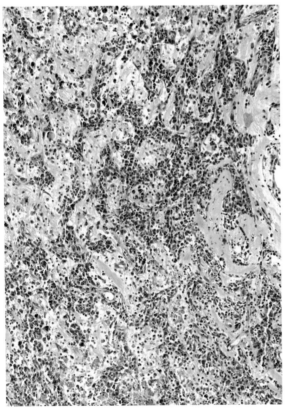

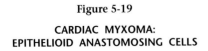

**Figure 5-19**

**CARDIAC MYXOMA: EPITHELIOID ANASTOMOSING CELLS**

The anastomosing nests of tumor cells are diffusely infiltrated by inflammatory cells.

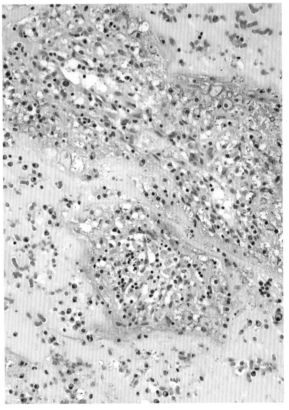

**Figure 5-20**

**CARDIAC MYXOMA: EPITHELIOID NESTS**

The ring-like structure is expanded to form a more sheet-like area of myxoma cells in a myxoid matrix infiltrated by inflammation.

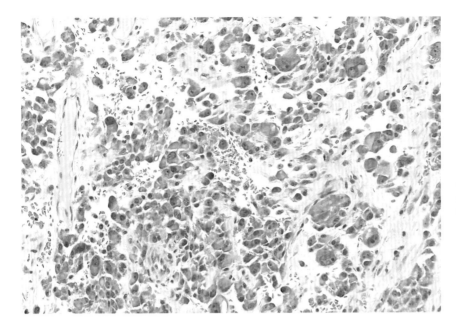

**Figure 5-21**

**CARDIAC MYXOMA:
EPITHELIOID TYPE
WITH ATYPIA**

The tumor cells are epithelioid, with abundant cytoplasm, but there is an admixture of lymphocytes and macrophages.

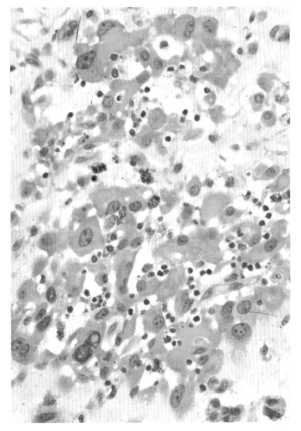

**Figure 5-22**

**CARDIAC MYXOMA: ATYPICAL**

At higher magnification, the tumor shown in figure 5-20 demonstrates epithelioid cells with focally enlarged nuclei and large intranuclear inclusions. Mitotic activity was minimal.

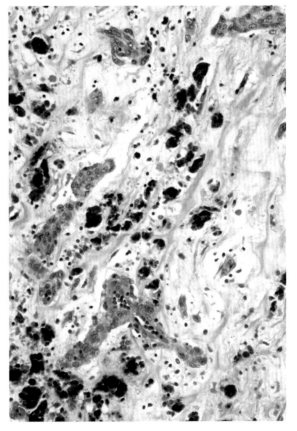

**Figure 5-23**

**CARDIAC MYXOMA**

Although hemosiderin-laden macrophages are almost always present to some degree, they may be extensive.

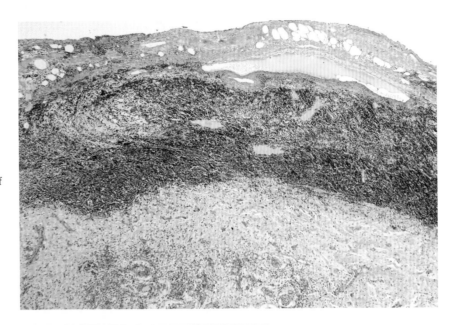

**Figure 5-24**

**CARDIAC MYXOMA: ATRIAL SEPTAL ATTACHMENT SITE**

In this case, there is a band of chronic inflammation.

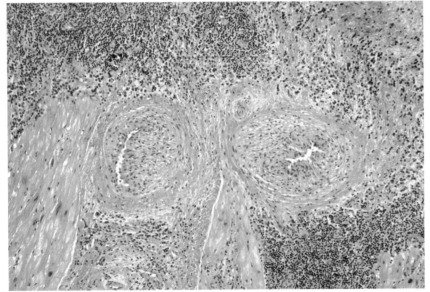

**Figure 5-25**

**CARDIAC MYXOMA: ATTACHMENT SITE**

Inflammation and prominent muscular arteries are typical at the interatrial septal attachment.

Other degenerative changes include ossification, which can include bone marrow, and Gamna-Gandy bodies. The latter, which represent iron encrustation of elastin fibers and are identical to those seen in spleens from patients with sickle cell disease, may compose the majority of the tumor, explaining reports in the literature of "Gamna body of the heart" (81). Gamna-Gandy bodies from cardiac myxomas are identified on cytologic preparations (82). Ossification occurs in less than 5 percent of tumors, more often on the right side (fig. 5-26). Extramedullary hematopoiesis is readily identified in about 5 percent of tumors (fig. 5-27) (33). The significance of this finding is unknown, but it has been associated with concurrent thalassemia (47).

An uncommon pattern of myxoma cell growth is that of the anastomosing cord pattern (fig. 5-28). Infiltration may occur at the base of the tumor (fig. 5-29). This feature is generally a reliable indicator of sarcoma, but in the presence of an otherwise typical histologic appearance and immunohistochemical profile of myxoma, does not exclude the diagnosis of myxoma.

Approximately 1 percent of cardiac myxomas contain glandular structures lined by mucin-laden

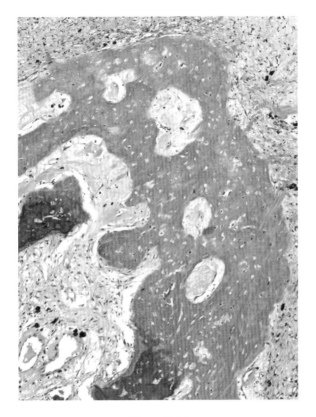

**Figure 5-26**

**CARDIAC MYXOMA: OSSIFICATION**

In some right atrial tumors, bone formation is extensive.

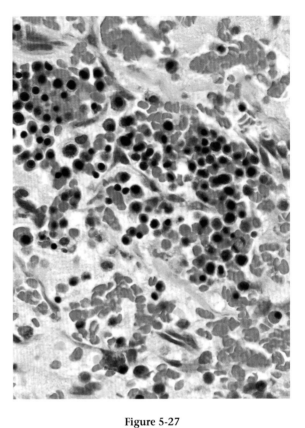

**Figure 5-27**

**CARDIAC MYXOMA: EXTRAMEDULLARY HEMATOPOIESIS**

This feature is found in 2 to 5 percent of myxomas, and is of no known clinical significance.

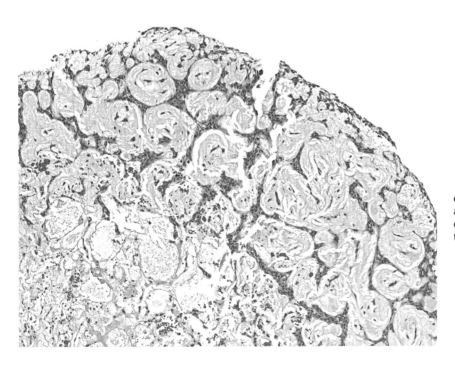

**Figure 5-28**

**CARDIAC MYXOMA: ANASTOMOSING PATTERN**

The cord-like pattern of cardiac myxoma often assumes an anastomosing lattice-like configuration, especially near the surface.

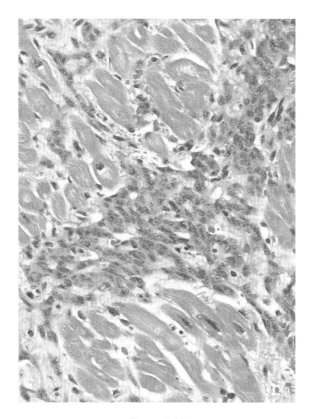

**Figure 5-29**

**CARDIAC MYXOMA:
INFILTRATION AT BASE OF TUMOR**

This feature is rare. Tumor cells course between bundles of cardiac atrial muscle.

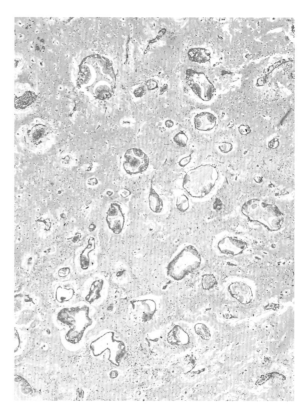

**Figure 5-30**

**CARDIAC MYXOMA: GLANDULAR DIFFERENTIATION**

Numerous ring-like structures of myxoma are seen.

cells that resemble the goblet cells of the gastrointestinal tract (figs. 5-30, 5-31). The mucin is periodic acid–Schiff (PAS) positive, diastase resistant, and the glands stain for cytokeratin and carcinoembryonic antigen by immunohistochemical techniques. The cytokeratin profile of the glandular elements share similarities with upper gastrointestinal glands, with expression of CK7 and CK20, and carcinoembryonic antigen (CEA) (83). The differential diagnosis of myxoma with glandular structures includes metastatic carcinoma, but there is no nuclear anaplasia or mitotic activity within the glands of myxoma and all reported cases are associated with the classic myxoma morphology in the same tumor. The first report of glandular myxoma was diagnosed as cystic glandular heterotopia of the atrium (84), and the myxomatous component mentioned descriptively. Rarely, the glandular component shows cytologic atypia (85).

Mucinous adenocarcinoma arising in the glandular variant has been reported (85a). Diffuse large B-cell lymphomas, some assocated with Epstein-Barr virus, have also been reported in the background of an otherwise classic cardiac myxoma (85b).

Cardiac myxomas may be composed predominantly of cysts that are lined by myxoma type cells, not mucinous cells (figs. 5-32, 5-33). We have encountered thymic rests in a single case of cardiac myxoma; these were present within the tumor itself. Two patients had neoplastic thymic tissue diagnostic of thymoma reported in left and right atrial myxomas (86).

Mononuclear inflammatory infiltrates are common in cardiac myxomas, and may consist of focal aggregates, infiltrates within the ring structures of the myxoma cells, or diffuse inflammation within the myxoid matrix. Dendritic cells, which express factor XIIIa, may be prominent in the stroma (figs. 5-33, 5-34) (87,88). So-called mesothelial/monocytic

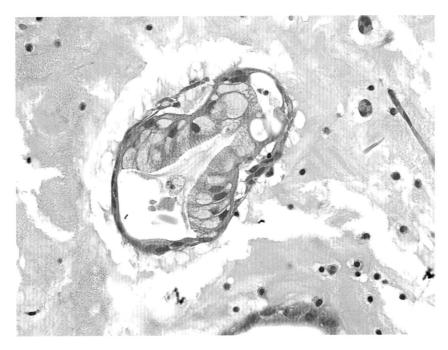

**Figure 5-31**

**CARDIAC MYXOMA:
GLANDULAR
DIFFERENTIATION**

The glands are focally and
segmentally lined by mucinous
epithelium (a higher-magnification view of figure 5-30).

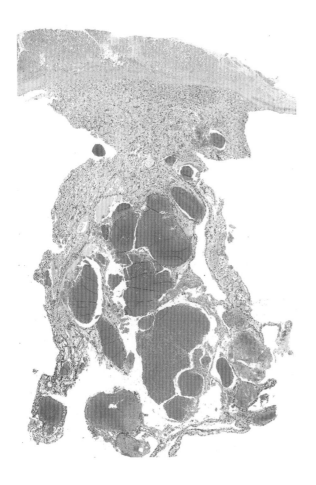

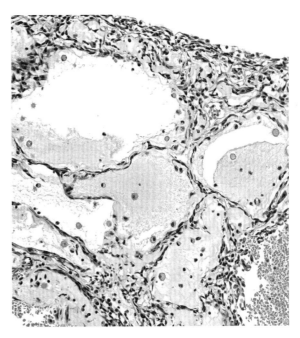

**Figure 5-32**

**CYSTIC CARDIAC MYXOMA**

Left: In rare examples, the tumor (same as seen in figure
5-29) is formed primarily by cysts, in this case filled with
blood and proteinaceous debris.

Above: At higher magnification, the cysts are seen lined
by myxoma cells.

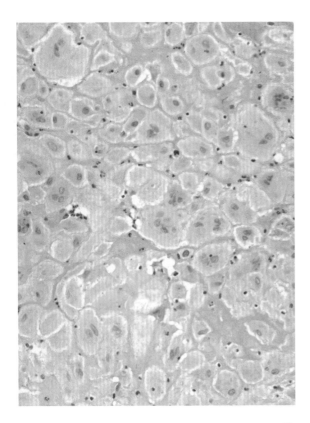 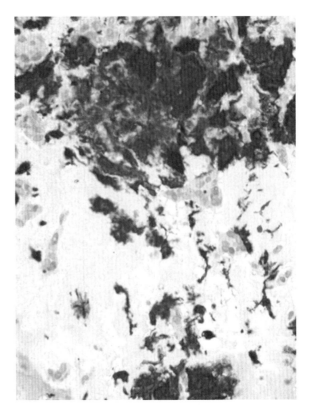

**Figure 5-33**

**CARDIAC MYXOMA: ABUNDANT DENDROCYTES**

Left: A sheet-like pattern is formed by an unusually large number of dendritic cells in the stroma.
Right: The epithelioid cells are strongly positive for factor XIIIa.

incidental cardiac excrescences (MICE) may occur on the surface of myxomas. The junction of the tumor and the interatrial septum is often characterized by lymphoid aggregates with or without germinal centers, smooth muscle bundles, occasional granuloma formation, and prominent thick-walled vessels, as noted above (figs. 5-24, 5-25).

## IMMUNOHISTOCHEMICAL FINDINGS

Myxoma cells express a variety of antigens, but consistently stain for calretinin (figs. 5-35–5-38). Calretinin has become a very useful marker and is expressed in most myxomas (89,90). Myxomas are generally cytokeratin negative, except in areas of glandular differentiation; S-100 protein, thrombomodulin, and smooth muscle actin have all been variably reported (91). The myxoma cells in ring structures usually express CD34, with less expression of CD31 restricted to the more differentiated inner capillary layer

(figs. 5-39–5-42). In some tumors, however, there is little difference in expression of CD31 and CD34. The mucins MUC1, MUC2, and MUC5AC are expressed, with the suggestion that MUC5AC-positive cases correlate with the rate of embolism. The rare glandular structures that are seen in myxomas express epithelial membrane antigen (EMA), polyclonal CEA, CA19.9, S-100 protein, CK7, CK20, and chromogranin in variable amounts (8,83,91–94). S-100 protein is also expressed in a subpopulation of myxoma cells in most tumors, but the significance of this finding is unclear. There is general, but not uniform, agreement that myxoma cells express vimentin, but the results of staining with antismooth muscle antigens have been variable (7,9,94,95).

Myxoma cells are positive for nonspecific histiocytic markers, such as lysozyme, alpha-1-antichymotrypsin, and alpha-1-antitrypsin, but do not express specific markers for histiocytic differentiation, such as CD68. These

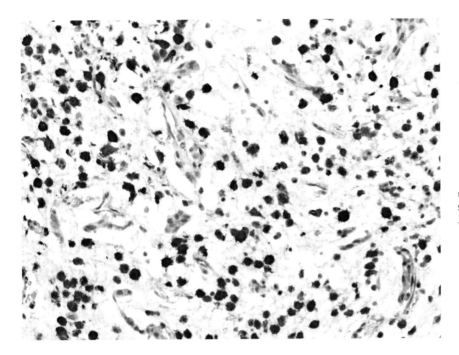

**Figure 5-34**

**CARDIAC MYXOMA: FACTOR XIIIA STAIN**

In tumors with otherwise unremarkable stroma, the interstitium contains numerous factor XIIIa macrophages.

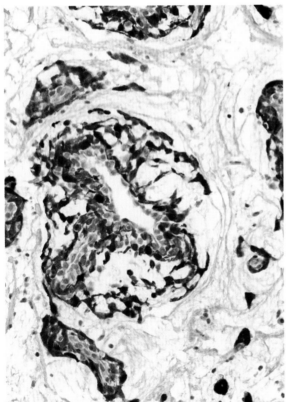

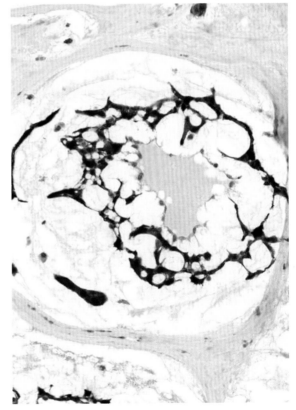

**Figure 5-35**

**CARDIAC MYXOMA: CALRETININ STAIN**

The ring and cord-like structures show diffuse calretinin staining.

**Figure 5-36**

**CARDIAC MYXOMA: CALRETININ STAIN**

Myxoma structures stain with calretinin, with the exception of the inner endothelial structure.

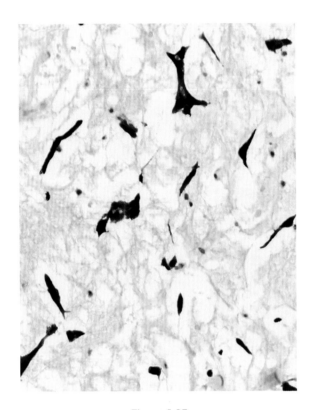

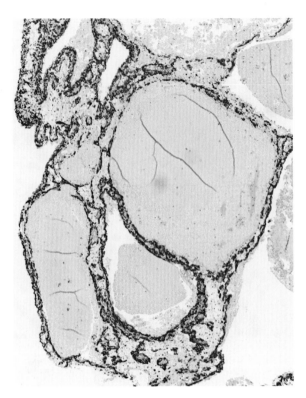

**Figure 5-37**

**CARDIAC MYXOMA: CALRETININ STAIN**

The cord-like structures are positive for calretinin.

**Figure 5-38**

**CARDIAC MYXOMA: CALRETININ STAIN**

The stain outlines the cysts in the cystic tumor illustrated in figure 5-33.

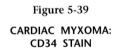

**Figure 5-39**

**CARDIAC MYXOMA: CD34 STAIN**

CD34 immunohistochemical staining tends to mirror that of calretinin, but the inner endothelial layer is also positive. When compared with figure 5-37, the difference is subtle, but note the center of the ring structure.

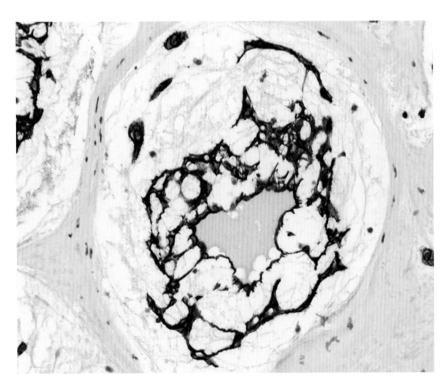

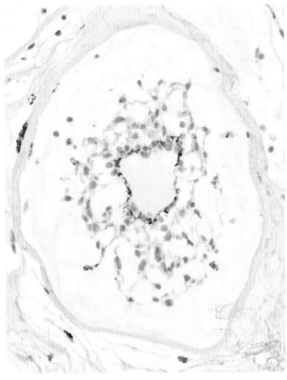

**Figure 5-40**

**CARDIAC MYXOMA: CD31 STAIN**

Only the more differentiated inner lining cells show endothelial cell differentiation by expressing CD31.

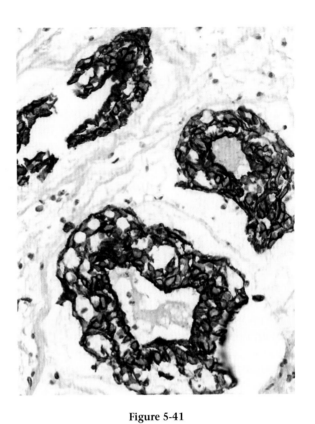

**Figure 5-41**

**CARDIAC MYXOMA: CD34 STAINING**

There is diffuse staining of all myxoma structure layers.

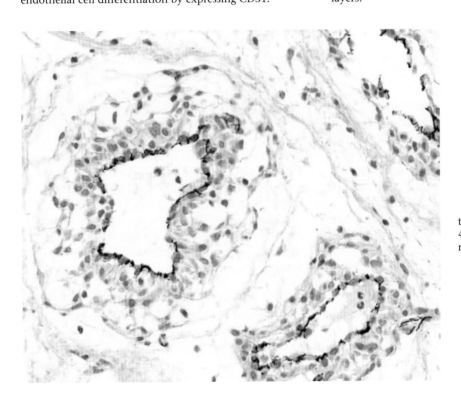

**Figure 5-42**

**CARDIAC MYXOMA: CD31 STAIN**

In this figure, corresponding to the field shown in figure 5-41, there is also CD31 staining restricted to the endothelial cells.

contradictory immunohistochemical findings corroborate the concept that myxomas arise from primitive cells that have the capacity to differentiate along many cell lines. The cardiomyocyte-specific transcription factors Nkx2.5/Csx, GATA-4, and eHAND, are demonstrated in these tumors, favoring cardiomyogenic differentiation. These markers are negative in cardiac sarcomas (17,96).

## DIFFERENTIAL DIAGNOSIS

**Malignant Tumors.** Sarcomas of the heart often occur in the left atrium and can be extensively myxoid, so-called myxoid imitators (97). There have been several examples of recurrent left atrial sarcomas that were initially erroneously diagnosed, radiologically and histologically, as myxoma (30). Many of these tumors have chondroid differentiation, which is rarely, if ever, present in myxoma. Most importantly, myxoid sarcomas lack ovoid or polygonal myxoma cells that form rings and cords, but are composed of atypical spindled cells. With sufficient sampling of the lesion, areas diagnostic of myxoid fibrosarcoma, chondrosarcoma, or malignant fibrous histiocytoma are found in most myxoid sarcomas. Mitotic figures are rare in myxomas and are confined to the surface of the tumor when present.

Although myxoid sarcomas are frequently misdiagnosed as myxoma, it is rare that myxomas are misdiagnosed as malignancies. Occasionally, myxomas have cellular areas on the tumor surface, and rarely, mitotic figures are found that suggest aggressive behavior. These findings are not indicative of future recurrence (4,33). We have seen two cases of myxoma with densely cellular areas suggestive of malignancy (33). These patients were without evidence of recurrence years after surgery, indicating that there may be pseudomalignant changes in a small subset of cardiac myxomas. The diagnosis of myxoma in both of these cases was made on the basis of areas of the tumor that were typical of myxoma, and the cellular areas in both cases were devoid of mitotic figures.

**Papillary Fibroelastoma.** Both myxoma and papillary fibroelastoma are endocardial lesions. In contrast to myxoma, papillary fibroelastomas often arise on valvular surfaces. The papillary fronds of papillary fibroelastoma are avascular, whereas a capillary network is always present in myxoma. Polygonal myxoma cells are absent in papillary fibroelastoma. Laminated elastic fibers are generally, but not always, present in papillary fibroelastoma and absent in myxoma.

**Mural Thrombus.** Occasionally, the pathologist encounters a cardiac mural fibrous mass without diagnostic areas of myxoma despite multiple sections. Occasionally, the distinction between organized thrombus and myxoma cannot be made, and a descriptive diagnosis is all that can be rendered. Because fibrotic myxomas rarely, if ever, recur, the distinction is probably not critical.

**Myxoma Emboli.** In the differential diagnosis of embolic myxoma is myxoid thrombus. Intraluminal organizing thrombi can elaborate myxoid ground substance from proliferating mesenchymal cells; however, myxoma cells and the structures they form are absent. The pathologist may receive a myxoid mass removed from a peripheral artery in a patient without a history of a cardiac mass (figs. 5-43, 5-44). Most cases contain typical myxoma cells within a myxoid background, and an echocardiogram will demonstrate an atrial tumor. Myxomas can embolize in toto, however, therefore, large embolic fragments with the histologic appearance of cardiac myxoma are best diagnosed as such, even if the subsequent echocardiogram is normal. As mentioned above, the differential diagnosis of myxoid material from embolectomies can be difficult, and may require immunohistochemical studies and comparison with the primary tumor (98).

Embolic sarcomas may also resemble embolic myxomas on histologic examination. We have seen examples of embolic chondrosarcoma, one originating in the aortic intima, which were initially misdiagnosed in an embolic site as cardiac myxoma. Again, the characteristic structures formed by myxoma cells are absent in embolic sarcoma, and occasional mitotic figures and the presence of chondroid differentiation favor a malignant diagnosis.

## SPREAD AND METASTASIS

The existence of "malignant" cardiac myxoma is controversial (99). From series of cardiac myxomas with follow-up data (46,100–103), there were two cases of sudden death, one death

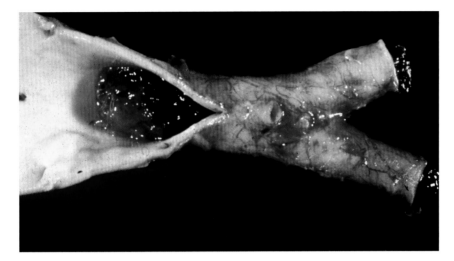

**Figure 5-43**

**CARDIAC MYXOMA: EMBOLIC**

A gelatinous tumor occludes the iliac bifurcation.

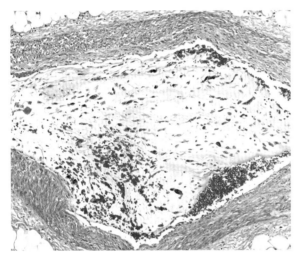

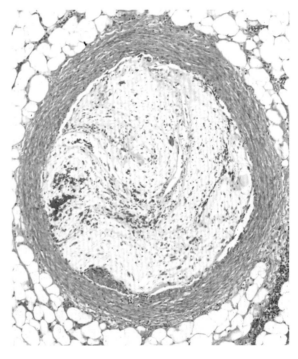

**Figure 5-44**

**CARDIAC MYXOMA: EMBOLIC**

Above: A coronary artery contains an occlusive myxoma embolus.

Right: A cross-section of the artery is seen.

related to multiple recurrences, and only one case of possible "malignant transformation" (101). More recent series have shown a low rate of postoperative deaths and recurrences, without documented malignant transformation in any case (37–40,104). We agree with a review (99) finding that malignant myxomas have been over-reported and that many are myxoid sarcomas that have been misdiagnosed as myxoma (97). The distinction between cerebral embolization and metastasis is somewhat blurred, as embolic deposits can persist with aneurysm formation, without significant infiltration of the parenchyma (105). There may be delayed metastases in the skin, but these have little tendency for extensive growth (106).

Although not true metastases, embolic myxomas have the capacity to grow into the arterial wall at the site of embolism, resulting in skin lesions (107), coronary insufficiency (108), and cerebral aneurysms (41,109–114). It has been suggested that embolism is related to tumor degradation by overexpression of matrix metalloproteinases (115).

Cerebral embolization occurs in about 12 percent of patients, and the symptoms are neurological, usually caused by ischemic cerebral infarct (116,117). There is no correlation with size; however, tumors resulting in emboli typically have a mobile component on transesophageal echocardiography. Histologically, embolic tumors tend to have abundant myxoid stroma and surface projections (33). Systemic embolization to the noncerebral circulation occurs in about one fifth of patients with cerebral symptoms. Aneurysmal dilatation with cerebral "metastasis" occurs only infrequently (118).

MRI of the brain has shown cerebral microbleeds (119) and multiple fusiform aneurysms (120) in myxoma patients with central nervous system symptoms. Long-term clinical follow-up in many patients with embolic myxoma is lacking (112), but these aneurysms may cause symptoms after removal of the primary tumor (112) or repeated embolization (121). Routine surveillance for cerebral aneurysms has been recommended (50). Embolic myxoma can persist as aneurysm in cerebral vessels or as nodules in pulmonary arteries for months or even years after excision of the primary tumor, but may also regress. A report of persistent coronary embolism emphasizes the long-term duration of myxoma deposits (108).

There are two convincing publications with adequate histologic confirmation of cardiac myxoma with bony deposits that resemble benign myxoma (99,122). However, these lesions did not cause the death of the patient and disseminated tumor was not present. Because embolic myxomas do not have the histologic characteristics of malignant neoplasms, and do not cause tumor deposits in viscera or lymph nodes, we do not interpret these deposits as true metastases or as evidence of malignant transformation.

Rarely, the entire tumor mass may embolize, resulting in a saddle aortic embolism without detectable cardiac tumor on imaging (125). In such cases, histologic evaluation of embolic material is required for the diagnosis. The differential diagnosis of myxoid material removed from embolectomy specimens includes myxoma and myxoid thrombus; identification of myxoma cells (often in concert with calretinin immunoperoxidase studies) and comparison of embolic material with primary tumor are useful. In some cases, it is impossible to make a definitive diagnosis (98).

## TREATMENT

Most patients with cardiac myxoma are cured by simple surgical excision, which can be minimally invasive (124). A biatrial approach with full-thickness excision of septum, necessitating repair of the resulting septal defect with a synthetic graft, is favored in some centers. The routine removal of the septum is not, however, necessary in all cases (37–40,102,125), and primary closure of the septum can be performed. It was previously believed that the risk of recurrence is increased if surgical excision is incomplete; currently, however, it is believed that the major factor in recurrence is the genetic predisposition to multiple and recurrent tumors (60,71). There is persistence of the belief that septal excision prevents recurrence (126).

As with coronary revascularization, recent surgical advances have allowed for minimally invasive surgery for myxoma resection (127,128). Complications of surgery include new onset atrial fibrillation, transient conduction disturbances, and perioperative mortality, which can be as high as 4 percent. In most series, there are no recurrences (129). Surgical mortality in other series is less than 1 percent (37,38,40,100–104). Right atrial tumors that have embolized may require, in addition to resection, pulmonary embolectomy (130). Left atrial tumors with cerebral ischemia pose the risk of operative anticoagulation extending the size of the infarct. Early surgery is recommended (131), and even thrombolytic therapy espoused for cerebral infarct (128). Myxomas on the mitral valve may necessitate valvuloplasty (132). In approximately 5 percent of cases, the mitral valve must be replaced or repaired because of tumor encroachment (101).

## RECURRENCE

The usual recurrence rate varies between 3 percent for sporadic cases and 22 percent for cases of Carney complex (105). Series of cardiac myxomas with long-term follow-up demonstrate a recurrence rate of less than 2 percent (46,100–103). In several recent series, there was an overall 1 percent recurrence rate (37–40,104,125).

The sites of recurrence within the heart are often distant from the site of the original tumor, indicating that recurrence is not usually related to incomplete excision. Patients with recurrent tumors are younger at age of presentation than patients with tumors that do not recur (33), and are more likely to be afflicted with the Carney complex.

## PROGNOSIS

The prognosis of patients with cardiac myxoma is excellent. As noted above, the rate of recurrence is low, generally with none or one patient in each series with a recurrence on follow-up (37–39,104,125). For most patients who survive surgery, the prognosis is excellent, with a median survival period of over 20 years (38,125). In one study, there was no difference in survival between patients with surgically excised myxomas and age-matched controls in the general population (38).

## REFERENCES

1. Dijkhuizen T, de Jong B, Meuzelaar JJ, Molenaar WM, van den Berg E. No cytogenetic evidence for involvement of gene(s) at 2p16 in sporadic cardiac myxomas: cytogenetic changes in ten sporadic cardiac myxomas. Cancer Genet Cytogenet 2001;126:162-165.

2. Dobin S, Speights VO Jr, Donner LR. Addition (1)(q32) as the sole clonal chromosomal abnormality in a case of cardiac myxoma. Cancer Genet Cytogenet 1997;96:181-182.

3. Dewald GW, Dahl RJ, Spurbeck JL, Carney JA, Gordon H. Chromosomally abnormal clones and nonrandom telomeric translocations in cardiac myxomas. Mayo Clin Proc 1987;62:558-567.

4. Seidman JD, Berman JJ, Hitchcock CL, et al. DNA analysis of cardiac myxomas: flow cytometry and image analysis. Hum Pathol 1991;22:494-500.

5. Amano J, Kono T, Wada Y, et al. Cardiac myxoma: its origin and tumor characteristics. Ann Thorac Cardiovasc Surg 2003;9:215-221.

6. Vaideeswar P, Butany JW. Benign cardiac tumors of the pluripotent mesenchyme. Semin Diagn Pathol 2008;25:20-28.

7. Curschellas E, Toia D, Borner M, Mihatsch MJ, Gudat F. Cardiac myxomas: immunohistochemical study of benign and malignant variants. Virchows Arch A Pathol Anat Histopathol 1991;418:485-491.

8. Goldman B, Frydman C, Harpaz N, Ryan S, Loiterman D. Glandular cardiac myxomas. Histologic, immunohistochemical, and ultrastructural evidence of epithelial differentiation. Cancer 1987;15:1767-1775.

9. Govoni E, Severi B, Cenacchi G, et al. Ultrastructural and immunohistochemical contribution to the histogenesis of human cardiac myxoma. Ultrastruct Pathol 1988;12:221-233.

10. Johansson L. Histogenesis of cardiac myxomas. An immunohistochemical study of 19 cases, including one with glandular structures, and review of the literature. Arch Pathol Lab Med 1989;113:735-741.

11. Krikler DM, Rode J, Davies MJ, Woolf N, Moss E. Atrial myxoma: a tumour in search of its origins. Br Heart J 1992;67:89-91.

12. Landon G, Ordonez NG, Guarda LA. Cardiac myxomas. An immunohistochemical study using endothelial, histiocytic, and smooth-muscle cell markers. Arch Pathol Lab Med 1986;110:116-120.

13. McComb RD. Heterogeneous expression of factor VIII/von Willebrand factor by cardiac myxoma cells. Am J Surg Pathol 1984;8:539-544.

14. Schuger L, Ron N, Rosenmann E. Cardiac myxoma. A retrospective immunohistochemical study. Pathol Res Pract 1987;182:63-66.

15. Tanimura A, Kitazono M, Nagayama K, Tanaka S, Kosuga K. Cardiac myxoma: morphologic, histochemical, and tissue culture studies. Hum Pathol 1988;19:316-322.

16. Markwald RR, Fitzharris TP, Manasek FJ. Structural development of endocardial cushions. Am J Anat 1977;148:85-119.

17. Kodama H, Hirotani T, Suzuki Y, Ogawa S, Yamazaki K. Cardiomyogenic differentiation in cardiac myxoma expressing lineage-specific transcription factors. Am J Pathol 2002;161:381-389

18. Orlandi A, Ciucci A, Ferlosio A, Genta R, Spagnoli LG, Gabbiani G. Cardiac myxoma cells exhibit embryonic endocardial stem cell features. J Pathol 2006;209:231-239.

19. Donato G, Conforti F, Zuccala V, et al. Expression of tenascin-c and CD44 receptors in cardiac myxomas. Cardiovasc Pathol 2009;18:173-177.

20. Sigurjonsson H, Andersen K, Gardarsdottir M, et al. Cardiac myxoma in Iceland: a case series with an estimation of population incidence. APMIS 2011;119:611-617.

21. Burke A, Virmani R. Tumors of the heart and hreat vessels. AFIP Atlas of Tumor Pathology, 3rd Series, Fascicle 16. Washington, DC: American Registry of Pathology; 1996:21-46.

22. Markel M, Waller B, Armstrong W. Cardiac myxoma. A review. Medicine (Baltimore) 1987; 66:114-125.

23. Mariano A, Pita A, Leon R, et al. Primary cardiac tumors in children: a 16-year experience. Rev Port Cardiol 2009;28:279-288.

24. Akyildiz EU, Tolgay E, Oz B, Yilmaz R, Koc S. Cardiac myxoma: an unusual cause of sudden death in childhood. Turk J Pediatr 2006;48:172-174.

25. Hovels-Gurich HH, Seghaye MC, Amo-Takyi BK, Hugel W, Duchateau J, von Bernuth G. Cardiac myxoma in a 6-year-old child—constitutional symptoms mimicking rheumatic disease and the role of interleukin-6. Acta Paediatr 1999;88:786-788.

26. Tsai TS, Chen YJ, Hsieh KS, Lee PC, Chi CS. Right ventricular myxoma in a 12-year-old child: a case report. Zhonghua Yi Xue Za Zhi (Taipei) 1994;54:447-451.

27. Kure K, Lingamfelter D, Taboada E. Large multifocal cardiac myxoma causing the sudden unexpected death of a 2-month-old infant—a rapidly growing, acquired lesion versus a congenital process?: A case report. Am J Forensic Med Pathol 2011;32:166-168.

28. Wu KH, Mo XM, Liu YL. Clinical analysis and surgical results of cardiac myxoma in pediatric patients. J Surg Oncol 2009;99:48-50.

29. Chan HS, Sonley MJ, Moes CA, Daneman A, Smith CR, Martin DJ. Primary and secondary tumors of childhood involving the heart, pericardium, and great vessels. A report of 75 cases and review of the literature. Cancer 1985;56:825-836.

30. Wold LE, Lie JT. Cardiac myxomas: a clinicopathologic profile. Am J Pathol 1980; 101:219-240.

31. Padalino MA, Basso C, Milanesi O, et al. Surgically treated primary cardiac tumors in early infancy and childhood. J Thorac Cardiovasc Surg 2005;129:1358-1363.

32. Padalino MA, Vida VL, Boccuzzo G, et al. Surgery for primary cardiac tumors in children: early and late results in a multicenter European Congenital Heart Surgeons Association study. Circulation 2012;126:22-30.

33. Burke AP, Virmani R. Cardiac myxoma. A clinicopathologic study. Am J Clin Pathol 1993;100:671-680.

34. Scott N, Veinot JP, Chan KL. Symptoms in cardiac myxoma. Chest 2003;124:2408.

35. Strotmann J. [Cardiac tumors—clinical symptoms, diagnostic approaches, and therapeutic aspects.] Med Klin (Munich) 2008;103:175-180. [German]

36. Vaughan CJ, Gallagher M, Murphy MB. Left ventricular myxoma presenting with constitutional symptoms and raised serum interleukin-6 both suppressed by naproxen. Eur Heart J 1997; 18:703.

37. Bossert T, Gummert JF, Battellini R, et al. Surgical experience with 77 primary cardiac tumors. Interact Cardiovasc Thorac Surg 2005;4:311-315.

37a. Maleszewski JJ, Larsen BT, Kip NS, et al. PRKAR1A in the development of cardiac myxoma: a study of 110 cases including isolated and syndromic tumors. Am J Surg Pathol 2014;38:1079-1087.

38. Elbardissi AW, Dearani JA, Daly RC, et al. Survival after resection of primary cardiac tumors: a 48-year experience. Circulation 2008;118:S7-15.

39. Kamiya H, Yasuda T, Nagamine H, et al. Surgical treatment of primary cardiac tumors: 28 years' experience in Kanazawa University Hospital. Jpn Circ J 2001;65:315-319.

40. Thomas-de-Montpreville V, Nottin R, Dulmet E, Serraf A. Heart tumors in children and adults: clinicopathological study of 59 patients from a surgical center. Cardiovasc Pathol 2007;16:22-28.

41. Price DL, Harris JL, New PF, Cantu RC. Cardiac myxoma. A clinicopathologic and angiographic study. Arch Neurol 1970;23:558-567.

42. Yokomuro H, Yoshihara K, Watanabe Y, Shiono N, Koyama N, Takanashi Y. The variations in the immunologic features and interleukin-6 levels for the surgical treatment of cardiac myxomas. Surg Today 2007;37:750-753.

43. Mendoza CE, Rosado MF, Bernal L. The role of interleukin-6 in cases of cardiac myxoma. Clinical features, immunologic abnormalities, and a possible role in recurrence. Tex Heart Inst J 2001;28:3-7.

44. Mendoza CE, Rosado MF, Pacheco P. Interleukin-6 production and recurrent cardiac myxoma. J Thorac Cardiovasc Surg 2001;121:395-396.

45. Morishima A, Marui A, Shimamoto T, Saji Y, Nishina T, Komeda M. A case of interleukin-6-producing cardiac myxoma resembling multicentric Castleman's disease. J Thorac Cardiovasc Surg 2009;138:499-501.

46. Larsson S, Lepore V, Kennergren C. Atrial myxomas: results of 25 years' experience and review of the literature. Surgery 1989;105:695-698.

47. Joukhadar R, De Las Casas LE, Lalude O, Gough D. Cardiac myxoma showing extramedullary hematopoiesis in a patient with beta thalassemia. South Med J 2009;102:769-771.

48. Charokopos NA, Rouska E, Pliakos C, et al. Atypical atrial myxomas in two asymptomatic patients: a case report. Cardiovasc Ultrasound 2009;7:45.

49. Grebenc ML, Rosado-de-Christenson ML, Green CE, Burke AP, Galvin JR. Cardiac myxoma: imaging features in 83 patients. Radiographics 2002; 22:673-689.

50. Stollberger C, Finsterer J. Patients with cardiac myxoma require surveillance for myxoma-related cerebral aneurysms. Eur J Neurol 2008;15: e110-111.

51. Turkmen N, Eren B, Fedakar R, Comunoglu N. An unusual cause of sudden death: cardiac myxoma. Adv Ther 2007;24:529-532.

52. Heck HA Jr, Gross CM, Houghton JL. Long-term severe pulmonary hypertension associated with right atrial myxoma. Chest 1992;102:301-303.

53. Virmani R, Clark MA, Posey DM, McAllister HA Jr. Right atrial myxoma causing pulmonary emboli and pulmonary hypertension. Am J Forensic Med Pathol 1982;3:249-252.

54. Dufkova B, Malek I, Vymetalova Y, et al. Myxoma of donor origin in a transplanted heart. J Heart Lung Transplant 2007;26:865-867.

55. Nishio Y, Ito Y, Iguchi Y, Sato H. MPO-ANCA-associated pseudovasculitis in cardiac myxoma. Eur J Neurol 2005;12:619-620.

56. Atherton D, Pitcher D, Wells R, MacDonald D. A syndrome of various cutaneous pigmented lesions, myxoid neurofibromata and atrial myxoma: The NAME syndrome. Br J Dermatol 1980;103:421-429.

57. Schweizer-Cagianut M, Salomon F, Hedinger CE. Primary adrenocortical nodular dysplasia with cushing's syndrome and cardiac myxomas. A peculiar familial disease. Virchows Arch A Pathol Anat Histol 1982;397:183-192.

58. Rhodes AR, Silverman RA, Harrist TJ, Perez-Atayde AR. Mucocutaneous lentigines, cardiomucocutaneous myxomas, and multiple blue nevi: the "LAMB" syndrome. J Am Acad Dermatol 1984;10:72-82.

59. Carney JA. The complex of myxomas, spotty pigmentation, and endocrine overactivity. Arch Intern Med 1987;147:418-419.

60. Carney J, Gordon H, Carpenter P, Shenoy B, Go V. The complex of myxomas, spotty pigmentation, and endocrine overactivity. Medicine (Baltimore) 1985;64:270-283.

61. McCarthy PM, Piehler JM, Schaff HV, et al. The significance of multiple, recurrent, and "complex" cardiac myxomas. J Thorac Cardiovasc Surg 1986;91:389-396.

62. van Gelder HM, O'Brien DJ, Staples ED, Alexander JA. Familial cardiac myxoma. Ann Thorac Surg 1992;53:419-424.

63. Wilkes D, McDermott DA, Basson CT. Clinical phenotypes and molecular genetic mechanisms of Carney complex. Lancet Oncol 2005;6:501-508.

64. Basson CT, MacRae CA, Korf B, Merliss A. Genetic heterogeneity of familial atrial myxoma syndromes (Carney complex). Am J Cardiol 1997;79:994-995.

65. Kirschner LS, Carney JA, Pack SD, et al. Mutations of the gene encoding the protein kinase A type I-alpha regulatory subunit in patients with the Carney complex. Nat Genet 2000;26:89-92.

66. Vargas-Alarcon G, Vargas-Barron J, Cruz-Robles D, et al. A deletion in the PRKAR1A gene is associated with Carney complex. J Pediatr Endocrinol Metab 2008;21:705-709.

67. Casey M, Mah C, Merliss AD, et al. Identification of a novel genetic locus for familial cardiac myxomas and Carney complex. Circulation 1998;98:2560-2566.

68. Casey M, Vaughan CJ, He J, et al. Mutations in the protein kinase A R1alpha regulatory subunit cause familial cardiac myxomas and Carney complex. J Clin Invest 2000;106:R31-38.

69. Matyakhina L, Pack S, Kirschner LS, et al. Chromosome 2 (2p16) abnormalities in Carney complex tumours. J Med Genet 2003;40:268-277.

70. Danoff A, Jormark S, Lorber D, Fleischer N. Adrenocortical micronodular dysplasia, cardiac myxomas, lentigines, and spindle cell tumors. Report of a kindred. Arch Intern Med 1987;147:443-448.

71. Farah MG. Familial cardiac myxoma. A study of relatives of patients with myxoma. Chest 1994;105:65-68.

72. Rahmanian PB, Castillo JG, Sanz J, Adams DH, Filsoufi F. Cardiac myxoma: preoperative diagnosis using a multimodal imaging approach and surgical outcome in a large contemporary series. Interact Cardiovasc Thorac Surg 2007;6:479-483.

73. Scohy TV, Lecomte PV, McGhie J, et al. Intraoperative real time three-dimensional transesophageal echocardiographic evaluation of right atrial tumor. Echocardiography 2008;25:646-649.

74. Tsuchiya F, Kohno A, Saitoh R, Shigeta A. CT findings of atrial myxoma. Radiology 1984;151: 139-143.

75. Grebenc ML, Rosado de Christenson ML, Burke AP, Green CE, Galvin JR. Primary cardiac and pericardial neoplasms: radiologic-pathologic correlation. Radiographics 2000;20:1073-1103; quiz 1110-1012.

76. Masui T, Takahashi M, Miura K, Naito M, Tawarahara K. Cardiac myxoma: identification of intratumoral hemorrhage and calcification on MR images. AJR Am J Roentgenol 1995;164:850-852.

77. Alter P, Grimm W, Rominger MB, et al. Right ventricular cardiac myxoma. Diagnostic usefulness of cardiac magnetic resonance imaging. Herz 2005;30:663-667.

78. Gonzalez-Ferrer JJ, Carnero M, Labayru VL, de Isla LP, Zamorano JL. Left atrial myxoma prolapsing through the foramen ovale. Eur J Echocardiogr 2008;9:595-597.

79. Shaikh AH, Khan G, Hanif B, Malik F, Bashir A. Biatrial myxoma. J Coll Physicians Surg Pak 2008;18:639-640.

80. Vitovskii RM, Isaenko VV, Zakharova VP, et al. [Observation of bilateral myxoma of interatrial septum.] Klin Khir 2008:59-60. [Russian]

81. Coard KC, Silver MD. Gamna body of the heart. Pathology 1984;16:459-461.

82. Jimenez Heffernan JA, Salas C, Tejerina E, Viguer JM. Gamna-Gandy bodies from cardiac myxoma on intraoperative cytology. Cytopathology 2010;21:203-205.

83. Pucci A, Bartoloni G, Tessitore E, Carney JA, Papotti M. Cytokeratin profile and neuroendocrine cells in the glandular component of cardiac myxoma. Virchows Arch 2003;443:618-624.

84. Honey M, Axelrad MA. Intracardiac endodermal heterotopia. Br Heart J 1962;24:667-670.

85. den Bakker MA, Dinjens WN, Bekkers JA. Cardiac myxoma with atypical glandular component, report of a case. Histopathology 2006;48:206-208.

85a. Berger MD, Schneider J, Ballmer PE, Eckhardt BP, Dommann-Scherrer C. Mucin-producing adenocarcinoma arising in an atrial myxoma. Ann Diagn Pathol 2013;17:104-107.

85b. Svec A, Rangaiah M, Giles M, Jaksa R, McAulay KA. EBV+ diffuse large B-cell lymphoma arising within atrial myxoma. An example of a distinct primary cardiac EBV+ DLBCL of immunocompetent patients. Pathol Res Pract 2012;208:172-176.

86. Miller DV, Tazelaar HD, Handy JR, Young DA, Hernandez JC. Thymoma arising within cardiac myxoma. Am J Surg Pathol 2005;29:1208-1213.

87. Berrutti L, Silverman JS. Cardiac myxoma is rich in factor xiiia positive dendrophages: Immunohistochemical study of four cases. Histopathology. 1996;28:529-535

88. Silverman JS, Berrutti L. Cardiac myxoma immunohistochemistry: value of CD34, CD31, and factor XIIIa staining. Diagn Cytopathol 1996;15:455-456.

89. Terracciano LM, Mhawech P, Suess K, et al. Calretinin as a marker for cardiac myxoma. Diagnostic and histogenetic considerations. Am J Clin Pathol 2000;114:754-759.

90. Acebo E, Val-Bernal JF, Gomez-Roman JJ. Thrombomodulin, calretinin and c-kit (CD117) expression in cardiac myxoma. Histol Histopathol 2001;16:1031-1036.

91. Pucci A, Gagliardotto P, Zanini C, Pansini S, di Summa M, Mollo F. Histopathologic and clinical characterization of cardiac myxoma: review of 53 cases from a single institution. Am Heart J 2000;140:134-138.

92. Lindner V, Edah-Tally S, Chakfe N, Onody T, Eisenmann B, Walter P. Cardiac myxoma with glandular component: Case report and review of the literature. Pathol Res Pract 1999;195:267-272.

93. Abenoza P, Sibley RK. Cardiac myxoma with glandlike structures. An immunohistochemical study. Arch Pathol Lab Med 1986;110:736-739.

94. Deshpande A, Venugopal P, Kumar AS, Chopra P. Phenotypic characterization of cellular components of cardiac myxoma: a light microscopy and immunohistochemistry study. Hum Pathol 1996;27:1056-1059.

95. Boxer ME. Cardiac myxoma: an immunoperoxidase study of histogenesis. Histopathology 1984;8:861-872+.

96. Kodama H, Inoue T, Watanabe R, et al. Cardiomyogenic potential of mesenchymal progenitors derived from human circulating CD14+ monocytes. Stem Cells Dev 2005;14:676-686.

97. Attum A, Johnson G, Masri Z, Girardet R, Lansing A. Malignant clinical behavior of cardiac myxomas and "myxoid imitators." Ann Thorac Surg 1987;44:217-222.

98. Dogan R, Dogan OF, Duman U, Duvan I, Terzioglu A, Firat P. Myxoid tissue fragments in femoral embolectomy material: Cardiac myxoma versus myxoid thrombus—a diagnostic dilemma. Anadolu Kardiyol Derg 2007;7:105-106.

99. Rupp G, Heyman R, Martinez A, Sekhar L, Jungreis C. The pathology of metastatic cardiac myxoma. Am J Clin Pathol 1989;91:221-227.

100. Dein JR, Frist WH, Stinson EB, et al. Primary cardiac neoplasms. Early and late results of surgical treatment in 42 patients. J Thorac Cardiovasc Surg 1987;93:502-511.

101. Blondeau P. Primary cardiac tumors—French studies of 533 cases. Thorac Cardiovasc Surg 1990;38(Suppl 2):192-195.

102. Murphy MC, Sweeney MS, Putnam JB Jr, et al. Surgical treatment of cardiac tumors: a 25-year experience. Ann Thorac Surg 1990;49:612-617; discussion 617-618.

103. Tazelaar HD, Locke TJ, McGregor CG. Pathology of surgically excised primary cardiac tumors. Mayo Clin Proc 1992;67:957-965.

104. Grande AM, Ragni T, Vigano M. Primary cardiac tumors. A clinical experience of 12 years. Tex Heart Inst J 1993;20:223-230.

105. Altundag MB, Ertas G, Ucer AR, et al. Brain metastasis of cardiac myxoma: case report and review of the literature. J Neurooncol 2005;75:181-184.

106. Terada Y, Wanibuchi Y, Noguchi M, Mitsui T. Metastatic atrial myxoma to the skin at 15 years after surgical resection. Ann Thorac Surg 2000;69:283-284.

107. Reed RJ, Utz MP, Terezakis N. Embolic and metastatic cardiac myxoma. Am J Dermatopathol 1989;11:157-165.

108. Milicevic G, Gavranovic Z, Cupic H, et al. Unremitting embolus from cardiac myxoma at circumflex artery trifurcation. Int J Cardiol 2008;126:424-426.

109. Branch CL Jr, Laster DW, Kelly DL Jr. Left atrial myxoma with cerebral emboli. Neurosurgery 1985;16:675-680.

110. Budzilovich G, Aleksic S, Greco A, Fernandez J, Harris J, Finegold M. Malignant cardiac myxoma with cerebral metastases. Surg Neurol 1979;11:461-469.

111. Damasio H, Seabra-Gomes R, da Silva JP, Damasio AR, Antunes JL. Multiple cerebral aneurysms and cardiac myxoma. Arch Neurol 1975;32:269-270.

112. Roeltgen DP, Weimer GR, Patterson LF. Delayed neurologic complications of left atrial myxoma. Neurology 1981;31:8-13.

113. Todo T, Usui M, Nagashima K. Cerebral metastasis of malignant cardiac myxoma. Surg Neurol 1992;37:374-379.

114. Frank RA, Shalen PR, Harvey DG, Berg L, Ferguson TB, Schwartz HG. Atrial myxoma with intellectual decline and cerebral growths on CT scan. Ann Neurol 1979;5:396-400.

115. Orlandi A, Ciucci A, Ferlosio A, Pellegrino A, Chiariello L, Spagnoli LG. Increased expression and activity of matrix metalloproteinases characterize embolic cardiac myxomas. Am J Pathol 2005;166:1619-1628.

116. Radoi MP, Stefanescu F, Arsene D. Brain metastases and multiple cerebral aneurysms from cardiac myxoma: case report and review of the literature. Br J Neurosurg 2012;26:893-895.

117. Elbardissi AW, Dearani JA, Daly RC, et al. Embolic potential of cardiac tumors and outcome after resection: a case-control study. Stroke 2009;40:156-162.

118. Lee VH, Connolly HM, Brown RD Jr. Central nervous system manifestations of cardiac myxoma. Arch Neurol 2007;64:1115-1120.

119. Vanacker P, Nelissen N, Van Laere K, Thijs VN. Images in neurology. Scattered cerebral microbleeds due to cardiac myxoma. Arch Neurol 2009;66:796-797.

120. Shinn SH, Chon SH, Kim HJ. Multiple cerebral aneurysms associated with cardiac myxoma in a patient with chronic renal failure: how can we resolve multiple cerebral aneurysms? Thorac Cardiovasc Surg 2009;57:47-48.

121. Li Q, Shang H, Zhou D, Liu R, He L, Zheng H. Repeated embolism and multiple aneurysms: central nervous system manifestations of cardiac myxoma. Eur J Neurol 2008;15:e112-113.

122. Seo IS, Warner TF, Colyer RA, Winkler RF. Metastasizing atrial myxoma. Am J Surg Pathol 1980;4:391-399.

123. Ohgo T, Yamamoto K, Furuno T. Complete detachment of cardiac myxoma causing aortic saddle embolization and cerebral infarction. Int J Cardiol 2008;127:e48-49.

124. Panos A, Myers PO. Video-assisted cardiac myxoma resection: basket technique for complete and safe removal from the heart. Ann Thorac Surg 2012;93:e109-110.

125. Bakaeen FG, Reardon MJ, Coselli JS, et at. Surgical outcome in 85 patients with primary cardiac tumors. Am J Surg 2003;186:641-647; discussion 647.

126. Durgut K, Gormus N, Ozulku M, Ozergin U, Ozpinar C. Clinical features and surgical treatment of cardiac myxoma: report of 18 cases. Asian Cardiovasc Thorac Ann 2002;10:111-114.

127. Kumar S. Minimally invasive approach for surgical management of cardiac myxoma. Heart Lung Circ 2006;15:280.

128. Marumoto A, Ashida Y, Maeta H, Ishiguro S, Kuroda H, Ohgi S. Surgical removal of left atrial myxoma through mini sternotomy and the superior transseptal approach. Jpn J Thorac Cardiovasc Surg 2001;49:185-187.

129. Ipek G, Erentug V, Bozbuga N, et al. Surgical management of cardiac myxoma. J Card Surg 2005;20:300-304.

130. Canale LS, Colafranceschi AS, Leal Botelho ES, de Oliveira Monteiro AJ. Surgical treatment of right atrial myxoma complicated with pulmonary embolism. Interact Cardiovasc Thorac Surg 2009;9:535-536.

131. Katz MG, Finkelshtein V, Raichman DB, Dekel H, Lampl Y, Sasson L. Surgical resection of left atrial myxoma presenting with acute multiple hemorrhagic cerebral infarctions: a case report. Heart Surg Forum 2008;11:E169-171.

132. Nomura K, Nakamura Y, Uno Y, Yamashiro M. Pediatric left atrial myxoma: surgical excision and mitral valve plasty. Ann Thorac Cardiovasc Surg 2007;13:65-67.

# 6 PAPILLARY FIBROELASTOMA

## DEFINITION

*Papillary fibroelastomas* are benign avascular papillary growths of the endocardium that have an uncertain histogenesis. Synonyms include *fibroelastic papilloma, papilloma of valves, giant Lambl excrescence, myxofibroma, myxoma of valves, hyaline fibroma,* and *fibroma of valves.* The term "papilloma" should probably be avoided since it is usually used within the context of papillary epithelial cell growths.

## GENERAL FEATURES

Papillary fibroelastomas arise in two settings: 1) sporadic without known cause, and 2) as an apparent response to hemodynamic disturbance caused either iatrogenically or by intrinsic cardiac disease (usually valvular). It is probably an exaggerated form of a Lambl excrescence, which is a reactive filiform growth that occurs at the sites of greatest hemodynamic stress, usually at the nodules of Arantius of the semilunar valves and along the lines of closure and free edges. The nodule of Arantius is a mid-cusp thickening located at the midscallop of the line of closure. In atrioventricular valves, Lambl excrescences are found at the site of valve closure on the atrial surface. In either site, they are thought to be age-related changes and may be a reaction to minor endothelial damage resulting from changes in hemodynamic shear stresses.

Unlike Lambl excrescences, papillary fibroelastomas become very large, and occur on any endocardium-lined surface (1–3). Thrombi may occur on the surface of the proliferation, and dislodged clots are responsible for embolic symptoms (4–7).

The pathogenesis of papillary fibroelastoma is unknown, and it is unclear whether it is a reactive or hamartomatous process. Because papillary fibroelastomas resemble Lambl excrescences, both grossly and microscopically, a shared histogenesis is probable.

Repetitive hemodynamic trauma may contribute to the development of papillary fibroelastomas, as they have been reported in association with diseases resulting in abnormal flow of blood in the heart, including rheumatic heart disease, hypertrophic cardiomyopathy, mitral valve prolapse, and atrial septal defect (8–16). The mechanisms by which such hemodynamic abnormalities contribute to papillary fibroelastoma growth are unclear.

There is increasing evidence that about 20 percent of papillary fibroelastomas develop as a result of iatrogenic factors (17,18), including thoracic irradiation and open-heart surgery (subaortic septal myectomy, valve repair, valve replacement, and repair of congenital defects) (17,19,20). In contrast to sporadic cases, which are most common on cardiac valves, iatrogenic papillary fibroelastomas tend to occur in a variety of nonvalvular endocardial surfaces, usually in close proximity to the predisposing iatrogenic factor, such as in the chamber most closely associated with the site of surgery. Multiplicity is especially common when the tumors arise in valves that are regurgitant or stenotic (21).

The true incidence of papillary fibroelastomas is unknown because they are often asymptomatic. They were previously considered rare: by 1991, only 132 cases had been published in the medical literature (22). With the increasing use of echocardiography, they are being more readily detected and recognized (23–25). In series of surgically resected cardiac tumors (26), papillary fibroelastomas were the second most common tumor, after myxoma. Among 102 benign tumors excised at the Mayo Clinic, 7 were papillary fibroelastomas, representing the second most common nonmyxoma benign tumor after fibroma (26). With the increased use of cardiac imaging, along with the improved resolution of such studies, it is likely that papillary fibroelastomas will become more common than cardiac

**Table 6-1**

**CLINICOPATHOLOGIC FEATURES OF PAPILLARY FIBROELASTOMA[a]**

| Clinicopathologic Feature | Percent |
|---|---|
| Male:female[b] (n = 44:72) | 38:62 |
| Mean age[c] | |
| Site | |
| Aortic valve (n=65) | 46 |
| Mitral valve (n=30) | 21 |
| Left ventricle (n=16) | 11 |
| Tricuspid valve (n=13) | 9 |
| Left atrium (n=8) | 6 |
| Right atrium (n=3) | 2 |
| Right ventricle (n=3) | 2 |
| Pulmonary valve (n=3) | 2 |
| Symptoms (percent of patients) | |
| None related to papillary fibroelastoma (incidental) | 26 |
| Chest pain, dyspnea | 17 |
| Syncope | 16 |
| Atrial fibrillation | 12 |
| Tachyarrhythmias | 10 |
| TIA[d]/stroke | 9 |
| Palpitations | 2 |
| Lower extremity embolization | 1 |
| Pulmonary embolism | 1 |

[a]141 cardiac papillary fibroelastomas excised from 129 patients from references 27, 31, and 85–87.
[b]In 12 patients multiple tumors were resected.
[c]Data available for 116 of the patients.
[d]TIA = transient ischemic attack.

myxomas in adults. In a more recent series of surgically resected heart tumors, 11 of 77 tumors were papillary fibroelastomas (27).

## CLINICAL FEATURES

Papillary fibroelastoma is more common in women, and there is a wide range of age at presentation, with a mean age of approximately 60 years (Table 6-1) (22,28–30). Most symptoms arise from left-sided lesions that shower surface thrombi or the papillary fronds themselves into the cerebral circulation or prolapse into the coronary orifice (31,32). The most common locations are the aortic and mitral valves or the left atrium, and tumors may be multiple (33–36). The most common symptoms are transient neurologic defects, myocardial ischemia (37,38), and rarely, sudden death (17,39,40). There is an association with abnormal heart valves, such as with rheumatic valvular disease (41). In a series of 41 cases reported by Edwards

et al. (28), 9 patients had congestive heart failure from unrelated causes, 2 patients had neurologic symptoms, 2 patients died suddenly, and the remainder were asymptomatic.

In 1991, 22 reports of papillary fibroelastoma causing embolic symptoms were compiled from the literature (42). All involved the left side of the heart, specifically the mitral valve (10 cases), aortic valve (9 cases), left ventricular papillary muscle (2 cases), and free wall (1 case). Embolism caused coronary occlusion (acute myocardial infarct, 13 cases), cerebral vascular occlusion (8 cases), and renal vascular occlusion (1 case). The diagnosis of papillary fibroelastoma is often made by echocardiography after the patient experiences transient ischemic attacks or stroke.

Right-sided papillary fibroelastomas, occurring primarily on the pulmonary and tricuspid valves, may also cause pulmonary embolism (43). The right atrium is an unusual site of origin resulting in recurrent pulmonary embolism (44). Multiple tumors on both the tricuspid and pulmonary valves may cause pulmonary symptoms.

Sudden death and ischemic heart disease are generally attributed to embolization or prolapse of tumors that are located on either the ventricular or aortic surfaces of the right or left cusps of the aortic valve (22,45–48). At least one illustration of a "myxoma" resulting in sudden death by embolism appears to represent a papillary fibroelastoma of the aortic valve (49). The cause of peripheral vascular occlusion is usually embolization of an adherent surface fibrin thrombus. It is uncommon for papillary fibroelastomas to cause significant valvular dysfunction or heart failure; however, these phenomena have been reported (50).

The diagnosis of papillary fibroelastoma is readily made clinically by two-dimensional echocardiography, and the tumor may be an incidental finding or detected after cerebral ischemia (47,51–57). If a diagnosis of papillary fibroelastoma is made prior to surgery, the tumor is simply excised, usually preserving the underlying valve architecture (58).

Papillary fibroelastomas of the cardiac valves demonstrate typical echocardiographic features (6,35). The size of the lesion is often greater by imaging than appreciated after excision, when the tumor collapses. Multiplicity occurs in 10 to 30 percent of cases (59); iatrogenically

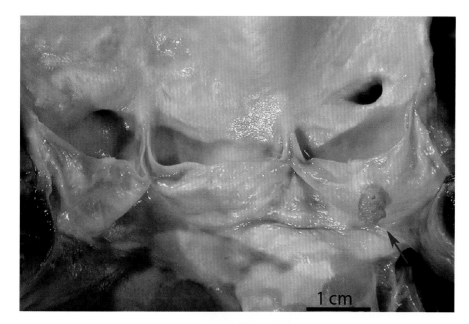

**Figure 6-1**

**PAPILLARY FIBROELASTOMA: AORTIC VALVE**

The polypoid lesion is on the ventricular surface of the left aortic cusp (arrow).

**Figure 6-2**

**PAPILLARY FIBROELASTOMA: MITRAL VALVE**

The polypoid lesion is on the closing surface of the anterior mitral valve leaflet (arrows). Insert shows higher-magnification view.

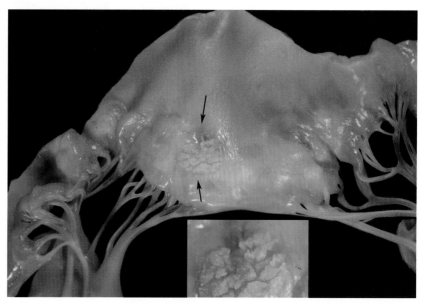

induced papillary fibroelastoma is more likely to be multiple (18,21,42,60–62). Transesophageal echocardiography is helpful in cases at rare sites, such as the venae cavae or atria (4,63).

Uchida et al. (64) reported a case of papillary fibroelastoma of the left ventricular outflow tract that lacked the typical frond-like appearance on echocardiography, indicating that the differential diagnosis between papillary fibroelastoma and myxoma is not always possible by imaging studies. Three-dimensional echocardiography may provide enhanced imaging (5,59).

## GROSS FINDINGS

Papillary fibroelastomas are invariably located on the endocardial surface, with 90 percent located on valve surfaces. They are filiform papillary tumors that open up to a somewhat spherical mass when placed under water (figs. 6-1–6-7). The appearance has been likened to that of a sea anemone, although most of the sea animals have thicker tentacles than the thin papillae of the cardiac tumor. Papillary fibroelastomas resemble large Lambl excrescences (fig. 6-5);

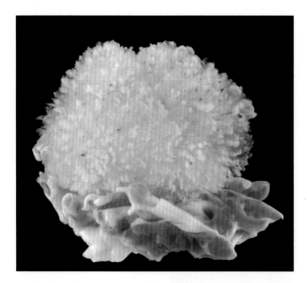

**Figure 6-3**

**PAPILLARY FIBROELASTOMA: LEFT VENTRICLE**

The specimen was excised at autopsy and immersed under water for photography. The tumor is arising from the apex of the left ventricle. Fine apical trabeculations can be seen below the tumor.

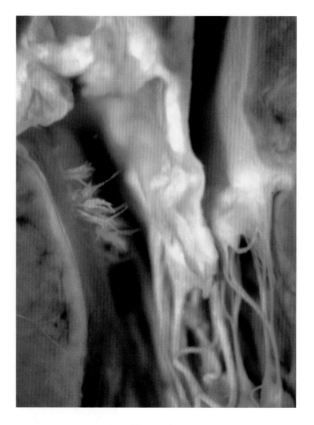

**Figure 6-4**

**PAPILLARY FIBROELASTOMA: LEFT VENTRICULAR OUTFLOW TRACT**

There is a frond-like filiform lesion of the ventricular outflow septum, just adjacent to the anterior leaflet of the mitral valve. The patient had marked cardiomegaly with features of hypertrophic cardiomyopathy.

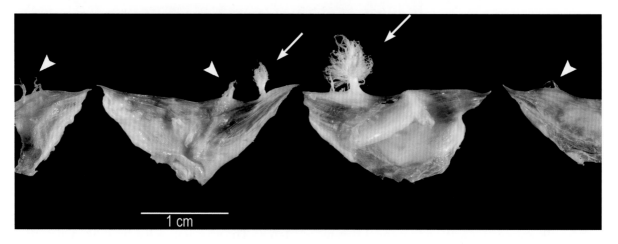

**Figure 6-5**

**MULTIPLE PAPILLARY FIBROELASTOMAS AND LAMBL EXCRESCENCES: AORTIC VALVE**

The papillary fibroelastomas (arrows) are larger and exhibit complex branching of the fronds. The Lambl excrescences, arising from the free edge, are shorter without significant branching (arrowheads).

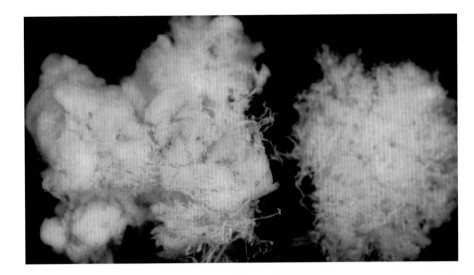

**Figure 6-6**

**PAPILLARY FIBROELASTOMA: MULTIPLE**

The patient had two lesions, both right-sided, on the pulmonary (left) and tricuspid valves (right). The gross appearance and size were remarkably similar.

**Figure 6-7**

**PAPILLARY FIBROELASTOMA: STENOTIC AORTIC VALVE**

The valve was resected in three pieces, corresponding to each cusp (top). A tumor was excised from the posterior cusp and submitted separately; when immersed, it showed features typical of a papillary fibroelastoma (bottom).

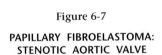

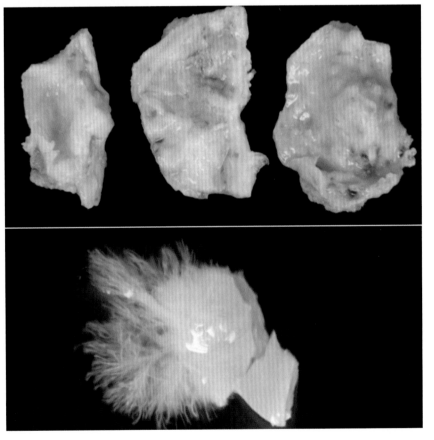

however, as mentioned, Lambl excrescences are specifically located at the lines of closure of the valve, whereas papillary fibroelastomas occur anywhere on the valvular surface. Moreover, Lambl excrescences typically do not exhibit the complex branching of the fronds that is usually seen in papillary fibroelastomas.

When papillary fibroelastomas occur on the atrioventricular valves, they have a predilection for the atrial surface, but there is no clear predilection for semilunar valves. The most common sites, especially for symptomatic lesions, are the aortic or mitral valve; right-sided tumors, such as those located on the tricuspid valve,

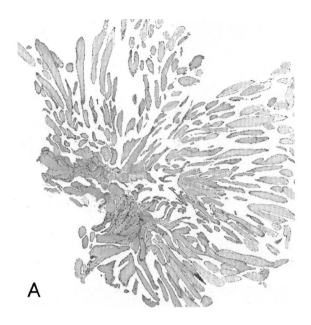

A

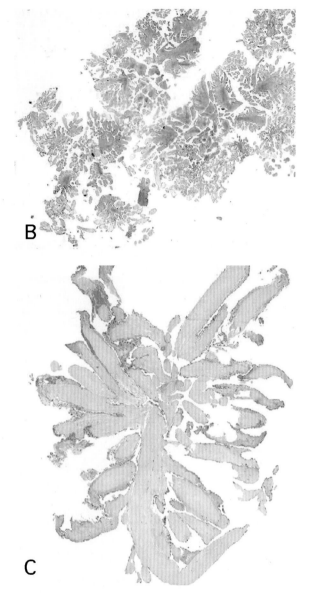

B

C

**Figure 6-8**

**PAPILLARY FIBROELASTOMA**

A: The papillae in this example are elongated and slender.

B: The central cores of the lesions are acellular and collagenous, with branching filiform papillae emanating from them.

C: In this case, the branching is not as fine and complex as in the prior two examples.

are often asymptomatic (65). Unusual nonvalvular sites include the papillary muscles, ostium of the right coronary artery (66), ventricular septum (50), left atrium (41), right atrium (44, 68,69), left ventricular outflow tract (fig. 6-6) (34,42,64,67,70), right ventricular outflow tract (71), tricuspid valve chordae (72), left ventricular endocardium (73), and Chiari network (38). A papillary fibroelastoma with two attachments by separate stalks on the anterior leaflet of the mitral valve and left ventricular outflow tract has been described (74).

Papillary fibroelastomas range in size from 2 to 50 mm in greatest dimension, and are usually

attached to the endocardial surface by a short single stalk. The lower end of the size spectrum is arbitrary, as the tumors overlap with Lambl excrescences, with which they form a spectrum.

## MICROSCOPIC FINDINGS

The papillary fronds of papillary fibroelastoma are usually narrow, elongated, and branching (figs. 6-8–6-15). The papillae resemble chordae tendineae. The matrix consists of mucopolysaccharides, elastic fibers, and rare spindle cells resembling smooth muscle cells or fibroblasts. A Movat pentachrome stain is useful for delineating these components (fig. 6-13), although

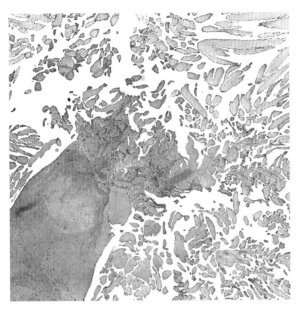

**Figure 6-9**

**PAPILLARY FIBROELASTOMA**

The fibrous core is thick, similar to a tree trunk.

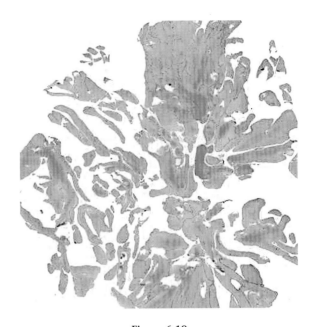

**Figure 6-10**

**PAPILLARY FIBROELASTOMA**

The stalk is inconspicuous in this case.

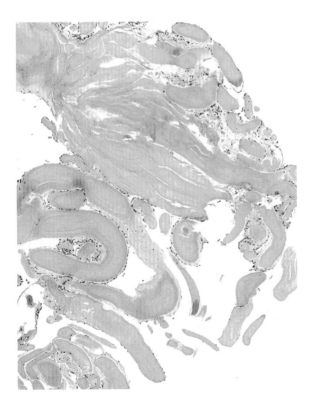

**Figure 6-11**

**PAPILLARY FIBROELASTOMA**

The papillae are uniform and thick, and lack vascularity or cellularity.

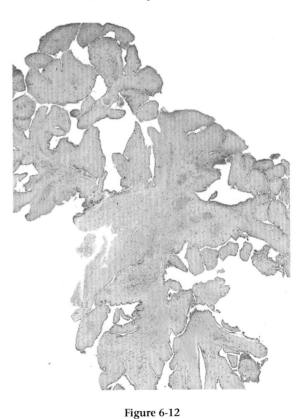

**Figure 6-12**

**PAPILLARY FIBROELASTOMA**

The cores are thick and stubby, but are avascular and paucicellular.

115

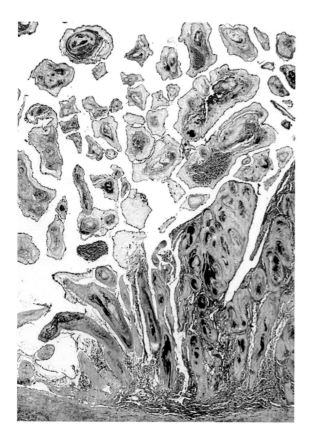

**Figure 6-13**

**PAPILLARY FIBROELASTOMA**

There is a variable amount of elastic tissue in the cores. Despite the name, these tumors frequently lack significant amounts of elastic tissue (Movat pentachrome stain).

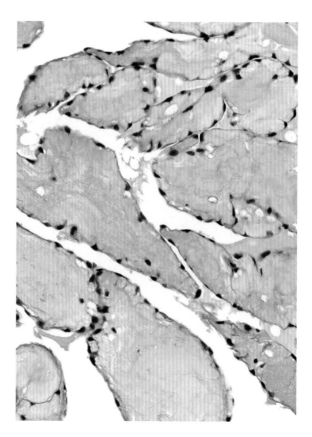

**Figure 6-14**

**PAPILLARY FIBROELASTOMA**

The tips of the cores are essentially acellular, lined by a single layer of endothelial cells.

elastic tissue is frequently absent or inconspicuous, despite the name of the tumor. In some cases, there may be simplification of the papillations, with rounding and a smoother surface. The papillae are avascular papillary structures lined by a single layer of endothelial cells (fig. 6-14). The surface may show fibrin (fig. 6-15), which may detach and account for embolic symptoms. The papillary cores contain a proteoglycan-rich stroma, and layers of elastic fibers and collagen are prominent near the base of the lesion. The cells covering the surface express vimentin, factor VIII-related antigen, and CD34, and the stroma is rich in collagen type IV (75).

## ULTRASTRUCTURAL FINDINGS

The connective tissue of papillary fibroelastoma contains mature collagen in which irregular elastic fibers are longitudinally oriented (29,50).

Fibroblasts and more primitive mesenchymal cells are present within the matrix. The surface endothelial cells are hyperplastic and possess numerous organelles and pinocytotic vesicles. Because the surface cells of papillary fibroelastoma ultrastructurally resemble endothelial cells, in contrast to atrial myxoma, Fishbein et al. (29) recommended the use of the term "endocardial papillary elastofibroma" for the designation of these tumors.

## DIFFERENTIAL DIAGNOSIS

There are few entities that can histologically be mistaken for papillary fibroelastoma. Tumors of the cardiac valves are rare; 73 percent are papillary fibroelastomas, and the remainder represent sarcomas, inflammatory myofibroblastic tumors, lipomatous hamartomas, myxomas, and hemangiomas (28,76). Myxomas are rarely located on

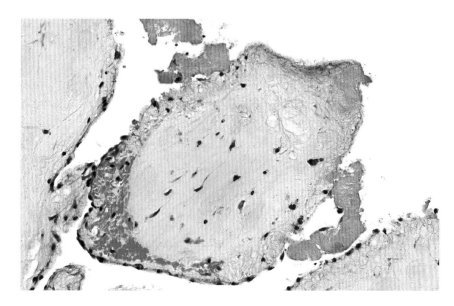

**Figure 6-15**

**PAPILLARY FIBROELASTOMA
WITH SURFACE THROMBUS**

Some of the papillae have areas of endothelial denudation and surface fibrin thrombi. Embolization can occur from a surface thrombus or the papillae themselves.

the valve surface, and many reported examples of valve myxomas are probably papillary fibroelastomas based on the histologic findings (77). Papillary fibroelastoma differs histologically from myxoma by the absence of vessels within papillae (these are always present in myxoma), the absence of polygonal "myxoma" cells within the papillae and on the surface of the tumor, the outer localization of myxoid matrix (diffuse in myxoma), and the presence of laminated elastic fibers. The last finding is variable; elastic tissue may be absent in papillary fibroelastoma, especially if only superficial portions of the tumor are sampled.

Another diagnostic problem is the overgrowth of papillary fibroelastoma by attached fibrin thrombi (marantic endocarditis). These vegetations may cause embolic symptoms, and the underlying tumor may be obscured by organizing thrombus. The gross appearance of papillary fibroelastoma can therefore mimic that of marantic endocarditis. For this reason, valvular excrescences should be routinely sampled for histologic evaluation.

Inflammatory myofibroblastic tumor is a rare tumor of cardiac valves that occurs primarily in children (76). In contrast to papillary fibroelastoma, this lesion is cellular, and generally contains inflammatory cells within a myofibroblast-rich matrix.

## TREATMENT

The treatment of symptomatic papillary fibroelastoma is simple excision, which is curative (78). Most often, the tumor is removed without excision of significant areas of surrounding endocardium or valve, with minimal repair of the valve leaflet (40,79). Valve-sparing excision produces good long-term results in most instances (25). Valve replacement, as was performed in the past, is rarely necessary currently (58,80).

Asymptomatic patients are treated surgically if the tumor is mobile on echocardiography, if left sided, or if over 1 cm (81); asymptomatic patients with nonmobile lesions can be followed closely with periodic clinical evaluation and echocardiography (6). Symptomatic lesions are always excised (82). If surgery is contraindicated or refused by the patient, anticoagulation is recommended, although specific guidelines are lacking.

## PROGNOSIS

Recurrences are rare, and valve-sparing minimally invasive surgery should be considered whenever possible, as regrowth of partially resected lesions does not occur (65,83,84). Although papillary fibroelastomas are benign, the long-term follow-up of patients who undergo surgery for resection shows increased mortality over the general population by a factor of 3, likely due to concurrent medical conditions (85). Long-term follow-up of resected heart tumors, in general, demonstrates that of all tumor types excised, only cardiac myxoma has no impact on long-term survival (85–87).

## REFERENCES

1. Butany J, Nair V, Ahluwalia MS, El Demellwy D, Siu S, Fiendel C. Papillary fibroelastoma of the interatrial septum: a case report. J Card Surg 2004;19:349-353.
2. Crestanello JA, Orszulak TA. Giant papillary fibroelastoma of the right atrium: an unusual presentation. Ann Thorac Surg 2002;74:1252-1254.
3. Sato Y, Yokoyama H, Satokawa H, Takase S, Maruyama Y. A report of a surgical case of papillary fibroelastoma in the left ventricular outflow tract. Ann Thorac Cardiovasc Surg 2003;9:270-273.
4. Baba Y, Tsuboi Y, Sakiyama K, et al. Cardiac papillary fibroelastoma as a cause of recurrent ischemic strokes: the diagnostic value of serial transesophageal echocardiography. Cerebrovasc Dis 2002;14:256-259.
5. Dichtl W, Muller LC, Pachinger O, Schwarzacher SP, Muller S. Images in cardiovascular medicine. Improved preoperative assessment of papillary fibroelastoma by dynamic three-dimensional echocardiography. Circulation 2002;106:1300.
6. Gowda RM, Khan IA, Nair CK, Mehta NJ, Vasavada BC, Sacchi TJ. Cardiac papillary fibroelastoma: a comprehensive analysis of 725 cases. Am Heart J 2003;146:404-410.
7. Kuroczynski W, Hake U, Pruefer D, Peivandi A, Heinemann M, Oelert H. Aortic valve papillary fibroelastoma. J Heart Valve Dis 2005;14:140-142.
8. Abad C, De la Rosa P. Right atrial papillary fibroelastoma associated with atrial septal defect, persistent superior vena cava, and coronary artery disease. J Thorac Cardiovasc Surg 2008; 136:538.
9. Taguchi M, Kaminishi Y, Konishi H, et al. [Cardiac papillary fibroelastomas: report of 2 cases.] Kyobu Geka 2005;58:1163-1165. [Japanese]
10. Watanabe T, Hosoda Y, Kikuchi N, Kawai S. Papillary fibroelastoma of the tricuspid valve in association with an atrial septal defect: report of a case. Surg Today 1996;26:831-833.
11. Shapira OM, Williamson WA, Dugan JM. Papillary fibroelastoma of the mitral valve. Cardiovasc Surg 1993;1:599-601.
12. Kobayashi Y, Saito S, Yamazaki K, Kurosawa H. Multiple papillary fibroelastoma in left ventricle associated with obstructive hypertrophic cardiomyopathy. Interact Cardiovasc Thorac Surg 2009;9:921-922.
13. Fuzellier JF, Brasselet C, Perotin S, Torossian PF, Metz D. Infected multiple fibroelastomas in hypertrophic cardiomyopathy. J Heart Valve Dis 2005;14:848-851.
14. Taniguchi I, Morimoto K, Miyasaka S, Marumoto A. Papillary fibroelastoma of the mitral valve associated with rheumatic mitral valve stenosis. Jpn J Thorac Cardiovasc Surg 2005;53:143-146.
15. Ohuchi S, Izumoto H, Kamata J, et al. [Aortic valve papillary fibroelastoma in a patient with mitral valve regurgitation.] Kyobu Geka 1999; 52:1124-1127. [Japanese]
16. Bedi HS, Sharma VK, Mishra M, Kasliwal RR, Trehan N. Papillary fibroelastoma of the mitral valve associated with rheumatic mitral stenosis. Eur J Cardiothorac Surg 1995;9:54-55.
17. Kurup AN, Tazelaar HD, Edwards WD, et al. Iatrogenic cardiac papillary fibroelastoma: a study of 12 cases (1990 to 2000). Hum Pathol 2002; 33:1165-1169.
18. Kumar TK, Kuehl K, Reyes C, Talwar S, Moulick A, Jonas RA. Multiple papillary fibroelastomas of the heart. Ann Thorac Surg 2009;88:e66-67.
19. Kim RW, Jeffery ME, Smith MJ, Wilensky RL, Woo EY, Woo YJ. Minimally invasive resection of papillary fibroelastoma in a high-risk patient. J Cardiovasc Med (Hagerstown) 2007;8:639-641.
20. Zamora RL, Adelberg DA, Berger AS, Huettner P, Kaplan HJ. Branch retinal artery occlusion caused by a mitral valve papillary fibroelastoma—correction. Am J Ophthalmol 1995;120:126.
21. Sydow K, Schrepfer S, Franzen O, et al. Coincidence of aortic valve stenosis and regurgitation and multiple cardiac papillary fibroelastomas in a young male adult. J Thorac Cardiovasc Surg 2007;133:564-565.
22. Amr SS, Abu al Ragheb SY. Sudden unexpected death due to papillary fibroma of the aortic valve. Report of a case and review of the literature. Am J Forensic Med Pathol 1991;12:143-148.
23. Kondoh H, Yamada T, Yoshida A, Arima R, Hatsuoka S, Shintani H. Rapid development of a papillary fibroelastoma in the aortic valve: report of a case. Surg Today 2009;39:713-716.
24. Biocic S, Puksic S, Vincelj J, Durasevic Z, Sutlic Z, Manojlovic S. Pulmonary valve papillary fibroelastoma diagnosed by echocardiography: a case report. Eur J Echocardiogr 2009;10:726-728.
25. Gopaldas RR, Atluri PV, Blaustein AS, Bakaeen FG, Huh J, Chu D. Papillary fibroelastoma of the aortic valve: operative approaches upon incidental discovery. Tex Heart Inst J 2009;36:160-163
26. Tazelaar HD, Locke TJ, McGregor CG. Pathology of surgically excised primary cardiac tumors. Mayo Clin Proc 1992;67:957-965.
27. Bossert T, Gummert JF, Battellini R, et al. Surgical experience with 77 primary cardiac tumors. Interact Cardiovasc Thorac Surg 2005;4:311-315.
28. Edwards FH, Hale D, Cohen A, Thompson L, Pezzella AT, Virmani R. Primary cardiac valve tumors. Ann Thorac Surg 1991;52:1127-1131.

29. Fishbein MC, Ferrans VJ, Roberts WC. Endocardial papillary elastofibromas. Histologic, histochemical, and electron microscopical findings. Arch Pathol 1975;99:335-341.

30. Heath D, Best PV, Davis BT. Papilliferous tumours of the heart valves. Br Heart J 1961;23:20-24.

31. Anastacio MM, Moon MR, Damiano RJ Jr, Pasque MK, Maniar HS, Lawton JS. Surgical experience with cardiac papillary fibroelastoma over a 15-year period. Ann Thorac Surg 2012;94:537-541.

32. Raju V, Srinivasan M, Padmanaban C, Soundararajan S, Kuppanna PJ. Left main coronary artery embolus: unusual presentation of papillary fibroelastoma of the aortic valve. Tex Heart Inst J 2010;37:365-367.

33. Dehnee AE, Brizendine S, Herrera CJ. Recurrent strokes in a young patient with papillary fibroelastoma: a case report and literature review. Echocardiography 2006;23:592-595.

34. Di Marco L, Al-Basheer A, Glineur D, Oppido G, Di Bartolomeo R, El-Khoury G. Aortic valve repair for papillary fibroelastoma. J Cardiovasc Med (Hagerstown) 2006;7:362-364.

35. Mohammadi S, Martineau A, Voisine P, Dagenais F. Left atrial papillary fibroelastoma: a rare cause of multiple cerebral emboli. Ann Thorac Surg 2007;84:1396-1397.

36. Yoda M, Tanabe H, Kanou H, Sawada H, Suma H. Multiple papillary fibroelastomas in rare locations of aortic valve and left ventricular outflow tract: a case report. J Heart Valve Dis 2009;18:575-577.

37. Bruno VD, Mariscalco G, De Vita S, Piffaretti G, Nassiacos D, Sala A. Aortic valve papillary fibroelastoma: a rare cause of angina. Tex Heart Inst J 2011;38:456-457.

38. Vivacqua A, Shafii A, Kalahasti V, Tan C, Gonzalez-Stawinski G. Images in cardiology. Ventricular outflow tract papillary fibroelastoma presenting with non-ST-segment elevation myocardial infarction. J Am Coll Cardiol 2010;55:2607.

39. Bottio T, Pittarello D, Bonato R, et al. Echocardiographic diagnosis of aortic valve papillary fibroelastoma. Tex Heart Inst J 2004;31:322-323.

40. Boulmier D, Ecke JE, Verhoye JP. Recurrent myocardial infarction due to obstruction of the RCA ostium by an aortic papillary fibroelastoma. J Invasive Cardiol 2002;14:686-688.

41. Kalman JM, Lubicz S, Brennan JB, Vernon-Roberts E, Calafiore P. Multiple cardiac papillary fibroelastomas and rheumatic heart disease. Aust N Z J Med 1991;21:744-746

42. Valente M, Basso C, Thiene G, et al. Fibroelastic papilloma: a not-so-benign cardiac tumor. Cardiovasc Pathol 1992;1:161-166.

43. Edwards WD. Pulmonary embolization of papillary fibroelastoma arising from the tricuspid valve. Tex Heart Inst J 1991;18:226-227.

44. Gabbieri D, Rossi G, Bavutti L, et al. Papillary fibroelastoma of the right atrium as an unusual source of recurrent pulmonary embolism. J Cardiovasc Med (Hagerstown) 2006;7:373-378.

45. Butterworth JS, Poindexter CA. Papilloma of cusp of the aortic valve. Report of a patient with sudden death. Circulation 1973;48:213-215.

46. Harris LS, Adelson L. Fatal coronary embolism from a myxomatous polyp of the aortic valve; an unusual cause of sudden death. Am J Clin Pathol 1965;43:61-64.

47. Richard J, Castello R, Dressler FA, et al. Diagnosis of papillary fibroelastoma of the mitral valve complicated by non-Q-wave infarction with apical thrombus: transesophageal and transthoracic echocardiographic study. Am Heart J 1993;126:710-712.

48. Rona G, Feeney N, Kahn DS. Fibroelastic hamartoma of the aortic valve producing ischemic heart disease. Associated pulmonary glomus bodies. Am J Cardiol 1963;12:869-874.

49. Puff M, Taff ML, Spitz WU, Eckert WG. Syncope and sudden death caused by mitral valve myxomas. Am J Forensic Med Pathol 1986;7:84-86.

50. Flotte T, Pinar H, Feiner H. Papillary elastofibroma of the left ventricular septum. Am J Surg Pathol 1980;4:585-588.

51. Matsumoto N, Sato Y, Kusama J, et al. Multiple papillary fibroelastomas of the aortic valve: case report. Int J Cardiol 2007;122:e1-3.

52. Shub C, Tajik AJ, Seward JB, et al. Cardiac papillary fibroelastomas. Two-dimensional echocardiographic recognition. Mayo Clin Proc 1981;56:629-633.

53. Frumin H, O'Donnell L, Kerin NZ, Levine F, Nathan LE Jr, Klein SP. Two-dimensional echocardiographic detection and diagnostic features of tricuspid papillary fibroelastoma. J Am Coll Cardiol 1983;2:1016-1018.

54. Fowles RE, Miller DC, Egbert BM, Fitzgerald JW, Popp RL. Systemic embolization from a mitral valve papillary endocardial fibroma detected by two-dimensional echocardiography. Am Heart J 1981;102:128-130.

55. Mann J, Parker DJ. Papillary fibroelastoma of the mitral valve: a rare cause of transient neurological deficits. Br Heart J 1994;71:6.

56. McFadden PM, Lacy JR. Intracardiac papillary fibroelastoma: an occult cause of embolic neurologic deficit. Ann Thorac Surg 1987;43:667-669.

57. Narang J, Neustein S, Israel D. The role of transesophageal echocardiography in the diagnosis and excision of a tumor of the aortic valve. J Cardiothorac Vasc Anesth 1992;6:68-69.

58. Marvasti MA, Obeid AI, Cohen PS, Giambartolomei A, Parker FB. Successful removal of papillary endocardial fibroma. Thorac Cardiovasc Surg 1983;31:254-255.

59. Le Tourneau T, Pouwels S, Gal B, et al. Assessment of papillary fibroelastomas with live three-dimensional transthoracic echocardiography. Echocardiography 2008;25:489-495.

60. Eslami-Varzaneh F, Brun EA, Sears-Rogan P. An unusual case of multiple papillary fibroelastoma, review of literature. Cardiovasc Pathol 2003;12:170-173.

61. Irie Y, Sato Y, Shioguchi S, et al. Multiple papillary fibroelastoma of the left ventricle. Asian Cardiovasc Thorac Ann 2004;12:184-185.

62. Gudgeon PG, Chow CM, Abramson B. Mitral and tricuspid valve papillary fibroelastomas: a rare cause of multiple intracardiac masses. Can J Cardiol 2009;25:e428.

63. Vora TR. Unusual presentation of papillary fibroelastoma: utility of serial transesophageal echocardiograms. Echocardiography 2004;21:69-71.

64. Uchida S, Obayashi N, Yamanari H, Matsubara K, Saito D, Haraoka S. Papillary fibroelastoma in the left ventricular outflow tract. Heart Vessels 1992;7:164-167.

65. Massarenti L, Benassi F, Gallerano A, Stefanelli G. Papillary fibroelastoma of the tricuspid anterior leaflet. J Cardiovasc Med (Hagerstown) 2009;10:933-935.

66. Boone S, Higginson LA, Walley VM. Endothelial papillary fibroelastomas arising in and around the aortic sinus, filling the ostium of the right coronary artery. Arch Pathol Lab Med 1992;116:135-137.

67. Saxena P, Shehatha J, Naran A, Rajaratnam S, Newman MA, Konstantinov IE. Papillary fibroelastoma of the interventricular septum: mimicking a cardiac myxoma. Tex Heart Inst J 2010;37:119-120.

68. Gallas MT, Reardon MJ, Reardon PR, DeFelice CA, Raizner AE, Mody DR. Papillary fibroelastoma. A right atrial presentation. Tex Heart Inst J 1993;20:293-295.

69. Schiller AL, Schantz A. Papillary endocardial excrescence of the right atrium: report of two cases. Am J Clin Pathol 1970;53:617-621.

70. Frolich ML, Davidsen ES, Lonnebakken MT, Gerdts E. An unusual location of a papillary fibroelastoma. Eur J Echocardiogr 2010;11:E10.

71. Chang YS, Chu PH, Jung SM, et al. Unusual cardiac papillary fibroelastoma in the right ventricular outflow tract. Cardiovasc Pathol 2005;14:104-106.

72. Totsugawa T, Kuinose M, Yoshitaka H, Tsushima Y, Ishida A, Minami H. Papillary fibroelastoma of the tricuspid valve chordae. Jpn J Thorac Cardiovasc Surg 2006;54:547-549.

73. Sa MI, Reis H, Lagarto V, et al. Papillary fibroelastoma located deep in the left ventricle: case

74. Burke AP, Virmani R. Tumors of the heart and great vessels. AFIP Atlas of Tumor Pathology, 3rd Series, Fascicle 16. Washington DC: American Registry of Pathology; 1996.

75. Rubin MA, Snell JA, Tazelaar HD, Lack EE, Austenfeld JL, Azumi N. Cardiac papillary fibroelastoma: an immunohistochemical investigation and unusual clinical manifestations. Mod Pathol 1995;8:402-407.

76. Burke A, Li L, Kling E, Kutys R, Virmani R, Miettinen M. Cardiac inflammatory myofibroblastic tumor: a "benign" neoplasm that may result in syncope, myocardial infarction, and sudden death. Am J Surg Pathol 2007;31:1115-1122.

77. Kim HY, Kwon SU, Jang WI, et al. A rare case of aortic valve myxoma: easy to confuse with papillary fibroelastoma. Korean Circ J 2012;42:281-283.

78. Topol EJ, Biern RO, Reitz BA. Cardiac papillary fibroelastoma and stroke. Echocardiographic diagnosis and guide to excision. Am J Med 1986;80:129-132.

79. Chavanon O, Hlal M, Bakkali A, et al. Multiple microthrombi on a papillary fibroelastoma of the aortic valve. Ann Thorac Surg 2012;93:304-306.

80. Georghiou GP, Shapira Y, Stamler A, et al. Surgical excision of papillary fibroelastoma for known or potential embolization. J Heart Valve Dis 2005;14:843-847.

81. Saloura V, Grivas PD, Sarwar AB, Gorodin P, Ledley GS. Papillary fibroelastomas: innocent bystanders or ignored culprits? Postgrad Med 2009;121:131-138.

82. Boodhwani M, Veinot JP, Hendry PJ. Surgical approach to cardiac papillary fibroelastomas. Can J Cardiol 2007;23:301-302.

83. Sumino S, Paterson HS. No regrowth after incomplete papillary fibroelastoma excision. Ann Thorac Surg 2005;79:e3-4.

84. Woo YJ, Grand TJ, Weiss SJ. Robotic resection of an aortic valve papillary fibroelastoma. Ann Thorac Surg 2005;80:1100-1102.

85. Elbardissi AW, Dearani JA, Daly RC, et al. Survival after resection of primary cardiac tumors: a 48-year experience. Circulation 2008;118:S7-15.

86. Bakaeen FG, Reardon MJ, Coselli JS, et al. Surgical outcome in 85 patients with primary cardiac tumors. Am J Surg 2003;186:641-647; discussion 647.

87. Strecker T, Rosch J, Weyand M, Agaimy A. Primary and metastatic cardiac tumors: imaging characteristics, surgical treatment, and histopathological spectrum: a 10-year-experience at a German heart center. Cardiovasc Pathol 2012;21:436-443.

study and literature review. Rev Port Cardiol 2006;25:605-609.

# 7 CARDIAC FIBROMA

## DEFINITION

*Cardiac fibroma* is a benign congenital tumor present within cardiac muscle, and composed of bland fibroblasts in a variably collagenized stroma.

## GENERAL FEATURES

Cardiac fibroma is not considered a true neoplasm, and has been reported with different names such as *fibromatosis* (1), *fibrous hamartoma* (2), and *fibroelastic hamartoma* (3). Because many fibromas occur in infants, and histologic changes are somewhat age-dependent, cardiac fibromas are most likely congenital lesions. Unlike rhabdomyoma, which is typically considered to be a hamartoma derived from cardiac myocytes, the term hamartoma is not consistently applied to fibromas. The term "hamartoma" has recently fallen out of favor as being nonspecific. We discourage the use of the term fibromatosis, as this suggests an aggressive, nonlocalized lesion, with distinct immunohistochemical and genetic profiles (4,5).

Cardiac involvement may rarely occur in congenital generalized fibromatosis (6), in which case the term is more appropriate. Because most fibromas of the heart do not appear to recur or grow aggressively, fibromas are most likely not neoplasms, although exceptional cases with recurrence have been reported (1).

## CLINICAL FEATURES

Cardiac fibromas are rare tumors: a recent review found fewer than 200 published cases (7). Most reports are single cases, small series, or a few examples in series of surgically resected heart tumors (1,3,8–12). Since 1995, fewer than 50 cases have been reported (4,5,13–17). In Elbardissi's series of resected heart tumors (18), there were 18 cases (6 percent of the total); the largest series consists of 23 cases from the 1990s (19).

Although rare, after rhabdomyoma, cardiac fibroma is the most common tumor of childhood encountered at autopsy (20–22). It is the most common surgically resected cardiac tumor in children in older series (3), and the second, after rhabdomyoma, in more recent reports (23–27). In several surgical series of patients of all ages, fibromas represent the second most common benign primary cardiac tumor after myxoma (28–31).

Eighty-six percent of cardiac fibromas occur in children, one third of whom are under 1 year of age (3,19). A series of heart tumors, mostly in adults, revealed a mean age of 22.5 years at diagnosis (18). Fewer than 10 percent of cases are diagnosed antenatally or in the neonatal period. In series of antenatally diagnosed tumors, fibromas account for few or none of the cases, and are single, unlike rhabdomyomas, which are multiple and encompass the vast majority (26,32). At the other extreme, there are reports of patients in the eighth and ninth decades of life with cardiac fibroma (7,33).

An early age at diagnosis has a direct correlation with overall survival, with an inherent bias of more severe cases being diagnosed earlier and not incidentally. In a recent review, there was a significant positive correlation between patient age and tumor diameter for patients younger than 17 years (7). In a series of 23 predominantly pediatric patients, the mean age at presentation was 13 years (19). There is a slight male predominance (7,19).

Approximately one third of patients present with heart failure or cyanosis, one third with arrhythmias or syncope, and one third are asymptomatic, with tumors discovered as incidental findings or as abnormalities on electrocardiogram (EKG) (34–38). In a series of 18 patients, 33 percent had palpitations, 33 percent ventricular tachycardia, 28 percent dyspnea, 28 percent syncope, 22 percent chest pain, 11 percent embolic symptoms, 6 percent constitutional symptoms, and in 17 percent, the tumor was an incidental finding (18). Incidental lesions are often identified by auscultation of murmurs at physical examination (39), by EKG abnormalities (38), by calcification or mild cardiomegaly on routine chest radiographs (40,41), or during evaluation for nevoid basal cell carcinoma syndrome (also known as Gorlin syndrome or basal cell nevus syndrome). Symptoms of heart failure may manifest as nonspecific failure to thrive (42). Sudden death may also be the initial presentation (19,43). Rarely, cardiac fibromas result in left ventricular outflow obstruction (44), pulmonary outflow obstruction (29), unexplained pericardial effusion (19), unexplained arrhythmias (45), and coronary insufficiency (28). Because of its propensity for the ventricular septum, fibromas may mimic hypertrophic cardiomyopathy (28,46). There is a correlation between the site in the ventricular septum and poor prognosis, presumably related to involvement of the conduction system (7).

There is little correlation between the type of presenting symptom and the location of the tumor in the heart. Arrhythmias can occur in patients with tumors in any location in the heart, including the right ventricle, left ventricle, and ventricular septum. Patients with heart failure generally have large, bulky tumors in either ventricle that are difficult to treat surgically (47–49).

Cardiac fibroma must be considered in the differential diagnosis of a child with unexplained congestive heart failure, arrhythmia, cardiomegaly, murmur, or pericardial effusion. Although rhabdomyomas are more common in the newborn period, they are usually multiple; fibromas are nearly always single lesions, with rare exceptions (50). The identification of tumoral calcification on imaging is a strong clue to the diagnosis, as rhabdomyomas rarely calcify (19,49,51,52). Calcification is not necessarily a sensitive diagnostic marker, since it occurs in less than a third of cases on chest radiography, but it can be more readily detected by magnetic resonance imaging (MRI) and computed tomography (CT) (19). Other calcified cardiac masses include myxoma and, very rarely, lipoma (28).

There is an increased risk of cardiac fibroma in patients with the nevoid basal cell carcinoma syndrome (19,53–56). The nevoid basal cell carcinoma syndrome is inherited in an autosomal dominant fashion and is characterized by enlarged occipital circumference, odontogenic keratocysts of the jaws, epidermal cysts, rib anomalies, multiple basal cell carcinomas of the skin, and several other manifestations (53,54). A mutation of the tumor suppressor gene *PTCH1* is the underlying cause of this syndrome (57). Cardiac fibromas are noted in less than 14 percent of patients with the syndrome but the association is not considered random (53,54,56). A suppressor role for the gene *PTCH1* has also been found in nonsyndromic cardiac fibromas (57). A patient with cardiac fibroma and multiple neural midline defects has also been described (58).

Cardiac fibroma is readily diagnosed by echocardiography (fig. 7-1), which is often performed for evaluation of arrhythmias or routine antenatal screening (38,46,59–61). Occasionally, the echocardiographic results are negative, in which case MRI is the more sensitive imaging modality (fig. 7-2) (46).

## GROSS FINDINGS

Based on two series, cardiac fibromas most commonly arise in the ventricular septum and then (in decreasing order of frequency) the free walls of the left and right ventricles, the right atrium, and the left atrium (19,39). In contrast, a recent review of all reported cases found the left ventricle to be the most common site, followed by the right ventricle and ventricular septum (Table 7-1) (7). A series of 18 cases showed that the left ventricle was involved in 15 and the right ventricle in the remaining 3 cases (18). In fewer than 10 percent of cases, fibromas involve more than one site of the myocardium. Atrial fibroma is rare (1,7,9). In some cases, fibromas are massive tumors that obliterate the ventricular cavities. Tumors arising at the ventricular septum are associated with a worse overall survival rate when compared to all other sites (7). Large tumors tend to be detected early in life.

Cardiac fibromas are rounded masses that, upon sectioning, are fibrous and white, with a whorled pattern, resembling leiomyomas from other sites (figs. 7-3–7-14). They are nearly always mural lesions, although a single polypoid fibroma resulting in subaortic stenosis in an

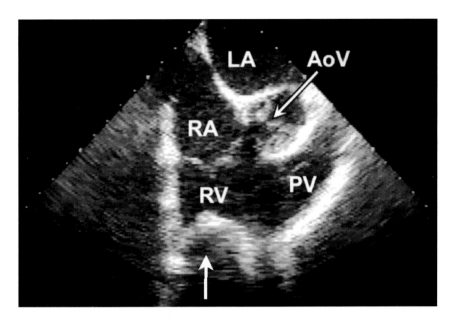

**Figure 7-1**

**CARDIAC FIBROMA**

The echocardiogram shows a mass in the right ventricle (lower arrow). (RA = right atrium; LA = left atrium; AoV = aortic valve [upper arrow]; PV = pulmonary valve.)

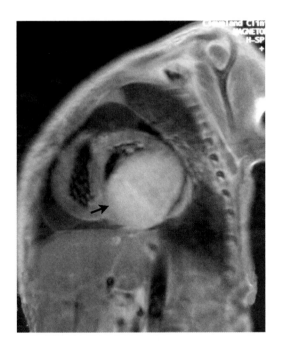

**Figure 7-2**

**CARDIAC FIBROMA**

Magnetic resonance imaging (MRI) shows the tumor in the inferior left ventricular wall. The arrow marks the junction with the interventricular septum.

**Table 7-1**

**CHARACTERISTICS OF CARDIAC FIBROMAS[a]**

| | |
|---|---|
| **Male:Female** | 26 patients:18 patients |
| **Age** (range) | 10.5 (0–51 years) |
| **Size** (range) | 5.5 cm (1–11 cm) |
| **Symptoms** | |
| Ventricular tachycardia | 26% |
| Dyspnea | 21% |
| Syncope | 19% |
| Neonatal cyanosis/heart failure | 18% |
| Chest pain | 16% |
| Palpitations | 15% |
| Cardiac arrest | 5% |
| Incidental finding | 3% |
| **Site** | |
| Left ventricle | 55% |
| Right ventricle | 21% |
| Interventricular septum | 18% |
| Atria | 6% |
| **Procedure** | |
| Complete resection | 72% |
| Transplant | 15% |
| Incomplete resection | 9% |
| Biopsy only | 4% |
| **Multiple Fibromas** | 4% |

[a]From references 18, 19, 26, 27, and 78.

infant has been described (44). It is unusual for these masses to result in outflow tract obstruction. Every reported case but one (34) has been single. In one series from a consultation service, the mean diameter was 5 cm (19), but tumors as large as 14 cm have been reported (7). Grossly, cardiac fibromas typically appear as well-circumscribed lesions.

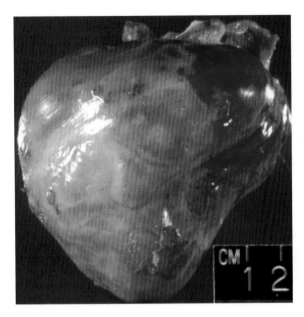

**Figure 7-3**

**CARDIAC FIBROMA**

The tumor bulges from the lateral wall of the left ventricle and has vaguely discernable bosselations.

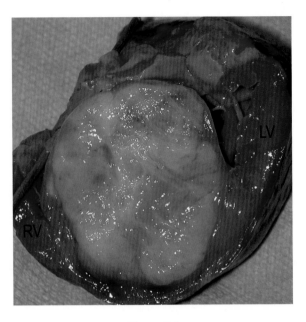

**Figure 7-4**

**CARDIAC FIBROMA**

The tumor replaces the ventricular septum. (LV = left ventricle; RV = right ventricle.)

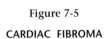

**Figure 7-5**

**CARDIAC FIBROMA**

The tumor is replacing the ventricular septum. (LV = left ventricle; Ao = aorta; LA = left atrium.)

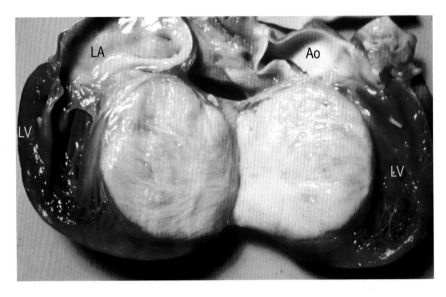

## MICROSCOPIC FINDINGS

Cardiac fibroma is a homogeneous proliferation of monomorphic fibroblasts that demonstrate little (if any) atypia (figs. 7-15–7-22). The degree of cellularity often decreases with the age of the patient, whereas the amount of collagen increases (19). This results in very collagenous cardiac fibromas in adults and older children. There may be a focally myxoid background (fig. 7-23). Mitoses are generally present only in tumors of patients less than a few months of age. Occasional perivascular aggregates of lymphocytes and histiocytes or sparse chronic inflammation is seen at the junction of the tumor and uninvolved myocardium.

Calcification is a common finding in fibromas from patients of all ages, and accounts for the calcification that is occasionally seen on

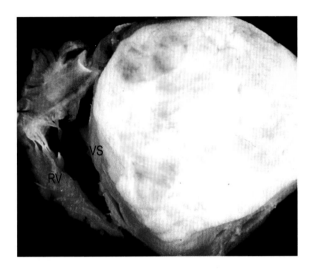

**Figure 7-6**

**CARDIAC FIBROMA**

The tumor replaces the ventricular septum. (VS = ventricular septum; RV = right ventricle.)

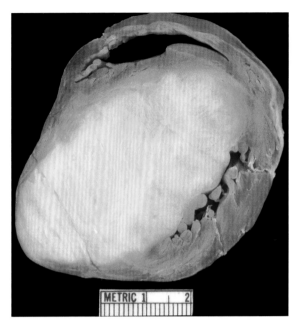

**Figure 7-7**

**CARDIAC FIBROMA**

The tumor replaces the ventricular septum.

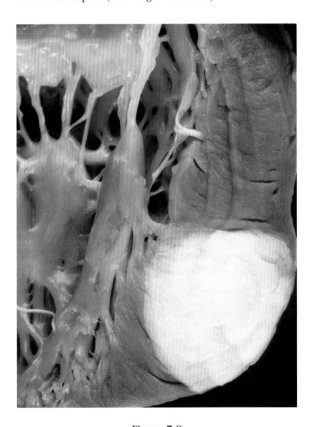

**Figure 7-8**

**CARDIAC FIBROMA**

The grossly well-circumscribed tumor is in the left ventricular free wall. The anterolateral papillary muscle is adjacent, and the posterior leaflet of the mitral valve above.

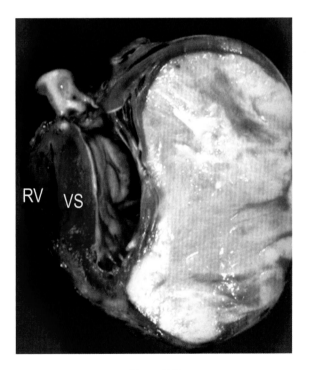

**Figure 7-9**

**CARDIAC FIBROMA**

There is a tumor larger than the heart itself, replacing the left ventricular free wall. (RV = right ventricle; VS = ventricular septum.)

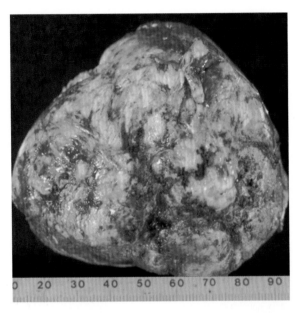
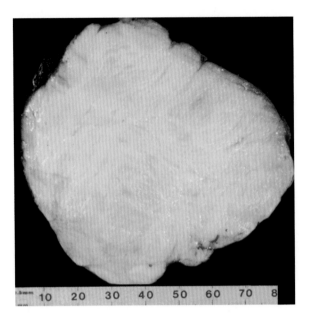

**Figure 7-10**

**CARDIAC FIBROMA**

Left: The surgical surface is irregular and somewhat variegated in this example.
Right: The cut surface of the tumor illustrated on the left shows a typical white whorled appearance.

**Figure 7-11**

**CARDIAC FIBROMA**

The cut surface resembles that of a leiomyoma or fibrous tumor of any site.

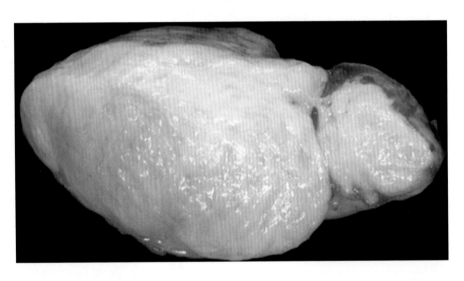

chest radiograph, MRI, or CT scan (fig. 7-24) (35,52,62). Variable numbers of elastic fibers may be present; this finding is independent of age (19). The presence of elastic fibers accounts for the occasional use of the term elastofibroma or fibroelastic hamartoma (3).

Despite the well-circumscribed gross appearance of these tumors, histologically they often exhibit intricate interdigitation with the adjacent myocardium. This phenomenon, which often results in positive margins, does not appear to affect the recurrence rate.

## IMMUNOHISTOCHEMICAL FINDINGS

There are few published reports on the immunohistochemical findings of cardiac fibromas. The tumor cells show myofibroblastic differentiation and are positive for vimentin and smooth muscle actin, whereas CD34, S-100 protein, and HMB-45 are negative (21,63–65).

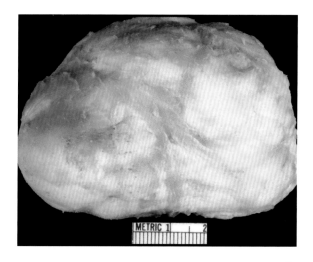
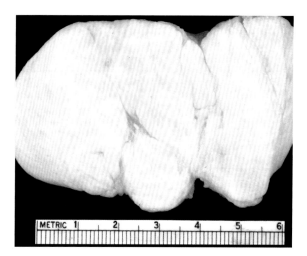

**Figure 7-12**

**CARDIAC FIBROMA**

Left: The surgical surface is irregular, with strands of cardiac muscle (brown).
Right: The cut surface of the tumor illustrated on the left shows a typical white whorled appearance.

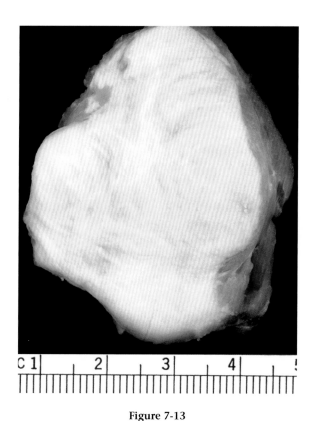

**Figure 7-13**

**CARDIAC FIBROMA**

There are vague strands of fibrous tissue that bulge from the cut surface.

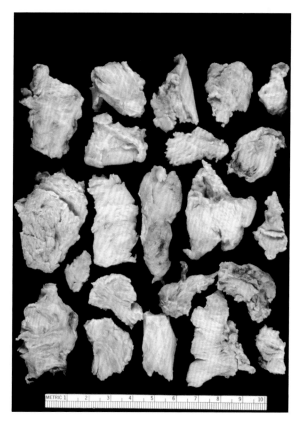

**Figure 7-14**

**CARDIAC FIBROMA**

This tumor was removed in pieces, as a morcellated specimen.

127

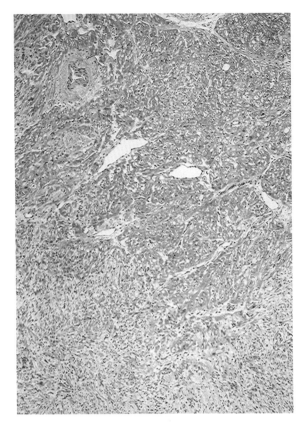

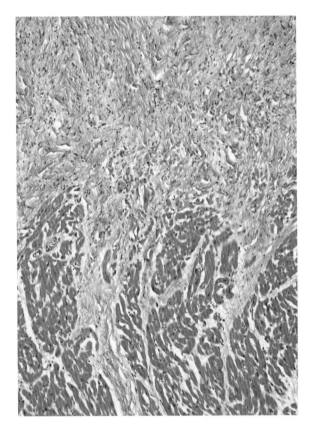

**Figure 7-15**

**CARDIAC FIBROMA**

This tumor infiltrates the junction with normal myocardium. Although grossly well circumscribed, the microscopic margin is indistinct and nonencapsulated. The myocardium is at the top.

**Figure 7-16**

**CARDIAC FIBROMA**

Fibrous strands of tumor insinuate among muscle bundles of the myocardium (bottom).

**Figure 7-17**

**CARDIAC FIBROMA**

This tumor, which is somewhat more cellular than those illustrated in figures 7-15 and 7-16, is seen insinuating among cardiomyocytes of normal myocardium.

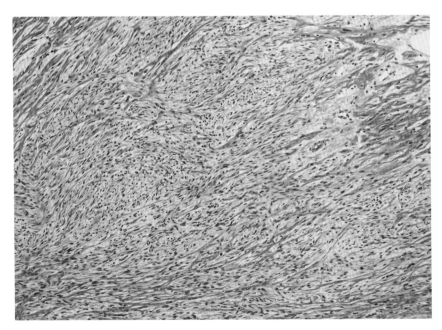

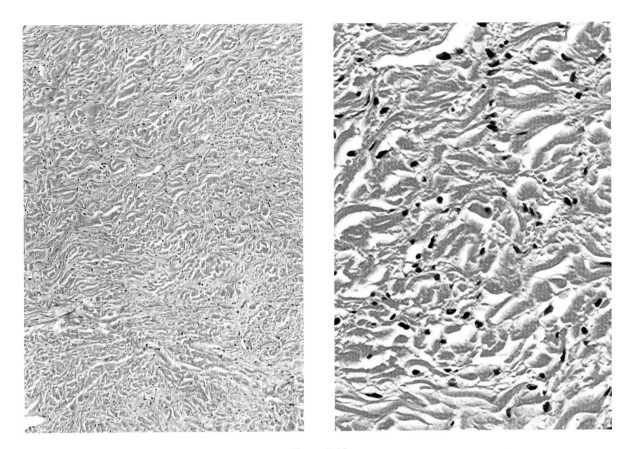

**Figure 7-18**

**CARDIAC FIBROMA: PAUCICELLULAR**

Left: Many fibromas, especially those excised from older individuals, are composed primarily of collagen.
Right: At higher magnification, dense collagen bundles with occasional fibroblast nuclei are seen.

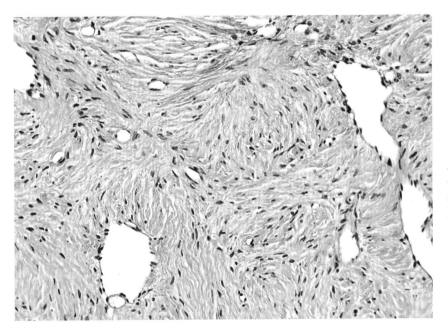

**Figure 7-19**

**CARDIAC FIBROMA:
MODERATELY CELLULAR**

This tumor has a somewhat whorled microscopic appearance, with looser collagen than that seen in figure 7-18. Occasionally, there is a fairly prominent vascular pattern.

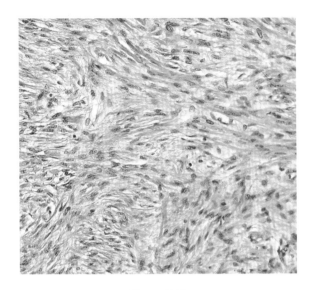

**Figure 7-20**

**CARDIAC FIBROMA: CELLULAR**

This cellular fibroma has little collagen, and fibroblastic tumor cells with plump nuclei. The tumor is acellular compared to cardiac sarcomas, which are rare in children.

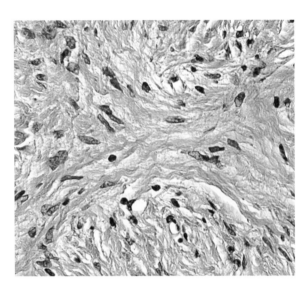

**Figure 7-21**

**CARDIAC FIBROMA: CELLULAR**

A storiform appearance is apparent. The tumor cells are bland, with interspersed, fairly uniform collagen bundles.

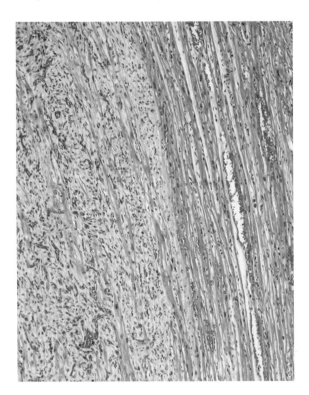

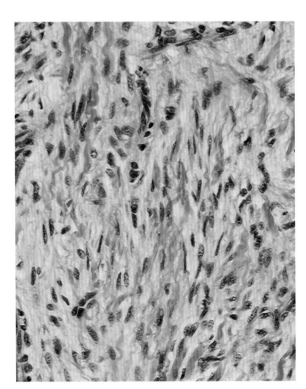

**Figure 7-22**

**CARDIAC FIBROMA: CELLULAR**

Left: The junction with normal myocardium (right) is fairly distinct.

Right: At higher magnification, the cellular tumor is composed of bland, uniform fibroblasts and collagen fibers in a sparsely myxoid matrix.

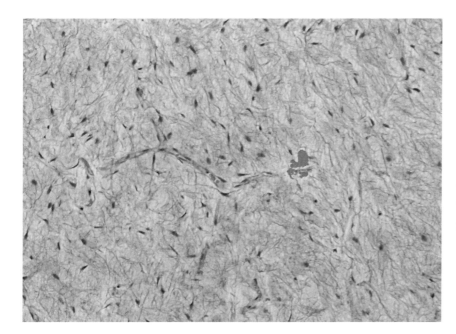

**Figure 7-23**

**CARDIAC FIBROMA: MYXOID**

Some tumors are in part myxoid. In contrast to myxomas (which are rare in children), this tumor is intramyocardial, and other features of myxoma (myxoma cells, hemorrhage, inflammation) are absent.

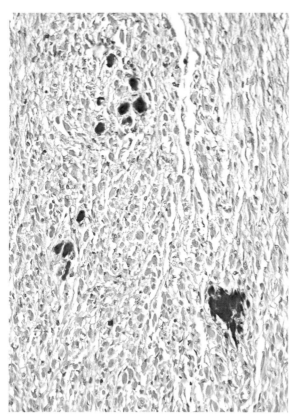

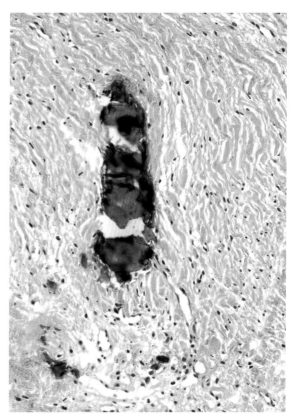

**Figure 7-24**

**CARDIAC FIBROMA: CALCIFICATION**

Left: Calcification is rare in rhabdomyoma, the other common heart tumor in children. When seen on imaging, calcification is highly suggestive of fibroma, especially if the tumor is single.

Right: At higher magnification, interstitial calcification is apparent.

## ULTRASTRUCTURAL FINDINGS

There have been several ultrastructural studies of cardiac fibroma with similar results (1,3,20,66,67). The tumor cells resemble fibroblasts with few cellular organelles, extensive endoplasmic reticulum, incompletely developed or absent basement membrane, ramifications of cytoplasmic processes, and a centrally placed, ovoid nucleus with a distinct nucleolus (1,66). Ultrastructurally, the predominant cell type is the fibroblast, although there may be a myofibroblastic component as well (1,3,66).

## MOLECULAR FINDINGS

The finding of chromosomal abnormalities in a case of cardiac fibroma is of considerable interest (68). Due to the morphologic similarities with fibromatosis of soft tissue, interest has been drawn to the histogenesis of these tumors. A recent genetic and immunohistochemical study tested their association, and did not show nuclear beta-catenin reactivity in cardiac hamartomas, nor did they show any beta-catenin exon 3 mutations, arguing against those lesions being identical processes (5). Scanlan et al. (57) performed conventional cytogenetic analysis and fluorescence in situ hybridization (FISH) studies on the *PTCH1* gene in three cardiac fibromas diagnosed in children and infants (57), since the *PTCH1* gene is the hallmark of the nevoid basal cell carcinoma syndrome (69). The authors found homozygous and heterozygous losses of the *PTCH1* gene, suggesting a tumor suppressor role for *PTCH1* in sporadic cardiac fibromas.

## DIFFERENTIAL DIAGNOSIS

The histologic diagnosis of cardiac fibroma is usually straightforward, and rests on finding a discrete mass within muscle, composed of partly or completely collagenized stroma with intervening fibroblasts. Occasionally, if the tumor is unresectable, the pathologist sees a wedge or needle biopsy specimen. The differential diagnosis then includes fibrosarcoma, which generally does not occur in the heart during the first few years of life. Histologically, the distinction between cellular fibromas of infants and fibrosarcoma is difficult, and is made on the basis of sparse mitotic activity in the fibroma. It is possible that rare examples of recurrent fibroma in infancy may in fact represent a low-grade fibrosarcoma (1). Fibromas in patients 6 months of age and older are fairly acellular, do not possess mitotic figures, and are, therefore, not histologically similar to fibrosarcoma.

Inflammatory myofibroblastic tumors (IMTs) have a much more prominent inflammatory infiltrate, and the tumor cells are stellate, rather than spindled, with the appearance of myofibroblasts. About two thirds of IMTs are positive for the ALK protein immunohistochemically, while there are no reports of ALK staining in cardiac fibromas to date. IMTs are more commonly endocardial based and often involve the cardiac valves, whereas fibromas are intramyocardial in location. Furthermore, IMTs tend to be multiple, unlike fibromas (65).

Also in the differential diagnosis is fibrous histiocytoma, an extremely rare cellular cardiac tumor that is composed of spindle cells and lipid-laden macrophages. In older patients, the tumor can histologically simulate a scar, but grossly, there is always a mass that results in thickening or bulging of the involved muscle, a feature of cardiac fibroma not encountered in healed infarcts of cardiac fibroma.

## TREATMENT

Cardiac fibromas have been successfully removed from infants as young as 1 month of age (28); however, some attempts at resection in infants younger than 4 months have resulted in operative deaths (19,37,39). There is evidence that tumors remain dormant for as long as 31 years (70), and spontaneous regression has been reported (71). For this reason, some patients are followed without surgery, especially if they are elderly (35). Some authors believe cardiac fibromas tend to grow in childhood along with the growth of the heart, and stop at puberty (7); others argue in favor of surgery in younger individuals.

The propensity for cardiac fibroma to cause arrhythmias is becoming increasingly evident (72). Surgery has been shown to ablate these, sometimes lethal, ventricular arrhythmias (18, 35,37). Successful resection with recurrence-free, long-term follow-up has been documented in over 40 patients (70,71,73–75). Even large tumors have been successfully resected without complications (76). Complete excision is not always possible, however, due to the encasement of critical structures (such as a coronary artery) (28). Despite incomplete excision with residual tumor that may be noted on echocardiography or chest radiography, patients usually remain asymptomatic (30,35,73). For adequate surgical removal, patch repair of the ventricular septum or free wall, valve replacement, or coronary artery grafting may be necessary (19).

In patients with large, unresectable tumors, refractory arrhythmias have been treated successfully with cardiac transplantation (1,74,77). An internal cardioverter-defibrillator was used as a bridge to transplantation in a teenager with significant ventricular arrhythmias (78). Another successful bridge-to-heart transplantation has been reported using a systemic-to-pulmonary shunt in a newborn who had significant right ventricular outflow tract obstruction (59).

## PROGNOSIS

In a long-term follow-up study, the median survival period for patients with cardiac fibroma after surgery was 27 years, which was equal or better than all other heart tumors studied (18). By multivariate analysis, however, the prognosis was poorer than that of myxoma and the control population because of the relatively young age at diagnosis (18). The prognosis is guarded for unresectable tumors treated by transplantation (26,79). Long-term complications of resection include mitral insufficiency that may necessitate valve replacement (80).

## REFERENCES

1. Turi GK, Albala A, Fenoglio JJ Jr. Cardiac fibromatosis: an ultrastructural study. Hum Pathol 1980;11:577-580.
2. Parks FR Jr, Adams F, Longmire WP Jr. Successful excision of a left ventricular hamartoma. Report of a case. Circulation 1962;26:1316-1320.
3. Feldman PS, Meyer MW. Fibroelastic hamartoma (fibroma) of the heart. Cancer 1976;38:314-323.
4. Miller DV, Edwards WD. Cardiovascular tumor-like conditions. Semin Diagn Pathol 2008;25:54-64.
5. Miller DV, Wang H, Fealey ME, Tazelaar HD. Beta-catenin mutations do not contribute to cardiac fibroma pathogenesis. Pediatr Dev Pathol 2008;11:291-294.
6. Shnitka TK, Asp DM, Horner RH. Congenital generalized fibromatosis. Cancer 1958;11:627-639.
7. Torimitsu S, Nemoto T, Wakayama M, et al. Literature survey on epidemiology and pathology of cardiac fibroma. Eur J Med Res 2012;17:5.
8. Nadas AS, Ellison RC. Cardiac tumors in infancy. Am J Cardiol 1968;21:363-366.
9. Iwa T, Kamata E, Misaki T, Ishida K, Okada R. Successful surgical ablation of reentrant ventricular tachycardia caused by myocardial fibroma. J Thorac Cardiovasc Surg 1984;87:469-473.
10. Kanemoto N, Usui K, Fusegawa Y. An adult case of cardiac fibroma. Intern Med 1994;33:10-12
11. Ackerman J, McKeown P, Gunasekaran S, Spicer D. Pathological case of the month. Cardiac fibroma. Arch Pediatr Adolesc Med 1995;149:199-200.
12. Busch U, Kampmann C, Meyer R, Sandring KH, Hausdorf G, Konertz W. Removal of a giant cardiac fibroma from a 4-year-old child. Tex Heart Inst J 1995;22:261-264.
13. Kobayashi D, L'Ecuyer TJ, Aggarwal S. Orthotopic heart transplant: a therapeutic option for unresectable cardiac fibroma in infants. Congenit Heart Dis 2012;7:E31-36.
14. Albaghdadi MS, Popescu A, Davidson CJ, McCarthy PM, Kansal P. Adult cardiac fibroma. J Am Coll Cardiol 2012;59:e15.
15. Teis A, Sheppard MN, Alpendurada F. Unusual location for a large cardiac fibroma. Circulation 2011;124:1481-1482.
16. Randhawa K, Ganeshan A, Hoey ET. Magnetic resonance imaging of cardiac tumors: part 1, sequences, protocols, and benign tumors. Curr Probl Diagn Radiol 2011;40:158-168.
17. Kumar N, Agarwal S, Ahuja A, Das P, Airon B, Ray R. Spectrum of cardiac tumors excluding myxoma: experience of a tertiary center with review of the literature. Pathol Res Pract 2011;207:769-774.
18. Elbardissi AW, Dearani JA, Daly RC, et al. Survival after resection of primary cardiac tumors: a 48-year experience. Circulation 2008;118:S7-15.
19. Burke AP, Rosado-de-Christenson M, Templeton PA, Virmani R. Cardiac fibroma: clinicopathologic correlates and surgical treatment. J Thorac Cardiovasc Surg 1994;108:862-870.
20. Marin-Garcia J, Fitch CW, Shenefelt RE. Primary right ventricular tumor (fibroma) simulating cyanotic heart disease in a newborn. J Am Coll Cardiol 1984;3:868-871.
21. Aliperta A, De Rosa N, Aliperta M, Palumbo A. [Double cardiac fibroma in a newborn infant.] Minerva Cardioangiol 1996;44:623-629. [Italian]

22. Mohammed W, Murphy A. Cardiac fibroma presenting as sudden death in a six-month-old infant. West Indian Med J 1997;46:28-29.

23. Kamiya H, Yasuda T, Nagamine H, et al. Surgical treatment of primary cardiac tumors: 28 years' experience in Kanazawa University Hospital. Jpn Circ J 2001;65:315-319.

24. Kosuga T, Fukunaga S, Kawara T, et al. Surgery for primary cardiac tumors. Clinical experience and surgical results in 60 patients. J Cardiovasc Surg (Torino) 2002;43:581-587.

25. Odim J, Reehal V, Laks H, Mehta U, Fishbein MC. Surgical pathology of cardiac tumors. Two decades at an urban institution. Cardiovasc Pathol 2003;12:267-270.

26. Padalino MA, Basso C, Milanesi O, et al. Surgically treated primary cardiac tumors in early infancy and childhood. J Thorac Cardiovasc Surg 2005;129:1358-1363.

27. Stiller B, Hetzer R, Meyer R, et al. Primary cardiac tumours: when is surgery necessary? Eur J Cardiothorac Surg 2001;20:1002-1006.

28. Reece IJ, Houston AB, Pollock JC. Interventricular fibroma. Echocardiographic diagnosis and successful surgical removal in infancy. Br Heart J 1983;50:590-591.

29. Murphy MC, Sweeney MS, Putnam JB Jr, et al. Surgical treatment of cardiac tumors: a 25-year experience. Ann Thorac Surg 1990;49:612-617; discussion 617-618.

30. Blondeau P. Primary cardiac tumors—French studies of 533 cases. Thorac Cardiovasc Surg 1990;38(Suppl 2):192-195.

31. Tazelaar HD, Locke TJ, McGregor CG. Pathology of surgically excised primary cardiac tumors. Mayo Clin Proc 1992;67:957-965.

32. Niewiadomska-Jarosik K, Stanczyk J, Janiak K, et al. Prenatal diagnosis and follow-up of 23 cases of cardiac tumors. Prenat Diagn 2010;30:882-887.

34. Otsuka T, Asano K, Murota Y, Fukuda S, Hada Y, Fujii J. Successful removal of a cardiac fibroma in an elderly patient. J Cardiovasc Surg (Torino) 1990;31:55-57.

34. Gonzalez-Crussi F, Eberts TJ, Mirkin DL. Congenital fibrous hamartoma of the heart. Arch Pathol Lab Med 1978;102:491-493.

35. Williams DB, Danielson GK, McGoon DC, Feldt RH, Edwards WD. Cardiac fibroma: long-term survival after excision. J Thorac Cardiovasc Surg 1982;84:230-236.

36. Tahernia AC, Bricker JT, Ott DA. Intracardiac fibroma in an asymptomatic infant. Clin Cardiol 1990;13:506-512.

37. Yamaguchi M, Hosokawa Y, Ohashi H, Imai M, Oshima Y, Minamiji K. Cardiac fibroma. Long-term fate after excision. J Thorac Cardiovasc Surg 1992;103:140-145.

38. Fazio G, Grassedonio E, Lo Re G, et al. A cardiac fibroma in a 7-year-old asymptomatic girl admitted for ECG anomalies. J Cardiovasc Med (Hagerstown) 2012;13:406-409.

39. Chan HS, Sonley MJ, Moes CA, Daneman A, Smith CR, Martin DJ. Primary and secondary tumors of childhood involving the heart, pericardium, and great vessels. A report of 75 cases and review of the literature. Cancer 1985;56:825-836.

40. Alotti N, Rashed A, Kecskes G, Sipos J. Cardiac fibroma on chest X-ray. Asian Cardiovasc Thorac Ann 2008;16:265.

41. Pozzi M, Deux JF, Kirsch M. Conservative management of left ventricle cardiac fibroma in an adult asymptomatic patient. Int J Cardiol 2012;161:e61-62.

42. Navarini S, Latzin P, Kadner A, Carrel T, Hutter D. Giant cardiac fibroma: an unusual cause of failure to thrive. Pediatr Cardiol 2013;34:1264-1266.

43. Istvan K, Toro K, Kardos M, Imre C, Gyorgy D, Agnes N. Sudden death due to infiltration of left bundle branches by interventricular septal cardiac fibroma. J Forensic Sci 2012;57:1669-1674.

44. Oliva PB, Breckinridge JC, Johnson ML, Brantigan CO, O'Meara OP. Left ventricular outflow obstruction produced by a pedunculated fibroma in a newborn: clinical, angiographic, echocardiographic and surgical observations. Chest 1978; 74:590-593.

45. Stratemann S, Dzurik Y, Fish F, Parra D. Left ventricular cardiac fibroma in a child presenting with ventricular tachycardia. Pediatr Cardiol 2008;29:223-226.

46. Nucifora G, Pasotti E, Pedrazzini G, Moccetti T, Faletra FF, Gallino A. Cardiac fibroma mimicking hypertrophic cardiomyopathy: role of magnetic resonance imaging in the differential diagnosis. Int J Cardiol 2012;154:e11-13.

47. Patane F, Zingarelli E, Verzini A, di Summa M. Vascular complications associated with a large cardiac fibroma. Eur J Cardiothorac Surg 2001;20: 636-638.

48. Ohashi T, Asakura T, Sakamoto N, Shimizu H, Yoshida T. Giant cardiac fibroma. Ann Thorac Surg 2006;82:1512-1513.

49. Parmley LF, Salley RK, Williams JP, Head GB 3rd. The clinical spectrum of cardiac fibroma with diagnostic and surgical considerations: noninvasive imaging enhances management. Ann Thorac Surg 1988;45:455-465.

50. Colmorn LB, Jensen T, Petersen BL, Helvind M, Jorgensen FS. Prenatal ultrasound diagnosis of a multiple atypical right atrial cardiac fibroma. Ultraschall Med 2012;33:85-86.

51. Brown IW, McGoldrick JP, Robles A, Curella GW, Gula G, Ross DN. Left ventricular fibroma: echocardiographic diagnosis and successful surgical excision in three cases. J Cardiovasc Surg (Torino) 1990;31:536-540.

52. Sugiyama H, Naito H, Tsukano S, Echigo S, Kamiya T. Evaluation of cardiac tumors in children by electron-beam computed tomography: rhabdomyoma and fibroma. Circ J 2005;69:1352-1356.

53. Gorlin RJ. Nevoid basal cell carcinoma (Gorlin) syndrome. Genet Med 2004;6:530-539.

54. Coffin CM. Congenital cardiac fibroma associated with Gorlin syndrome. Pediatr Pathol 1992; 12:255-262.

55. Doede T, Seidel J, Riede FT, Vogt L, Mohr FW, Schier F. Occult, life-threatening, cardial tumor in syndactylism in Gorlin Goltz syndrome. J Pediatr Surg 2004;39:e17-19.

56. Kopp BT, Rosen KL, O'Donovan JC, Sheikh S. Cardiac fibroma, anomalous pulmonary venous course, and persistent pneumonia in a patient with Gorlin syndrome. Pediatr Pulmonol 2014;49:E7-9.

57. Scanlan D, Radio SJ, Nelson M, et al. Loss of the PTCH1 gene locus in cardiac fibroma. Cardiovasc Pathol 2008;17:93-97.

58. de Leon GA, Zaeri N, Donner RM, Karmazin N. Cerebral rhinocele, hydrocephalus, and cleft lip and palate in infants with cardiac fibroma. J Neurol Sci 1990;99:27-36.

59. Waller BR, Bradley SM, Crumbley AJ 3rd, Wiles HB, McQuinn TC, Bennett AT. Cardiac fibroma in an infant: single ventricle palliation as a bridge to heart transplantation. Ann Thorac Surg 2003; 75:1306-1308.

60. Lee C, Kim SJ, Kim YM. Cardiac fibroma in an infant: complete resection after a Blalock-Taussig shunt as initial palliation. Ann Thorac Surg 2010; 90:1011-1014.

61. Vander Salm TJ. Unusual primary tumors of the heart. Semin Thorac Cardiovasc Surg 2000; 12:89-100.

62. Numata K, Tomita H. [Cardiac fibroma in an infant: comparison of echocardiographic findings with cardiac rhabdomyoma.] J Cardiol 1994;24: 71-76. [Japanese]

63. Vougiouklakis T, Goussia A, Ioachim E, Peschos D, Agnantis N. Cardiac fibroma. A case presentation. Virchows Arch 2001;438:635-636.

64. Viswanathan S, Gibbs JL, Roberts P. Clonal translocation in a cardiac fibroma presenting with incessant ventricular tachycardia in childhood. Cardiol Young 2003;13:101-102.

65. de Montpreville VT, Serraf A, Aznag H, Nashashibi N, Planche C, Dulmet E. Fibroma and inflammatory myofibroblastic tumor of the heart. Ann Diagn Pathol 2001;5:335-342.

66. Fine G, Osamura RY, Lee MW. Ultrastructure of the myocardial fibroma. Arch Pathol Lab Med 1979;103:11-17.

67. Valente M, Cocco P, Thiene G, et al. Cardiac fibroma and heart transplantation. J Thorac Cardiovasc Surg 1993;106:1208-1212.

68. Ferguson HL, Hawkins EP, Cooley LD. Infant cardiac fibroma with clonal t(1;9)(q32;q22) and review of benign fibrous tissue cytogenetics. Cancer Genet Cytogenet 1996;87:34-37.

69. Takahashi C, Kanazawa N, Yoshikawa Y, et al. Germline PTCH1 mutations in Japanese basal cell nevus syndrome patients. J Hum Genet 2009; 54:403-408.

70. Charuzi Y, Mills H, Buchbinder NA, Marshall LA. Primary intramural cardiac tumor: long-term follow-up. Am Heart J 1983;106:414-419.

71. Filiatrault M, Beland MJ, Neilson KA, Paquet M. Cardiac fibroma presenting with clinically significant arrhythmias in infancy. Pediatr Cardiol 1991;12:118-120.

72. Lee YC, Singleton RT, Tang CK. Benign mesenchymal tumor of the heart. Spontaneous regression and disappearance of pulmonary artery stenosis. Chest 1982;82:503-505.

73. Ceithaml EL, Midgley FM, Perry LW, Dullum MK. Intramural ventricular fibroma in infancy: survival after partial excision in 2 patients. Ann Thorac Surg 1990;50:471-472.

74. Sharma K, Rohlicek C, Cecere R, Tchervenkov CI. Malignant arrhythmias secondary to a cardiac fibroma requiring transplantation in a teenager. J Heart Lung Transplant 2007;26:639-641.

75. Nwachukwu H, Li A, Nair V, Nguyen E, David TE, Butany J. Cardiac fibroma in adults. Cardiovasc Pathol 2010;20:e146-152.

76. Antonio MT, Powell AJ, del Nido PJ. Successful surgical excision of a large left ventricular fibroma in a child. Cardiol Young 2011;21:595-597.

77. Jamieson SW, Gaudiani VA, Reitz BA, Oyer PE, Stinson EB, Shumway NE. Operative treatment of an unresectable tumor of the left ventricle. J Thorac Cardiovasc Surg 1981;81:797-799.

78. Sharma K, Rohlicek C, Cecere R, Tchervenkov CI. Malignant arrhythmias secondary to a cardiac fibroma requiring transplantation in a teenager. J Heart Lung Transplant 2007;26:639-41.

79. Cho JM, Danielson GK, Puga FJ, et al. Surgical resection of ventricular cardiac fibromas: early and late results. Ann Thorac Surg 2003;76:1929-1934.

80. Thomas-de-Montpreville V, Nottin R, Dulmet E, Serraf A. Heart tumors in children and adults: clinicopathological study of 59 patients from a surgical center. Cardiovasc Pathol 2007;16:22-28.

# 8 CARDIAC RHABDOMYOMA

## DEFINITION

*Cardiac rhabdomyoma* is a hamartoma that occurs exclusively in the heart, often as multiple nodules composed of altered cardiac myocytes with large vacuoles and abundant intracellular glycogen. There is a strong association with the tuberous sclerosis complex (TSC) (1–3).

## GENERAL FEATURES

Although it was once considered a glycogen storage disease (4), or a true neoplasm (5), current opinion is that cardiac rhabdomyoma is a hamartoma (2,6,7). Unlike most neoplasms, rhabdomyomas are often multiple, lack mitotic activity, and are congenital rather than acquired (2). The focal nature of the lesions, absence of biochemical evidence of an enzyme deficiency, and lack of extracardiac involvement are incompatible with a glycogen storage disease. Ultrastructural studies demonstrate that the tumor cells are altered cardiac myocytes (2,6–11). Tumors with similar morphology have been found in the hearts of domestic swine, guinea pigs, sheep, deer, and dogs (12–16).

Although rare, rhabdomyoma is the most common cardiac tumor in infancy and childhood (5,17,18), accounting for 50 to 75 percent of pediatric tumors. There were 7 cases among 11,000 autopsies in Boston Children's Hospital Medical Center (5) and 8 cases at The Hospital for Sick Children in Toronto over a 62-year interval (17). In surgical series, cardiac rhabdomyomas are the most frequently encountered heart tumors in children (19), although fibromas are more likely to be excised (20).

Over 90 percent of intracardiac tumors discovered in intrauterine life are rhabdomyomas (21). When detected in utero, these tumors are commonly associated with TSC, a disease that may manifest in multiple organs including the brain, kidney, pancreas, retina, and skin. In autopsy series, cardiac rhabdomyomas were found in 30 to 50 percent of patients with TSC (22–24). In prenatal ultrasound studies, the incidence appears to be higher, and the presence of multiple rhabdomyomas prenatally is a strong predictor of TSC (25–28).

About 80 percent of children with cardiac rhabdomyoma have a clinical, radiologic, or family history of TSC, and more than 50 percent of patients with tuberous sclerosis have cardiac masses (29,30). Multiplicity of cardiac tumors is associated with TSC, which exhibits an autosomal dominant inheritance. A family history is positive in slightly less than half the cases, due to sporadic mutations in the majority. There are two genes involved: *TSC1* at chromosome 9q34 and *TSC2* at chromosome 16p13 (1,26). The *TSC1* and *TSC2* genes encode the proteins hamartin and tuberin, respectively. The two proteins work in conjunction to help regulate cell growth and size. The proteins act as tumor suppressors and form a complex that activates the GTPase-activating protein Rheb to inhibit the mammalian target of rapamycin (mTOR), which is a highly conserved protein kinase that regulates protein synthesis and cellular metabolism, differentiation, growth, and migration. Constitutive activation of mTOR results in the abnormal cellular proliferation and differentiation that is thought to be responsible for the hamartomatous lesions of TSC (31).

## CLINICAL FEATURES

Cardiac rhabdomyomas are seen primarily in fetuses, neonates, and children. It is a rare diagnosis in patients older than 10 years (32). Those with TSC have intracranial hamartomas, facial angiofibromas, subungual fibromas, linear epidermal nevi, renal angiomyolipomas, and other hamartomas. In these patients, symptoms related to extracardiac manifestations often dominate the clinical findings. In a series of Stiller et al. (20), 6 of 13 infants with rhabdomyomas had TSC, as did 10 of 32 in a series by Padalino et al. (19) and 4 of 9 in a study by Thomas-de-Montpreville (33).

**Table 8-1**

**CLINICOPATHOLOGIC FEATURES OF CARDIAC RHABDOMYOMA**[a]

| Feature | Frequency/Characteristics |
|---|---|
| Male:Female | 1:1 |
| Age | Prenatal – 6 years |
| | Mean, 2 weeks |
| Tuberous sclerosis | 56% |
| Multiplicity | 65% |
| Surgically resected | 75% |
| Site in heart | |
|   RV[b] | 38% |
|   LV | 36% |
|   Biventricular | 25% |
|   RA | 4% |
|   LA | 3% |
| Symptoms | Related to tuberous sclerosis (especially prenatal) |
| | Congestive heart failure, related to ventricular outflow tract obstruction or large ventricular masses |
| | Cyanosis |
| | Arrhythmias, especially supraventricular tachycardia |
| | SVC[c] syndrome |
| | Bronchial compression |
| | Related to associated congenital heart defects |
| Good prognostic features | Multiple small tumors without outflow tract obstruction |
| | Single moderate sized tumors, with outflow obstruction amenable to resection |
| Bad prognostic features | Associated anomalies (TSC or congenital heart defects) |
| | Large unresectable tumor causing heart failure |

[a]Adapted from references 20, 33, 34, 43, 73, and 74. Frequencies are approximate as not all data presented.
[b]RV = right ventricle; LV = left ventricle; RA = right atrium; LA = left atrium.
[c]SVC = superior vena cava; TSC = tuberous sclerosis complex.

Cardiac rhabdomyomas are detected by imaging for the evaluation of arrhythmias or for cardiac symptoms of hemodynamic instability related to ventricular outflow tract obstruction (Table 8-1). The lesions are congenital, and most patients are diagnosed in infancy or prenatally, although the diagnosis may be first discovered in older children (34). There is no gender predilection. The symptomatic presentation is varied, including manifestations of hydrops, congestive heart failure, supraventricular arrhythmias, murmurs, cyanosis, outflow tract obstruction, and sudden cardiac death (1,20,32–40). In contrast to patients with TSC, which usually manifests as multiple cardiac masses, approximately 50 percent of sporadic cardiac rhabdomyomas are single lesions. This group of patients most often benefits from surgical excision, which can be curative (17,19,40–44).

Cardiac rhabdomyomas should always be investigated in patients with family history of TSC, and detection of a cardiac mass in infancy should raise the possibility of TSC. The prevalence of cardiac rhabdomyomas in patients with TSC is dependent on age. Most infants with TSC have cardiac masses consistent with rhabdomyomas by echocardiography (18,45–47), although only 60 percent of children and less than 25 percent of adults with the syndrome have cardiac masses (43,46,48–50).

The decrease in incidence of cardiac rhabdomyoma with age in patients with TSC is not only a function of better survival of patients without cardiac tumors, but is also due to the propensity of these lesions to spontaneously regress (18,50,51). The rate of regression is from 30 to 65 percent (49,52). With the use of more advanced imaging modalities, magnetic resonance imaging (MRI) in particular, patients with TSC are now being screened and there is a slight increase in the detection of small intracardiac masses compatible with cardiac rhabdomyomas (36,49,53).

There is no sex predilection for patients with cardiac rhabdomyoma and TSC. The presenting symptom is usually related to TSC or fetal hydrops (2). Patients with cardiac rhabdomyomas and TSC who survive the first few weeks of life usually have no cardiac symptoms because the tumors in these patients are usually intramural and do not obstruct blood flow (2). There have been reports of cardiac rhabdomyoma associated with glomerulocystic disease and megacystic-microcolon-intestinal hypoperistalsis syndrome (54,55), which may be unusual manifestations of TSC.

About 50 percent of infants and children with cardiac rhabdomyoma have no evidence of TSC. These patients are more likely to be diagnosed in postnatal life than those with TSC, and the lesions are more likely to be single obstructive lesions amenable to surgery. In a series of Stiller et al. (20), four of six infants with sporadic rhabdomyomas presented with ventricular outflow tract obstruction (three right, two left), and surgery was performed in two, with the others regressing without excision (20). In a series of Thomas-de-Montpreville et al. (33), the indication for tumor excision was left ventricular outflow obstruction (most frequent), right ventricular outflow obstruction, bronchial compression, or superior vena cava obstruction. The age at presentation ranged from birth to 15 years of age, and there was no sex predilection. In a recent series of 89 primary cardiac tumors in children who had surgery, 32 were rhabdomyomas (36 percent) and of those, 11 had evidence of TSC and 80 percent had some symptoms or abnormal electrocardiographic findings (19). In another series of 120 children with surgically resected heart tumors, 42 were rhabdomyomas (35 percent), and all but 3 neonates survived (34). In this series the mean age was 7 months, although the oldest patient with cardiac rhabdomyoma was 6 years. The most common presenting symptoms were murmurs and supraventricular tachycardia.

Cardiac rhabdomyomas have been described in individuals with a number of congenital heart defects: hypoplastic left heart syndrome, transposition of the great arteries, ventricular septal defect, endocardial fibroelastosis, subaortic stenosis, Ebstein anomaly, hypoplastic tricuspid valve, double outlet right ventricle, aortic atresia, and pulmonary atresia (1,2,5,43,56,57). In some cases there are chromosomal defects including trisomy 21 (43). In these cases, tuberous sclerosis is not usually present, and the clinical features are dominated by the congenital heart disease.

In most patients, echocardiography provides adequate information for diagnosis and clinical management, thus obviating the need for additional imaging tests. MRI is reserved for selected patients in whom the tumor type is questionable after echocardiography or when additional anatomic or functional information is required (58). Rhabdomyomas appear as well-circumscribed masses, usually in the ventricles, but they can be found anywhere in the heart, and cause a hyperintense signal on T1- and T2-weighted MRIs (59). Compared with the signal from uninvolved myocardium, the masses are hypointense on postgadolinium imaging. The lack of tumor enhancement is a feature that helps distinguish cardiac rhabdomyomas from cardiac fibromas in selected cases (60).

## GROSS FINDINGS

The most common locations for rhabdomyomas are the left ventricle and ventricular septum, although 30 percent involve the atrium or right ventricle (18,19). In a series of 42 patients, surgically resected rhabdomyomas were distributed evenly between the two ventricles, often with outflow tract obstruction (34). Most cases diagnosed in utero or in early infancy are multiple (20,43), and 40 percent are multiple in surgical series including older children (34). Tumors may extend from the right ventricle into the right atrium, and to a lesser extent, left ventricle into left atrium; tumors isolated to the atria are rare (34).

Rhabdomyomas are firm, white-tan, well-circumscribed lobulated nodules that occur in any location in the heart, but are more common in the ventricular walls (figs. 8-1–8-7). When multiple, they may consist of numerous miliary nodules measuring less than 1 mm (32,63,64), a feature termed *rhabdomyomatosis* (63,64). In a pathology-based series of cardiac rhabdomyomas, the size range was 0.3 to 9.0 cm, with a mean of 3.4 cm (1). One case of a "giant" rhabdomyoma measuring 5.5 cm

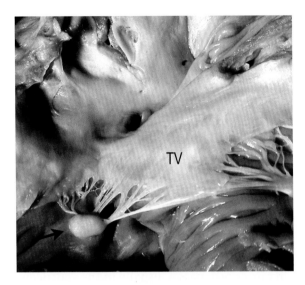

**Figure 8-1**

**CARDIAC RHABDOMYOMA**

Above: The heart is opened from the right side, with the anterior leaflet of the tricuspid valve (TV) and right atrium above. A subendocardial yellow nodule (arrow) is seen, which was histologically rhabdomyoma. The tumor is near the membranous septum and septal chordal insertions of the septal and anterior tricuspid valve leaflets.

Right: At higher magnification, the endocardial-based nature of this lesion is seen.

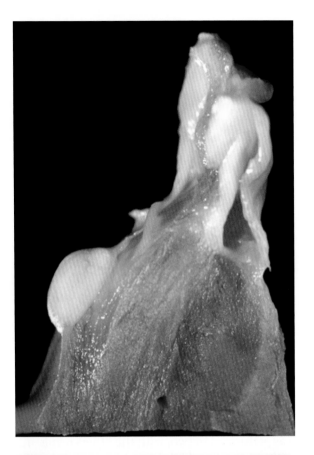

**Figure 8-2**

**CARDIAC RHABDOMYOMA**

Left atrium autopsy specimen from a 12-year-old child shows a sporadic tumor (arrow) just above the annulus of the mitral valve, anterior leaflet.

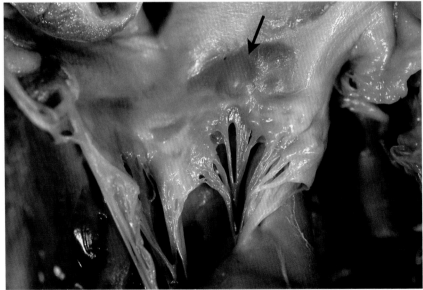

treated surgically has been recently reported (60). Large tumors may obliterate and distort the ventricular cavity (fig. 8-5) (65).

Resected tumors show the nondescript findings of a homogeneous tumor mass, usually with irregular surgical margins (fig. 8-8). Occasionally, fragments of cardiac muscle and endocardium are present (fig. 8-7). Surgical margins are unnecessary to report, because incomplete resection offers relief of obstructive symptoms, usually

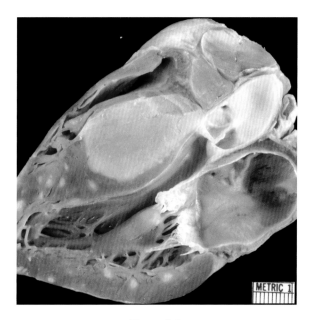

**Figure 8-3**

**CARDIAC RHABDOMYOMAS**

There are large intramural masses within the ventricular septum and multiple, minute tumors toward the apex and at the left ventricular free wall. This pattern of involvement is typical in patients with tuberous sclerosis. (Courtesy of Dr. W.D. Edwards, Rochester, MN.)

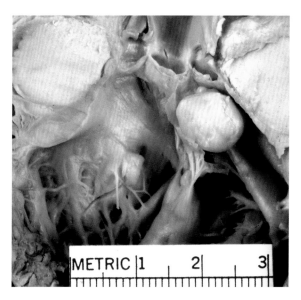

**Figure 8-4**

**MULTIPLE CARDIAC RHABDOMYOMAS**

The left ventricle is opened and there are homogenous tumor nodules in the endocardium on the mitral valve and filling both ventricular outflow tracts. There are large round and tan masses both intramurally and projecting into the ventricular cavities. The aortic valve (middle) is spared by a tumor causing subaortic stenosis. (Courtesy of Dr. W.D. Edwards, Rochester, MN.)

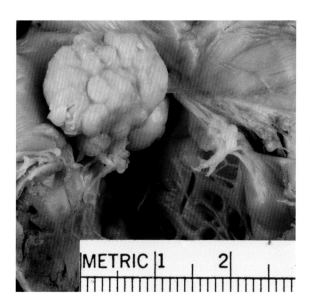

**Figure 8-5**

**RIGHT VENTRICULAR RHABDOMYOMA
EXTENDING INTO RIGHT ATRIUM**

There is a large mass obstructing the tricuspid valve. Tumors that project into a cavity, such this one, are typical of sporadic cases. (Courtesy of Dr. W.D. Edwards, Rochester, MN.)

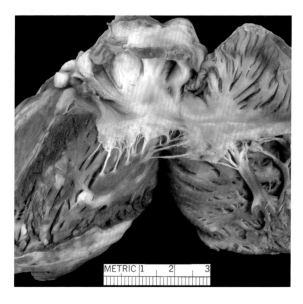

**Figure 8-6**

**MULTIPLE RHABDOMYOMAS**

An adult has multiple tumors, some of which stud the epicardial surface. Endocardial-based tumors are in the right ventricle, the largest at the apex. (Courtesy of Dr. W.D. Edwards, Rochester, MN.)

### Figure 8-7

**RHABDOMYOMA**

A surgically excised tumor (asterisk) includes a portion of endocardium (arrow) and myocardium (arrows). The patient was a 7-day-old girl with a transatrial cardiac tumor embedded in the posterior wall of the right ventricle. Surgery included resuspension of the tricuspid valve, enlargement of the right atrium, closure of an atrial septal defect, and Blalock-Taussig shunt. There was no evidence of tuberous sclerosis clinically.

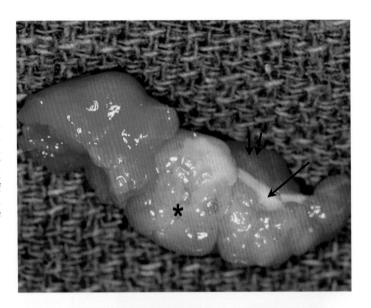

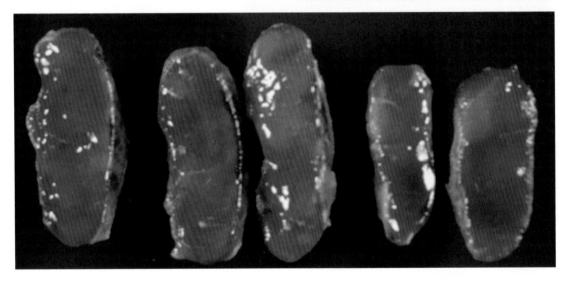

### Figure 8-8

**RHABDOMYOMA**

The tumor was serially sectioned after removal from a 6-month-old girl who presented with cardiac arrest. A magnetic resonance image (MRI) showed a 4-cm left ventricular mass; the chest X ray was normal.

without recurrence. Repeat resection may be necessary in cases of multiple tumors, but is the exception (1 of 42 patients in a series by Bielefeld et al. [34]).

## MICROSCOPIC FINDINGS

Cardiac rhabdomyomas are distinctive, and unlikely to be confused with other entities. The tumors are characterized by large round or polygonal cells with cytoplasmic clearing and small centrally placed nuclei (figs. 8-9–8-13). The vacuoles in the cytoplasm may be abundant and cause invaginations of the cytoplasmic membrane, giving the typical cell appearance often referred to as "spider cells." Mitoses and necrosis are absent. Calcification is typically absent, unlike a large proportion of fibromas. There is a strong reaction with periodic acid–Schiff (PAS) reagent, reflecting the abundant glycogen content of rhabdomyoma cells.

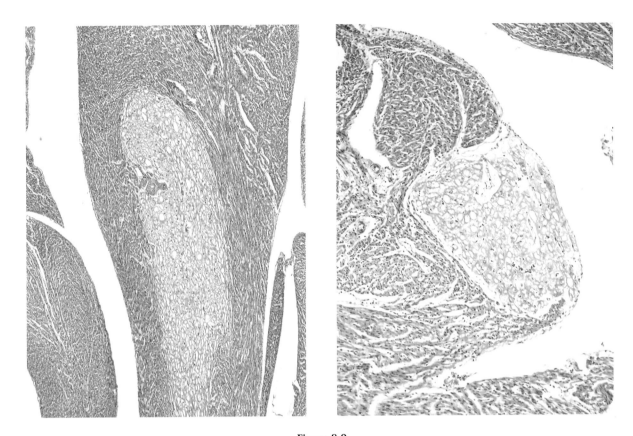

**Figure 8-9**

**RHABDOMYOMA: SUBENDOCARDIAL**

Left: On low magnification, there are discrete areas of vacuolated cells in the right ventricular trabeculae.

Right: A different area demonstrates a separate nodule of diffuse cytoplasmic clearing. The minute tumor involves one of the papillary muscles. The patient had multiple tumors and tuberous sclerosis complex.

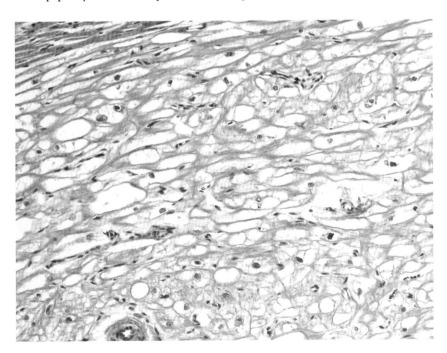

**Figure 8-10**

**RHABDOMYOMA: CYTOPLASMIC CLEARING**

The tumor cells are myocytes that cause diffuse clearing of the cytoplasm. There are a few "spider cells" in this field.

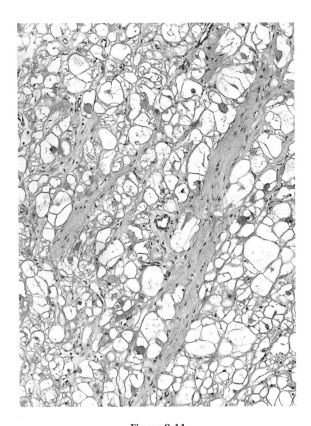

**Figure 8-11**

**RHABDOMYOMA: SPIDER CELLS**

Masses of eosinophilic cytoplasm with strands of cytoplasm moving toward the periphery characterize the classic cell of cardiac rhabdomyoma.

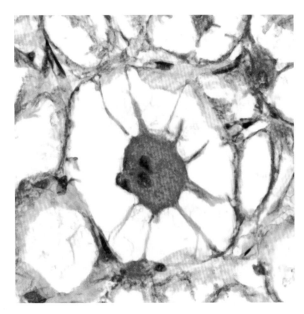

**Figure 8-12**

**RHABDOMYOMA: SPIDER CELL**

There is central cytoplasmic condensation with strands of cytoplasm emanating toward the periphery.

## ULTRASTRUCTURAL AND IMMUNOHISTOCHEMICAL FINDINGS

There have been several ultrastructural studies of cardiac rhabdomyomas (2,6–11). Electron microscopy shows, in some cases, well-formed Z-bands, with occasional actin myosin filaments as well as mitochondria, primitive T-tubules, lipid droplets, and zebra-like bodies. The ultrastructural features are those of myocyte origin. In one study, two types of cells were identified by electron microscopy in a single tumor examined: spider cells, with few contractile elements and abundant glycogen, and other cells with abundant myofibrils and autophagic membrane-bound glycogen vacuoles (9). These findings, together with the lack of developed T-tubules, led the authors to conclude that rhabdomyomas are the result of localized arrests in cardiomyocyte cell development (9).

By immunohistochemistry, cardiac rhabdomyoma cells reflect their myogenic derivation, exhibiting reactivity with antibodies directed against actin, desmin, and myoglobin (fig. 8-13) (1,66,67). The proliferative (Ki-67) index is close to zero (68). Hamartin and tuberin, the protein products of the genes associated with TSC, are positive in rhabdomyomas, with some evidence pointing to a down-regulation status of these proteins in rhabdomyoma cells when compared to normal myocytes (68).

## DIFFERENTIAL DIAGNOSIS

The diagnosis of cardiac rhabdomyoma is rarely problematic; indeed, in patients with TSC, a tissue diagnosis is considered unnecessary if multiple cardiac masses are present. Histologically, the differential diagnosis includes lipoma, granular cell tumor, glycogen storage diseases, and histiocytoid cardiomyopathy. Lipomas lack myofibers and are located primarily on the epicardial surface. Lipomatous hypertrophy of the atrial septum is a localized process composed of brown fat cells, mature fat cells, and an admixed population of enlarged but mature atrial myocytes. Granular cell tumors are

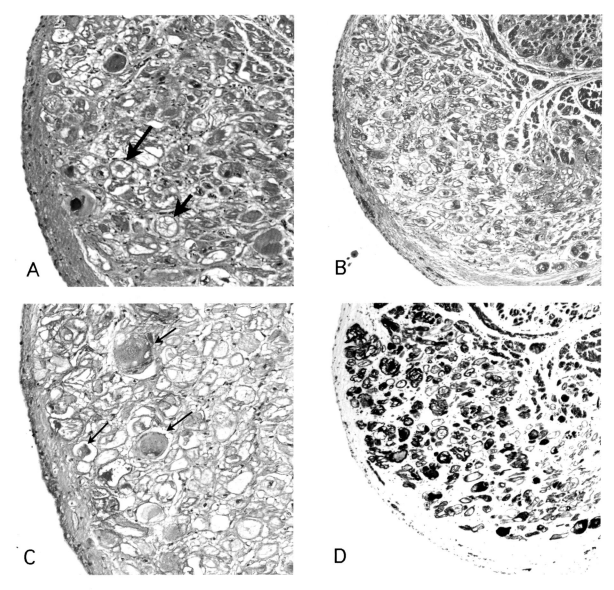

**Figure 8-13**

**SUBENDOCARDIAL RHABDOMYOMA**

A: In this example from an older child, many of the tumor cells have abundant cytoplasm. The arrows point to scattered spider cells.

B: The Masson trichrome stains the cytoplasm of rhabdomyoma cells in a similar way to cardiac muscle.

C: Although ultrastructurally the vacuoles are composed largely of glycogen, many of the tumor cells are artifactually empty. There are scattered periodic acid–Schiff (PAS)-positive cells (arrows).

D: The residual cytoplasm of the rhabdomyoma cells contains striated muscle, which stains for desmin.

small lesions that are generally present on the epicardial surface, and lack the vacuolated cells of rhabdomyoma. Granular cell tumors do not possess myofibers, and are S-100 protein positive and desmin and myoglobin negative, unlike rhabdomyomas. Glycogen storage diseases can mimic the vacuolated appearance of cardiac rhabdomyoma, and possess abundant intracytoplasmic glycogen like cardiac rhabdomyoma. They do not form well-circumscribed nodules, however, and ultrastructurally the cells show intact polar intercalated discs of mature myocytes.

Histiocytoid cardiomyopathy has been termed a form of rhabdomyomatosis; in contrast to rhabdomyoma, however, tumor nodules are small, and there is fine granularity to the cells without large vacuoles and spider cells.

## TREATMENT

Patients with cardiac rhabdomyomas and arrhythmias or cardiac murmurs are treated surgically, with excellent outcome (1,19,48,52,69). Most patients are under 1 year of age, although there was a single 9-year-old (1) and a 6-year-old (34) reported. Most patients undergoing surgical procedures have sporadic single masses or conditions that require immediate surgical intervention, such as ventricular outflow tract obstruction (35,70,71). Surgery may be advocated even in the absence of symptoms, if significant dysrhythmia or hemodynamic abnormalities are noted on electrocardiography or imaging (19). As noted above, incomplete resection is common, and is generally curative without recurrence.

Because surgical treatment is not always possible, pharmacologic treatments have been investigated. Mutations in genes related to TSC lead to the production of hamartin and tuberin heterodimers that inhibit mTOR, which controls the cell proliferation and growth in normal circumstances (72). Everolimus has been approved by the Food and Drug Administration for pancreatic progressive neuroendocrine tumors, tuberous sclerosis–associated inoperable subependymal giant cell astrocytoma (SEGA), and progressive renal cell carcinoma, and it is a promising therapy under investigation as a treatment option for tumors associated with TSC, including cardiac rhabdomyomas (31,52,72). One of these reports described regression of a cardiac rhabdomyoma while the patient was in treatment with everolimus for SEGA (31). The other two reports were of patients receiving primary treatment with everolimus for cardiac rhabdomyoma with favorable results (52,72).

## PROGNOSIS

Although the prognosis of children with cardiac rhabdomyoma in the setting of TSC was poor in the past (4,17), currently, the prognosis for such patients is good, with regression of cardiac lesions common (18,52,73). The prognosis for patients with an in utero diagnosis of cardiac rhabdomyoma (often with TSC), however, is poor because of frequent extracardiac defects and central nervous system involvement (43). Features that are associated with poor neonatal outcome include the size of the tumor, and the presence of fetal arrhythmia and hydrops (74).

Approximately 10 percent of fetuses with the diagnosis die in utero, often from the manifestations of TSC, and approximately 50 percent of live-born infants diagnosed in utero die in the neonatal period. Patients who survive have multiple small tumors without hemodynamic consequences that eventually regress, or (less likely) more localized tumors that cause outflow tract obstruction that can be excised or partly resected (43). Surgery to relieve outflow tract obstruction is effective even when the tumors are only partially resected. In one series, although only 46 percent of tumors could be completely resected, subsequent regression and sustained symptom-free survival was typical, with no late deaths and only one death due to postoperative brain hemorrhage (19). In the series of Stiller et al. (20), all of the infants with cardiac masses and TSC were followed without surgery and in all the tumors regressed or vanished.

It is difficult to establish definitively a prenatal diagnosis of TSC if a cardiac tumor is diagnosed by ultrasound, although most patients are ultimately diagnosed with TSC. More than half of fetuses with prenatal diagnosis of presumed cardiac rhabdomyoma do not survive until term, and one third have neurologic sequelae after birth even if the prenatal brain imaging is normal (36). The rate of neurologic complications is two thirds if prenatal ultrasound is suggestive of central nervous systemic involvement by TSC (36).

## REFERENCES

1. Burke AP, Virmani R. Cardiac rhabdomyoma: a clinicopathologic study. Mod Pathol 1991;4:70-74.
2. Fenoglio JJ Jr, McAllister HA Jr, Ferrans VJ. Cardiac rhabdomyoma: a clinicopathologic and electron microscopic study. Am J Cardiol 1976;38:241-251.
3. Yu K, Liu Y, Wang H, Hu S, Long C. Epidemiological and pathological characteristics of cardiac tumors: a clinical study of 242 cases. Interact Cardiovasc Thorac Surg 2007;6:636-649.
4. Kidder LA. Congenital glycogenic tumors of the heart. AMA Arch Pathol 1950;49:55-62.
5. Padalino MA, Basso C, Milanesi O, et al. Surgically treated primary cardiac tumors in early infancy and childhood. J Thorac Cardiovasc Surg 2005;129:1358-1363.
6. Fenoglio JJ Jr, Diana DJ, Bowen TE, McAllister HA Jr, Ferrans VJ. Ultrastructure of a cardiac rhabdomyoma. Hum Pathol 1977;8:700-706.
7. Silverman JF, Kay S, McCue CM, Lower RR, Brough AJ, Chang CH. Rhabdomyoma of the heart: ultrastructural study of three cases. Lab Invest 1976;35:596-606.
8. Arciniegas E, Hakimi M, Farooki ZQ, Truccone NJ, Green EW. Primary cardiac tumors in children. J Thorac Cardiovasc Surg 1980;79:582-591.
9. Bruni C, Prioleau PG, Ivey HH, Nolan SP. New fine structural features of cardiac rhabdomyoma: report of a case. Cancer 1980;46:2068-2073.
10. Kim CJ, Cho JH, Chi JG, Kim YJ. Multiple rhabdomyoma of the heart presenting with a congenital supraventricular tachycardia—report of case with ultrastructural study. J Korean Med Sci 1989;4:143-147.
11. Trillo AA, Holleman IL, White JT. Presence of satellite cells in a cardiac rhabdomyoma. Histopathology 1978;2:215-223.
12. Kobayashi T, Kobayashi Y, Fukuda U, et al. A cardiac rhabdomyoma in a Guinea pig. J Toxicol Pathol 2010;23:107-110
13. Radi ZA, Metz A. Canine cardiac rhabdomyoma. Toxicol Pathol 2009;37:348-350.
14. Tanimoto T, Ohtsuki Y. The pathogenesis of so-called cardiac rhabdomyoma in swine: a histological, immunohistochemical and ultrastructural study. Virchows Arch 1995;427:213-221
15. Bradley R, Wells GA, Arbuckle JB. Ovine and porcine so-called cardiac rhabdomyoma (hamartoma). J Comp Pathol 1980;90:551-558.
16. Kolly C, Bidaut A, Robert N. Cardiac rhabdomyoma in a juvenile fallow deer (Dama dama). J Wildl Dis 2004;40:603-606.
17. Chan HS, Sonley MJ, Moes CA, Daneman A, Smith CR, Martin DJ. Primary and secondary tumors of childhood involving the heart, pericardium, and great vessels. A report of 75 cases and review of the literature. Cancer 1985;56:825-836.
18. Smythe JF, Dyck JD, Smallhorn JF, Freedom RM. Natural history of cardiac rhabdomyoma in infancy and childhood. Am J Cardiol 1990;66:1247-1249.
19. Padalino MA, Vida VL, Boccuzzo G, et al. Surgery for primary cardiac tumors in children: early and late results in a multicenter European Congenital Heart Surgeons Association study. Circulation 2012;126:22-30.
20. Stiller B, Hetzer R, Meyer R, et al. Primary cardiac tumours: when is surgery necessary? Eur J Cardiothorac Surg 2001;20:1002-1006.
21. Groves AM, Fagg NL, Cook AC, Allan LD. Cardiac tumours in intrauterine life. Arch Dis Child 1992;67:1189-1192.
22. Byard RW. The potential significance of occult cardiac rhabdomyomas at autopsy in traumatic death. Forensic Sci Med Pathol 2011;7:367-368.
23. Jain D, Maleszewski JJ, Halushka MK. Benign cardiac tumors and tumorlike conditions. Ann Diagn Pathol 2010;14:215-230.
24. Parames F, Freitas I, Martins JD, Trigo C, Pinto MF. Cardiac tumors: the 17-year experience of pediatric cardiology department. Rev Port Cardiol 2009;28:929-940.
25. Markov D, Pavlova E, Pavlova M, et al. [Congenital rhabdomyoma—prenatal diagnosis with three-dimensional ultrasound of two cases with different pregnancy outcome.] Akush Ginekol (Sofiia) 2010;49:59-63. [Bulgarian]
26. Burke A, Virmani R. Pediatric heart tumors. Cardiovasc Pathol 2008;17:193-198.
27. O'Callaghan MG, House M, Ebay S, Bhadelia R. Rhabdomyoma of the head and neck demonstrated by prenatal magnetic resonance imaging. J Comput Assist Tomogr 2005;29:130-132.
28. Bossert T, Gummert JF, Battellini R, et al. Surgical experience with 77 primary cardiac tumors. Interact Cardiovasc Thorac Surg 2005;4:311-315.
29. Beghetti M, Gow RM, Haney I, Mawson J, Williams WG, Freedom RM. Pediatric primary benign cardiac tumors: a 15-year review. Am Heart J 1997;134:1107-1114.
30. Tworetzky W, McElhinney DB, Margossian R, et al. Association between cardiac tumors and tuberous sclerosis in the fetus and neonate. Am J Cardiol 2003;92:487-489.

31. Tiberio D, Franz DN, Phillips JR. Regression of a cardiac rhabdomyoma in a patient receiving everolimus. Pediatrics 2011;127:e1335-1337.

32. Shrivastava S, Jacks JJ, White RS, Edwards JE. Diffuse rhabdomyomatosis of the heart. Arch Pathol Lab Med 1977;101:78-90.

33. Thomas-de-Montpreville V, Nottin R, Dulmet E, Serraf A. Heart tumors in children and adults: clinicopathological study of 59 patients from a surgical center. Cardiovasc Pathol 2007;16:22-28.

34. Bielefeld KJ, Moller JH. Cardiac tumors in infants and children: study of 120 operated patients. Pediatr Cardiol 2013;34:125-128.

35. Gupta A, Narula N, Mahajan R, Rohit M. Sudden death of a young child due to cardiac rhabdomyoma. Pediatr Cardiol 2010;31:894-896.

36. Saada J, Hadj Rabia S, Fermont L, et al. Prenatal diagnosis of cardiac rhabdomyomas: incidence of associated cerebral lesions of tuberous sclerosis complex. Ultrasound Obstet Gynecol 2009; 34:155-159.

37. Kusano KF, Ohe T. Cardiac tumors that cause arrhythmias. Card Electrophysiol Rev 2002;6:174-177.

38. Case CL, Gillette PC, Crawford FA. Cardiac rhabdomyomas causing supraventricular and lethal ventricular arrhythmias in an infant. Am Heart J 1991;122:1484-1486.

39. Golding R, Reed G. Rhabdomyoma of the heart. Two unusual clinical presentations. N Engl J Med 1967;276:957-959.

40. Reece IJ, Cooley DA, Frazier OH, Hallman GL, Powers PL, Montero CG. Cardiac tumors. Clinical spectrum and prognosis of lesions other than classical benign myxoma in 20 patients. J Thorac Cardiovasc Surg 1984;88:439-446.

41. Blondeau P. Primary cardiac tumors—French studies of 533 cases. Thorac Cardiovasc Surg 1990;38(Suppl 2):192-195.

42. Murphy MC, Sweeney MS, Putnam JB Jr, et al. Surgical treatment of cardiac tumors: a 25-year experience. Ann Thorac Surg 1990;49:612-617; discussion 617-618.

43. Niewiadomska-Jarosik K, Stanczyk J, Janiak K, et al. Prenatal diagnosis and follow-up of 23 cases of cardiac tumors. Prenat Diagn 2010;30:882-887.

44. Carvalho SR, Marcolin AC, Cavalli RC, et al. [Fetal cardiac rhabdomyoma: Analysis of five cases.] Rev Bras Ginecol Obstet 2010;32:156-162. [Portuguese]

45. Diamant S, Sharaz J, Holtzman M, Laniado S. Echocardiographic diagnosis of cardiac tumors in symptomatic tuberous sclerosis patients. Clin Ped 1983;22:297-299.

46. Smith HC, Watson GH, Patel RG, Super M. Cardiac rhabdomyomata in tuberous sclerosis: their course and diagnostic value. Arch Dis Child 1989;64:196-200.

47. Calhoun BC, Watson PT, Hegge F. Ultrasound diagnosis of an obstructive cardiac rhabdomyoma with severe hydrops and hypoplastic lungs. A case report. J Reprod Med 1991;36:317-319.

48. Pucci A, Botta G, Sina N, et al. Life-threatening tumors of the heart in fetal and postnatal age. J Pediatr 2013;162:964-969.

49. Lee KA, Won HS, Shim JY, Lee PR, Kim A. Molecular genetic, cardiac and neurodevelopmental findings in cases of prenatally diagnosed rhabdomyoma associated with tuberous sclerosis complex. Ultrasound Obstet Gynecol 2013;41:306-311.

50. Watson GH. Cardiac rhabdomyomas in tuberous sclerosis. Ann N Y Acad Sci 1991;615:50-57.

51. Durairaj M, Mangotra K, Makhale CN, Shinde R, Mehta AC, Sathe AS. Cardiac rhabdomyoma in a neonate: application of serial echocardiography. Echocardiography 2006;23:510-512.

52. Kocabas A, Ekici F, Cetin II, et al. Cardiac rhabdomyomas associated with tuberous sclerosis complex in 11 children: presentation to outcome. Pediatr Hematol Oncol 2013;130:e243-247.

53. Kivelitz DE, Muhler M, Rake A, Scheer I, Chaoui R. MRI of cardiac rhabdomyoma in the fetus. Eur Radiol 2004;14:1513-1516.

54. Wu SS, Collins MH, de Chadarevian JP. Study of the regression process in cardiac rhabdomyomas. Pediatr Dev Pathol 2002;5:29-36.

55. Chao AS, Chao A, Wang TH, et al. Outcome of antenatally diagnosed cardiac rhabdomyoma: case series and a meta-analysis. Ultrasound Obstet Gynecol 2008;31:289-295.

56. Couper RT, Byard RW, Cutz E, Stringer DA, Durie PR. Cardiac rhabdomyomata and megacystis-microcolon-intestinal hypoperistalsis syndrome. J Med Genet 1991;28:274-276.

57. Saguem MH, Laarif M, Remadi S, Bozakoura C, Cox JN. Diffuse bilateral glomerulocystic disease of the kidneys and multiple cardiac rhabdomyomas in a newborn. Relationship with tuberous sclerosis and review of the literature. Pathol Res Pract 1992;188:367-373; discussion 373-364.

58. Watanabe T, Hojo Y, Kozaki T, Nagashima M, Ando M. Hypoplastic left heart syndrome with rhabdomyoma of the left ventricle. Pediatr Cardiol 1991;12:121-122.

59. Charbonneau S, Giroux L, Vauclair R, Allaire G, Robert F. [Cardiac rhabdomyomas and aortic valve atresia: an unusual association.] Ann Pathol 1986;6:206-210. [French]

60. Berkenblit R, Spindola-Franco H, Frater RW, Fish BB, Glickstein JS. MRI in the evaluation and management of a newborn infant with cardiac rhabdomyoma. Ann Thorac Surg 1997;63:1475-1477.

61. Grebenc ML, Rosado de Christenson ML, Burke AP, Green CE, Galvin JR. Primary cardiac and pericardial neoplasms: radiologic-pathologic correlation. Radiographics 2000;20:1073-1103.
62. Padalino MA, Vida VL, Bhattarai A, et al. Giant intramural left ventricular rhabdomyoma in a newborn. Circulation 2011;124:2275-2277.
63. Uzun O, McGawley G, Wharton GA. Multiple cardiac rhabdomyomas: tuberous sclerosis or not? Heart 1997;77:388.
64. Uzun O, Wilson DG, Vujanic GM, Parsons JM, De Giovanni JV. Cardiac tumours in children. Orphanet J Rare Dis 2007;2:11.
65. Salinas-Martin MV, Munoz-Repeto I, Pavon-Delgado A. [Cardiac rhabdomyomatosis associated with tuberous sclerosis.] Med Clin (Barc) 2008;130:638. [Spanish]
66. Bussani R, Rustico MA, Silvestri F. Fetal cardiac rhabdomyomatosis as a prenatal marker for the detection of latent tuberous sclerosis. An autopsy case report. Pathol Res Pract 2001;197:559-561.
67. Burke AP, Virmani R. Tumors of the heart and great vessels. AFIP Atlas of Tumor Pathology, 3rd Series, Fascicle 16. Washington DC: American Registry of Pathology; 1996.
68. Neri M, Di Donato S, Maglietta R, et al. Sudden death as presenting symptom caused by cardiac primary multicentric left ventricle rhabdomyoma, in an 11-month-old baby. An immunohistochemical study. Diagn Pathol 2012;7:169.
69. Guschmann M, Entezami M, Becker R, Vogel M. Intrauterine rhabdomyoma of the heart. A case report. Gen Diagn Pathol 1997;143:255-259.
70. Kotulska K, Larysz-Brysz M, Grajkowska W, et al. Cardiac rhabdomyomas in tuberous sclerosis complex show apoptosis regulation and mTOR pathway abnormalities. Pediatr Dev Pathol 2009;12:89-95.
71. Karnak I, Alehan D, Ekinci S, Buyukpamukcu N. Cardiac rhabdomyoma as an unusual mediastinal mass in a newborn. Pediatr Surg Int 2007;23:811-814.
72. Ilina MV, Jaeggi ET, Lee KJ. Neonatal rhabdomyoma causing right ventricular inflow obstruction with duct-dependent pulmonary blood flow: successful stenting of PDA. Catheter Cardiovasc Interv 2007;69:881-885.
73. Mandke JV, Kinare SG, Phatak AM. Congenital diffuse rhabdomyomatosis of the heart with biventricular outflow obstruction. Indian Heart J 1992;44:187-188.
74. Demir HA, Ekici F, Yazal Erdem A, Emir S, Tunc B. Everolimus: a challenging drug in the treatment of multifocal inoperable cardiac rhabdomyoma. Pediatrics 2012;130:e243-247.
75. Kamiya H, Yasuda T, Nagamine H, et al. Surgical treatment of primary cardiac tumors: 28 years' experience in Kanazawa University Hospital. Jpn Circ J 2001;65:315-319.
76. Kosuga T, Fukunaga S, Kawara T, et al. Surgery for primary cardiac tumors. Clinical experience and surgical results in 60 patients. J Cardiovasc Surg (Torino) 2002;43:581-587.

# 9 HISTIOCYTOID CARDIOMYOPATHY

## DEFINITION

*Histiocytoid cardiomyopathy* is a congenital, multicentric hamartoma of oncocytic cardiac myocytes. Synonyms include *Purkinje cell tumor, cardiac hamartoma, histiocytoid nodule,* and *oncocytic cardiomyopathy*. It is currently considered a form of genetic cardiomyopathy according to the American Heart Association (1).

## GENERAL FEATURES

The cell of origin of histiocytoid cardiomyopathy is an altered cardiac myocyte with an accumulation of mitochondria. The earliest descriptions were likely reported as rhabdomyomas (2,3). For several years the lesions were interpreted as nests of glycogenated cells (4–7). Also once thought to be a histiocytic reaction (8), the myocytic nature of the cells has been firmly established, along with the fact that the cytoplasmic changes are due to the accumulation of mitochondria and not glycogen.

The term histiocytoid cardiomyopathy was first used in 1977 by Bruton et al. (9). The finding of cholinesterase in tumor cells led to the theory that the tumors were of Purkinje cell origin (10). There is a close association between histiocytoid cardiomyopathy and the conduction system since many tumors involve the conduction tissues, and the clinical symptoms are often dominated by arrhythmias (11,12). Because they are multicentric aggregates of modified cells occurring exclusively in infants, the clusters of cells in histiocytoid cardiomyopathy are currently believed to be hamartomas. A sequela of rubella infection has also been considered, but there is little clinical and morphologic evidence for this theory (12). This unique "tumor" has for decades straddled the entities of cardiomyopathy on one hand and benign multicentric hamartoma on the other (13,14).

Historically, histiocytoid cardiomyopathy has been considered a hamartomatous growth of oncocytic myocytes with abundant mitochondria, and not an intrinsic mitochondrial disorder (12). Currently, there is a theory that histiocytoid cardiomyopathy falls within the spectrum of primary mitochondrial diseases, despite the fact that there are discrete tumorlike lesions (15). The basis for this lies largely in case reports. There have been reports of patients with histiocytoid cardiomyopathy with steatosis of the liver and the mitochondrial A8344G transition, associated with reduced activity of complexes I and IV of the respiratory chain (16). Another case report demonstrated a G15498A mitochondrial cytochrome b mutation, resulting in the amino acid exchange of glycine with aspartic acid at position 251 in a patient with histiocytoid cardiomyopathy (17). An additional patient with histiocytoid cardiomyopathy demonstrated X-linked cytogenetic abnormalities, lactic acidosis, and agenesis of the corpus callosum (18). Yet another infant had skeletal muscle myopathy with decreased cytochrome c oxidase activity (19). Biochemical studies of cardiomyocytes in cases of histiocytoid cardiomyopathy have shown decreased succinate-cytochrome c and NADH-cytochrome c reductase, reflecting defects of complex III of the respiratory chain (20). Although compelling, these reports fail to convincingly prove that mitochondrial defects underlie the condition, and are not secondary (12).

## CLINICAL FEATURES

The incidence of histiocytoid cardiomyopathy is unknown because not all cases are documented pathologically. In 1994, 53 cases had been reported (12); by 2013, 75 to 85 were reported, depending on the inclusion of early cases reported under various designations (21–26). The largest pathologic series included a series of biopsies from infants with tachyarrhythmias and ablative procedures (27).

### Table 9-1

**CLINICAL FINDINGS IN 74 PATIENTS WITH HISTIOCYTOID CARDIOMYOPATHY[a]**

| Findings | Frequency |
|---|---|
| Male:female (n) | 13:61 |
| Mean age (range) | 10 months (birth – 30 months) |
| Diagnosis made first at autopsy (n, %) | 60 (81%) |
| Biopsy diagnosis (n, %) | 14 (19%) |
| Arrhythmias as presenting symptom[b] (n) | |
| Ventricular tachycardia | 18 |
| Supraventricular tachycardia | 16 |
| Sudden cardiac death | 17 |
| Wolff-Parkinson-White syndrome | 5 |

[a]Data from 74 reported cases presented in references 12, 16, 17, 19, 23, 25, 26, 29–31, 33, 35, 36, 43–45, and 47; some data extracted from reviews in references 12 and 47.
[b]Four patients died suddenly with a prior history of episodic ventricular tachycardia. Data were not available in all cases.

### Table 9-2

**CONDITIONS ASSOCIATED WITH HISTIOCYTOID CARDIOMYOPATHY**

| | |
|---|---|
| Central nervous system | agenesis of the corpus callosum cerebellar malformation hydrocephalus |
| Head and neck | cleft palate laryngeal webs |
| Eyes | microphthalmia oblong pupils hazy/cloudy corneas/Peter anomaly aphakia |
| Endocrine | oncocytic collections in glands |
| Renal | cysts tubular calcifications |
| Ovary | hypoplasia, cysts |
| Cardiac | atrial septal defect ventricular septal defect left ventricular noncompaction endocardial fibroelastosis hypoplastic left heart syndrome |

The age range at presentation is birth to 4 years (mean, 10 to 13 months) (11,12,28). There is a female predominance of 4 to 1. The most common presenting feature is an arrhythmia, followed by sudden death (29–35), seizures, cyanosis, and dyspnea. Heart failure is uncommon but may necessitate transplantation (36).

The specific arrhythmias and conduction disturbances in patients with histiocytoid cardiomyopathy include ventricular tachycardia and fibrillation (19), supraventricular tachycardias, premature ventricular contractions, Wolff-Parkinson-White syndrome (9,37), heart block, and Lown-Ganong-Levine syndrome (Table 9-1) (38). The diagnosis is often made clinically, based on the finding in infants of incessant ventricular tachycardia (occurring 10 to 90 percent of the day), with or without other cardiac complications. These include cardiac arrest, often after digitalis administration for presumed supraventricular tachycardia; congestive heart failure; and Wolff-Parkinson-White syndrome. The rate of incessant ventricular tachycardia averages 260 beats/min with a QRS duration from 0.06 to 0.11 second. The most common electrocardiographic pattern (just under 50 percent) is right bundle branch block with left axis deviation, but other right and left bundle branch block patterns are observed (28).

Associated cardiac and extracardiac anomalies affect approximately 25 percent of patients (Table 9-2). These include atrial and ventricular septal defect, left ventricular noncompaction (22–24,39), hypoplastic left heart syndrome, endocardial fibroelastosis (30), ovarian cysts, midline defects of the central nervous system, malformations of the eyes, and oncocytic changes in glands (12). The association of noncompaction and histiocytoid cardiomyopathy has also been reported in a cat (40).

The diagnosis of histiocytoid cardiomyopathy is frequently made at autopsy in infants with sudden unexplained death, which clinically may resemble sudden infant death syndrome. In children with recurrent tachyarrhythmias, the diagnosis is suspected and confirmed by endomyocardial biopsy (11,21,41,42). In series of surgically excised heart tumors, histiocytoid cardiomyopathy represents less than 1 percent of cardiac tumors in children, with most series reporting none (42).

Jain and Chopra (25) reported a case of histiocytoid cardiomyopathy diagnosed in a fetus terminated for trisomy 21. In this case, the heart weight and gross findings were unremarkable, and the lesions were found histologically in the subendocardium of the ventricular septum.

## GROSS FINDINGS

At autopsy, the heart is almost always larger than expected, and usually there is significant cardiomegaly (Table 9-3). In over one third of cases, the heart is grossly normal, even with evaluation by dissecting microscope (43). There may be irregularities of the epicardial surface if there is involvement in this region (44). More commonly, there are endocardial nodules, typically at the base of the heart near the valves, that are raised and yellowish. Their size ranges from 1 mm to 1.5 cm, but lesions are usually smaller than 2 mm (fig. 9-1) (43,45). The left ventricle is always involved, but right ventricular and atrial nodules are also common. There is a predilection for subendocardial regions at the base of the ventricular septum.

## MICROSCOPIC FINDINGS

Histiocytoid cardiomyopathy is characterized by clusters of foamy cells that are well demarcated from the adjacent normal myocardium (figs. 9-2–9-7). There have been at least five reports of biopsy diagnosis, totaling 14 cases (11,27,41,42,46). In these cases, surgery was performed to resect endocardial nodules, subepicardial nodules, or both, at approximately equal frequencies.

Histiocytoid cardiomyopathy is usually a diagnosis made at autopsy. The tumors may be located anywhere in the heart, but typically endocardium, valves, and/or conduction system is involved (27,31,33,43). In a literature review,

it was found that one third of patients had nodules limited to the endocardium, epicardium, or valves, and in two thirds the lesions were dispersed throughout (12). Occasionally, the tumors result in atrioventricular and nodoventricular connections (31), sometimes referred to as Mahaim fibers (38), which may account for the supraventricular arrhythmias. The tumor nests have a propensity for the atrioventricular nodal region within the atrioventricular septum (fig. 9-3), but often do not involve the nodal fibers themselves (44).

### Table 9-3

**GROSS AND MICROSCOPIC FINDINGS, OF HISTIOCYTOID CARDIOMYOPATHY[a]**

| Finding | Frequency |
|---|---|
| **Gross Findings** | |
| Cardiomegaly | 61% |
| Grossly seen lesions | 60% |
| **Microscopic Findings** | |
| Endocardial lesions | 100% |
| Epicardial lesions | 63% |
| Conduction system involvement | 86% |
| Left ventricular involvement | 95% |
| Right ventricular involvement | 74% |
| Interventricular septal involvement | 57% |
| Valvular involvement | 49% |
| Inflammation | 53% |

[a]Data from 74 reported cases presented in references 12, 16, 17, 19, 23, 25, 26, 29–31, 33, 35, 36, 43–45, and 47; some data extracted from reviews in references 12 and 47.

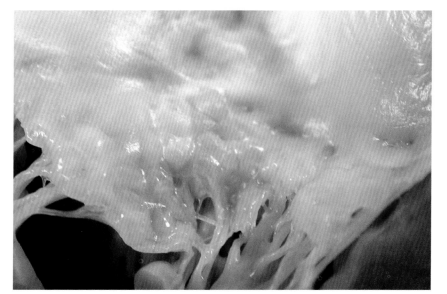

**Figure 9-1**

**HISTIOCYTOID CARDIOMYOPATHY**

A 22-month-old girl was found dead. There were multiple confluent brown-tan nodules, 1 to 2 mm in diameter, on the atrial surface of anterior mitral valve leaflet, of aggregate measurement 8 x 6 x 2 mm.

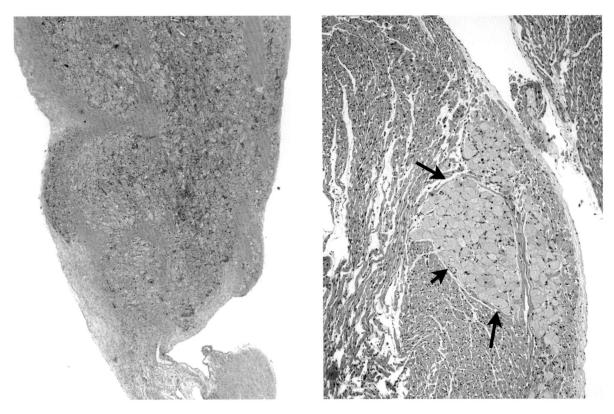

**Figure 9-2**

**HISTIOCYTOID CARDIOMYOPATHY**

Left: On low magnification, there is a vaguely nodular appearance to the myocytes under the valve annulus.
Right: At higher magnification of a different area, demarcated areas of cytoplasmic pallor (arrows) are seen.

**Figure 9-3**

**HISTIOCYTOID
CARDIOMYOPATHY**

The arrows surround an area
of tumor, which is located at the
crest of the ventricular septum
near the branching bundles.

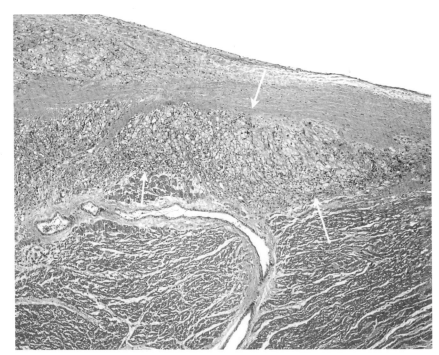

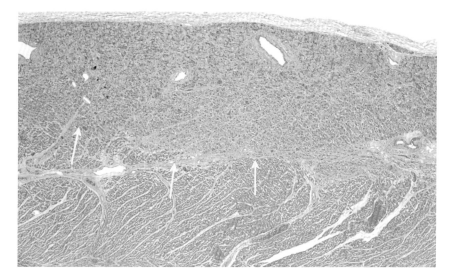

**Figure 9-4**

**HISTIOCYTOID CARDIOMYOPATHY**

The subendocardium is a common location for nests of histiocytoid cardiomyopathy. In this example of the endocardial area of the left ventricular outflow tract, there is a fairly discrete demarcation between normal myocardium and tumor (arrows).

**Figure 9-5**

**HISTIOCYTOID CARDIOMYOPATHY**

The demarcation between tumor and normal muscle is not distinct. At this magnification, an inflammatory process could not be excluded.

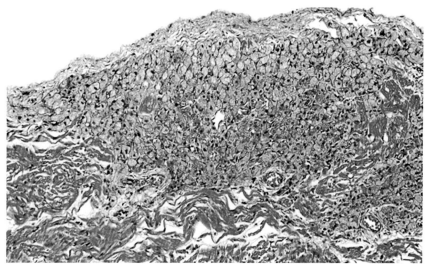

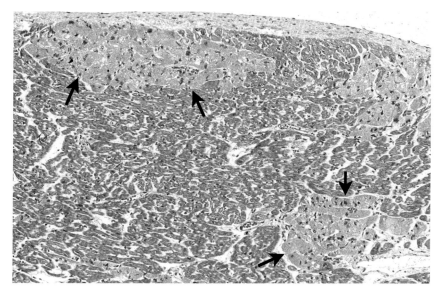

**Figure 9-6**

**HISTIOCYTOID CARDIOMYOPATHY: MULTIFOCAL**

There are multiple patches of pale myocytes (arrows).

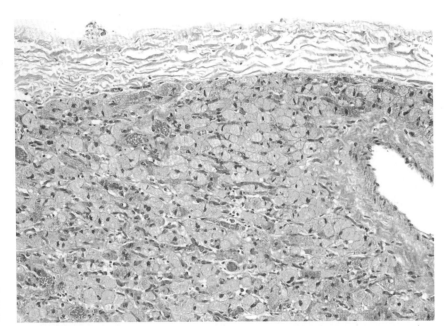

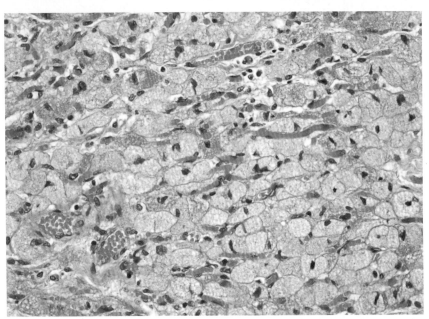

**Figure 9-7**

**HISTIOCYTOID CARDIOMYOPATHY**

Top: The myocytes are finely vacuolated. The process extends around a branch of coronary artery (incomplete section, right).

Bottom: At higher magnification, the fine vacuoles within the myocytes, which ultrastructurally correspond to mitochondria, have an epithelioid appearance.

The abnormal cells are large and pale, and rounded to oval (figs. 9-7–9-13). They are often surrounded by thin collagen fibers, and stain faintly with periodic acid–Schiff (PAS). Morphologically, there is a striking overlap with Purkinje cells (see fig. 1-17). In contrast to rhabdomyoma, large vacuoles and cytoplasmic streaming are absent (27). There may be a linear arrangement to the affected myocytes (figs. 9-14, 9-15). Associated endocardial fibroelastosis may also be present (fig. 9-16).

## IMMUNOHISTOCHEMICAL FINDINGS

By immunohistochemical techniques, the cells are negative for histiocytic markers, such as CD68, lysozyme, and alpha-1-antitrypsin (23,29,45) and positive for myoglobin, actin, desmin, and myosin (19,23,29,32,33,45). Ki-67 immunostaining shows no proliferative activity (33). Most studies show negative staining for S-100 protein (45). Terminal deoxynucleotidyl-transferase dUTP nick end labeling (TUNEL) has

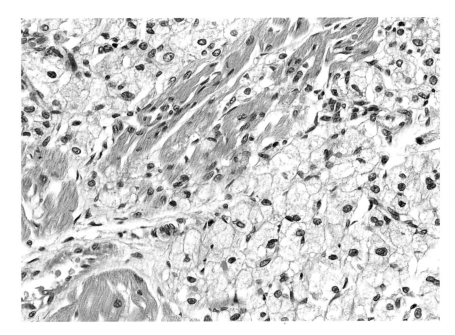

**Figure 9-8**

**HISTIOCYTOID CARDIOMYOPATHY**

The tumor cells look very much like histiocytes with interspersed cardiac muscle bundles.

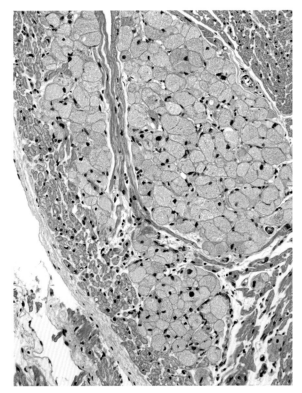

**Figure 9-9**

**HISTIOCYTOID CARDIOMYOPATHY**

Macrophage-like collections of myocytes have interspersed normal muscle.

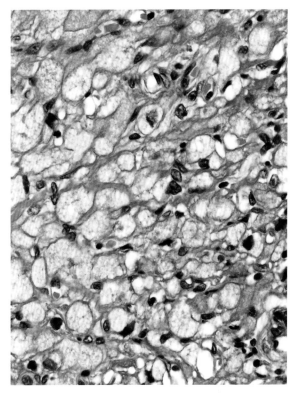

**Figure 9-10**

**HISTIOCYTOID CARDIOMYOPATHY**

A higher magnification of figure 9-5 demonstrates compressed tumor nuclei that may mimic lymphocytes, almost giving the impression of a lymphohistiocytic infiltrate. A sparse inflammatory reaction is reported in half of the cases of histiocytoid cardiomyopathy.

157

**Figure 9-11**

**HISTIOCYTOID CARDIOMYOPATHY**

At highest magnification, it can almost be appreciated that the finely vacuolated flocculent cytoplasm is caused by mitochondria.

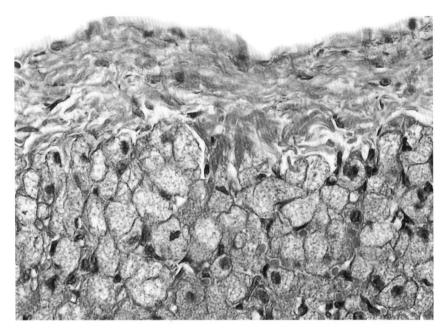

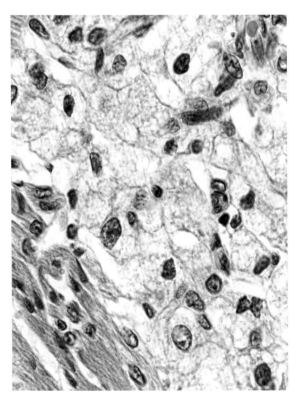

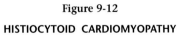

**Figure 9-12**

**HISTIOCYTOID CARDIOMYOPATHY**

In this example, which is a higher magnification of figure 9-8, the resemblance to macrophages is striking. If necessary, confirmatory immunohistochemical studies show positivity for muscle markers and negativity for CD68 and other histiocytic markers.

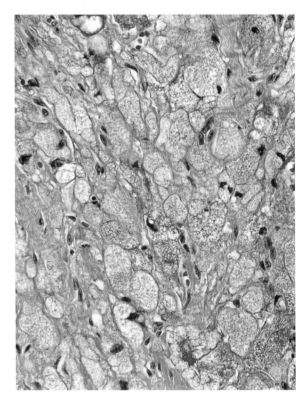

**Figure 9-13**

**HISTIOCYTOID CARDIOMYOPATHY**

The mitochondria are appreciated as fine intracellular vacuole-like spaces. There is a small amount of interstitial collagen.

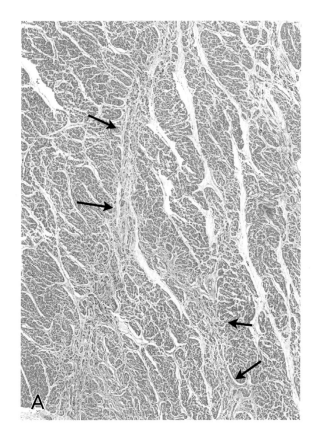

**Figure 9-14**

**HISTIOCYTOID CARDIOMYOPATHY**

A: As opposed to clusters or nodules, the tumor cells may be arranged in cords, sometimes resulting in nodo-ventricular or atrioventricular connections if present near the atrioventricular node. In this case, there were cords of cells in the myocardium of the ventricular septum (arrows).

B: A different area of the tumor shows an interstitial location.

C: Another area of the tumor shows sparse collagen fibers surrounding the tumor cells.

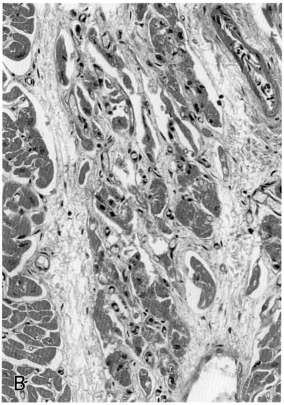

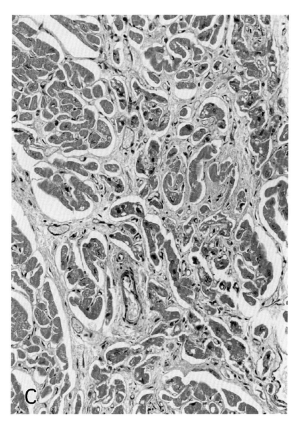

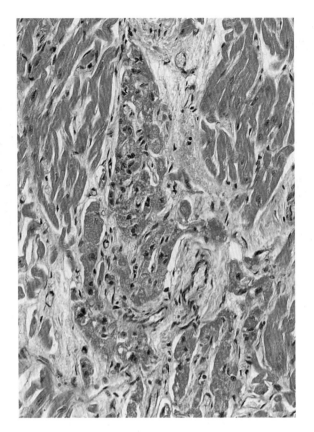

**Figure 9-15**

**HISTIOCYTOID CARDIOMYOPATHY**

The cells are smaller and less vacuolated than is typically seen. In other areas of the lesion the histologic appearance was more typical.

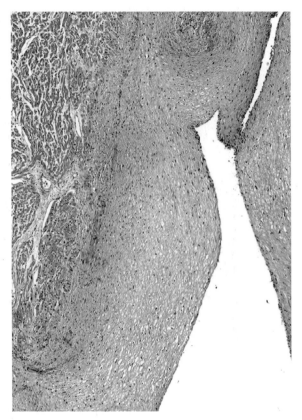

**Figure 9-16**

**HISTIOCYTOID CARDIOMYOPATHY: ENDOCARDIAL FIBROELASTOSIS**

The endocardium near the myocardium illustrated in figure 9-14A shows endocardial fibrosis, a nonspecific finding that may be secondary to heart failure.

shown that the tumor cells undergo apoptotic cell death (23). In one case, immunohistochemical staining for lymphocytes documented a sparse lymphocytic reaction (43), a finding that has been frequently reported based on light microscopic observations (12). One recent case interestingly found positivity for the skeletal muscle transcription factor MyoD1 (22).

## ULTRASTRUCTURAL FINDINGS

Histiocytoid cells have few or no myofibrils, marked mitochondriosis, an absence of T-tubules, limited numbers of desmosomes, rare intercalated discs, and occasional leptomeric fibers (12,20,32). Nonspecific findings such as fat, variable glycogen deposits, and leptomeric myofibrils have been reported, as well as poorly developed intercellular junctions (16,

19,33). Although the presence of increased mitochondria is a constant feature (fig. 9-17), it is unclear whether there are significant morphologic abnormalities (fig. 9-18) (19,32,47). Specifically, reported inclusions are similar to artifacts seen with suboptimal fixation and processing, and convincing cristal morphologic abnormalities have not been documented (16, 19,29,33,43,45,47).

The ultrastructural findings are similar to those of rhabdomyoma, except that in histiocytoid cardiomyopathy mitochondria are extremely numerous, glycogen is not significantly increased as in rhabdomyoma, and cellular junctions are less developed. The absence of T-tubules is characteristic of Purkinje cells; however, the lack of glycogenosis, lack of complex intercellular junctions with nexus formation,

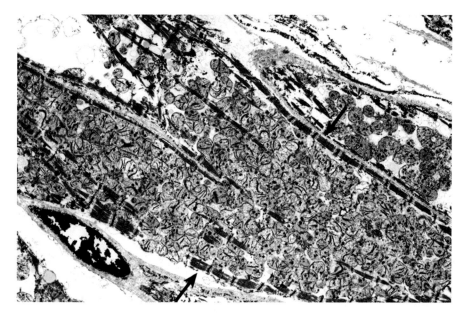

**Figure 9-17**

**HISTIOCYTOID CARDIOMYOPATHY**

Electron microscopy shows that the tumor cells contain abundant mitochondria, with only sparse myofibrils with Z-bands (arrows).

**Figure 9-18**

**HISTIOCYTOID CARDIOMYOPATHY**

By electron microscopy, the mitochondria show artifactual changes in the cristae, but giant mitochondria and cristal abnormalities are not seen.

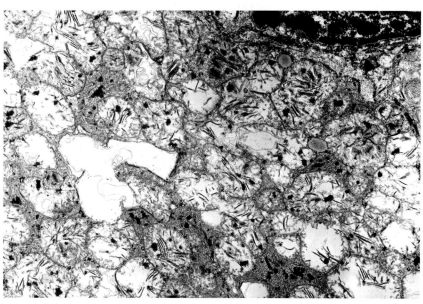

and increased mitochondria are not. The lack of T-tubules has been explained by the paucity of myofibrils, and does not necessarily indicate a Purkinje cell origin.

## MOLECULAR FINDINGS

A genetic basis for histiocytoid cardiomyopathy has been proposed, including both autosomal recessive (48) and X-linked (47) transmission. As noted above, mitochondrial mutations have been demonstrated (16,17,19). Recently, Shehata et al. (49) demonstrated that RNA and DNA extracted from paraffin sections of histiocytoid cardiomyopathy showed down-regulated genes in two clusters. The first included the genes *S100A8*, *S100A9*, and *S100A12* at 1q21.3c, and the second included genes *IL1RL1 (ST2)*, *IL18R1*, and *IL18RAP* at 2q12.1a. In addition, there was down-regulation of interleukin 33.

Most cases of histiocytoid cardiomyopathy are sporadic, indicating that there is no increased risk in subsequent pregnancies. However, histiocytoid cardiomyopathy has been reported in two sets of siblings (50).

## TREATMENT AND PROGNOSIS

In patients with refractory arrhythmias, electrophysiologic mapping with cryoablation or surgical excision has been successful in ameliorating symptoms (41,46). Although most cases present as cardiac arrest or sudden death, prolonged survival of up to 7 years has been achieved after surgical excision (46). In a series by Kearney et al. (27), the majority of children with surgically excised lesions were alive up to 30 months after treatment. Successful cardiac transplantation for heart failure has been reported (36).

## REFERENCES

1. Maron BJ, Towbin JA, Thiene G, et al. Contemporary definitions and classification of the cardiomyopathies: an American Heart Association Scientific Statement from the Council on Clinical Cardiology, Heart Failure and Transplantation Committee; Quality of Care and Outcomes Research and Functional Genomics and Translational Biology Interdisciplinary Working Groups; and Council on Epidemiology and Prevention. Circulation 2006;113:1807-1816.
2. Wegman ME, Egbert DS. Congenital rhabdomyoma of the heart associated with arrhythmia. J Pediatr 1935;10:818-824.
3. Voth D. [On arachnocytosis of the myocardium (a contribution to the problem of rhabdomyoma of the heart).] Frankf Z Pathol 1962;71:646-656. [German]
4. Olsen RE, Cooper RJ. Congenital nodular glycogenic degeneration of the myocardium. Am J Pathol 1941;17:125-128.
5. Batchelor TM, Maun ME. Congenital glycogenic tumors of the heart. Arch Pathol 1945;39:67-73.
6. Kidder LA. Congenital glycogenic tumors of the heart. AMA Arch Pathol 1950;49:55-62.
7. Sussman W, Stasney J. Congenital glycogenic tumor of the heart. Am Heart J 1950;40:312-315.
8. Reid JD, Hajdu SI, Attah E. Infantile cardiomyopathy: a previously unrecognized type with histiocytoid reaction. J Pediatr 1968;73:335-339.
9. Bruton D, Herdson PB, Becroft DM. Histiocytoid cardiomyopathy of infancy: an unexplained myofibre degeneration. Pathology 1977;9:115-122.
10. Zimmermann A, Diem P, Cottier H. Congenital "histiocytoid" cardiomyopathy: evidence suggesting a developmental disorder of the Purkinje cell system of the heart. Virchows Arch A Pathol Anat Histol 1982;396:187-195.
11. Gelb AB, Van Meter SH, Billingham ME, Berry GJ, Rouse RV. Infantile histiocytoid cardiomyopathy—myocardial or conduction system hamartoma: what is the cell type involved? Hum Pathol 1993;24:1226-1231.
12. Malhotra V, Ferrans VJ, Virmani R. Infantile histiocytoid cardiomyopathy: three cases and literature review. Am Heart J 1994;128:1009-1021.
13. Ferrans VJ, McAllister HA Jr, Haese WH. Infantile cardiomyopathy with histiocytoid change in cardiac muscle cells. Report of six patients. Circulation 1976;53:708-719.
14. Amini M, Bosman C, Marino B. Histiocytoid cardiomyopathy in infancy: a new hypothesis? Chest 1980;77:556-558.
15. Finsterer J. Histiocytoid cardiomyopathy: a mitochondrial disorder. Clin Cardiol 2008;31:225-227.
16. Vallance HD, Jeven G, Wallace DC, Brown MD. A case of sporadic infantile histiocytoid cardiomyopathy caused by the A8344G (MERRF) mitochondrial DNA mutation. Pediatr Cardiol 2004;25:538-540.
17. Andreu AL, Checcarelli N, Iwata S, Shanske S, DiMauro S. A missense mutation in the mitochondrial cytochrome b gene in a revisited case with histiocytoid cardiomyopathy. Pediatr Res 2000;48:311-314.
18. Kutsche K, Werner W, Bartsch O, von der Wense A, Meinecke P, Gal A. Microphthalmia with linear skin defects syndrome (MLS): a male with a mosaic paracentric inversion of Xp. Cytogenet Genome Res 2002;99:297-302.
19. Otani M, Hoshida H, Saji T, Matsuo N, Kawamura S. Histiocytoid cardiomyopathy with hypotonia in an infant. Pathol Int 1995;45:774-780.
20. Papadimitriou A, Neustein HB, Dimauro S, Stanton R, Bresolin N. Histiocytoid cardiomyopathy of infancy: deficiency of reducible cytochrome b in heart mitochondria. Pediatr Res 1984;18:1023-1028.
21. Labombarda F, Maragnes P, Jokic M, Jeanne-Pasquier C. [Sudden death due to histiocytoid cardiomyopathy.] Rev Esp Cardiol 2011;64:837-838. [Spanish]

22. Planas S, Ferreres JC, Balcells J, et al. Association of ventricular noncompaction and histiocytoid cardiomyopathy: case report and review of the literature. Pediatr Dev Pathol 2012;15:397-402.

23. Edston E, Perskvist N. Histiocytoid cardiomyopathy and ventricular non-compaction in a case of sudden death in a female infant. Int J Legal Med 2009;123:47-53.

24. Finsterer J, Stollberger C. Is mitochondrial disease the common cause of histiocytoid cardiomyopathy and non-compaction? Int J Legal Med 2009;123:507-508.

25. Jain D, Chopra P. Histiocytoid cardiomyopathy: does it exist in the fetal-age group? Cardiovasc Pathol 2011;20:386-387.

26. Coulibaly B, Piercecchi-Marti MD, Fernandez C, et al. [A rare cause of sudden cardiac failure: histiocytoid cardiomyopathy.] Ann Pathol 2011; 31:93-97. [French]

27. Kearney DL, Titus JL, Hawkins EP, Ott DA, Garson A Jr. Pathologic features of myocardial hamartomas causing childhood tachyarrhythmias. Circulation 1987;75:705-710.

28. Garson A Jr, Smith RT Jr, Moak JP, et al. Incessant ventricular tachycardia in infants: myocardial hamartomas and surgical cure. J Am Coll Cardiol 1987;10:619-626.

29. Boissy C, Chevallier A, Michiels JF, et al. Histiocytoid cardiomyopathy: a cause of sudden death in infancy. Pathol Res Pract 1997;193:589-593; discussion 595-586.

30. Grech V, Ellul B, Montalto SA. Sudden cardiac death in infancy due to histiocytoid cardiomyopathy. Cardiol Young 2000;10:49-51.

31. Koponen MA, Siegel RJ. Histiocytoid cardiomyopathy and sudden death. Hum Pathol 1996; 27:420-423.

32. Prahlow JA, Teot LA. Histiocytoid cardiomyopathy: case report and literature review. J Forensic Sci 1993;38:1427-1435.

33. Ruszkiewicz AR, Vernon-Roberts E. Sudden death in an infant due to histiocytoid cardiomyopathy. A light-microscopic, ultrastructural, and immunohistochemical study. Am J Forensic Med Pathol 1995;16:74-80.

34. Saffitz JE, Ferrans VJ, Rodriguez ER, Lewis FR, Roberts WC. Histiocytoid cardiomyopathy: a cause of sudden death in apparently healthy infants. Am J Cardiol 1983;52:215-217.

35. Aksglaede L, Graem N, Jacobsen JR. [Histiocytoid cardiomyopathy. A rare cause of ventricular tachycardia and sudden cardiac death in small children.] Ugeskr Laeger 2006;168:61-62. [Danish]

36. Zangwill SD, Trost BA, Zlotocha J, Tweddell JS, Jaquiss RD, Berger S. Orthotopic heart transplantation in a child with histiocytoid cardiomyopathy. J Heart Lung Transplant 2004;23:902-904.

37. Cabana MD, Becher O, Smith A. Histiocytoid cardiomyopathy presenting with Wolff-Parkinson-White syndrome. Heart 2000;83:98-99.

38. Rossi L, Piffer R, Turolla E, Frigerio B, Coumel P, James TN. Multifocal Purkinje-like tumor of the heart. Occurrence with other anatomic abnormalities in the atrioventricular junction of an infant with junctional tachycardia, Lown-Ganong-Levine syndrome, and sudden death. Chest 1985;87:340-345.

39. Burke A, Mont E, Kutys R, Virmani R. Left ventricular noncompaction: a pathological study of 14 cases. Hum Pathol 2005;36:403-411.

40. Gelberg HB. Purkinje fiber dysplasia (histiocytoid cardiomyopathy) with ventricular noncompaction in a savannah kitten. Vet Pathol 2009;46: 693-697.

41. Ott DA, Garson A Jr, Cooley DA, Smith RT, Moak J. Cryoablative techniques in the treatment of cardiac tachyarrhythmias. Ann Thorac Surg 1987;43:138-143.

42. Tazelaar HD, Locke TJ, McGregor CG. Pathology of surgically excised primary cardiac tumors. Mayo Clin Proc 1992;67:957-965.

43. Heifetz SA, Faught PR, Bauman M. Pathological case of the month. Histiocytoid (oncocytic) cardiomyopathy. Arch Pediatr Adolesc Med 1995; 149:464-465.

44. Ottaviani G, Matturri L, Rossi L, Lavezzi AM, James TN. Multifocal cardiac Purkinje cell tumor in infancy. Europace 2004;6:138-141.

45. Baillie T, Chan YF, Koelmeyer TD, Cluroe AD. Test and teach. Ill-defined subendocardial nodules in an infant. Histiocytoid cardiomyopathy. Pathology 2001;33:230-234.

46. McGregor CG, Gibson A, Caves P. Infantile cardiomyopathy with histiocytoid change in cardiac muscle cells: successful surgical intervention and prolonged survival. Am J Cardiol 1984; 53:982-983.

47. Shehata BM, Patterson K, Thomas JE, Scala-Barnett D, Dasu S, Robinson HB. Histiocytoid cardiomyopathy: three new cases and a review of the literature. Pediatr Dev Pathol 1998;1:56-69.

48. Gilbert-Barness E. Review: metabolic cardiomyopathy and conduction system defects in children. Ann Clin Lab Sci 2004;34:15-34.

49. Shehata BM, Bouzyk M, Shulman SC, et al. Identification of candidate genes for histiocytoid cardiomyopathy (HC) using whole genome expression analysis: analyzing material from the hc registry. Pediatr Dev Pathol 2011;14:370-377.

50. Suarez V, Fuggle WJ, Cameron AH, French TA, Hollingworth T. Foamy myocardial transformation of infancy: an inherited disease. J Clin Pathol 1987;40:329-334.

# 10 CARDIAC HEMANGIOMA AND LYMPHANGIOMA

## HEMANGIOMA

**Definition.** *Hemangiomas* are benign tumors of blood vessels that resemble capillaries (*capillary hemangioma*), dilated capillary-like channels (*cavernous hemangioma*), or dysplastic malformed arteries and veins (*arteriovenous hemangioma* or *malformation*). The tumor cells may have abundant cytoplasm (epithelioid or histiocytoid features). *Epithelioid hemangioma* and *epithelioid hemangioendothelioma* are separate and distinct entities, the former reactive and the latter a low-grade sarcoma.

**General Features.** Hemangiomas have some features of malformations and neoplasms. Although they may recur, especially after incomplete resection (1), they do not behave aggressively, and may regress after anti-inflammatory treatment (2). A subset of cardiac hemangiomas demonstrates the histologic features of intramuscular hemangiomas of skeletal muscle, suggesting that some cardiac hemangiomas and intramuscular hemangiomas are related lesions.

Hemangiomas of the heart and pericardium are rare: fewer than 200 cases have been reported to date, with about 100 in the last decade. As recently as 1993, only 23 cases had been reported (3). In series of resected tumors, 0 to 20 percent of tumors in children are hemangiomas (4–9), with a similar frequency in adults (8,10–14).

**Clinical Features.** Cardiac hemangiomas occur in patients of all ages, from newborns (7,15) to the seventh decade (7,15,16). Approximately 10 percent occur in children, and 10 percent are diagnosed in utero or in infants (Table 10-1). The mean age at diagnosis is during the fifth and sixth decades (17,18–21). There have been several reviews of cardiac hemangioma (17,22–24). There is a small male predominance.

In adults, hemangiomas are often diagnosed as incidental findings, after abnormalities in screening electrocardiograms, chest X rays, or preoperative echocardiograms are noted (23,25–31). Many patients present with palpitations or syncopal episodes (32–37). Specific rhythm disturbances attributed to cardiac hemangiomas include complete atrioventricular block (38,39), paroxysmal atrial fibrillation (40), ventricular tachycardia (41–43) and supraventricular tachycardia (44,45). Other symptoms may be related to pericardial effusions (46–50) and congestive heart failure (6,17,51–53). When in the ventricles, there may be symptoms related to left or right outflow tract obstruction (54–56). Anginal chest pain secondary to coronary insufficiency has been reported (57,58). Two patients with cardiac hemangioma and embolization, to the coronary and cerebral circulation (57) and to the brain alone (59) have been reported. Occasionally, the presenting symptom is sudden cardiac death (24,60,61) or sudden onset heart failure with cardiovascular collapse (62). Hemangiomas causing sudden cardiac death generally cause conduction disturbances in the heart, and may be located in the region of the atrioventricular node or in close association with the coronary arteries (24,60–63). There has been a report of cardiac hemangioma causing palpitations during pregnancy (34), and a report of recurrent pericardial tamponade from an atrial hemangioma (64).

There is an occasional association of cardiac hemangiomas with extracardiac hemangiomas of the gastrointestinal tract (21) and port wine stain of the face (65). Giant cardiac hemangiomas may result in thrombosis and coagulopathies (Kasabach-Merritt syndrome) (66,67).

In children, cardiac hemangiomas result in symptoms similar to those of adults, including ventricular tachycardia (42), syncope (68), and dyspnea on exertion (69). In a series of pediatric heart tumors with tissue diagnosis, 3 of 26 were hemangiomas (6). Cardiac hemangiomas in children occur in all cardiac chambers, and may cause right ventricular outflow tract obstruction (42,70) or are mobile, pedunculated tumors within the ventricular cavity (68).

There are increasing reports of intrauterine or neonatal diagnosis of cardiac hemangioma

**Table 10-1**

**CLINICAL AND PATHOLOGIC FINDINGS OF CARDIAC HEMANGIOMA[a]**

| Finding | Infants and Fetuses (n=10) | Children (n=10) | Adults (n=81) |
|---|---|---|---|
| Male:female | 5:3 (2 not stated) | 5:5 | 45:35 |
| Age (range) | 7 in utero<br>1 newborn<br>2 and 7 months | mean, 11 (4-16) | 52 (20-86) |
| Procedure | Resections 6<br>Incomplete resections 2<br>Biopsies 2 | Resection 7<br>Biopsy 2<br>Biopsy, subsequent resection 1 | Resection 79<br>Biopsy and subsequent resection 1<br>Autopsy 1 |
| Site | RA[b] 6<br>Pericardium 2<br>RA pericardium 1<br>LV lateral wall 1 | RV 4<br>RV 2<br>LV 2<br>MV 1<br>LA 1 | LV 24<br>RA 14<br>Valves 14[c]<br>LA 14<br>RV 7<br>IAS 5<br>VS 1<br>Biatrial 1<br>Pericardium 3[d] |
| Clinical features[e] | Prenatal effusions 4<br>Prenatal effusion with impending tamponade 2<br>Effusion with early hydrops 1<br>Prenatal effusion with RA mass 1<br>Neonatal cyanosis and tachypnea 1<br>Fever 2 | Incidental (asymptomatic) 2<br>Syncope, ventricular tachycardia 2<br>Murmur 3<br>Palpitations 2<br>Dyspnea on exertion 1<br>Angina 1<br>Pericardial effusion 1 | Asymptomatic 44%<br>Dyspnea, SOB 32%<br>Chest pain 22%<br>Palpitations 19%<br>Dysrhythmia 12%[f]<br>Syncope 7%<br>Symptomatic pericardial effusion 4%[g]<br>Cerebral ischemia 4% |
| Size in cm, range | 2.7, 1.9 – 3; 5 cases not stated | 2.5, 1 – 4.5; 3 cases not stated | 4.5, 0.8 – 13; 12 cases not stated |
| Gross findings | Infiltrative 4<br>Discrete 3<br>Not stated 3 | Discrete endocardial mass 3<br>Exophytic with stalk 1<br>Infiltrative 2<br>Not stated 4 | Endocardial 74%<br>Endocardial with stalk 6%<br>Endocardial with infiltrating base 2%<br>Predominantly infiltrating 11% |
| Microscopic type | Capillary 3<br>Cavernous 3<br>Hemangioendothelioma 1<br>Not stated 3 | Capillary 2<br>Capillary-cavernous 1<br>Cavernous 1<br>Not stated 6 | Cavernous 43%<br>Capillary 11%<br>Mixed 21%<br>Arteriovenous malformation 5%<br>Intramuscular 8%[h] |

[a]101 recently reported cardiac hemangiomas, 2000-2012. Data from references of fetal and infantile cardiac hemangiomas (2,15,22,48,71–75,82,134), childhood hemangiomas (6,14,42,68–70,82,131,132), and adult hemangiomas (1,14,17,23–26,28–39,41,43–45,49,53,55,57,62,64,76,77,79,83,85,86,88,89,91,96,97,99,100–104,106–108,110–112,124,126,128,155–162).
[b]RA = right atrium; LA = left atrium; LV = left ventricle; RV = right ventricle; MV = mitral valve; IAS = interatrial septum; VS = ventricular septum; SOB = shortness of breath.
[c]6 mitral, 5 tricuspid, 2 aortic, 1 pulmonic.
[d]Also with atrial or ventricular involvement.
[e]Multiple symptoms may overlap among patients; data available in 76 adult patients.
[f]3 supraventricular tachycardia, 2 atrioventricular block, 3 ventricular tachycardia, 1 new onset atrial fibrillation.
[g]Seen only in left and right atrial tumors.
[h]Seen only in left ventricular tumors.

(46–50). Fetal echocardiography may demonstrate the tumor mass (71). In neonates, the diagnosis is usually suspected based on pericardial effusion on fetal sonography (49,71–73).

In infants and children, the finding of a hemangioma may raise the possibility of a systemic syndrome. In most reported cases of infantile cardiac hemangioma, there are no extracardiac lesions, however. In neonates, most cardiac hemangiomas occur in the right atrium or pericardium (15,71–75). Although infantile hemangiomatosis often results in heart failure, cardiac involvement by a vascular tumor is rare (52). Hepatic hemangiomas have been found in adults with cardiac hemangioma (76,77), but there is a high prevalence of vascular liver tumors.

Most cardiac hemangiomas are diagnosed as a cardiac mass based on transthoracic echocardiography. Echocardiography is a sensitive, noninvasive method for detecting cardiac masses, including hemangiomas (17,53,57,61,78–80). Often, transesophageal echocardiograms, typically during surgery, help pinpoint the extent and location of the mass. Cardiac magnetic resonance imaging (MRI) may suggest the diagnosis of hemangioma based on an intermediate or increased signal on T1-weighted images, and a high signal on T2-weighted images (43,75,81). A T2-weighted spin echo sequence is useful for distinguishing vascular tumors, such as hemangiomas, from avascular tumors, such as fibromas (82). The lack of signal homogeneity, with diffuse echodensities on echocardiograms, is also characteristic (83). An angiogram typically demonstrates tumor "blush" from feeder vessels (84–86), but this finding is not always present (49).

The specific diagnosis of hemangioma is made preoperatively by cardiac catheterization (87) and prenatally by ultrasound. More recently FDG (fludeoxyglucose)positron emission tomography (PET)/computerized tomography (CT) has been added as a valuable imaging method for detecting and evaluating cardiac masses; hemangiomas as vascular tumors are readily identifiable and mediastinal disease is excluded (69,88,89). Due to a higher spatial resolution and multiple images of very thin sliced thickness, MRI is currently much more precise in locating cardiac masses than echocardiography (89).

Endoluminal hemangiomas that are attached to the endocardium by a stalk may appear as mobile masses on echocardiography (23,90–92).

**Gross Findings.** Hemangiomas may occur in any location in the heart (Table 10-1). Of 45 cases (20,21), 15 were located in the atria, 12 in the left ventricle or ventricular septum, 11 in the right ventricle, 6 in the pericardium or on the epicardium, and 1 on the mitral valve. Hemangiomas of the heart range in size from less than 1 cm to 8 cm or larger (20). A tumor with a maximum dimension of 13 cm has been reported (93).

Approximately 80 percent of cardiac hemangiomas are endoluminal tumors (figs. 10-1–10-3) that are frequently described as circumscribed or even "encapsulated" by surgeons (64,76,77,86,92). A "hemangioma" of the tricuspid valve that has been illustrated as a circumscribed, demarcated blue dome, is likely a large blood cyst (94). Some cardiac hemangiomas are infiltrative (fig. 10-4) and extend transmurally through the ventricular wall into the epicardium (45).

Upon palpation, hemangiomas are often described as "spongy," most of which are of the cavernous histologic subtype (84,95–97).

**Microscopic Findings.** Although there is overlap, the primary histologic patterns of hemangioma are *capillary, cavernous, arteriovenous,* and *epithelioid* (98). In the heart, the most frequent type is cavernous, followed by mixed cavernous-capillary and capillary (Table 10-1).

The histologic appearance of cardiac hemangioma is similar to that of extracardiac hemangioma. Cavernous hemangiomas are composed of thin- or thick-walled capillary or venous structures filled with blood, and are more likely mural tumors (figs. 10-5–10-10). In contrast, capillary hemangiomas are composed of lobules of endothelial cells, with scattered pericytes and fibroblasts (figs. 10-11–10-13). There may be open capillary lumens, especially at the periphery of the tumor, and cavernous and capillary channels may coexist (figs. 10-14–10-18). There are no clinical differences in capillary, cavernous, or mixed tumors, and the designation is often somewhat arbitrary.

In approximately 10 percent of cardiac hemangiomas, there are areas of dysplastic, irregularly thickened arterial and venous structures, typical of arteriovenous malformations, or *arteriovenous hemangiomas* (figs. 10-19–10-23). These hemangiomas are mural tumors that are likely to be poorly circumscribed. Histologically, they may contain fibrous tissue and fat, have areas indistinguishable from capillary hemangioma, and be similar in appearance to intramuscular hemangiomas of skeletal muscle.

Cardiac hemangiomas with adipocytes similar to intramuscular hemangiomas have been reported infrequently (21,81,99,100). Intramuscular cardiac hemangiomas are uncommon (41,101,102), and all have been reported in the left ventricle or interventricular septum. Those

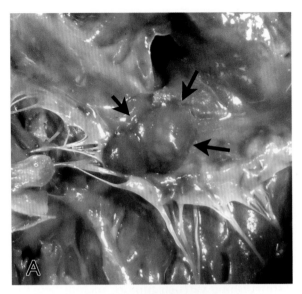

**Figure 10-1**

**CARDIAC HEMANGIOMA: TRICUSPID VALVE**

A: The finding was unexpected at autopsy. Echocardiogram and cardiac magnetic resonance imaging (MRI) performed for the evaluation of cardiomyopathy shortly before death demonstrated thickening of the valve. There is a nodule on the surface of the septal leaflet toward the annulus (arrows). The coronary sinus is above.

B: A cross section shows the atrial septum and the valve leaflet, with a nodule on the surface of the leaflet.

C: A subgross histologic section is seen.

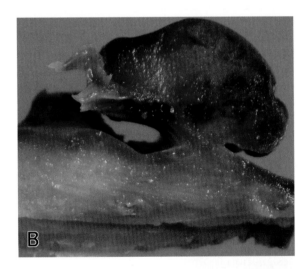

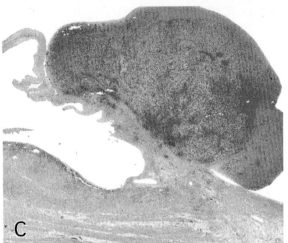

**Figure 10-2**

**CARDIAC HEMANGIOMA**

The tumor is lobulated and circumscribed. Cardiac hemangiomas are often spongy to palpation, as this was. The tumor was endocardial based and removed from the right ventricle.

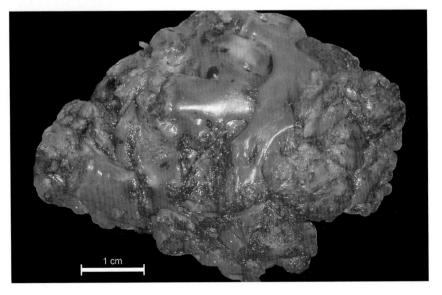

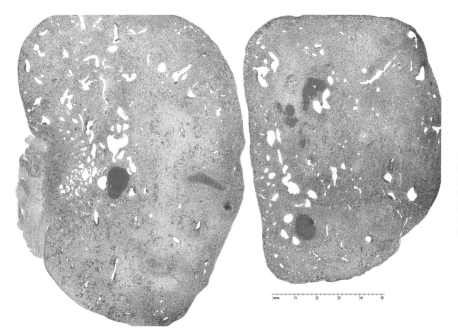

**Figure 10-3**

**CARDIAC HEMANGIOMA**

A subgross histologic section of the a right atrial mass found incidentally in a 70-year old man. Most cardiac hemangiomas are endocardial-based tumors that are sessile or pedunculated, and amenable to resection.

**Figure 10-4**

**CARDIAC HEMANGIOMA: INTRAMURAL**

Some cardiac hemangiomas are intramuscular; these are seldom excised surgically.

Inset: There is an irregular area of scarring, corresponding to blue staining with the Masson trichrome stain.

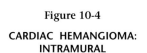

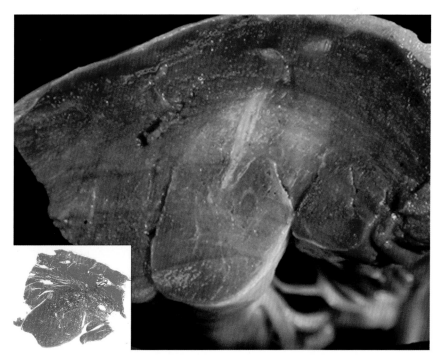

with venous vessels (59,64,103,104) are more frequent in the right ventricle or right atrium.

Right atrial hemangiomas may be diagnostically challenging because the trabeculations of the atrial wall may be lined with tumor cells, and the distinction from organizing thrombus difficult (fig. 10-24). A similar problem may occur in the left atrium, although the endocardial surface is generally smoother (fig. 10-25). Inflammation is frequent in cardiac hemangiomas (fig. 10-26), especially those in children, and may account for the response to anti-inflammatory treatment (20,49,77).

The tumor cells of hemangiomas, especially capillary tumors with a more crowded growth pattern, may possess abundant cytoplasm. This

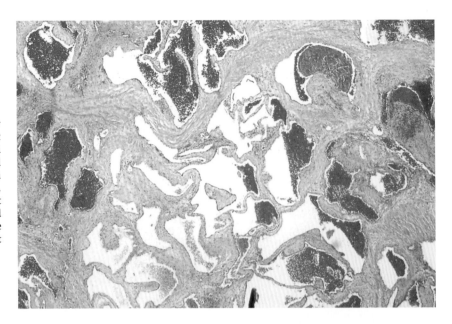

**Figure 10-5**

**CARDIAC HEMANGIOMA: CAVERNOUS TYPE**

Dilated channels are partly filled with blood. The patient was a middle-aged man with a heart murmur. Transesophageal echocardiogram showed a 3-cm mass in the interatrial septum, extending into right atrium; it measured 5 cm on chest computed tomography (CT). At surgery, the mass was immediately adjacent to the sinoatrial node.

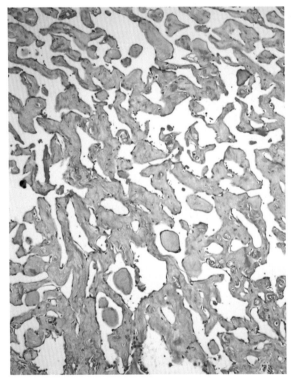

**Figure 10-6**

**CARDIAC HEMANGIOMA: CAVERNOUS TYPE**

There are dilated and anastomosing channels. The patient was a middle-aged male with a 3 x 3 x 5-cm mass centered in the atrial septum and extending into both atria, as seen on CT.

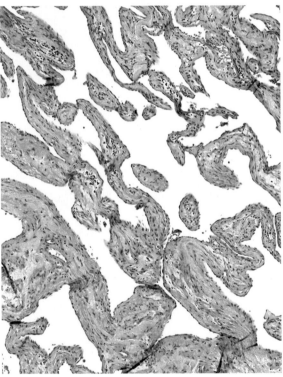

**Figure 10-7**

**CARDIAC HEMANGIOMA: CAVERNOUS TYPE**

An elderly woman with iron deficiency anemia and weight loss was found to have cardiomegaly on chest X ray; the echocardiogram showed a large mass in the left atrium deforming the interatrial septum and protruding into the right atrium. At surgery, a 10-cm circumscribed mass was removed "like a large egg" per surgical report. There are dilated and anastomosing channels.

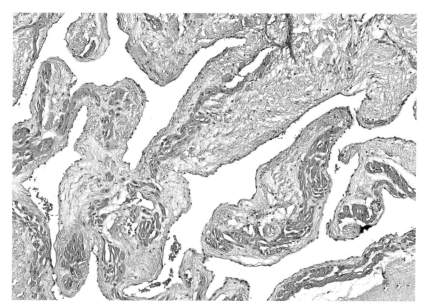

**Figure 10-8**

**CARDIAC HEMANGIOMA: WITH INTERSPERSED CARDIAC MUSCLE**

The patient was a 19-year-old man who died from presumed drowning. A 3-cm mass was found in the interventricular septum near the atrioventricular node. The tumor is formed by dilated channels with intervening cardiac muscle, typical of infiltrating intramuscular cardiac hemangiomas of the left ventricle and ventricular septum.

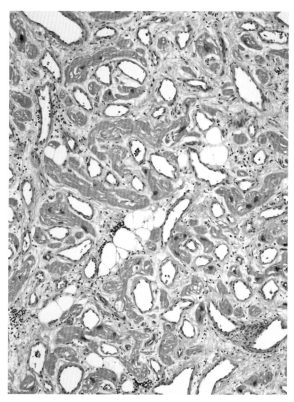

**Figure 10-9**

**CARDIAC HEMANGIOMA: WITH INTERSPERSED CARDIAC MUSCLE**

A 59-year-old man with coronary artery disease underwent bypass grafting. Prior to surgery, a right ventricular tumor was noted on angiography, with a tumor "blush" in the right ventricle near the apex. The tumor, measuring 3 x 2.5 x 2 cm, was partly removed.

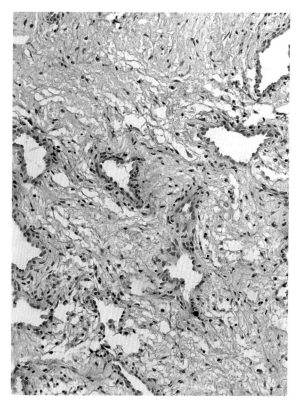

**Figure 10-10**

**CARDIAC HEMANGIOMA: CAVERNOUS, WITH MYXOID STROMA**

A 3-year-old girl had a left atrial tumor partly excised shortly after birth, after presenting with pericardial effusion. The repeat resection showed a vascular tumor with a bland myxoid stroma.

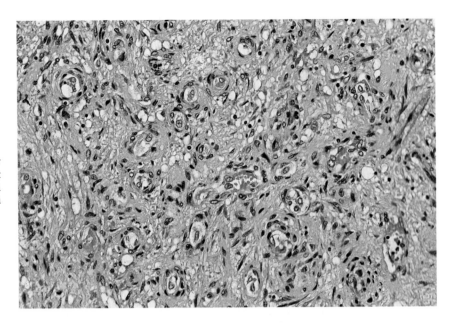

**Figure 10-11**

**CARDIAC HEMANGIOMA: CAPILLARY TYPE**

The tumor was predominantly of capillary type, with prominent pericytes. The tumor is shown grossly and at low magnification in figure 10-1.

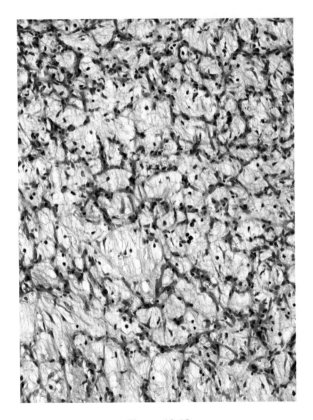
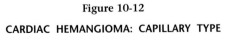

**Figure 10-12**

**CARDIAC HEMANGIOMA: CAPILLARY TYPE**

A 73-year-old man with aortic stenosis and coronary artery disease underwent valve replacement and bypass grafting. The preoperative angiogram and echocardiogram demonstrated a left ventricular endoluminal mass near the cardiac apex. The tumor has a prominent myxoid matrix.

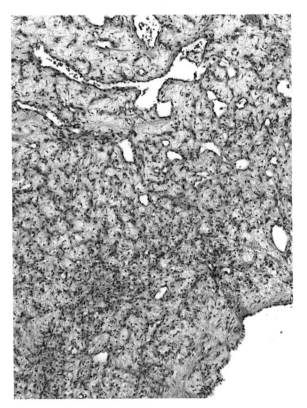

**Figure 10-13**

**CARDIAC HEMANGIOMA: CAPILLARY TYPE**

There is a myxoid background, and a sparse chronic inflammatory infiltrate.

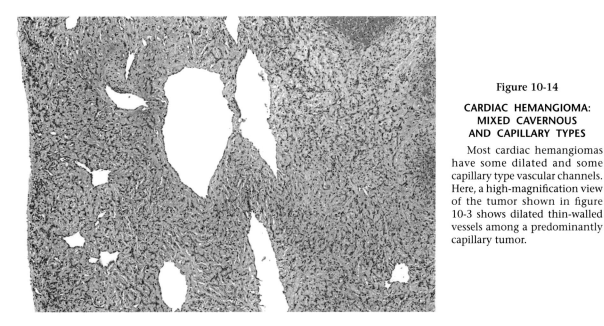

**Figure 10-14**

**CARDIAC HEMANGIOMA: MIXED CAVERNOUS AND CAPILLARY TYPES**

Most cardiac hemangiomas have some dilated and some capillary type vascular channels. Here, a high-magnification view of the tumor shown in figure 10-3 shows dilated thin-walled vessels among a predominantly capillary tumor.

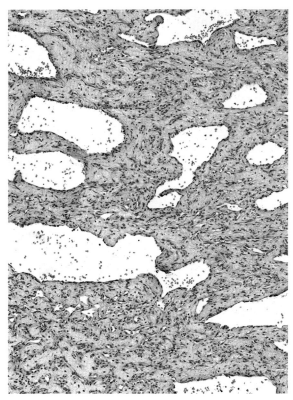

**Figure 10-15**

**CARDIAC HEMANGIOMA: MIXED CAVERNOUS AND CAPILLARY TYPE**

The tumor was removed from the left ventricular outflow tract of a young pregnant woman with Marfan syndrome.

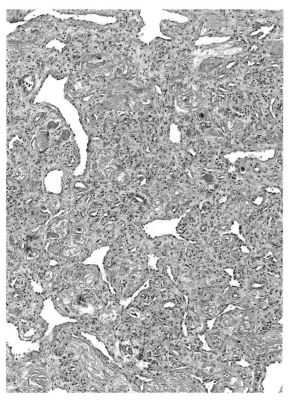

**Figure 10-16**

**CARDIAC HEMANGIOMA: MIXED CAVERNOUS AND CAPILLARY TYPE**

The tumor infiltrating cardiac muscle was surgically resected from a young man, who had a mass discovered in the posterior interventricular septum after complaining of palpitations.

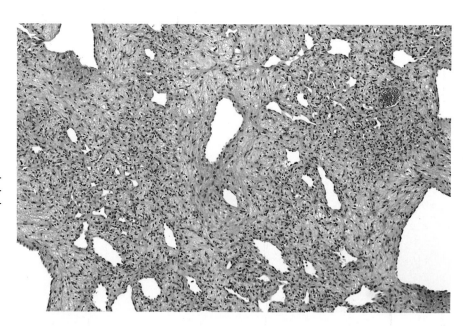

**Figure 10-17**

**CARDIAC HEMANGIOMA: MIXED CAVERNOUS AND CAPILLARY TYPE**

Dilated thin-walled channels are interspersed in a background of capillary hemangioma.

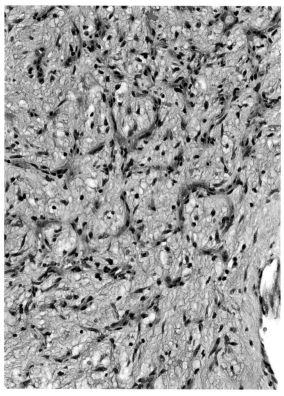

**Figure 10-18**

**CARDIAC HEMANGIOMA: MIXED CAVERNOUS AND CAPILLARY TYPE**

In most cases of cardiac hemangioma, there is a prominent pericytic component surrounding the capillary vascular channels. This finding contrasts starkly with cardiac myxoma, which may share a myxoid background with hemangioma, but which lacks well-formed vascular channels.

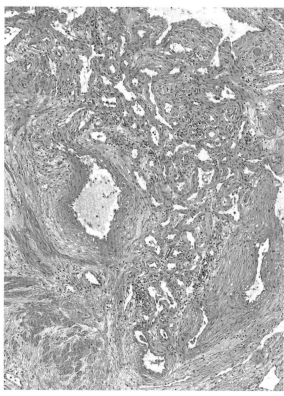

**Figure 10-19**

**CARDIAC HEMANGIOMA: INTRAMUSCULAR WITH ARTERIOVENOUS FEATURES**

There are vessels of various sizes, some with prominent media. The patient was a middle-aged woman with a mass noted on chest X ray; the mass had recently enlarged.

characteristic has been designated "epithelioid" or "histiocytoid," and is more frequent in pediatric hemangiomas (21,73,83,105). The term "hemangioendothelioma" has also been used for angiomas with abundant cytoplasm (22), but should not be confused with "epithelioid hemangioendothelioma," a low-grade angiosarcoma.

**Immunohistochemical Findings.** Many studies have supported the endothelial nature of hemangioma with the demonstration of vessels expressing endothelial markers (CD31, CD34, factor VIII, and lectins) (figs. 10-28, 10-29) (23,94,106–112). These markers, however, are not helpful in diagnosis, as capillaries are present in a variety of tumors, including myxomas. More helpful for diagnosis, and far less frequently documented, is the presence of actin-positive pericytes, the presence of which differentiates hemangioma from myxoma (fig. 10-30) (41,70,108). Immunohistochemical stains usually are not necessary for diagnosis, unless the distinction from myxoma, in endocardial myxoid hemangioma, is needed.

**Differential Diagnosis.** Cardiac hemangioma is rarely misdiagnosed histologically. There are two main entities in the differential diagnosis: myxoma and angiosarcoma. Intracavitary cardiac hemangiomas may possess a myxoid background, and the erroneous diagnosis of myxoma may be made. There are no myxoma cells or ring structures in cardiac hemangioma,

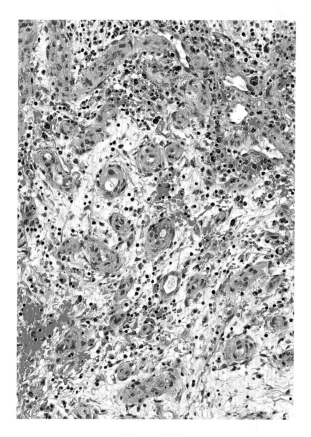

**Figure 10-20**

**CARDIAC HEMANGIOMA: EPITHELIOID FEATURES**

Many of the vessels are composed of endothelial cells with abundant cytoplasm. The tumor was removed from the right atrium of a 12-year-old boy.

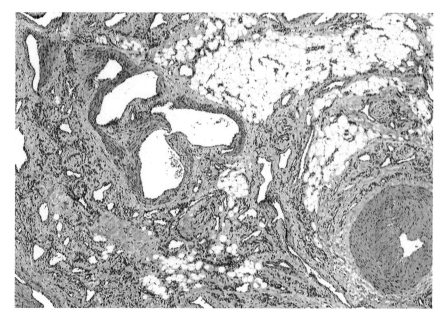

**Figure 10-21**

**CARDIAC HEMANGIOMA: INFILTRATING INTRAMUSCULAR TYPE**

In some cardiac hemangiomas involving the left ventricle or interventricular septum, the histologic appearance resembles that of intramuscular hemangioma of skeletal muscle, with fat and polymorphous vascular channels that range from larger arterial-like vessels to capillaries. (Fig. 4.16 from Tazelaar H, Burke AP, Wantanabe G, Basson T. Haemangioma. In: WHO classification of tumours, pathology and genetics of tumours of the lung, pleura, thymus and heart. Lyon: IARC Press, Lyon 2004:267.)

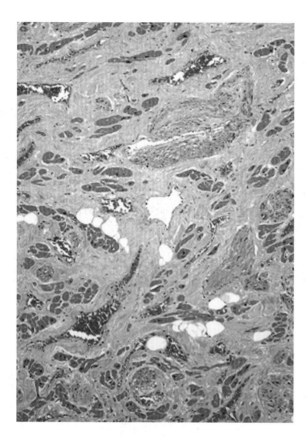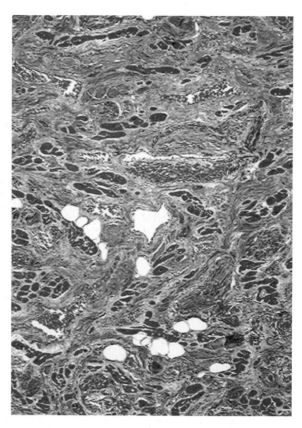

**Figure 10-22**

**CARDIAC HEMANGIOMA: INFILTRATING INTRAMUSCULAR TYPE**

Left: A middle-aged man was found dead sitting in a chair. At autopsy, there was no explanation for the death other than a poorly circumscribed mass in the anterior left ventricle. Histologically, the tumor consisted of thick walled vessels, collagen, and some adipocytes.

Right: A Masson trichrome stain shows the collagen in the tumor.

**Figure 10-23**

**CARDIAC HEMANGIOMA: ARTERIOVENOUS TYPE**

This tumor was excised from a man who presented with angina. A transthoracic echocardiogram showed a tumor near the mitral annulus at the posterior junction of the anterior and posterior leaflets. The mitral valve was repaired without need for replacement. A Movat pentachrome stain demonstrates irregular thick-walled vessels that resemble dysplastic arteries.

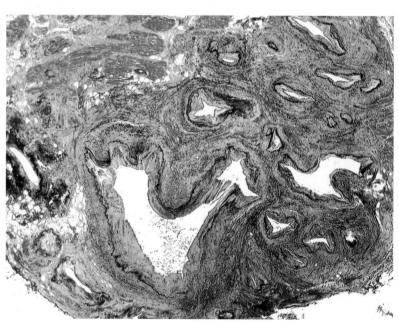

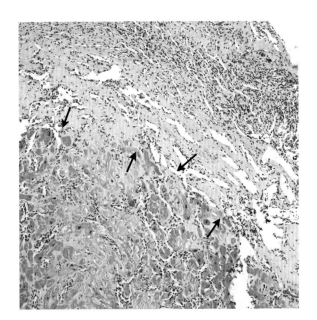
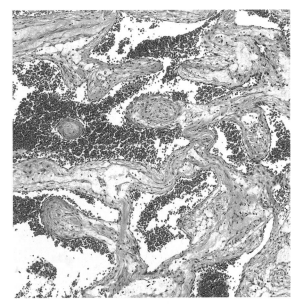

**Figure 10-24**

**CARDIAC HEMANGIOMA**

Left: This right atrial tumor is endoluminal, with a sparse collagen background (upper right). It infiltrates the atrial muscle (bottom left). The junction of the two growth patterns is demarcated by arrows. The patient was a 24-year-old man who presented with a cerebrovascular accident and presumed atrial thrombus by imaging.

Right: Anastomosing channels are lined by endothelial cells within cardiac muscle. The pattern can be difficult to distinguish from anastomosing trabeculations in the atrial appendage.

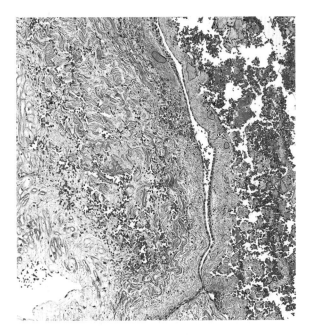
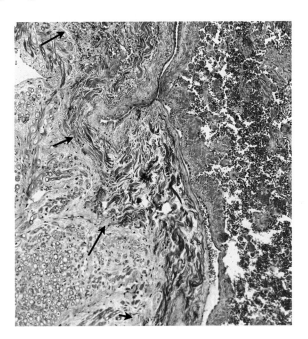

**Figure 10-25**

**CARDIAC HEMANGIOMA**

Left: The tumor was found incidentally in the left atrium. There was prominent papillary endothelial hyperplasia (top).

Right: A Masson trichrome stain shows the collagenized background of the tumor and normal atrium below. The junction between tumor and atrium is marked by arrows.

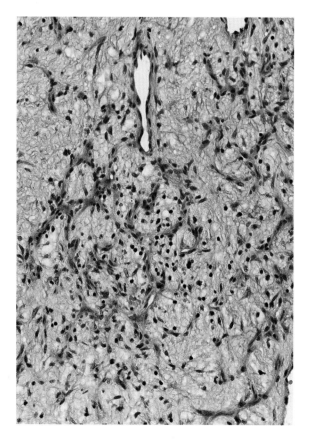

**Figure 10-26**

**CARDIAC HEMANGIOMA: CHRONIC INFLAMMATION**

Scattered inflammatory cells are seen in a capillary hemangioma with a myxoid background (same tumor as in fig. 10-3). In children, anti-inflammatory treatment is given in conjunction with surgical treatment and may hasten regression of hemangiomas.

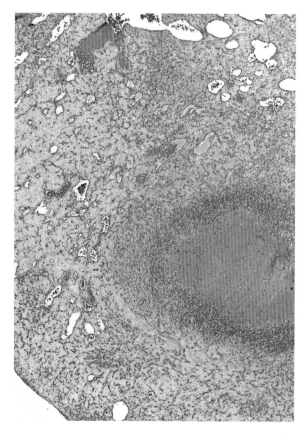

**Figure 10-27**

**CARDIAC HEMANGIOMA: ORGANIZING THROMBUS**

A different area of the tumor shown in figure 10-15 shows a hematoma within the tumor. The organizing clot shows granulation tissue and papillary endothelial hyperplasia.

however, and cellular areas with numerous capillaries are usually present. In addition, cardiac hemangiomas are rarely attached to the fossa ovalis of the left atrium (108,113).

Papillary endothelial hyperplasia (20,21) is a reactive, unusually exuberant form of endothelial proliferation that may be a component of an organizing thrombus or hemangioma and may mimic angiosarcoma (fig. 10-27). This finding is more common in hemangiomas with larger cavitary spaces (59,76,89,89). This lesion has been confused with angiosarcoma, but there is no atypia or mitotic figures, and spindled areas or solid growth are absent. Unlike angiosarcoma, necrosis and marked nuclear atypia are absent, and there is usually organizing fibrin thrombus within the papillae (114). However,

with complete tumor sampling, angiosarcoma is readily excluded, because most of the cardiac hemangioma is composed of bland vascular structures lacking endothelial atypia; such areas are absent in angiosarcoma.

The epithelioid or histiocytoid cells of hemangioma are of endothelial origin, as shown by immunohistochemical or ultrastructural methods (115). There is confusion with epithelioid hemangioma, or angiolymphoid hyperplasia with eosinophilia, which is probably a reactive process with reactive lymphoid hyperplasia (116,117). There is further confusion with mesothelial-monocyte incidental cardiac excrescence, a tumor-like collection of macrophages, mesothelial cells, and lymphocytes (118). The left atrial hemangioma described by Kuo et al. (115) is unique, in that it shares histologic features with epithelioid hemangioendothelioma, but

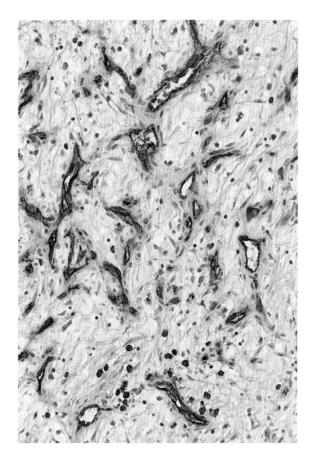

**Figure 10-28**

**CARDIAC HEMANGIOMA**

The endothelial cells lining the channels stain for CD31, with no staining in the pericytes. CD31 staining is nonspecific, as myxoma, often in the differential diagnosis, is also positive.

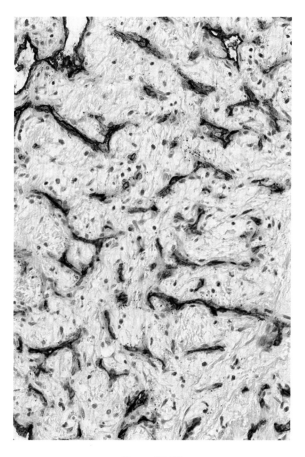

**Figure 10-29**

**CARDIAC HEMANGIOMA**

The endothelial cells lining the channels stain for CD34, while the pericytes are negative. CD34 staining is nonspecific.

is associated with peripheral eosinophilia, suggestive of epithelioid hemangioma.

**Treatment.** After cardiac evaluation with imaging is performed, most children and adults with cardiac hemangiomas are successfully treated. There have been about 100 reports of surgically resected cardiac hemangiomas since 2000 and several before then (21,54,67,114,119–123).

Often, intraoperative consultation with frozen section is sought, and occasionally a deferred diagnosis delays curative surgery (124). In the majority of these cases, complete excision is possible, even with large tumors (125). In some cases, however, complete resection is not possible because of growth into surrounding structures (103). Nevertheless, the majority of adult hemangiomas are exophytic lesions that project into the cavity

and are amenable to complete resection with a rim of normal cardiac muscle. Occasionally, the surgeon will ablate the base of the tumor with cryotechniques to ensure adequacy of excision (99). Adequacy of excision with inking margins is recommended if possible.

In atrial tumors in particular, cardiac hemangiomas may infiltrate the wall of the chamber and extend into the pericardial space. In such cases, reconstruction of ventricular outflow with Dacron grafts may be necessary (21,49,77,95,124). In rare examples, extensive atrial infiltration requires temporary cardiac explantation, removal of the tumor, and reimplantation of the heart (autotransplantation) (126). Although most ventricular hemangiomas can be excised, in one case, a right ventricular

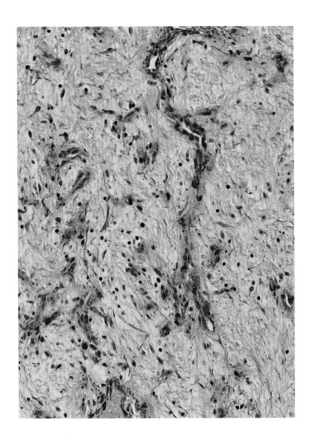 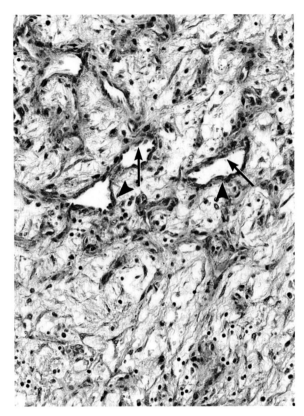

**Figure 10-30**

**CARDIAC HEMANGIOMA**

Left: In contrast to myxoma, the vascular structures of hemangioma are lined by smooth muscle actin-positive pericytes.

Right: At higher magnification, the actin-positive pericytes (arrowheads) and actin-negative endothelial cells (arrows) that are positive for CD31 and CD34 are seen.

outflow tract reconstruction with a Gore-Tex stent was performed postoperatively (127). Sudden death has been reported after partial removal of cardiac hemangioma (93). In some patients, postoperative antiarrhythmic mediations or indwelling pacemakers in case of postsurgical atrioventricular block (38,102) are necessary. Although most valvular hemangiomas are treated with excision and valve replacement, valve-sparing surgery may be performed if the tumor is readily excisable (128).

In rare instances, massive, unresectable cardiac hemangiomas are found in relatively asymptomatic individuals (129). Although more frequently documented in children, cardiac hemangiomas can regress in adults (130), and follow-up without surgery has been contemplated. There is a single reported case of angiosarcoma developing 7 years after surgical excision of a cardiac hem-

angioma (105); it is unclear whether there was a second primary or whether the initial tumor was indeed an angiosarcoma.

Although the postoperative prognosis in children is excellent, one child died years after excision of progressive heart failure (14). Postoperative heart block may occur if the excision is near the membranous septum (131,132). Cryoablation has been used, as in adults, after excision of sessile lesions to ensure complete excision (68). Valve repair may be successful after removal of a tumor near the annulus, with reimplantation of the valve leaflet (132). If a biopsy demonstrates a hemangioma in a child with an unresectable tumor, there may be conservative management with follow-up or anti-inflammatory steroid treatment (69,82). There are sporadic reports of cardiac hemangioma with chromosomal abnormalities, including Turner syndrome (133).

In fetuses, treatment may include intrauterine pericardiocentesis (93,94) and cesarean section if there is impending tamponade. Because it is generally believed that the course of congenital hemangioma is that of regression (75,134), the treatment of infants is often conservative, including medical treatment with steroids or interferon (82). Surgery may be necessary for relief of hemodynamic obstruction or pericardial effusions (48,72,74), although often only incomplete resection is possible (95,97). Atrial reconstruction after resection of large tumors at the base of the heart may be necessary and the reported long-term results have been good (48).

In adults, surgical resection is usually possible with limited imaging studies, such as transthoracic and intraoperative transesophageal echocardiograms. In these instances, a specific diagnosis is often not made preoperatively, and the differential diagnosis involves other lesions, especially cardiac myxoma and thrombus (57).

**Prognosis.** The surgical excision of hemangioma is generally successful. In a review by Brizard et al. (3) 20 years ago, there was only 1 postoperative death among 15 patients, the remainder living with up to 6 years follow-up. More recent studies have shown a single late death (11 years postoperatively) in a boy (14), but otherwise good long-term survival (6,135). Elbardissi (136) found that patients with surgically resected cardiac hemangiomas had decreased long-term survival rates compared to controls and patients with myxoma, although they were included in a group with other benign tumors.

## LYMPHANGIOMA

**Definition.** *Lymphangioma* is a localized mass of dilated lymphatic vessels. Because of frequent occurrence in neonates, it is often considered a congenital hamartoma or malformation as opposed to a true neoplasm. Cardiac lymphangioma is by definition located within the pericardium, either attached to the epicardium, or within the cardiac chambers.

**General Features.** Cardiac lymphangioma is rare, and generally not represented in series of heart tumors. As of 2013, fewer than 20 had been reported, making the lesion about 10 times less common than cardiac hemangioma (137). A series of mediastinal lymphangiomas of adults revealed only 1 of 19 intrapericardial

tumors (138). By imaging, it is often difficult to ascertain if lymphangiomas of the middle mediastinum are within or outside the pericardium; indeed, some reports do not clarify the exact location (139,140).

**Clinical Features.** Approximately 30 percent of cardiac lymphangiomas occur in children or neonates, and the remainder in adults. The mean age is approximately 25 years at presentation (137,139–154). In children, pericardial effusion and cardiac symptoms are common, including respiratory distress and cyanosis (143,145). The diagnosis has been made in utero (139,140). In adults, the tumor may be an incidental discovery (144,147), cause chest pain (137,141,153), or result in heart failure (142). Tumors causing symptoms are more likely intracavitary than pericardial. Pericardial tumors cause symptoms by compression of the cardiac chambers (especially right atrium and ventricle) or by the formation of effusions. There is a slight female predominance (60 percent of patients). Imaging demonstrates the cystic nature of the tumor, and the relationship to cardiac structures (fig. 10-31).

**Gross Findings.** Of 15 cardiac lymphangiomas reported in the last 10 years, 9 were predominantly intrapericardial, and the remainder within the cardiac cavities (137,139–149,151, 152). Infiltrating lesions have a propensity for the right atrium, and several have been reported growing around the right coronary artery (145,146,153). Lesions may be either circumscribed masses that are excised completely (fig. 10-32), or may invade the wall of the cardiac chamber, making complete excision difficult. Grossly, lymphangiomas are multicystic, spongy masses with few firm or solid areas. Hemorrhage, calcification and necrosis are absent.

**Microscopic Findings.** Cardiac lymphangiomas are similar to those of soft tissue (figs. 10-33, 10-34). Those that are composed of large, grossly visible cysts are referred to as "hygromas" and those composed of smaller microscopic cysts as "cavernous lymphangiomas." The cysts are irregular, and lined by flattened endothelial cells. The septa typically are thick, and contain disorganized muscle bundles. Lymphoid aggregates are common, typically around the periphery of the tumor.

**Immunohistochemical Findings.** The endothelial lining cells express CD31 and CD34, with

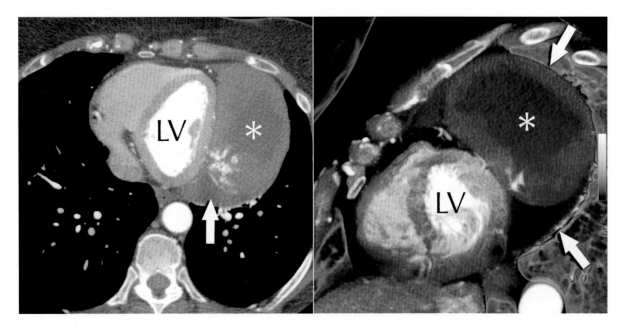

**Figure 10-31**

**CARDIAC LYMPHANAGIOMA**

Left: Contrast-enhanced ECG-gated axial CT image demonstrates a thick-walled, smoothly marginated and heterogeneously enhancing ovoid mass with central low attenuation (*). It exerts extrinsic mass effect upon the left ventricle (LV) and is partly rimmed by pericardial effusion (arrow), thus presumably centered in the pericardium.

Right: Contrast-enhanced ECG-gated cardiac CT, short axis 3-dimensional reconstruction, shows a large pericardial mass (*) partly compressing the left ventricle (LV) and draped by pericardium (arrows).

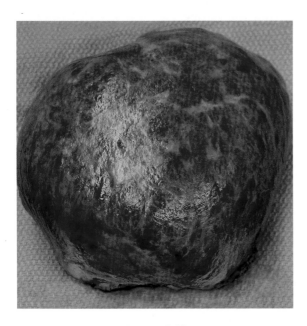

**Figure 10-32**

**CARDIAC LYMPHANGIOMA**

Resected specimen of the tumor illustrated in the previous figure was a well-encapsulated smooth-surfaced intrapericardial lymphangioma measuring 11 cm.

patchy positivity for factor VIII related antigen. Expression of lymphatic markers, such as D2-40, has been documented in extracardiac lymphangioma, and there has been a report of podoplanin positivity in a cardiac lymphangioma (153).

**Differential Diagnosis.** The diagnosis of lymphangioma is generally straightforward. In contrast to cavernous hemangioma, the tumor typically does not contain blood, has abundant smooth muscle in the septa, and demonstrates frequent lymphoid aggregates. Expression of lymphatic markers distinguishes lymphangioma from hemangioma.

**Treatment and Prognosis.** Cardiac lymphangiomas are generally treated by excision, if primarily pericardial. Complete excision is curative (137,139–142,144–147,151,152). Infiltrative tumors may require reconstruction of valves or coronary arteries (141,149). In many cases, complete resection is impossible (143,153). No case has been reported to recur, however. One patient with arrhythmias was only biopsied, with implantation of an automated defibrillator to control ventricular tachyarrhythmias (148).

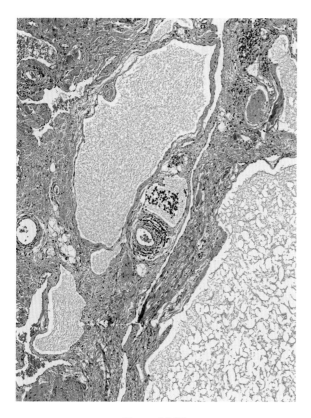

**Figure 10-33**

**LYMPHANGIOMA**

There are anastomosing endothelial-lined spaces, some of which are filled with proteinaceous lymph fluid.

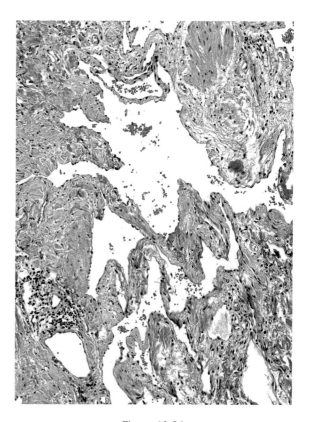

**Figure 10-34**

**LYMPHANGIOMA**

Smooth muscle bundles are typically prominent.

## REFERENCES

1. Colli A, Budillon AM, DeCicco G, et al. Recurrence of a right ventricular hemangioma. J Thorac Cardiovasc Surg 2003;126:881-883.
2. Wu G, Jones J, Sequeira IB, Pepelassis D. Congenital pericardial hemangioma responding to high-dose corticosteroid therapy. Can J Cardiol 2009;25:e139-140.
3. Brizard C, Latremouille C, Jebara VA, et al. Cardiac hemangiomas. Ann Thorac Surg 1993;56:390-394.
4. Wang JN, Yao CT, Chen JS, Yang YJ, Tsai YC, Wu JM. Cardiac tumors in infants and children. Acta Paediatr Taiwan 2003;44:215-219.
5. Uzun O, Wilson DG, Vujanic GM, Parsons JM, De Giovanni JV. Cardiac tumours in children. Orphanet J Rare Dis 2007;2:11.
6. Stiller B, Hetzer R, Meyer R, et al. Primary cardiac tumours: when is surgery necessary? Eur J Cardiothorac Surg 2001;20:1002-1006.
7. Sallee D, Spector ML, van Heeckeren DW, Patel CR. Primary pediatric cardiac tumors: a 17 year experience. Cardiol Young 1999;9:155-162.
8. Thomas-de-Montpreville V, Nottin R, Dulmet E, Serraf A. Heart tumors in children and adults: clinicopathological study of 59 patients from a surgical center. Cardiovasc Pathol 2007;16:22-28.
9. Qiu LS, Sun YJ, Ding WX, Xu ZW, Liu JF. [Treatment strategies for pediatric patients with primary cardiac tumors.] Zhonghua Wai Ke Za Zhi. 2011;49:227-231. [Chinese]
10. Kosuga T, Fukunaga S, Kawara T, et al. Surgery for primary cardiac tumors. Clinical experience and surgical results in 60 patients. J Cardiovasc Surg (Torino) 2002;43:581-587.
11. Grande AM, Ragni T, Vigano M. Primary cardiac tumors. A clinical experience of 12 years. Tex Heart Inst J 1993;20:223-230.

12. Endo A, Ohtahara A, Kinugawa T, et al. Characteristics of 161 patients with cardiac tumors diagnosed during 1993 and 1994 in Japan. Am J Cardiol 1997;79:1708-1711.

13. Agarwal V, Agarwal SK, Srivastava AK, Kapoor S. Primary cardiac tumors: Surgical experience and follow-up. Indian Heart J 2003;55:632-636.

14. Kamiya H, Yasuda T, Nagamine H, et al. Surgical treatment of primary cardiac tumors: 28 years' experience in Kanazawa University Hospital. Jpn Circ J 2001;65:315-319.

15. Baird C, Bengur R, Blalock S, Ikemba C. Right atrial hemangioma in the newborn: utility of fetal imaging. Ann Pediatr Cardiol 2012;5:81-84.

16. Grebenc ML, Rosado de Christenson ML, Burke AP, Green CE, Galvin JR. Primary cardiac and pericardial neoplasms: radiologic-pathologic correlation. Radiographics 2000;20:1073-1103.

17. Han Y, Chen X, Wang X, Yang L, Zeng Y, Yang J. Cardiac capillary hemangioma: a case report and brief review of the literature. J Clin Ultrasound 2014;42:53-56.

18. Karangelis D, Tagarakis G, Bouliaris K, Tsilimingas N. Cardiac hemangioma; facing a dilemma in treatment. Interact Cardiovasc Thorac Surg 2011;12:519.

19. Pigato JB, Subramanian VA, McCaba JC. Cardiac hemangioma. A case report and discussion. Tex Heart Inst J 1998;25:83-85.

20. Abad C. Cardiac hemangioma. Ann Thorac Surg 1994;57:1373-1374.

21. Burke A, Johns JP, Virmani R. Hemangiomas of the heart. A clinicopathologic study of ten cases. Am J Cardiovasc Pathol 1990;3:283-290.

22. Gasparovic H, Anic D, Saric D, Gasparovic V, Djuric Z, Jelic I. Surgical excision of a hemangioendothelioma of the left ventricle. Ann Thorac Surg 2002;74:914-916.

23. Kojima S, Sumiyoshi M, Suwa S, et al. Cardiac hemangioma: a report of two cases and review of the literature. Heart Vessels 2003;18:153-156.

24. Ray R, Rishi A, Venugopal P, Chopra P. Hemangioma of the tricuspid valve: a report of two cases with review of literature. Cardiovasc Pathol 2004;13:120-122.

25. Ayadi-Kaddour A, Abid M, Harrath Y, Smati B, Kilani T, El Mezni F. Asymptomatic hemangioma of the interatrial septum. J Thorac Cardiovasc Surg 2006;132:691-692.

26. Cannata A, Russo CF, Merlanti B, et al. Cavernous hemangioma replacing the septal leaflet of the tricuspid valve. J Card Surg 2010;25:524-527.

27. Lin CT, Lee CY, Hong GJ, et al. Cardiac hemangioma located at the apex of the left ventricle: a rare case report. Acta Chir Belg. 2012;112:453-456.

28. Murthy A, Jain A, Nappi AG. Tumor blush: left ventricular cardiac hemangioma with supply from both the left anterior descending and circumflex arteries. J Invasive Cardiol 2012;24:138-139.

29. Newcomb AE, Pelenghi S, Karski J, Butany J, David TE. Cardiac papillary muscle hemangioma. J Thorac Cardiovasc Surg 2007;134:1345-1346.

30. Oshima H, Hara M, Kono T, Shibamoto Y, Mishima A, Akita S. Cardiac hemangioma of the left atrial appendage: CT and MR findings. J Thorac Imaging 2003;18:204-206.

31. Thomas JE, Eror AT, Kenney M, Caravalho J Jr. Asymptomatic right atrial cavernous hemangioma: a case report and review of the literature. Cardiovasc Pathol 2004;13:341-344.

32. Marrone G, Sciacca S, D'Ancona G, Pilato M, Luca A, Gridelli B. A rare case of left ventricular intramural hemangioma diagnosed using 1.5-T cardiac MRI with histopathological correlation and successfully treated by surgery. Cardiovasc Intervent Radiol 2010;33:164-168.

33. Nair KS, Lawrence DR, Smith PL. An unusual cause of mixed mitral valve disease. Heart 2002; 88:560.

34. Nye SW, Orsinelli DA, Baker PB, Brown DA. Surgical treatment of a hemangioma of the mitral valve. Ann Thorac Surg 2001;71:345-347.

35. Perk G, Yim J, Varkey M, Colvin SB, Tunick PA, Kronzon I. Cardiac cavernous hemangioma. J Am Soc Echocardiogr 2005;18:979.

36. Thung KH, Wan IY, Yip G, Underwood MJ. Cardiac tumor masquerading as obstructive sleep apnea syndrome. Interact Cardiovasc Thorac Surg 2008;7:358-359.

37. Yuan SM, Shinfeld A, Kuperstein R, Raanani E. Cavernous hemangioma of the right atrium. Kardiol Pol 2008;66:974-976.

38. Huang CL, Feng AN, Chuang YC, et al. Malignant presentation of cardiac hemangioma: a rare cause of complete atrioventricular block. Circ Cardiovasc Imaging 2008;1:e1-3.

39. Turak O, Ozcan F, Basar FN, et al. Cavernous hemangioma of the right atrium: a very rare case of complete atrioventricular block. J Am Coll Cardiol 2012;60:1204.

40. Lev-Ran O, Matsa M, Paz Y. Cavernous hemangioma of the heart. Eur J Cardiothorac Surg 2000; 18:371.

41. Abu-Omar Y, Mezue K, Ali A, Kneeshaw JD, Goddard M, Large SR. Intractable ventricular tachycardia secondary to cardiac hemangioma. Ann Thorac Surg 2010;90:1347-1349.

42. Bonney WJ, Ceresnak SR, Ira S, Hordof A, Liberman L. Verapamil sensitive ventricular tachycardia associated with a cardiac hemangioma in the right ventricular outflow tract. Indian Pacing Electrophysiol J 2009;9:355-359.

43. Ainsworth CD, Salehian O, Nair V, Whitlock RP. A bloody mass: rare cardiac tumor as a cause of symptomatic ventricular arrhythmias. Circulation 2012;126:1923-1931.

44. Verunelli F, Amerini A, D'Alfonso A, et al. Left atrial cardiac hemangioma: a report of two cases. Ital Heart J 2004;5:299-301.

45. Rammos KS, Ketikoglou DG, Hatzibougias IG. Large left ventricular capillary hemangioma with cavernous areas. Tex Heart Inst J 2007;34:128-129.

46. Cartagena AM, Levin TL, Issenberg H, Goldman HS. Pericardial effusion and cardiac hemangioma in the neonate. Pediatr Radiol 1993;23:384-385.

47. Chao JC, Reyes CV, Hwang MH. Cardiac hemangioma. South Med J 1990;83:44-47.

48. Laga S, Gewillig MH, Van Schoubroeck D, Daenen W. Imminent fetal cardiac tamponade by right atrial hemangioma. Pediatr Cardiol 2006; 27:633-635.

49. Ramasubbu K, Wheeler TM, Reardon MJ, Dokainish H. Visceral pericardial hemangioma: unusual location for a rare cardiac tumor. J Am Soc Echocardiogr 2005;18:981.

50. Thorp JA, Geidt A, Gelatt M, Gowdamarajan R. Decompression of fetal cardiac tamponade caused by congenital capillary hemangioma of the pericardium. Obstet Gynecol 2000;96:816-817.

51. Hosono S, Ohno T, Kimoto H, et al. Successful transcutaneous arterial embolization of a giant hemangioma associated with high-output cardiac failure and Kasabach-Merritt syndrome in a neonate: a case report. J Perinat Med 1999;27:399-403.

52. Lopriore E, Markhorst DG. Diffuse neonatal haemangiomatosis: new views on diagnostic criteria and prognosis. Acta Paediatr 1999;88:93-97.

53. Abad C, de Varona S, Limeres MA, Morales J, Marrero J. Resection of a left atrial hemangioma. Report of a case and overview of the literature on resected cardiac hemangiomas. Tex Heart Inst J 2008;35:69-72.

54. Reiss N, Theissen P, Feaux de Lacroix W. Right-ventricular hemangioma causing serious outflow-tract obstruction. Thorac Cardiovasc Surg 1991;39:234-236.

55. Iba Y, Watanabe S, Akimoto T, Abe K, Koyanagi H. Pedicled cardiac hemangioma with right ventricular outflow tract obstruction. Jpn J Thorac Cardiovasc Surg 2005;53:269-271.

56. Kann BR, Kim WJ, Cilley JH Jr, Marra SW, DelRossi AJ. Hemangioma of the right ventricular outflow tract. Ann Thorac Surg 2000;70:975-977.

57. Kocak H, Ozyazicioglu A, Gundogdu C, Sevimli S. Cardiac hemangioma complicated with cerebral and coronary embolization. Heart Vessels 2005; 20:296-297.

58. Kemme DJ, Rainer WG. Subendocardial arteriovenous malformation in a patient with unstable angina. Clin Cardiol 1991;14:82-84.

59. Kipfer B, Englberger L, Stauffer E, Carrel T. Rare presentation of cardiac hemangiomas. Ann Thorac Surg 2000;70:977-979.

60. Krous HF, Chapman AJ, Altshuler G. Cardiac hemangioma: a rare (or possible) cause of sudden death in children. J Forensic Sci 1978;23:375-378.

61. Nakamura K, Funabashi N, Miyauchi H, et al. Hemangioma located just above the left main coronary artery, in a subject who had cardiac arrest due to ventricular fibrillation, led to a diagnosis of brugada syndrome. Int J Cardiol 2008;127:437-441.

62. Marmade L, Laaroussi M, Elkouache M, et al. [Haemangioma of the right atrium revealed by cardiogenic shock.] Arch Mal Coeur Vaiss 2005; 98:337-341. [French]

63. Patel J, Sheppard MN. Sudden death owing to right atrial hemangioma. J Forensic Sci 2011;56: 529-530.

64. Sata N, Moriyama Y, Hamada N, Horinouchi T, Miyahara K. Recurrent pericardial tamponade from atrial hemangioma. Ann Thorac Surg 2004; 78:1472-1475.

65. Weston CF, Hayward MW, Seymour RM, Stephens MR. Cardiac haemangioma associated with a facial port-wine stain and recurrent atrial tachycardia. Eur Heart J 1988;9:668-671.

66. Gengenbach S, Ridker PM. Left ventricular hemangioma in Kasabach-Merritt syndrome. Am Heart J 1991;121:202-203.

67. Dein JR, Frist WH, Stinson EB, et al. Primary cardiac neoplasms. Early and late results of surgical treatment in 42 patients. J Thorac Cardiovasc Surg 1987;93:502-511.

68. Tomasian A, Iv M, Lai C, Jalili M, Krishnam MS. Cardiac hemangioma: features on cardiovascular magnetic resonance. J Cardiovasc Magn Reson 2007;9:873-876.

69. Martinez-Rodriguez I, Banzo I, Quirce R, et al. F-18 FDG PET/CT uptake by a cardiac hemangioma. Clin Nucl Med 2010;35:330-331.

70. Moniotte S, Geva T, Perez-Atayde A, Fulton DR, Pigula FA, Powell AJ. Images in cardiovascular medicine. Cardiac hemangioma. Circulation 2005;112:e103-104.

71. Sebastian V, Einzig S, D'Cruz C, Costello C, Kula M, Campbell A. Cardiac hemangioma of the right atrium in a neonate: fetal management and expedited surgical resection. Images Paediatr Cardiol 2005;7:5-9.

72. Kitagawa N, Ohhama Y, Fukuzato Y, et al. Pericardial hemangioma presenting fetal cardiac tamponade and postnatal bronchostenosis. Pediatr Surg Int 2004;20:376-377.

73. Tansel T, Aydogan U, Yilmazbayhan D, Bilgic B, Demiryont M, Onursal E. Epithelioid hemangioendothelioma of the heart in infancy. Ann Thorac Surg 2005;79:1402-1405.

74. Eichler T, Paul T, Schneider HE. Hemangioma as a rare cause of a neonatal cardiac tumor resulting in inflow obstruction of the tricuspid valve. Clin Res Cardiol 2011;100:469-470.

75. Puligandla PS, Kay S, Morin L, et al. Pericardial hemangioma presenting as thoracic mass in utero. Fetal Diagn Ther 2004;19:178-181.

76. Kan CD, Yae CT, Yang YJ. Left ventricular haemangioma with papillary endothelial hyperplasia and liver involvement. Heart 2004;90:e49.

77. Esmaeilzadeh M, Jalalian R, Maleki M, Givtaj N, Mozaffari K, Parsaee M. Cardiac cavernous hemangioma. Eur J Echocardiogr 2007;8:487-489.

78. Gonzalez Lopez MT, Aranda Granados PJ, Delange Segura L, Gutierrez de Loma J. An unexpected left atrial cavernous hemangioma: the cardiac surgeon needs an optimal preoperative study! Interact Cardiovasc Thorac Surg 2011;13:529-531.

79. Farinelli A, Ferrara E, Cirillo M, Zorzi F. [Right ventricular cavernous hemangioma: A rare cardiac primary neoplasia.] Ital Heart J Suppl 2005; 6:498-501. [Italian]

80. Cunningham T, Lawrie GM, Stavinoha J Jr, Quinones MA, Zoghbi WA. Cavernous hemangioma of the right ventricle: echocardiographic-pathologic correlates. J Am Soc Echocardiogr 1993;6: 335-340.

81. Alsaileek A, Tepe SM, Alveraz L, Miller DV, Tajik J, Breen J. Diagnostic features of cardiac hemangioma on cardiovascular magnetic resonance, a case report. Int J Cardiovasc Imaging 2006;22: 699-702.

82. Kiaffas MG, Powell AJ, Geva T. Magnetic resonance imaging evaluation of cardiac tumor characteristics in infants and children. Am J Cardiol 2002;89:1229-1233.

83. Dod HS, Burri MV, Hooda D, et al. Two- and three-dimensional transthoracic and transesophageal echocardiographic findings in epithelioid hemangioma involving the mitral valve. Echocardiography 2008;25:443-445.

84 Lo LJ, Nucho RC, Allen JW, Rohde RL, Lau FY. Left atrial cardiac hemangioma associated with shortness of breath and palpitations. Ann Thorac Surg 2002;73:979-981.

85. Matsumoto Y, Watanabe G, Endo M, Sasaki H. Surgical treatment of a cavernous hemangioma of the left atrial roof. Eur J Cardiothorac Surg 2001;20:633-635.

86. Arjomand H, Van Decker W, Fyfe B, Nixon T, Wolf NM, Sokil AB. Right ventricular hemangioma causing right ventricular inflow obstruction and right heart failure. J Am Soc Echocardiogr 2004;17:186-188.

87. Sulayman R, Cassels DE. Myocardial coronary hemangiomatous tumors in children. Chest 1975;68:113-115.

88. Chiappini B, Gregorini R, Vecchio L, et al. Cardiac hemangioma of the left atrial appendag: a case report and discussion. J Card Surg 2009;24:522-523.

89. Langer C, Korfer J, Peterschroder A, et al. Right atrial hemangioma in modern cardiac imaging. Clin Res Cardiol 2006;95:482-487.

90. Di Valentino M, Menafoglio A, Mazzucchelli L, Siclari F, Gallino A. Rapid-growing left intraventricular cardiac hemangioma. J Am Soc Echocardiogr 2006;19:939, e935-937.

91. Eftychiou C, Antoniades L. Cardiac hemangioma in the left ventricle and brief review of the literature. J Cardiovasc Med (Hagerstown) 2009;10:565-567.

92. Perez-Sanz TM, Fulquet E, Neilan TG, Rollan MJ, Mar de la Torre M, Bratos JL. A case report of a round cystic tumor in the left ventricular outflow tract. J Am Soc Echocardiogr 2006;19:1402. e1409-1402 e1411.

93. Zanati SG, Hueb JC, Cogni AL, et al. Cardiac hemangioma of the right atrium. Eur J Echocardiogr 2008;9:52-53.

94. Lapenna E, De Bonis M, Torracca L, La Canna G, Dell'Antonio G, Alfieri O. Cavernous hemangioma of the tricuspid valve: minimally invasive surgical resection. Ann Thorac Surg 2003;76:2097-2099.

95. Gersak B, Sostaric M, Dolenc-Strazar Z, Staric F, Kozelj M. Cavernous hemangioma in the junction between the left atrium and the aorta: case report. Heart Surg Forum 2005;8:E72-74.

96. Turkoz R, Gulcan O, Oguzkurt L, Atalay H, Bolat B, Sezgin A. Surgical treatment of a huge cavernous hemangioma surrounding the right coronary artery. Ann Thorac Surg 2005; 79:1765-1767.

97. Wang HJ, Lin JL, Lin FY. Images in cardiovascular medicine. Cardiac hemangioma. Circulation 2002;106:2520.

98. Lee KJ, Shin JH, Choi JH, et al. A case of arteriovenous type cardiac hemangioma. Korean J Intern Med 1998;13:123-126.

99. Tomizawa Y, Endo M, Nishida H, Kikuchi C, Koyanagi H. Reconstruction of the left ventricle in a patient with cardiac hemangioma at the apex. Ann Thorac Surg 2001;71:2032-2034.

100. Rajab TK, Khalpey Z, Cohn LH, Gallegos RP. Cardiac hemangioma presenting with angina pectoris. J Card Surg 2010;25:664-666.

101. Zhang B, Xu Z, Tang H. Intermuscular hemangioma of the left ventricle. J Card Surg 2012; 27:572-575.

102. Velthuis BO, van Es J, van Houwelingen G, Toes GJ, Wagenaar L. Extensive left ventricular hemangioma. J Am Coll Cardiol 2012;60:e35.

103. Tillett RL, Jiskoot PM, Glenville BE. Case report: cardiac hemangioma. Heart Surg Forum 2001;4:247-250.

104. Vaideeswar P. Cardiac sub-pulmonary arteriovenous hemangioma. Indian J Pathol Microbiol 2011;54:646-647.

105. Chalet Y, Mace L, Franc B, Neveux JY, Lancelin B. Angiosarcoma 7 years after surgical excision of histiocytoid haemangioma in left atrium. Lancet 1993;341:1217.

106. Floria M, Guedes A, Buche M, Deperon R, Marchandise B. A rare primary cardiac tumour: cavernous hemangioma of the tricuspid valve. Eur J Echocardiogr 2011;12:477.

107. Nemati MH, Astaneh B, Joubeh A. Cardiac hemangioma presenting with neurological manifestations. Gen Thorac Cardiovasc Surg 2009;57:155-158.

108. Val-Bernal JF, Cuadrado M, Garijo MF, Revuelta JM. Incidental in vivo detection of an isolated hemangioma of the aortic valve in a man with a history of renal transplantation. Virchows Arch 2006;449:121-123.

109. Novitzky D, Rose AG, Morgan JA, Barnard CN. Primary cardiac haemangiomas. A report of 2 cases. S Afr Med J 1984;66:267-270.

110. Roser M, Hamdan A, Komoda T, et al. Images in cardiovascular medicine. Left ventricular cardiac hemangioma presenting with atypical chest pain. Circulation 2008;117:2958-2960.

111. Vivirito M, Boldorini R, Rossi L, Caimmi PP, Bernardi M, Teodori G. Capillary hemangioma of the aortic valve: false preoperative diagnosis of endocarditis. J Thorac Cardiovasc Surg 2006;132:690-691.

112. Yaganti V, Patel S, Yaganti S, Victor M. Cavernous hemangioma of the mitral valve: A case report and review of literature. J Cardiovasc Med (Hagerstown) 2009;10:420-422.

113. Rose AG. Venous malformations of the heart. Arch Pathol Lab Med 1979;103:18-20.

114. Abad C, Campo E, Estruch R, et al. Cardiac hemangioma with papillary endothelial hyperplasia: report of a resected case and review of the literature. Ann Thorac Surg 1990;49:305-308.

115. Kuo TT, Hsueh S, Su IJ, Gonzalez-Crussi F, Chen JS. Histiocytoid hemangioma of the heart with peripheral eosinophilia. Cancer 1985;55:2854-2861.

116. Rosai J. Angiolymphoid hyperplasia with eosinophilia of the skin. Its nosological position in the spectrum of histiocytoid hemangioma. Am J Dermatopathol 1982;4:175-184.

117. Kanavaros P, Lavergne A, Dellagi K, Elaerts J, Ouzan J, Piwnica A. [Histiocytoid hemangioma of the heart. Histological and immunohistochemical study of a case.] Ann Pathol 1988;8:228-233. [French]

118. Luthringer DJ, Virmani R, Weiss SW, Rosai J. A distinctive cardiovascular lesion resembling histiocytoid (epithelioid) hemangioma. Evidence suggesting mesothelial participation. Am J Surg Pathol 1990;14:993-1000.

119. Vander Salm TJ. Unusual primary tumors of the heart. Semin Thorac Cardiovasc Surg 2000;12:89-100.

120. Manasse E, Nicolini F, Canziani R, Gallotti R. Left ventricular hemangioma. Eur J Cardiothorac Surg 1999;15:864-866.

121. Parker JR, Knott-Craig C, Min KW, Uzelmeier WJ. Cellular hemangioma of the posterior mediastinum: unusual presentation of a rare vascular neoplasm. J Okla State Med Assoc 1997;90:7-9.

122. Galli R, Albanese S, Pilato E, et al. [The surgical treatment of a rare primary cardiac tumor: hemangioma. A report of 2 cases.] Cardiologia 1997;42:89-93. [Italian]

123. Caires G, Canada M, Gouveia R, et al. [Hemangioma of the right ventricle.] Rev Port Cardiol 1997;16:561-567. [Portuguese]

124. Solum AM, Romero SC, Ledford S, Parker R, Madani MM, Coletta JM. Left atrial hemangioma presenting as cardiac tamponade. Texas Heart Instit J 2007;34:126-127.

125. Takahashi A, Sakurai M, Fujikawa T. Resection of a giant cardiac hemangioma. Gen Thorac Cardiovasc Surg 2013;61:353-355.

126. Novitzky D, Guglin M, Sheffield C. Cardiac autotransplantation for removal of left atrial hemangioma and a review of the literature. Heart Surg Forum 2009;12:E279-284.

127. Sogawa M, Fukuda T, Tayama M, Moro H, Ishihara N. Reconstruction of the right ventricular outflow tract after surgical removal of a cardiac hemangioma. Gen Thorac Cardiovasc Surg 2012;60:661-663.

128. Muzzi L, Davoli G, Specchia L, Chiavarelli M. Primary hemangioma of the mitral valve: an unusual presentation. J Heart Valve Dis 2007; 16:209-211.

129. Grenadier E, Margulis T, Palant A, Safadi T, Merin G. Huge cavernous hemangioma of the heart: a completely evaluated case report and review of the literature. Am Heart J 1989;117: 479-481.

130. Palmer TE, Tresch DD, Bonchek LI. Spontaneous resolution of a large, cavernous hemangioma of the heart. Am J Cardiol 1986;58:184-185.

131. Ugras S, Bayram I. Cavernous haemangioma of the mitral valve in a child: report of a case and review of the literature. Pathology 2005;37:396-398.

132. Kutay V, Yakut C, Ekim H. Mitral annular tumors: report of two cases in childhood. J Card Surg 2006;21:191-194.

133. Orakzai RH, Nalawadi S, Cuk O, et al. Multimodality evaluation of a rare intracardiac tumor: Cardiac hemangioma. Am J Med 2011;124:e3-4.

134. Robinson HA, Keeton BR, Moore IE. Critical obstruction of the right ventricular outflow tract by a primary hemangioendothelioma in a seven month old. Cardiol Young 1999;9:185-188.

135. Padalino MA, Vida VL, Boccuzzo G, et al. Surgery for primary cardiac tumors in children: early and late results in a multicenter european congenital heart surgeons association study. Circulation 2012;126:22-30.

136. Elbardissi AW, Dearani JA, Daly RC, et al. Survival after resection of primary cardiac tumors: a 48-year experience. Circulation 2008;118:S7-15.

137. Huang Z. Lymphangioma of the left ventricle. J Card Surg 2013;28:24-6.

138. Shaffer K, Rosado-de-Christenson ML, Patz EF Jr, Young S, Farver CF. Thoracic lymphangioma in adults: CT and MR imaging features. AJR Am J Roentgenol 1994;162:283-9.

139. Pham NM, Alexander PM, Chow CW, Jones BO, d'Udekem Y, Konstantinov IE. Anterior mediastinal lymphangioma in an infant: diagnosis and surgical management. Heart Lung Circ 2012;21:289-91.

140. Adaletli I, Towbin AJ, Ozbayrak M, Madazli R. Anterior mediastinal lymphangioma: pre- and postnatal sonographic findings. J Clin Ultrasound 2013;41:383-5.

141. Cailleba L, Labrousse L, Marty M, Montaudon M, Gerbaud E. Pericardial cystic lymphangioma. Eur Heart J Cardiovasc Imaging 2013;14:246.

142. Biskupski A., Waligórski S, Mokrzycki K, Biskupska K, Brykczyóski M. Cardiac lymphangioma in the right atrium. Ann Thorac Surg 2013;96:328.

143. Zakaria RH, Barsoum NR, El-Basmy AA, El-Kaffas SH. Imaging of pericardial lymphangioma. Ann Pediatr Cardiol 2011;4:65-7.

144. Shroff GS, Lata AL, Parks GE, Entrikin DW. Giant pericardial lymphangioma—imaging, surgical, and pathologic correlations. J Comput Assist Tomogr 2011;35:642-4.

145. Almarsafawy H, Matter M, Elgamal MA, Zalata K. Cardiac lymphangioma in an infant. Pediatr Cardiol 2011;32:1253-5.

146. Naz I, Lone I. Cystic lympnagioma of the heart. Internet J Pathol 2009;10.

147. Kim SJ, Shin ES, Kim SW, et al. A case of cardiac lymphangioma presenting as a cystic mass in the right atrium. Yonsei Med J 2007;48:1043-7.

148. Pennec PY, Blanc JJ. Cardiac lymphangioma: a benign cardiac tumour. Eur Heart J 2006;27:2913.

149. Florchinger B, Rümmele P, Lehane C, Schmid FX, Birnbaum DE. Mitral prolapse caused by lymphangioma. Thorac Cardiovasc Surg 2005;53:180-3.

150. Soler R, Rodríguez E, Remuiñán C, Castro JM. Mediastinal lymphangioma involving the heart: CT and MR findings. Clin Radiol 2002;57:415-8.

151. Kaji T, Takamatsu H, Noguchi H, et al., Cardiac lymphangioma: case report and review of the literature. J Pediatr Surg 2002;37:E32.

152. Jougon, J., Laborde MN, Parrens M, MacBride T. Cystic lymphangioma of the heart mimicking a mediastinal tumor. Eur J Cardiothorac Surg 2002;22:476-8.

153. Sinzelle, E., Duong Van Huyen JP, Breiteneder-Geleff S, et al. Intrapericardial lymphangioma with podoplanin immunohistochemical characterization of lymphatic endothelial cells. Histopathology 2000;37:93-4.

154. Hatipoglu A. Intrapericardial and cardiac lymphangiomas. Pediatr Cardiol 1998;19:192.

155. Chen X, Lodge AJ, Dibernardo LR, Milano CA. Surgical treatment of a cavernous haemangioma of the heart. Eur J Cardiothorac Surg 2012;41:1182-1183.

156. Fan D, Yarnall C, Parmet JL, et al. Resection of a large atrial hemangioma using a bloodless surgical technique: a case report. Heart Surg Forum 2007;10:E87-89.

157. Fathala A. Left ventricular cardiac cyst: unusual echocardiographic appearance of a cardiac hemangioma. Circulation 2012;125:2171-2172.

158. Jo SH, Choi YJ, Cho GY, Lee WY. Huge cardiac hemangioma. Eur J Cardiothorac Surg 2008;34:1108.

159. Kaza AK, Buchanan SA, Parrino GP, Fiser SM, Long SM, Tribble CG. Cardioscope-assisted excision of a left ventricular tumor—a case report. Heart Surg Forum 2002;5:75-76.

160. Pasquino S, Balucani C, di Bella I, et al. Cardiac hemangioma of the right atrium: A possible cause of cerebellar stroke. Cerebrovasc Dis 2007;24:154-155.

161. Rizzoli G, Bottio T, Pittarello D, Napodano M, Thiene G, Basso C. Atrial septal mass: Transesophageal echocardiographic assessment. J Thorac Cardiovasc Surg 2004;128:767-769.

162. Serri K, Schraub P, Lafitte S, Roudaut R. Cardiac hemangioma presenting as atypical chest pain. Eur J Echocardiogr 2007;8:17-18.

# 11 BENIGN TUMORS OF FATTY TISSUE

## LIPOMATOUS HYPERTROPHY OF THE ATRIAL SEPTUM

**Definition.** *Lipomatous hypertrophy of the atrial septum* is a nonencapsulated mass of mature fat, adipose cells resembling fetal fat cells (brown fat), and enlarged cardiac myocytes. Synonyms include *lipomatous hamartoma of the atrial septum* (1,2) and *massive fatty deposits of the atrial septum* (3).

Any deposit of fat in the atrial septum at the level of the fossa ovalis that exceeds 2 cm in transverse dimension is lipomatous hypertrophy (3). The upper limit of normal fat has alternately been defined as 1.5 cm in young adults, with increasing limits as age progresses (4,5). The increase in mass in the atrial septum is likely secondary to an increased number of fat cells (adipocyte hyperplasia), as opposed to hypertrophied adipocytes or myocytes. Therefore, the word "hypertrophy" in lipomatous hypertrophy is a misnomer (1–3). In the surgical literature, true cardiac lipomas are typically not distinguished from lipomatous hypertrophy of the atrial septum and often, reported atrial "lipomas" are frequently lipomatous hypertrophy.

**General Features.** The precise nature of lipomatous hypertrophy of the atrial septum is unknown. Because there is an association between it and obesity, advanced age, and cardiomegaly (3,6), it may be related to underlying metabolic disturbances and has been described in association with cerebrotendinous xanthomatosis (7), mediastinoabdominal lipomatosis (8,9), and cutaneous lipomatosis (10). It also has been described as a complication of parenteral nutrition (11). Although linked to obesity in most large studies (3,12), not all patients with lipomatous hypertrophy are obese (13). Some have proposed that it represents a hamartomatous process while others have suggested that it represents ectopia resulting from misplaced embryonic mesenchyme during atrial septation (12).

The true incidence of lipomatous hypertrophy of the atrial septum is difficult to pinpoint, because most cases are incidental findings and may be overlooked at autopsy. In one series, the estimated incidence was 1.1 percent in over 7,000 autopsies, but these were selected cases because of underlying cardiovascular disease (18). A more contemporary study has shown an incidence of 2.2 percent by prospective imaging (computerized tomography [CT] scans) (12).

**Clinical Findings.** The mean age of 218 patients from seven combined series of lipomatous hypertrophy of the atrial septum was 69 years (3,4,6,12–15); there were 134 men and 84 women, with an age range of 22 to 91 years. No race predilection has been described (3). Over one third of patients are obese (14) and there is an association between increased body weight and increased thickness of the atrial septum (13). The mean body weight of patients with fatty accumulations in the atrial septum of greater than 3 cm does not differ significantly from those with fatty accumulations of greater than 2 cm but less than 3 cm (3). An association with starvation or anemia has not been reported, which is significant because of the known association between fetal fat deposition and cachexia.

The association between atrial arrhythmias and fatty infiltrates of the atrium was initially made in 1969 (16) and has been corroborated by other investigators (17,18). The incidence of atrial arrhythmias in autopsy cases of lipomatous hypertrophy of the atrial septum ranges from 40 to 70 percent (3,4,14). Although both advancing age and coronary artery disease contribute to atrial arrhythmias in many patients, Shirani et al. (3) provide convincing statistical evidence that lipomatous hypertrophy is in itself causatory. The types of arrhythmias described in patients with lipomatous hypertrophy of the atrial septum include atrial fibrillation, atrial premature complexes, junctional rhythms, and ectopic atrial rhythms.

Although it is impossible to prove that this lesion is capable of causing sudden death, lipomatous hypertrophy is generally accepted as a presumptive cause of fatal arrhythmias. Lipomatous hypertrophy was the only finding to explain sudden death in three cases in the series published by McAllister and Fenoglio (15). In addition to arrhythmias or sudden death, lipomatous hypertrophy can compress the superior vena cava (19), and massive tumors may cause congestive heart failure, requiring surgical removal (13,17,20,21). There is a single report, without histologic documentation, of an atrial "lipoma," which may actually represent lipomatous hypertrophy, that resulted in recurrent embolization necessitating amputation of the left arm (22).

When lipomatous hypertrophy is diagnosed during life, resection is the treatment modality. The first antemortem diagnosis occurred in 1982 (18). Today, magnetic resonance imaging (MRI) and transesophageal echocardiography are used to make the diagnosis prior to surgery (23,24). The fat densities seen on cardiac MRI are characteristic (figs. 11-1, 11-2).

Even though the tumor is intra-atrial, it tends to result in a right atrial mass (13). In a series of 323 surgically resected tumors, 6 of 8 resected lipomatous tumors occurred in the atrium (25). In recent surgical series 5 of 605 tumors were atrial lipomas; the clinical presentation included syncope and incidental findings (25–30). In the largest surgical series of 11 cases (13), 8 were women, with an average age of 63 years; 3 were incidentally found, and the other patients had symptoms related to atrial fibrillation, congestive heart failure, palpitations and dizziness, supraventricular tachycardia, and obstruction of the superior vena cava. Uncommon complications include pericardial effusion with constrictive pericarditis (21).

**Gross Findings.** Grossly, the atrial septum (particularly the limbus of the fossa ovalis) is thickened up to several centimeters (fig. 11-3), and the fatty mass generally projects into the right atrial cavity (6). The thickness of the posterior limbus is typically greater than that of the anterior portion, but they may be roughly equivalent, imparting a dumbbell shape to the septum (fig. 11-4) (3).

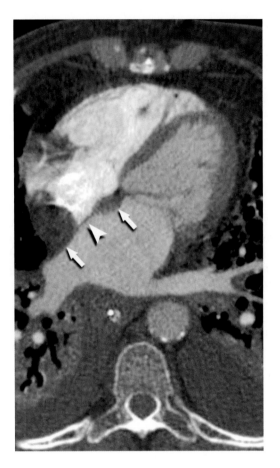

**Figure 11-1**

**LIPOMATOUS HYPERTROPHY OF THE ATRIAL SEPTUM**

Contrast-enhanced axial computerized tomography (CT) image demonstrates a dumbbell-shaped homogeneous lesion of fat attenuation (arrows) centered in the interatrial septum with sparing of the fossa ovalis (arrowhead).

These tumors can achieve great dimensions, even up to 15 cm (19). Although grossly the lesions appear to be well-circumscribed, with a bulging endocardial surface (fig. 11-3), histologically they have a more infiltrative character. The valve of the fossa ovalis is usually spared, although there can be mild fatty infiltration at this site.

**Microscopic Findings.** Histologically, the lesion is characteristic, and contains a mixture of fat and cardiac myocytes (figs. 11-5, 11-6). The fatty areas contain both mature adipocytes as well as brown fat, sometimes referred to as "fetal fat." In most cases, the interspersed cardiac myocytes are bizarre and greatly enlarged (fig. 11-7). Mitoses are absent. Abundant vacuolated fat cells and atypical myocytes with a nuclear

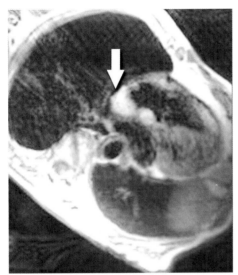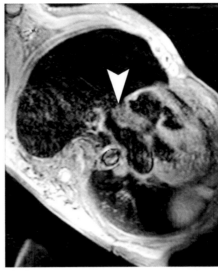

**Figure 11-2**

**LIPOMATOUS HYPERTROPHY OF THE ATRIAL SEPTUM**

T1-weighted magnetic resonance image (MRI), horizontal long-axis, without (left) and with (right) fat saturation.

Left: The interatrial mass shows high signal intensity (arrow), matching the subcutaneous fat in the chest wall.

Right: With fat saturation, the mass decreases in signal intensity (arrowhead) thus confirming its fatty composition.

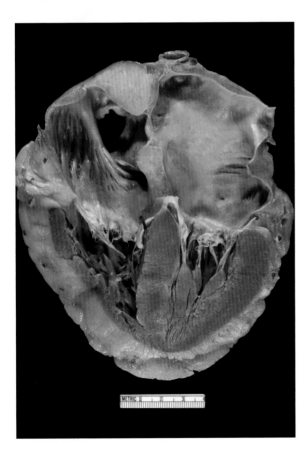

**Figure 11-3**

**LIPOMATOUS HYPERTROPHY OF THE ATRIAL SEPTUM**

There is a nearly spherical fatty mass projecting into the right atrium at the posterior region of the limbus of the fossa ovalis. The anterior limb (located beneath the valve of the fossa ovalis in this image) is also thickened, although to a much lesser extent.

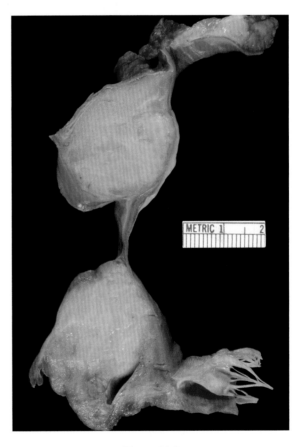

**Figure 11-4**

**LIPOMATOUS HYPERTROPHY OF THE ATRIAL SEPTUM**

Near equal involvement throughout the limbus of the fossa ovalis causes the atrial septum to assume a dumbbell shape.

191

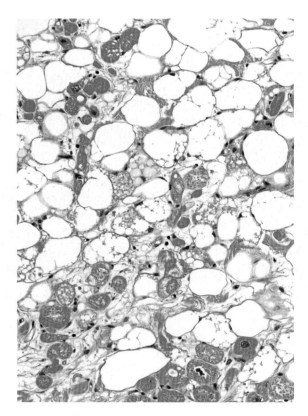

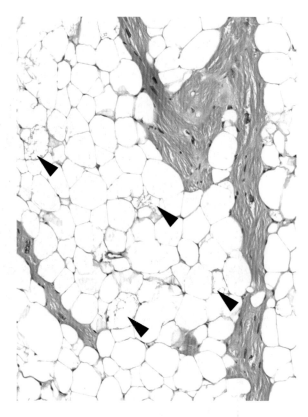

**Figure 11-5**

**LIPOMATOUS HYPERTROPHY OF THE ATRIAL SEPTUM**

There is a mixture of mature (white) fat, brown fat, and hypertrophied myocytes.

**Figure 11-6**

**LIPOMATOUS HYPERTROPHY OF THE ATRIAL SEPTUM**

There are white fat cells, brown fat (arrowheads), and hypertrophied cardiac myocytes.

length exceeding 40 μm are significantly more prevalent in cases of lipomatous hypertrophy than in controls, independent of age (13).

There is an association between the interatrial thickness of the lesion and cardiomegaly and obesity (3,13). Although some have proposed an association between lipomatous hypertrophy of the atrial septum and coronary atherosclerosis (3), this has not been substantiated in more recent studies (5,13). Increased epicardial fat is commonly associated with lipomatous hypertrophy (fig. 11-3).

**Differential Diagnosis.** The differential diagnosis of lipomatous hypertrophy includes liposarcoma and other sarcomas, especially if there is a large mass resected surgically. The brown fat cells in lipomatous hypertrophy are sometimes mistaken for lipoblasts of liposarcoma. Unlike lipoblasts, the fat cells in lipomatous hypertrophy do not form signet ring structures and do not have enlarged, hyperchromatic indented

nuclei, as does liposarcoma. The hyperchromatic, enlarged myocytes are also sometimes mistaken for malignant cells, but the lack of mitotic figures and the other features of lipomatous hypertrophy point to the correct diagnosis. Moreover, similar enlarged and bizarre cardiac myocytes are seen in both dilated and hypertrophic forms of cardiomyopathy.

Rarely, the diagnosis is made on the basis of an endomyocardial biopsy (31). In such instances, clinical and radiologic correlation is essential, given the small size of these biopsies. The imaging features, together with the presence of mature fat, is strongly suggestive of the diagnosis.

**Treatment and Prognosis.** Once, lipomatous hypertrophy of the atrial septum was only diagnosed at autopsy; now, it is a recognized radiologic and surgical entity. The short-term outcome of resection is excellent (13,17,19,21,27), although one study showed a

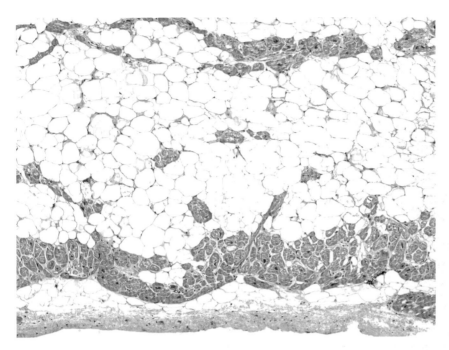

**Figure 11-7**

**LIPOMATOUS HYPERTROPHY OF THE ATRIAL SEPTUM**

At low magnification, the infiltrative appearance of the fat is appreciated, with the entrapped myocytes throughout.

long-term survival period shorter than that for patients with operative myxomas (25).

Surgery includes open biopsy with frozen section to confirm a benign diagnosis in cases of incidentally found lesions (13). If complete resection is the goal, then pericardial patch repair is frequently required (13). Indications for surgical intervention include heart failure or intractable arrhythmias (32). In many cases, there is resolution of the atrial arrhythmia or improvement of cardiac function postoperatively.

## LIPOMA

**Definition.** *Lipomas* of the heart are, like lipomas of extracardiac soft tissue, benign neoplasms of mature adipocytes. In distinction to lipomatous hypertrophy of the atrial septum, there is no brown fat or interspersed cardiomyocytes.

**General Features.** Lipomas of the heart are rare. There were 17 examples in Mahaim's monograph on cardiac tumors (33). In general, surgical series of heart tumors show few or no lipomas (excluding lipomatous hypertrophy): only 1 percent of 634 resected tumors are lipomas (25–30,34). Heath (35) stated that 30 cases had been reported by 1968. It is difficult to determine, however, the proportion of these cases that were, in reality, lipomatous hypertrophy of the atrial septum. Eight cardiac and five pericardial lipomas were reported in the second edition of this

series (15). A recent, large retrospective study reported that of 323 surgically resected cardiac tumors, 3 percent were atrial cardiac lipomas that were presumably lipomatous hypertrophy but less than 1 percent were fatty tumors found outside the atria (25).

**Clinical Features.** In contrast to lipomatous hypertrophy, lipomas are usually found on the epicardial surfaces and are generally asymptomatic. Nevertheless, several large epicardial lipomas have caused preoperative left ventricular dysfunction (22,36), and one tumor infiltrated the soft tissue surrounding an epicardial coronary artery, necessitating complex surgery (37). These reports indicate that cardiac lipomas are not always innocent lesions. One case of multiple lipomas of the posterior wall in the right ventricle in a patient with a partial atrioventricular canal has been reported (38), as well as multiple tumors in patients with tuberous sclerosis (15). A preoperative diagnosis can be made with MRI, which shows hyperintensity on the T1-weighted sequence (38,39).

**Molecular Findings.** Cardiac lipomas have not, to date, been shown to be associated with the same molecular genetic underpinnings that extracardiac lipomas frequently exhibit, namely, chromosome 12 abnormalities. A single report, however, of a large invasive epicardial lipoma arising in association with lipomatosis was

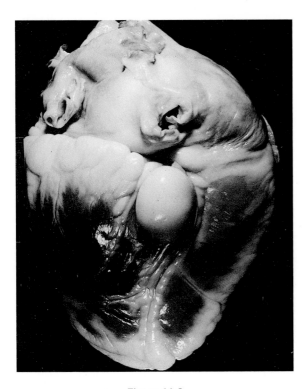

**Figure 11-8**

**CARDIAC LIPOMA**

There is a circumscribed mass on the inferior aspect of the heart at the base.

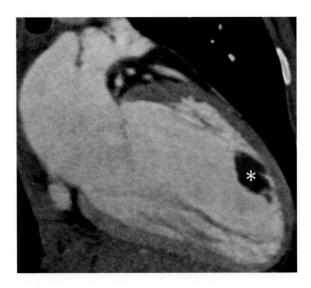

**Figure 11-9**

**CARDIAC LIPOMA**

Contrast-enhanced echocardiogram (ECG)-gated cardiac CT angiographic image, two-chamber view reconstruction, shows a nonenhancing ovoid lesion of fat attenuation (asterisk) within the left ventricular chamber attached to papillary muscle fibers.

demonstrated to have a novel translocation, t(2;19)(p13;p13.2) (8). A single case report has described a right atrial lipoma arising in association with Cowden syndrome, confirmed by a demonstrable mutation in the *PTEN* gene (40). Several cases of cardiac lipoma associated with tuberous sclerosis have been reported (41,42).

**Gross Findings.** Most cardiac lipomas are epicardial lesions (fig. 11-8), although intracavitary lesions have been described (43,44). They occur on the surface or within the cavity of both atria and both ventricles (figs. 11-9, 11-10), where they usually manifest as well-circumscribed tan-yellow lesions (fig. 11-11). Most reported cases have been single, with the exception of those that have arisen in association with tuberous sclerosis (45). Multiple lipomas have also been documented in association with congenital heart defects (45).

**Microscopic Findings.** Histologically, cardiac lipomas are composed essentially of mature adipocytes, although there may be entrapped myocytes at the base of the tumor (figs. 11-12,

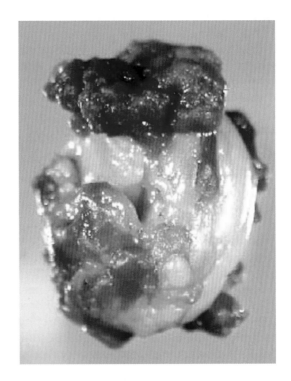

**Figure 11-10**

**CARDIAC LIPOMA**

At surgery, a 2.4 x 1.3-cm left ventricular lipoma was resected from the anterolateral papillary muscle.

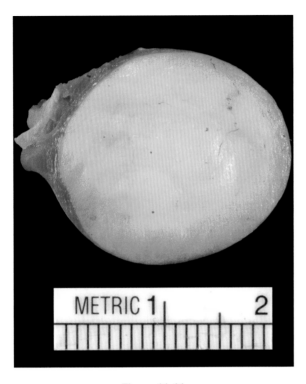

**Figure 11-11**

**CARDIAC LIPOMA**

An intracavitary right atrial lipoma that was surgically resected from the crista terminalis shows the well-circumscribed nature of the mass.

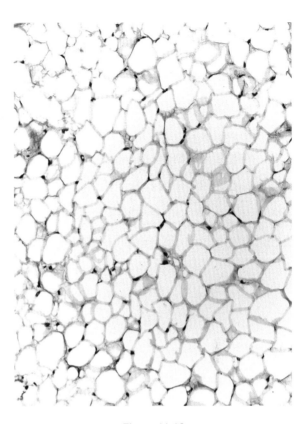

**Figure 11-12**

**CARDIAC LIPOMA**

High-power view of a cardiac lipoma characterized almost entirely by mature adipocytes.

11-13). A capsule is usually present (15), although it may be focally absent or attenuated. There is a single report of a mural, incidental angiolipoma infiltrating the posterior wall of the left ventricle (46). Its location, infiltrative nonencapsulated appearance, and the large number of vessels, described as veins, capillaries, and arterioles within the tumor, suggest to us that the lesion is best classified as a hemangioma. Cardiac hemangiomas are typically mural, rather than epicardial lesions, and may contain significant accumulations of fat (see chapter 7).

**Treatment.** Reports of surgical excision of cardiac lipomas show no significant complications (22,37,45,47–50).

## LIPOMATOUS HAMARTOMA OF CARDIAC VALVES

There have been at least nine reports of *lipomatous tumors involving the atrioventricular valves*, with roughly equal frequency between the mitral and tricuspid valves (6,51–58). The patients range from 2 to 76 years at presentation (53,54), and no sex predilection is apparent. At least one patient was obese (55).

Patients present with the symptoms of valve incompetence, and the preoperative diagnosis is facilitated by echocardiography and CT (51). The tumors may be multiple, and valve replacement may be necessary because of involvement of the papillary muscle or adjacent atrial tissue (51,53,55).

Histologically, the lesions are composed of varying proportions of mature fat and fibrous tissue. While they have been reported to have an infiltrative border with the adjacent myocardium, this is not necessarily indicative of malignant behavior (57). They are considered to be hamartomas, because there is often an admixture of fibrous tissue and a lack of encapsulation (54).

**Figure 11-13**

**CARDIAC LIPOMA**

The well-circumscribed border that lipomas typically exhibit with the adjacent myocardium is seen, although some fat is present superficially in the interstitium.

## THE FATTY HEART

Although not tumors, fat may occur diffusely in the epicardial surfaces, with areas of infiltration of the myocardium. The *fatty heart* or *lipomatous infiltration of the heart* is not a discrete lesion. There is a large increase in fat in the atrioventricular sulci, over both ventricles, and occasionally within the ventricular walls (figs. 11-14, 11-15). Occasionally, fatty replacement of scar tissue is seen with old myocardial injury, such as infarction.

There is no clear definition of an abnormal accumulation of epicardial fat. Five percent of hearts in a large autopsy series had extensive fat deposits, resulting in "floating" hearts when immersed in water (59). In all cases, the fatty infiltration was an incidental finding, associated with obesity and lipomatous infiltration of the atrial septum (59). Rarely, lipomatous infiltration that is not limited to the atrial septum causes sudden death (60). Histologically, the fatty deposits are composed of mature fat, which may diffusely infiltrate the ventricles.

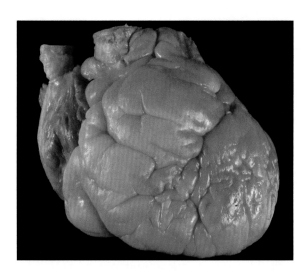

**Figure 11-14**

**FATTY HEART**

This heart exhibits marked epicardial fat that was, in this case, not associated with obesity.

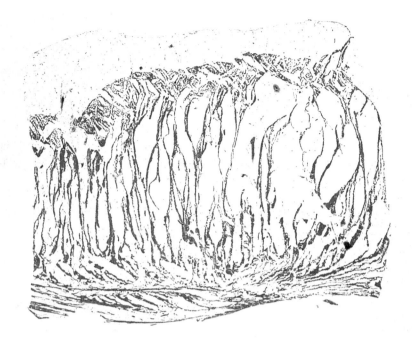

**Figure 11-15**

**MASSIVE FATTY INFILTRATION, RIGHT VENTRICLE**

The patient was a 50-year-old obese woman who died suddenly. At autopsy, there was severe coronary atherosclerosis, as well as marked thickening of the right ventricular wall, up to 2 cm.

## REFERENCES

1. Agbamu DA, McMahon RF. Lipomatous hamartoma of the interatrial septum. Am J Cardiovasc Pathol 1993;4:371-373.
2. Inoue TM, Mohri N, Nagahara T, Takanashi R. A case report of "lipomatous hypertrophy of the cardiac interatrial septum" with a proposal for a new term "lipomatous hamartoma of the cardiac atrial septum." Acta Pathol Jpn 1988;38:1583-1585.
3. Shirani J, Roberts W. Clinical, electrocardiographic and morphologic features of massive fatty deposits ("lipomatous hypertrophy") in the atrial septum. J Am Coll Cardiol 1993;22:226-238.
4. Page D. Lipomatous hypertrophy of the cardiac interatrial septum: Its development and probable clinical significance. Hum Pathol 1970;1:151-163.
5. Agmon Y, Meissner I, Tajik AJ, et al. Clinical, laboratory, and transesophageal echocardiographic correlates of interatrial septal thickness: a population-based transesophageal echocardiographic study. J Am Soc Echocardiogr 2005;18:175-182.
6. Crocker D. Lipomatous infiltrates of the heart. Arch Pathol Lab Med 1978;102:69-72.
7. Dotti MT, Mondillo S, Plewnia K, Agricola E, Federico A. Cerebrotendinous xanthomatosis: evidence of lipomatous hypertrophy of the atrial septum. J Neurol 1998;245:723-726.
8. Vaughan CJ, Weremowicz S, Goldstein MM, et al., A t(2;19)(p13;p13.2) in a giant invasive cardiac lipoma from a patient with multiple lipomatosis. Genes Chromosomes Cancer 2000;28:133-137.
9. Enzi G, Busetto L, Ceschin E, Coin A, Digito M, Pigozzo S. Multiple symmetric lipomatosis: clinical aspects and outcome in a long-term longitudinal study. Int J Obes Relat Metab Disord 2002;26:253-261.
10. Takayama S, Sukekawa H, Arimoto T, et al. Lipomatous hypertrophy of the interatrial septum with cutaneous lipomatosis. Circ J 2007;71:986-989.
11. Beau PM, Michel P, Coisne D, Morichau-Beauchant M. Lipomatous hypertrophy of the cardiac interatrial septum: An unusual complication in long-term home parenteral nutrition in adult patients. J Parenteral Enteral Nutrition 1991;15:659-662.
12. Heyer CM, Kagel T, Lemburg SP, Bauer TT, Nicolas V. Lipomatous hypertrophy of the interatrial septum: a prospective study of incidence, imaging findings, and clinical symptoms. Chest 2003;124:2068-2073.

13. Burke AP, Litovsky S, Virmani R. Lipomatous hypertrophy of the atrial septum presenting as a right atrial mass. Am J Surg Pathol 1996;20:678-685.

14. Reyes C, Jablokow V. Lipomatous hypertrophy of the cardiac interatrial septum. A report of 38 cases and review of the literature. Am J Clin Pathol 1979;72:785-788.

15. McAllister HA, Fenoglio JJ Jr. Tumors of the cardiovascular system. Atlas of Tumor Pathology, 2nd Series, Fascicle 15. Washington DC: Armed Forces Institute of Pathology; 1978.

16. Kluge WF. Lipomatous hypertrophy of the interatrial septum. Northwest Med 1969;68:25-30.

17. Fisher MS, Edmonds P. Lipomatous hypertrophy of interatrial septum. Diagnosis by magnetic resonance imaging. J Comput Tomogr 1988; 12:267-269.

18. Isner JM, Swan CS 2nd, Mikus JP, Carter BL. Lipomatous hypertrophy of the interatrial septum. In vivo diagnosis. Circulation 1982;66:470-473.

19. Case Records of the Massachusetts General Hospital. Weekly clinicopathological exercises. Case 10-1989. A 60-year-old man with a large right atrial mass. N Engl J Med 1989;320:652-660.

20. Bhattacharjee M, Neligan M, Dervan P. Lipomatous hypertrophy of the interatrial septum: an unusual intraoperative finding. Br Heart J 1991;65:49-50.

21. Tschirkov A, Stegaru B. Lipomatous hypertrophy of interatrial septum presenting as recurring pericardial effusion and mistaken for constrictive pericarditis. Thorac Cardiovasc Surg 1979; 27:400-403.

22. Verkkala K, Kupari M, Maamies T, et al. Primary cardiac tumours—operative treatment of 20 patients. Thorac Cardiovasc Surg 1989;37:361-364.

23. Levine RW, Weyman AE, Dinsmore RE, et al. Noninvasive tissue characterization: diagnosis of lipomatous hypertrophy of the atrial septum by nuclear magnetic resonance imaging. J Am Coll Cardiol 1986;7:688-692.

24. Pochis WT, Saeian K, Sagar KB. Usefulness of transesophageal echocardiography in diagnosing lipomatous hypertrophy of the atrial septum with comparison to transthoracic echocardiography. Am J Cardiol 1992;70:396-398.

25. Elbardissi AW, Dearani JA, Daly RC, et al. Survival after resection of primary cardiac tumors: a 48-year experience. Circulation 2008;118(14 Suppl):S7-15.

26. Bakaeen FG, Reardon MJ, Coselli JS, et al. Surgical outcome in 85 patients with primary cardiac tumors. Am J Surg 2003;186:641-647; discussion 647.

27. Bossert T, Gummert JF, Battellini R, et al. Surgical experience with 77 primary cardiac tumors. Interact Cardiovasc Thorac Surg 2005;4:311-315.

28. Kamiya H, Yasuda T, Nagamine H, et al. Surgical treatment of primary cardiac tumors: 28 years' experience in Kanazawa University Hospital. Jpn Circ J 2001;65:315-319.

29. Odim J, Reehal V, Laks H, Mehta U, Fishbein MC. Surgical pathology of cardiac tumors. Two decades at an urban institution. Cardiovasc Pathol 2003;12:267-270.

30. Thomas-de-Montpreville V, Nottin R, Dulmet E, Serraf A. Heart tumors in children and adults: clinicopathological study of 59 patients from a surgical center. Cardiovasc Pathol 2007;16:22-28.

31. Stone GW, O'Kell RT, Good TH, Hartzler GO. Lipomatous hypertrophy of the interatrial septum: diagnosis by percutaneous transvenous biopsy. Am Heart J 1990;119(Pt 1):406-468.

32. Zeebregts CJ, Hensens AG, Timmermans J, Pruszczynski MS, Lacquet LK. Lipomatous hypertrophy of the interatrial septum: indication for surgery? Eur J Cardiothorac Surg 1997;11:785-787.

33. Mahaim I. Les tumeurs et les polypes du cœur: étude anatomoclinique. Paris: Masson et Cie; 1945.

34. Grande AM, Ragni T, Vigano M. Primary cardiac tumors. A clinical experience of 12 years. Tex Heart Inst J 1993;20:223-230.

35. Heath D. Pathology of cardiac tumors. Am J Cardiol 1968;21:315-327.

36. Rokey R, Mulvagh SL, Cheirif J, Mattox KL, Johnston DL. Lipomatous encasement and compression of the heart: antemortem diagnosis by cardiac nuclear magnetic resonance imaging and catheterization. Am Heart J 1989;117:952-953.

37. Reece IJ, Cooley DA, Frazier OH, Hallman GL, Powers PL, Montero CG. Cardiac tumors. Clinical spectrum and prognosis of lesions other than classical benign myxoma in 20 patients. J Thorac Cardiovasc Surg 1984;88:439-446.

38. Tuna IC, Julsrud PR, Click RL, Tazelaar HD, Bresnahan DR, Danielson GK. Tissue characterization of an unusual right atrial mass by magnetic resonance imaging. Mayo Clin Proc 1991;66:498-501.

39. Auger D, Pressacco J, Marcotte F, Tremblay A, Dore A, Ducharme A. Cardiac masses: an integrative approach using echocardiography and other imaging modalities. Heart 2011;97:1101-1109.

40. Ceresa F, Calarco G, Franzì E, Patanè F. Right atrial lipoma in patient with Cowden syndrome. Interact Cardiovasc Thorac Surg 2010;11:803-804.

41. Jabir S, Al-Hyassat S, Histological diagnosis of cardiac lipoma in an adult with tuberous sclerosis. BMJ Case Rep 2013;Jan.

42. Winterkorn EB, Dodd JD, Inglessis I, Holmvang G, Thiele EA. Tuberous sclerosis complex and myocardial fat-containing lesions: a report of four cases. Clin Genet 2007;71:371-373.

43. Tanzola RC, Allard R, Hamilton A. Intraoperative transesophageal echocardiography for an intracavitary left ventricular lipoma. Anesth Analg 2009;108:786-787.

44. Grebenc ML, Rosado de Christenson ML, Burke AP, Green CE, Galvin JR. Primary cardiac and pericardial neoplasms: radiologic-pathologic correlation. Radiographics 2000;20:1073-1103; quiz 1110-1112.

45. Tazelaar HD, Locke TJ, McGregor CG. Pathology of surgically excised primary cardiac tumors. Mayo Clin Proc 1992;67:957-965.

46. Kiaer HW, Myocardial angiolipoma. Acta Pathol Microbiol Immunol Scand A 1984;92:291-292.

47. Blondeau P. Primary cardiac tumors—French studies of 533 cases. Thorac Cardiovasc Surg 1990;38(Suppl 2):192-195.

48. Murphy MC, Sweeney MS, Putnam JB Jr, et al. Surgical treatment of cardiac tumors: a 25-year experience. Ann Thorac Surg 1990;49:612-617; discussion 617-618.

49. Zhu SB, Zhu J, Liu Y, Wang RP. Surgical treatment of a giant symptomatic cardiac lipoma. J Thorac Oncol 2013;8:1341-2.

50. Singh B, Bhairappa S, Shankar SK, Prasad NM, Manjunath CN. Cardiac lipoma at unusual location—mimicking atrial myxoma. Echocardiography 2013;30:E72-4.

51. Anderson DR, Gray MR. Mitral incompetence associated with lipoma infiltrating the mitral valve. Br Heart J 1988;60:169-171.

52. Barberger-Gateau P, Paquet M, Desaulniers D, Chenard J. Fibrolipoma of the mitral valve in a child. Clinical and echocardiographic features. Circulation 1978;58:955-958.

53. Behnam R, Williams G, Gerlis L, Walker D, Scott O. Lipoma of the mitral valve and papillary muscle. Am J Cardiol 1983;51:1459-1460.

54. Crotty TB, Edwards WD, Oh JK, Rodeheffer RJ. Lipomatous hamartoma of the tricuspid valve: echocardiographic-pathologic correlations. Clin Cardiol 1991;14:262-266.

55. Dollar AL, Wallace RB, Kent KM, Burkhart MW, Roberts WC. Mitral valve replacement for mitral lipoma associated with severe obesity. Am J Cardiol 1989;64:1405-1407.

56. Harth M, Ruemmele P, Knuechel-Clarke R, Elsner D, Riegger G. Sclerosed lipoma of the mitral valve. J Heart Valve Dis 2003;12:722-725.

57. Jyrala A, Kay GL. Mitral valve lipomatous hamartoma infiltrating myocardium. J Thorac Cardiovasc Surg 2010;140:e11-12.

58. Vadmal MS, Hajdu SI. Lipoma of the mitral valve in a child. Ann Clin Lab Sci 1998;28:242-245.

59. Roberts WC, Roberts JD. The floating heart or the heart too fat to sink: analysis of 55 necropsy patients. Am J Cardiol 1983;52:1286-1289.

60. Voigt J, Agdal N. Lipomatous infiltration of the heart. An uncommon cause of sudden, unexpected death in a young man. Arch Pathol Lab Med 1982;106:497-498.

# 12 CARDIAC PARAGANGLIOMA

## DEFINITION

*Cardiac paraganglioma* is a neoplasm of paraganglion cells situated in or around the heart. These tumors are derived from atrial paraganglial tissue or aortic body tissue found at the base of the great vessels.

Paraganglial tissues function as baroreceptors, and are present in the aortic bodies, carotid bodies, and atria as part of the atrial stretch reflex. Arterial or high-pressure baroreceptors are most concentrated in the aortic bodies and carotid sinuses; low-pressure receptors (cardiopulmonary) are present in the walls of the atria, especially right atrium, veins, and less frequently, ventricles.

Aortic bodies are present along the aortic arch, the outer curvature of the aorta; the term *aorticopulmonary body* is sometimes used to encompass paraganglial tissue around the pulmonary trunk as well. Tumors from these cells may be partially intrapericardial but surround the ascending aorta, and sometimes the pulmonary trunk, with little or no involvement of the atria. Carotid body paragangliomas are more common than those derived from other baroreceptors, but are located outside the pericardium at the bifurcation of the carotid artery. This chapter discusses paragangliomas that arise from paraganglial tissue within the atria, and more rarely, ventricles, and tumors of the proximal great arteries that arise within the pericardium. In larger tumors the precise site of origin (aortic body receptor in the ascending aorta, atrial paraganglial tissue) may not be discernable, as mediastinal paragangliomas are generally near the heart or great arteries (1).

There are a variety of synonyms for paraganglioma. Extra-adrenal paragangliomas that secrete catecholamines have been termed *chromaffin paraganglioma*, or *extra-adrenal pheochromocytoma* (obsolete term). Tumors of similar morphology that occur in the region of the carotid body and aortic body are sometimes called *chemodectomas*. Paragangliomas of the carotid body and jugulotympanic region have been termed *glomus jugulare* and *glomus tympanicum tumors*, respectively.

The terms *pheochromocytoma* (2–5) and *chemodectoma* (6) are used for cardiac paragangliomas that are functional and nonfunctional, respectively, but the latter term is generally reserved for tumors in the head and neck. There are no consistent histologic differences between functioning and nonfunctioning paragangliomas, and the chromaffin reaction does not reliably separate these tumors. Therefore, the use of the term paraganglioma has been recommended for extra-adrenal paragangliomas of soft tissue regardless of secretory status.

## GENERAL FEATURES

The cells of origin of cardiac paraganglioma are most likely those of the intrinsic cardiac paraganglia, which are located in the atria, along the atrioventricular groove, and near the roots of the great vessels. Neoplasms arising from paraganglial cells are rare. Paraganglia are very rare in the ventricles, accounting for the rarity of ventricular paragangliomas (7–9). The cardiac atria (including the atrial septum) are innervated by visceral autonomic paraganglia, as opposed to aorticopulmonary paragangliomas, which are derived from branchial arch structures (4). As noted above, paragangliomas of the heart are termed pheochromocytomas (10,11), when there is clinical evidence of catecholamine secretion, or chemodectomas.

Pheochromocytoma and other paragangliomas are part of the multiple endocrine neoplasia (MEN) syndrome, specifically types 2a and 2b. Cardiac paraganglioma as part of this syndrome is rare (12). Susceptibility genes for paraganglioma include the proto-oncogene *RET* (associated with MEN2) and the tumor-suppressor gene *VHL* (associated with von Hippel-Lindau disease). The genes for succinate dehydrogenase subunit D (*SHD*) and succinate dehydrogenase

**Table 12-1**

**CLINICAL FEATURES OF CARDIAC PARAGANGLIOMAS**[a]

| Feature | Frequency |
|---|---|
| Male:female | 37:45 |
| Functionally active ("pheochromocytomas") | 79% |
| Invasive into myocardium | 64% |
| Age, years, ± SD[b] (total) | 39 ± 15 |
|     Functionally active (elevated serum catecholamines) | 35 ± 14 |
|     Functionally inactive | 47 ± 10 |
|     Invasive | 36 ± 12 |
|     Noninvasive | 46 ± 17 |
| Symptom, at diagnosis | |
|     Refractory hypertension | 53% |
|     Chest pain | 14% |
|     Shortness of breath | 12% |
|     Palpitations, headache, sweating | 11% |
|     Asymptomatic | 9% |
|     Syncope | 1% |
| Size, cm ± SD | 5.7 ± 2.2 |
| Site in heart | |
|     Left atrium | 39% |
|     Right atrium | 19% |
|     AP window | 18% |
|     Left ventricle | 8% |
|     Atrioventricular groove | 6% |
|     Interatrial septum | 5% |
| Tumor involves pericardial space | 69% |
| Tumor entirely myocardial | 31% |
| Tumor blood supply | |
|     Right coronary artery | 49% |
|     Left coronary artery | 48% |
|     Noncoronary arteries | 3% |

[a]Data retrieved from case reports from reference 63 of 82 surgically resected cardiac paragangliomas.
[b]SD = standard deviation.

subunits B and C (*SDHB* and *SDHC*) recently have been associated with paragangliomas (13), the latter reported in a patient with cardiac paraganglioma (14). A case of cardiac paraganglioma as part of Carney-Stratakis syndrome (pulmonary chondroma and gastrointestinal stromal tumor) has been reported (15).

Cardiac paragangliomas are rare tumors. Approximately 75 cases have been reported in the English language literature at the time of this writing. Only 5 percent of surgically resected paragangliomas occur within the pericardium (16–21). Although 10 to 50 percent of parasympathetic paragangliomas are familial, there are only rare familial cardiac paragangliomas (22,23).

## CLINICAL FEATURES

Most intrapericardial paragangliomas developing within the atria, are benign, and are functional, resulting in systemic hypertension (Table 12-1) (6,24–26). Distinct from head and neck paragangliomas, the cardiac variety is usually functional, while fewer than 5 percent of extracardiac paragangliomas are clinically functional. Most patients with cardiac paraganglioma are young or middle aged, with an age range at diagnosis from 15 to 60 years (mean, 39 years). There may be a slight female predominance (1). Patients as young as 15 years have been reported with cardiac paraganglioma (27,28). Slightly more than 50 percent of patients present with paroxysmal hypertension and symptoms of pheochromocytoma (27,29), and most have hypertension (1), indicating that these tumors are functional. An elevated 24-hour urinary norepinephrine level (1) is an indication of catecholamine secretion by the tumor. Other symptoms include palpitations, chest pain (18,30,31), headache (32), shortness of breath (33), murmurs, angina (34,35), acute myocardial infarction (36), and mitral regurgitation (37). Gestational hypertension has been reported as an initial symptom of cardiac paraganglioma (38). Embolic stroke may occur due to left ventricular mural thrombus (39).

Cardiac paraganglioma may be an incidental finding (40). Rarely, the feeder artery is prominent angiographically and results in aneurysm (40). There has been one report of mediastinal paracardiac paraganglioma as part of the Carney triad (1).

Rare malignant cardiac paragangliomas have been reported (41–43). Unfortunately, these reports lack a detailed histologic description. The malignant nature was documented in these cases by bone metastasis (41) and lymph node metastasis (43).

Echocardiography (44), computed tomography (CT), and magnetic resonance imaging (MRI) have been successfully used to characterize cardiac paragangliomas preoperatively (8,45–47). Somatostatin-receptor nuclear imaging provides functionally specific imaging (48). $^{131}$I-metaiodobenzylguanidine scintigraphy is also useful for the localization of mediastinal paragangliomas (1,4). Positron emission tomography (PET) in conjunction with CT is used, as

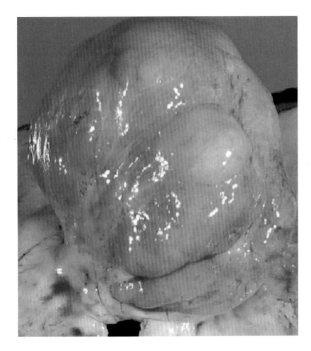

**Figure 12-1**

**CARDIAC PARAGANGLIOMA**

Rarely, cardiac paraganglioma is a polypoid intracavitary lesion. This tumor arose from the interatrial septum and projected into the left atrial cavity. The tumor was 8 cm in greatest dimension. The patient was a middle-aged man who presented with fatigue and shortness of breath. Imaging studies, including echocardiography, computerized tomography (CT), and magnetic resonance imaging (MRI), demonstrated a cardiac mass involving the left atrium that protruded into the right atrium through the oval fossa. There was no history of hypertension. The preoperative diagnosis was biatrial myxoma.

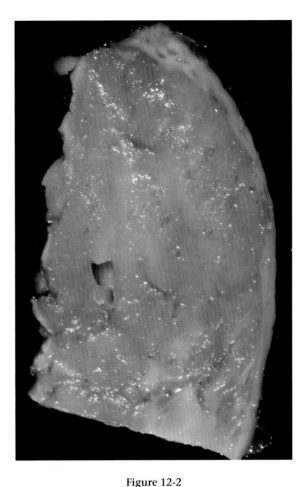

**Figure 12-2**

**CARDIAC PARAGANGLIOMA**

The cut surface is homogeneous and copper tan, with minimal scarring. The tumor was a large lesion at the base of the heart, involving both atria and extending into the pericardium.

with other tumors (49). Preoperative angiography may show feeder arteries that guide the surgical approach (18).

## GROSS FINDINGS

Paragangliomas are poorly circumscribed, large (5 to 15 cm) masses (29) that are typically most prominent in the atria. Approximately two thirds are invasive (Table 12-1), which may necessitate aggressive surgical treatment. Either the right atrium (27,50) or left atrium (51,52) is the primary tumor site, and biatrial cardiac paragangliomas occur (53). Although the tumor typically grows into the atrial wall, left atrial paragangliomas are occasionally intraluminal, mimicking cardiac myxoma (51). Sites of extension through the atrial wall include the mediastinum (54) and pericardial space (55). Right

atrial tumors may compress the superior vena cava, causing inflow obstruction to the right atrium (18). Compression of the pulmonary veins has been reported in tumors arising in the left atrium (34). Left ventricular paragangliomas are very rare (6,9).

Most cardiac paragangliomas are located on the epicardial surface of the base of the heart or atria; less commonly, they are intracavitary atrial lesions that may present as polypoid lesions and mimic myxomas (fig. 12-1), or appear to arise from within the atrial septum (37,56). On cut section, they are usually uniformly tan-yellow and homogeneous (figs. 12-2, 12-3), although there may be areas of gross hemorrhage.

**Figure 12-3**

**CARDIAC PARAGANGLIOMA**

The cut surface is homogeneous with focal scarring. The tumor arose from the right atrioventricular groove in a young woman with severe hypertension. Urine metanephrines and norepinephrines were markedly increased. The patient required right ventricular reconstruction with tricuspid valve replacement and coronary artery bypass surgery. (Courtesy Dr. H. Tazelaar, Rochester, MN.)

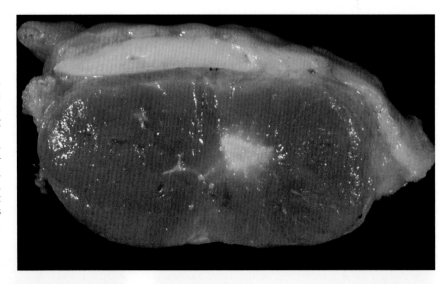

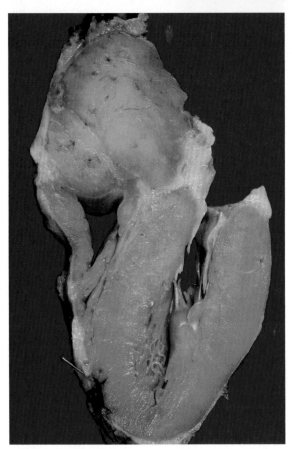

**Figure 12-4**

**CARDIAC PARAGANGLIOMA**

The tumor was located between the proximal ascending aorta and pulmonary trunk, and was unresectable (same tumor as shown in figure 12-2). The patient required a heart transplant.

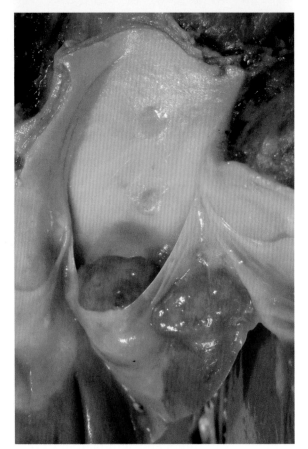

**Figure 12-5**

**CARDIAC PARAGANGLIOMA**

The tumor illustrated in figure 12-4 is seen growing through the pulmonary artery into the pulmonary valve.

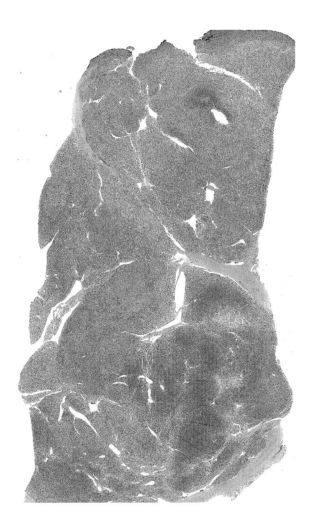

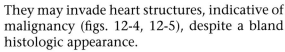

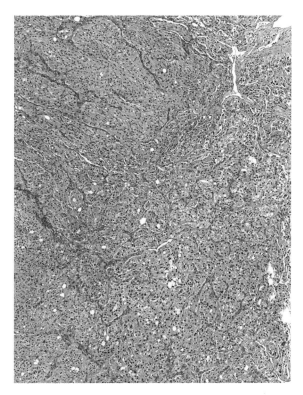

**Figure 12-6**

**CARDIAC PARAGANGLIOMA**

Left: At low magnification, the tumor illustrated in figure 12-2 is homogenous and cellular, with rare fibrous strands.

Above: At slightly higher magnification, the typical trabecular and organoid pattern of paraganglioma is seen.

They may invade heart structures, indicative of malignancy (figs. 12-4, 12-5), despite a bland histologic appearance.

## MICROSCOPIC FINDINGS

Cardiac paragangliomas are histologically similar to extracardiac paragangliomas and adrenal pheochromocytomas. Paragangliomas are fairly homogeneous cellular tumors (fig. 12-6). Although unencapsulated, there is often a fibrous band around the tumor (figs. 12-7–12-9) that may be infiltrated by tumor cells, analogous to capsular invasion (fig. 12-10). Cardiac paragangliomas almost always consist of tumor cell nests in an organoid pattern (figs. 12-11–12-14). Anastomosing cords and trabeculae are less frequent (fig. 12-15). Sustentacular cells are of variable prominence (figs. 12-16, 12-17). There is typically a prominent vascular pattern, but hemangiopericytoma-like branching vessels are

unusual. There may be mild cytologic atypia (figs. 12-18, 12-19). Hemorrhage may be present between the cell nests, similar to extracardiac paragangliomas (fig. 12-20). Cytoplasmic clearing is often a prominent feature in cardiac paraganglioma (figs. 12-21–12-23). Pseudoinclusions and intracytoplasmic hyaline globules are not as frequent in cardiac paragangliomas as in paragangliomas of the adrenal gland (pheochromocytomas). Ganglioneuromatous differentiation, as has been described in extracardiac sites, has not been reported in the heart. A pigmented cardiac paraganglioma has been reported (57).

There are no histologic criteria that predict aggressive behavior in cardiac paraganglioma. Nuclear pleomorphism is common in tumors with a benign course (figs. 12-24–12-26), and not an indication of malignancy. The histologic features associated with aggressive behavior in extracardiac paragangliomas include necrosis,

205

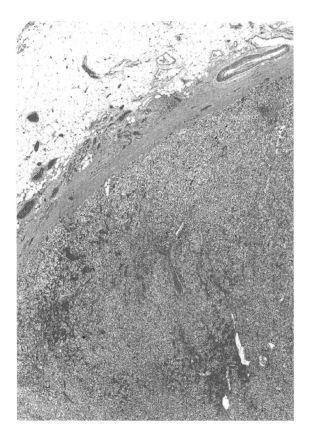 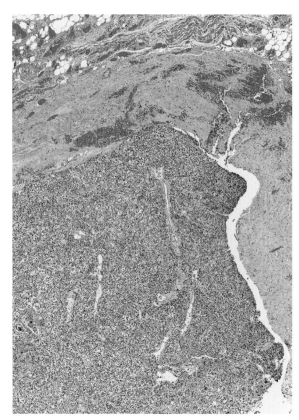

**Figure 12-7**

**CARDIAC PARAGANGLIOMA**

Left: A fibrous capsule separates the tumor from the surrounding fat. This tumor has focal hemorrhage.
Right: A different area shows the junction between the tumor and the left atrial fat, with an interface of fibrous tissue.

**Figure 12-8**

**CARDIAC PARAGANGLIOMA**

The interface between the tumor and the atrial tissue is generally distinct, but the tumor is not discretely encapsulated.

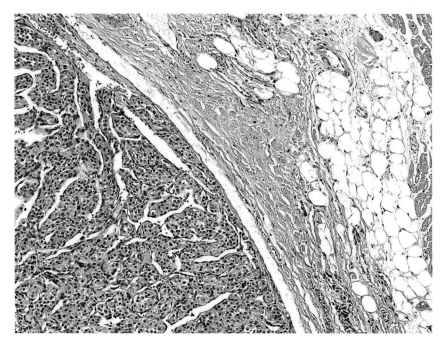

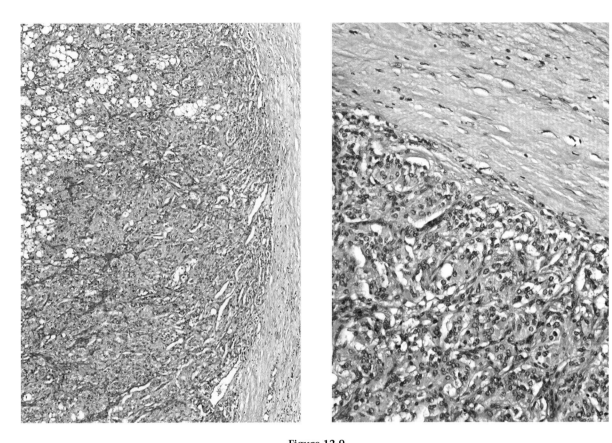

**Figure 12-9**

**CARDIAC PARAGANGLIOMA**

Left: The interface between the tumor and the fibrous capsule is usually intact, as in this section.

Right: At higher magnification, the periphery of the tumor shows a circumscribed border. If there is infiltration along the edge, this may be a sign of aggressive behavior and is worthy of mention in the diagnostic report.

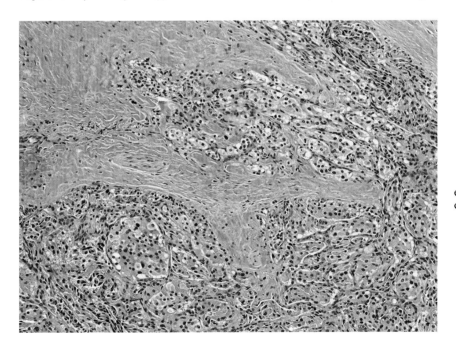

**Figure 12-10**

**CARDIAC PARAGANGLIOMA**

The broad fibrous bands extend from the periphery to the central portion of the tumor.

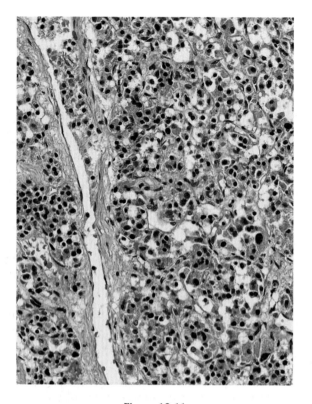

**Figure 12-11**

**CARDIAC PARAGANGLIOMA: ORGANOID APPEARANCE**

The cell nests are subtle, with little intervening fibrous tissue or vascularity.

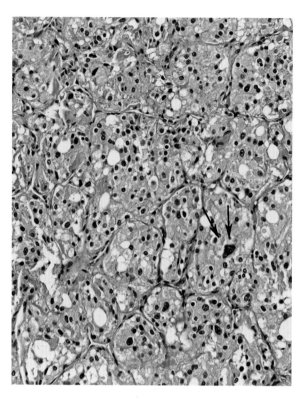

**Figure 12-12**

**CARDIAC PARAGANGLIOMA: ORGANOID APPEARANCE**

The cell nests are fairly discrete and surrounded by delicate fibrovascular septa. There is moderate nuclear pleomorphism (arrows).

**Figure 12-13**

**CARDIAC PARAGANGLIOMA: ORGANOID APPEARANCE**

Fibrous bands separate the cell nests. In addition, there is patchy cytoplasmic clearing.

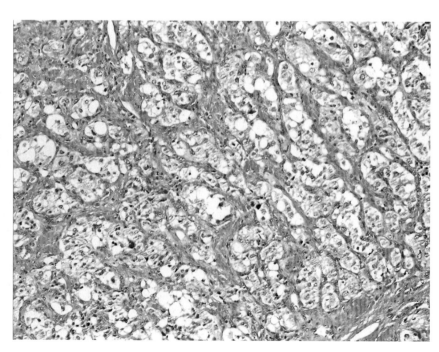

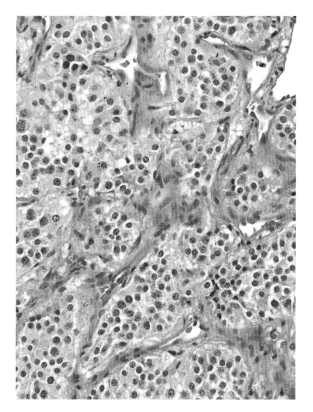

**Figure 12-14**

**CARDIAC PARAGANGLIOMA: ORGANOID APPEARANCE**

The nests are separated by fibrovascular septa.

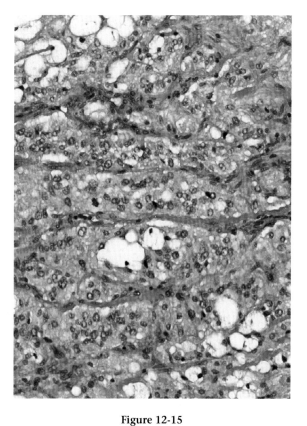

**Figure 12-15**

**CARDIAC PARAGANGLIOMA:
TRABECULAR GROWTH PATTERN**

There is often a combined organoid and trabecular growth pattern. There are intervening fibrovascular septa.

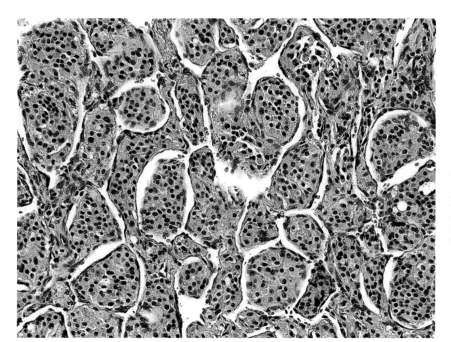

**Figure 12-16**

**CARDIAC PARAGANGLIOMA:
ORGANOID APPEARANCE**

There are artifactual spaces between the nests of cells, resulting in the prominence of the lining sustentacular cells. The epithelioid tumor cells are very monotonous and uniform in this example.

**Figure 12-17**

**CARDIAC PARAGANGLIOMA: ORGANOID APPEARANCE**

This tumor shows a septal framework, with prominent sustentacular cells, equal in cellularity to the epithelioid cell nests.

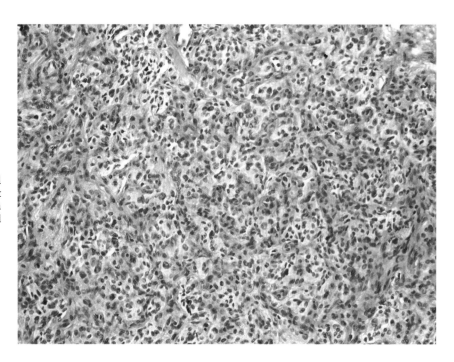

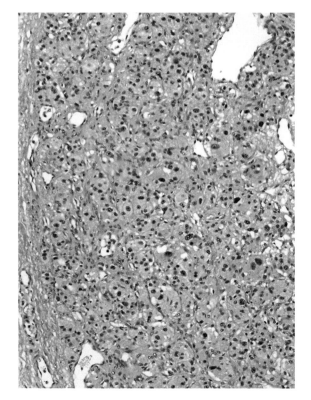

**Figure 12-18**

**CARDIAC PARAGANGLIOMA: VASCULAR PATTERN**

Although a staghorn hemangiopericytoma-like vascular pattern is not usual, there may be dilated irregular vessels in cardiac paragangliomas.

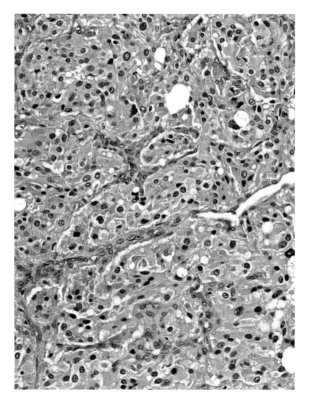

**Figure 12-19**

**CARDIAC PARAGANGLIOMA: VASCULAR PATTERN**

More typically, the vessels within the septa are not markedly dilated, but lined by prominent endothelial cells.

210

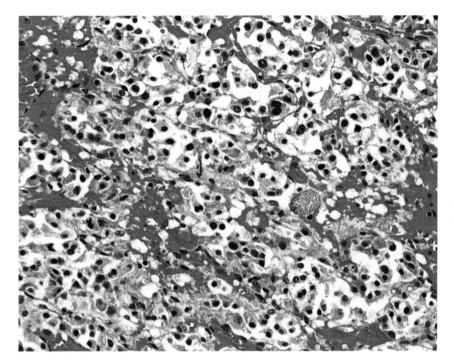

**Figure 12-20**

**CARDIAC PARAGANGLIOMA: SEPTAL HEMORRHAGE**

As in noncardiac paragangliomas, hemorrhage within the septal planes may be evident.

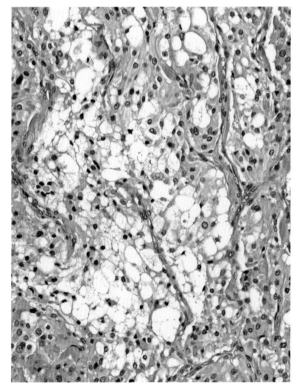

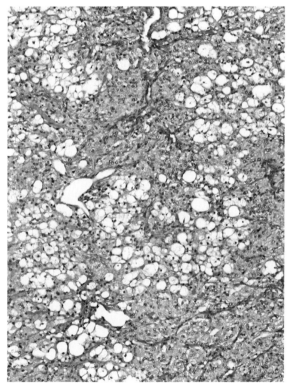

**Figure 12-21**

**CARDIAC PARAGANGLIOMA: CYTOPLASMIC CLEARING**

Cytoplasmic vacuoles are a common feature.

**Figure 12-22**

**CARDIAC PARAGANGLIOMA: CYTOPLASMIC CLEARING**

The cytoplasmic vacuoles are large and affect zones of tumor cells. Again, the vascular pattern is present, without significant vascular dilatation.

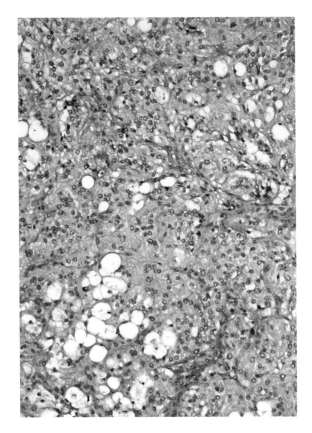

**Figure 12-23**

**CARDIAC PARAGANGLIOMA: CYTOPLASMIC CLEARING**

A higher-magnification view of figure 12-21 shows areas of marked cytoplasmic vacuolization.

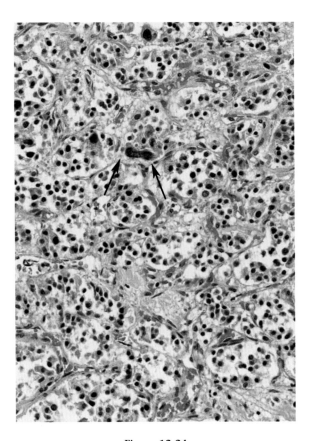

**Figure 12-24**

**CARDIAC PARAGANGLIOMA: NUCLEAR PLEOMORPHISM**

There are scattered tumor cells that are many times the size of other tumor cells (arrows). The tumor otherwise has the typical organoid appearance of paraganglioma.

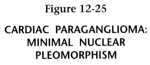

**Figure 12-25**

**CARDIAC PARAGANGLIOMA: MINIMAL NUCLEAR PLEOMORPHISM**

In this example, there is the typical organoid pattern of cell growth, with intervening fibrovascular septa. The tumor cells have round nuclei, which vary in size.

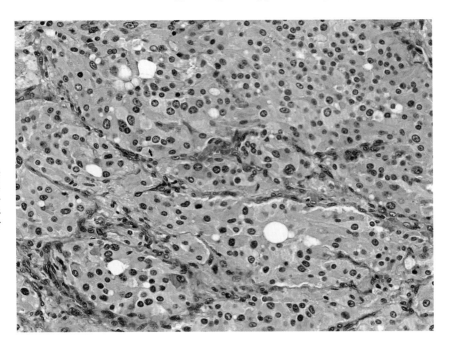

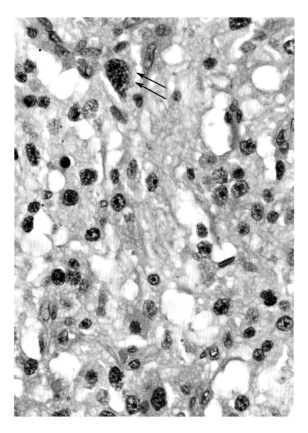

**Figure 12-26**

**CARDIAC PARAGANGLIOMA: NUCLEAR PLEOMORPHISM**

The nuclei are round and fairly uniform, with dispersed nuclear chromatin without prominent chromocenters or nucleoli. There are occasional nuclei that are far larger than surrounding ones (arrows).

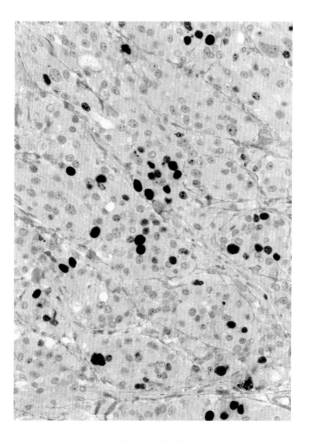

**Figure 12-27**

**CARDIAC PARAGANGLIOMA**

A small proportion of tumor cells demonstrates nuclear positivity for Ki-67, in this case, 16 percent by morphometric analysis.

presence of any mitotic figures, vascular or capsular invasion, and a high rate of Ki-67 immunoreactivity (fig. 12-27) (58). Extracardiac paragangliomas are metastatic only in a small proportion of cases, and metastases are mostly confined to regional lymph nodes.

In the few malignant cardiac paragangliomas reported, the pathologic data are not given in detail. Jirari et al. (43) described micrometastases at the time of surgery for resection of an aorticopulmonary paraganglioma, but no histologic description was given. The malignant paraganglioma of Arai et al. (41) was diagnosed only by functional imaging studies without histologic confirmation. The malignant mediastinal paraganglioma in the series of Brown et al. (1) does not disclose histologic information. Cruz (42) reported a spinal metastasis 2 years after resec-

tion of a left ventricular paraganglioma but detailed histologic features were not provided.

Although the diagnosis is readily made by routine staining to highlight the endocrine or "Zellballen" appearance of tumor nests, the immunohistochemical expression of chromogranin or other neuroendocrine markers may be helpful in the diagnosis. Typically, the sustentacular cells are S-100 protein and glial fibrillary acidic protein (GFAP) positive (59), and the epithelioid cells are chromogranin and synaptophysin positive, although the biphasic population is not always evident (figs. 12-28–12-33). Similar to most extracardiac paragangliomas, epithelial markers, including cytokeratins, are negative. As with extracardiac paragangliomas, cardiac paragangliomas are positive for chromogranin, neuron-specific enolase, and often met-enkephalin. Endocrine

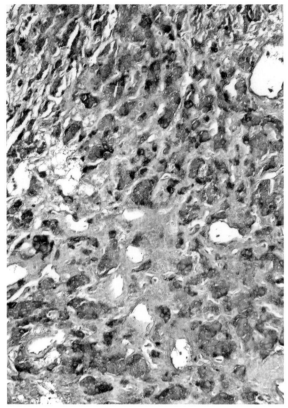

**Figure 12-28**

**CARDIAC PARAGANGLIOMA**

There is diffuse cytoplasmic staining for chromogranin in the tumor cells.

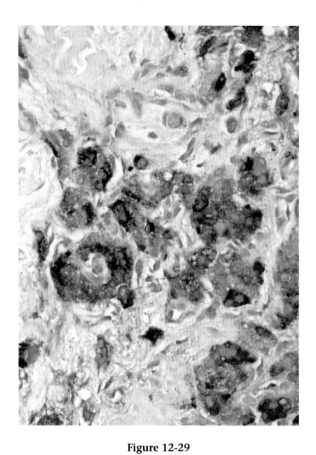

**Figure 12-29**

**CARDIAC PARAGANGLIOMA**

A higher-magnification view of figure 12-28 shows cytoplasmic staining for chromogranin.

**Figure 12-30**

**CARDIAC PARAGANGLIOMA**

Tumor islands are clearly delineated by chromogranin positivity.

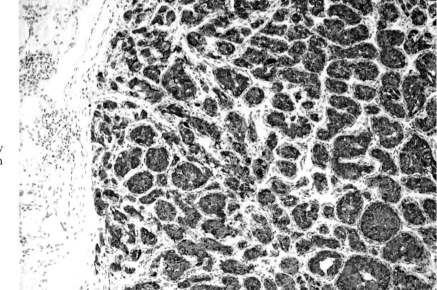

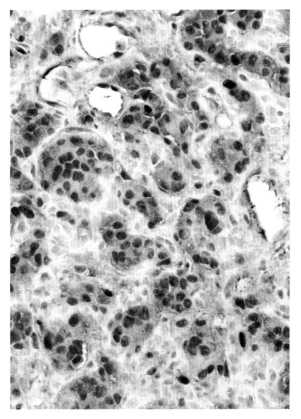

**Figure 12-31**

**CARDIAC PARAGANGLIOMA**

The sustentacular cells are quite numerous. There is nuclear and cytoplasmic staining for S-100 protein. There is wide variation regarding the extent of S-100 protein positivity in paragangliomas (compare with figure 12-33).

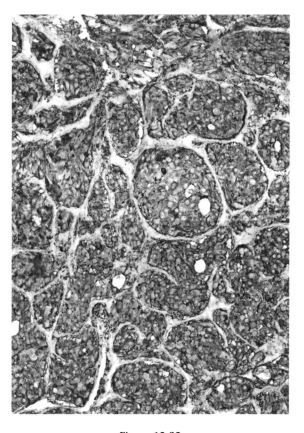

**Figure 12-32**

**CARDIAC PARAGANGLIOMA**

Strong cytoplasmic positivity for synaptophysin highlights the Zellballen pattern.

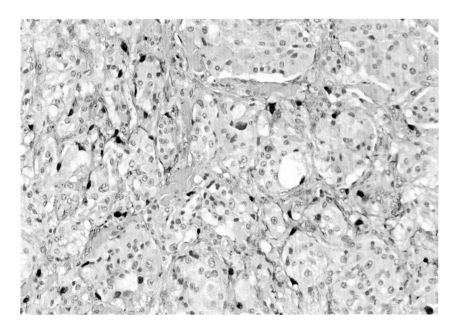

**Figure 12-33**

**CARDIAC PARAGANGLIOMA**

These typical S-100-positive sustentacular cells present around tumor nests and show a dendritic appearance.

polypeptides have not been demonstrated within tumor cells, in contrast to carcinoid tumors (59). Ultrastructurally, both epinephrine- and norepinephrine-type granules have been demonstrated, although the latter predominate (59).

## DIFFERENTIAL DIAGNOSIS

There are few entities in the histologic differential diagnosis of cardiac paraganglioma, especially if the tumor is in the atria at the base of the heart. Carcinoid tumor, which is possibly the most similar histologic mimicker, does not usually occur in the myocardium, unless there is widespread metastatic disease. In contrast to paraganglioma, carcinoid tumor stains for cytokeratins. Granular cell tumors are rare, generally smaller, and may have a similar organoid pattern, but have distinct histologic features (see chapter 13). Metastatic malignant melanoma may have some characteristics of paraganglioma, but should show mitotic activity, cellular pleomorphism, and necrosis. Theoretically, malignant paraganglioma of the heart would be difficult to separate from melanoma, and the distinction would necessitate the lack of melanocytic markers immunohistochemically and the presence of two cell types (sustentacular and epithelioid) substantiating the diagnosis of paraganglioma. Tumors of myocyte origin may share some features of paraganglioma, such as circumscription and cytoplasmic clearing, but the age of the patient, site in the heart, and other histologic features should separate paraganglioma from rhabdomyoma.

## TREATMENT AND PROGNOSIS

Complete surgical excision is recommended for all cardiac paragangliomas, often with an atrial graft repairing the removed portion of atrium or atrial septum. Functional tumors have been successfully removed with remission of symptoms (1). Normalization of blood pressure is usual in patients with preoperative hypertension (1,60). In the case of functional paragangliomas, special anesthetic procedures to control catecholamine release have been recommended (61). Left atrial reconstruction (62), repair of pulmonary veins (32), and right atrial and ventricular reconstruction with bypass grafting (28) may be required for bulky tumors. Cardiac transplantation may be necessary for invasive tumors (see fig. 12-4) (63,64).

Although treatment is primarily surgical, chemotherapeutic agents such as adriamycin have been given as adjuvant treatment (52). Malignant tumors are rare, and have been treated with combination chemotherapy and radiation therapy (41–43).

Cardiac paragangliomas are generally benign, and patients survive for long periods with partial excision. Rare intraoperative deaths have been reported: of 35 reports of surgical excision, there were 4 postoperative deaths (1,5,24,28, 29,33,65).

## REFERENCES

1. Brown ML, Zayas GE, Abel MD, Young WF Jr, Schaff HV. Mediastinal paragangliomas: the Mayo clinic experience. Ann Thorac Surg 2008; 86:946-951.
2. David TE, Lenkei SC, Marquez-Julio A, Goldberg JA, Meldrum DA. Pheochromocytoma of the heart. Ann Thorac Surg 1986;41:98-100.
3. Renoult E, Danchin N, Mathieu P, et al. Intrapericardial phaeochromocytoma associated with two intercarotid paragangliomas: diagnostic considerations. Postgrad Med J 1992;68:842-843.
4. Shapiro B, Sisson J, Kalff V, et al. The location of middle mediastinal pheochromocytomas. J Thorac Cardiovasc Surg 1984;87:814-820.
5. Gupta N, Karwande S, Gupta S. Primary cardiac pheochromocytoma. J Am Coll Cardiol 2009; 53:732.
6. Gopalakrishnan R, Ticzon AR, Cruz PA, et al. Cardiac paraganglioma (chemodectoma): a case report and review of the literature. J Thorac Cardiovasc Surg 1978;76:183-189.

7. Gabhane SK, Gangane NM, Sinha RT. Pentalogy of Fallot and cardiac paraganglioma: a case report. Cases J 2009;2:9392.

8. Alghamdi AA, Sheth T, Manowski Z, Djoleto OF, Bhatnagar G. Utility of cardiac CT and MRI for the diagnosis and preoperative assessment of cardiac paraganglioma. J Card Surg 2009;24:700-701.

9. Lorusso R, De Cicco G, Tironi A, Gelsomino S, De Geest R. Giant primary paraganglioma of the left ventricle. J Thorac Cardiovasc Surg 2009;137:499-500.

10. Meunier JP, Tatou E, Bernard A, Brenot R, David M. Cardiac pheochromocytoma. Ann Thorac Surg 2001;71:712-713.

11. Pickering TG, Isom OW, Bergman GW, Barbieri JM. Pheochromocytoma of the heart. Am J Cardiol 2000;86:1288-1289.

12. Imperatori A, De Monte L, Rotolo N, et al. Hypertension and intrapericardial paraganglioma: an exceptional presentation of multiple endocrine neoplasia type IIa syndrome. Hypertension 2011;58:e189-190.

13. Schiavi F, Boedeker CC, Bausch B, et al. Predictors and prevalence of paraganglioma syndrome associated with mutations of the SDHC gene. JAMA 2005;294:2057-2063.

14. Illouz F, Pinaud F, De Brux JL, Mirebeau-Prunier D, Rodien P. Long-delayed localization of a cardiac functional paraganglioma with SDHC mutation. Ann Intern Med 2012;157:222-223.

15. Vaughan P, Pabla L, Hobin D, Barron DJ, Parikh D. Cardiac paraganglioma and gastrointestinal stromal tumor: a pediatric case of Carney-Stratakis syndrome. Ann Thorac Surg 2011;92:1877-1878.

16. Boumzebra DA, Charifchefchaouni ZS, Belhadj SA, Maazouzi WA, Al-Halees ZY. Intrapericardial paraganglioma. Saudi Med J 2002;23:1278-1280.

17. Grebenc ML, Rosado de Christenson ML, Burke AP, Green CE, Galvin JR. Primary cardiac and pericardial neoplasms: radiologic-pathologic correlation. Radiographics 2000;20:1073-1103.

18. Hawari M, Yousri T, Hawari R, Tsang G. Intrapericardial paraganglioma directly irrigated by the right coronary artery. J Card Surg 2008;23:780-782.

19. Pacheco Gomez N, Marcos Gomez G, Garciperez de Vargas FJ, Perez Calvo C. Intrapericardial paraganglioma. Rev Esp Cardiol 2010;63:116-117.

20. Rosamond TL, Hamburg MS, Vacek JL, Borkon AM. Intrapericardial pheochromocytoma. Am J Cardiol 1992;70:700-702.

21. Somasundar P, Krouse R, Hostetter R, Vaughan R, Covey T. Paragangliomas—a decade of clinical experience. J Surg Oncol 2000;74:286-290.

22. Ginocchio G, Garavelli G, Boari L, Tenca P, Casiglia E, Pessina AC. [Familial pheochromocytoma: a family studied for 3 generations.] G Ital Cardiol 1995;25:281-288. [Italian]

23. Aguilo F, Tamayo N, Vazquez-Quintana E, et al. Pheochromocytoma: a twenty year experience at the University Hospital. P R Health Sci J 1991;10:135-142.

24. Abad C, Jimenez P, Santana C, et al. Primary cardiac paraganglioma. Case report and review of surgically treated cases. J Cardiovasc Surg (Torino) 1992;33:768-772.

25. Lupinski RW, Shankar S, Agasthian T, Lim CH, Mancer K. Primary cardiac paraganglioma. Ann Thorac Surg 2004;78:e43-44.

26. Sook M, Hamoir E, de Leval L, et al. Cardiac paraganglioma: diagnostic work up and review of the literature. Acta Chir Belg 2012;112:310-313.

27. Yuan WQ, Wang WQ, Su TW, et al. A primary right atrium paraganglioma in a 15-year-old patient. Endocrine 2007;32:245-248.

28. Zhou J, Chen HT, Xiang J, Qu XH, Zhou YQ, Zang WF. Surgical treatment of cardiac pheochromocytoma: a case report. Ann Thorac Surg 2009;88:278-281.

29. Aravot DJ, Banner NR, Cantor AM, Theodoropoulos S, Yacoub MH. Location, localization and surgical treatment of cardiac pheochromocytoma. Am J Cardiol 1992;69:283-285.

30. Tahir M, Noor SJ, Herle A, Downing S. Right atrial paraganglioma: a rare primary cardiac neoplasm as a cause of chest pain. Tex Heart Inst J 2009;36:594-597.

31. Turley AJ, Hunter S, Stewart MJ. A cardiac paraganglioma presenting with atypical chest pain. Eur J Cardiothorac Surg 2005;28:352-354.

32. Ceresa F, Sansone F, Rinaldi M, Patane F. Left atrial paraganglioma: diagnosis and surgical management. Interact Cardiovasc Thorac Surg 2010;10:1047-1048.

33. Hong SN, Srichai MB, Morgan JA, Dimitrova K, Galloway AC. Cardiac pheochromocytoma presenting as shortness of breath. Am J Med 2009; 122:e1-2.

34. Rana O, Gonda P, Addis B, Greaves K. Image in cardiovascular medicine. Intrapericardial paraganglioma presenting as chest pain. Circulation 2009;119:e373-375.

35. Khalid TJ, Zuberi O, Zuberi L, Khalid I. A rare case of cardiac paraganglioma presenting as anginal pain: a case report. Cases J 2009;2:72.

36. Hayek ER, Hughes MM, Speakman ED, Miller HJ, Stocker PJ. Cardiac paraganglioma presenting with acute myocardial infarction and stroke. Ann Thorac Surg 2007;83:1882-1884.

37. Hui G, McAllister H, Angelini P. Left atrial paraganglioma: report of a case and review of the literature. Am Heart J 1987;113:1230-1234.

38. Dhanasopon AP, Shemin RJ, Yeh MW. Cardiac paraganglioma presenting as gestational hypertension. Surgery 2010;147:459-461.

39. Buchbinder NA, Yu R, Rosenbloom BE, Sherman CT, Silberman AW. Left ventricular thrombus and embolic stroke caused by a functional paraganglioma. J Clin Hypertens (Greenwich) 2009; 11:734-737.

40. Lee CC, Chua S, Huang SC, Lee FY, Chung SY. Intrapericardial paraganglioma with intratumoral coronary arterial aneurysm and an arteriovenous fistula. J Am Soc Echocardiogr 2009;22:211.e1-3.

41. Arai A, Naruse M, Naruse K, et al. Cardiac malignant pheochromocytoma with bone metastases. Intern Med 1998;37:940-944.

42. Cruz PA, Mahidhara S, Ticzon A, Tobon H. Malignant cardiac paraganglioma: follow-up of a case. J Thorac Cardiovasc Surg 1984;87:942-944.

43. Jirari A, Charpentier A, Popescu S, Boidin P, Eisenmann B. A malignant primary cardiac pheochromocytoma. Ann Thorac Surg 1999;68:565-566.

44. Osranek M, Bursi F, Gura GM, Young WF Jr, Seward JB. Echocardiographic features of pheochromocytoma of the heart. Am J Cardiol 2003; 91:640-643.

45. Didier D, Meyer P, Philippe J. Multislice gated-computed tomography of cardiac paragangliomas. J Am Coll Cardiol 2010;55:2509.

46. Conti VR, Saydjari R, Amparo EG. Paraganglioma of the heart. The value of magnetic resonance imaging in the preoperative evaluation. Chest 1986;90:604-606.

47. Orr LA, Pettigrew RI, Churchwell AL, Jennings HS 3rd, Petracek MR, Vansant JP. Gadolinium utilization in the MR evaluation of cardiac paraganglioma. Clin Imaging 1997;21:404-406.

48. Cottin Y, Berriolo A, Guy F, et al. Somatostatin-receptor scintigraphy identifies a cardiac pheochromocytoma. Circulation 1999;100:2387-2388.

49. Tomasian A, Lai C, Ruehm S, Krishnam MS. Cardiovascular magnetic resonance and PET-CT of left atrial paraganglioma. J Cardiovasc Magn Reson 2010;12:1.

50. Kennelly R, Aziz R, Toner M, Young V. Right atrial paraganglioma: an unusual primary cardiac tumour. Eur J Cardiothorac Surg 2008;33:1150-1152.

51. Imren Y, Tasoglu I, Benson AA, Sinci V. A rare intracardiac mass: cardiac paraganglioma. Heart Lung Circ 2007;16:116-117.

52. Jimenez JF, Warren ET, Shroff RK, Stolz GA. Primary cardiac paraganglioma. J Ark Med Soc 2005;101:362-364.

53. Maxey TS, Grow P, Morris CD, Patton KT, Guyton RA. Biatrial primary cardiac paraganglioma: a rare finding. Cardiovasc Pathol 2007;16:179-182.

54. Leo F, Furia S, Duranti L, Pastorino U. Extraluminal cardiac paraganglioma: unexpected diagnosis of a large mediastinal mass. Eur J Cardiothorac Surg 2010;37:1470.

55. Vicente CC, Rodriguez E, Aragoncillo P, et al. Images in cardiovascular medicine. Paracardiac nonfunctioning paraganglioma in a young woman. Circulation 2008;118:574-575.

56. Kawasuji M, Matsunaga Y, Iwa T. Cardiac phaeochromocytoma of the interatrial septum. Eur J Cardiothorac Surg 1989;3:175-177.

57. Gonnella C, Messa FC, Confessore P, Greco C. Angiographic evidence of pigmented cardiac paraganglioma. J Cardiovasc Med (Hagerstown) 2008;9:319.

58. Kimura N, Watanabe T, Noshiro T, Shizawa S, Miura Y. Histological grading of adrenal and extra-adrenal pheochromocytomas and relationship to prognosis: a clinicopathological analysis of 116 adrenal pheochromocytomas and 30 extra-adrenal sympathetic paragangliomas including 38 malignant tumors. Endocr Pathol 2005;16:23-32.

59. Johnson TL, Shapiro B, Beierwaltes WH, et al. Cardiac paragangliomas. A clinicopathologic and immunohistochemical study of four cases. Am J Surg Pathol 1985;9:827-834.

60. Hodgson S, Sheps S, Subramanian R, Lie J, Carney J. Catecholamine-secreting paraganglioma of the interatrial septum. Am J Med 1984;77:157-161.

61. Ng JM. Desflurane and remifentanil use during resection of a cardiac pheochromocytoma. J Cardiothorac Vasc Anesth 2004;18:630-631.

62. Petersen J, Cooper G, Drew P, Silverstein B, Beave T. Paraganglioma resection requiring left atrial reconstruction. Clin Cardiol 2010;33:E75-77.

63. Khan MF, Datta S, Chisti MM, Movahed MR. Cardiac paraganglioma: clinical presentation, diagnostic approach and factors affecting short and long-term outcomes. Int J Cardiol 2013;166:315-320.

64. Goldstein DJ, Oz MC, Rose EA, Fisher P, Michler RE. Experience with heart transplantation for cardiac tumors. J Heart Lung Transplant 1995; 14:382-386.

65. Knop G, Margaria R. Cardiac pheochromocytoma: a new case reported. J Thorac Cardiovasc Surg 2006;132:1230-1231.

# 13 MISCELLANEOUS BENIGN SOFT TISSUE TUMORS

## HAMARTOMA OF MATURE CARDIAC MYOCYTES

**Definition.** *Hamartoma of mature cardiac myocytes* is a tumor of disorganized, enlarged cardiac muscle cells. The term, as initially defined, is applied to tumors composed predominantly of striated muscle.

**General Features.** Hamartoma of mature cardiac myocytes was initially described in 1998 in two publications. One reported the biopsy findings from a distal ventricular septal mass in a 24-year-old man with palpitations; histologically, the tumor was composed of hypertrophied myocytes and fat (1). That year a series of three patients, one presenting with sudden death, was also published (2). In this report, the histologic similarity between the newly described entity and hypertrophic cardiomyopathy was emphasized. The largest series to date has also illustrated the histologic similarity between hamartoma of mature cardiac myocytes and the myofiber disarray seen in hypertrophic cardiomyopathy (3). Since these publications, the term has been applied to other hamartomas with a proliferation of thick-walled vessels, prominent fibrous tissue, and fat. Fibrolipomatous tumors with prominent, thick-walled vessels, should probably best be classified as hemangiomas, because they resemble intramuscular hemangiomas of skeletal muscle (see chapter 10) (4–8). The term "hamartoma" has been used for a variety of different heart tumors, including histiocytoid cardiomyopathy and cardiac fibroma, in addition to rhabdomyoma. Unfortunately, the true nature of reported hamartomas of the heart is often difficult to ascertain without histologic documentation.

**Clinical Features.** Hamartomas of mature cardiac myocytes are rare: fewer than 15 cases have been reported that fit the histologic definition (Table 13-1). There is a male predominance. The age at presentation of reported cases is strikingly broad, from infancy to late adulthood. For this reason, it is unclear whether the tumor is

| Table 13-1 HAMARTOMA OF MATURE CARDIAC MYOCYTES[a] | |
|---|---|
| Male:female ratio | 10:5 |
| Age, mean (range) | 25 years (0.5-76) |
| Site (number) | |
| Left ventricle | 6 |
| Right atrium | 3 |
| Interventricular septum | 2 |
| Right ventricle | 2 |
| Multiple | 2 |
| Size: mean[b] | 5.0 cm |
| range | Microscopic (in multiple tumors) to 9 cm |
| Symptoms | |
| Incidental | 7[c] |
| Palpitations | 1 |
| Palpitations and chest pain | 2 |
| Chest pain | 1 |
| Dyspnea | 1 |
| Syncope | 1 |
| Sudden death | 2 |
| Diagnostic pathologic procedure | |
| Autopsy | 6 |
| Complete resection | 3 |
| Partial resection | 1 |
| Frozen section biopsy and partial resection | 1 |
| Biopsy, open | 3 |
| Endomyocardial biopsy | 1 |
| Histologic features | |
| Myocyte vacuolization | 6 of 15 (focal only) |
| Interstitial fibrosis | None (2), mild (5), moderate (8) |
| Interstitial fat | 4 of 15 |
| Thickened vessels | Arteries (1), arterioles (2), none described or illustrated (12) |

[a]Review of reported cases as defined by a discrete mass composed primarily of myocytes with hypertrophy or disarray (1–3,9,10,15,107). Two cases reported by Menon et al. (6) are included in the series of Fealey et al. (3).
[b]In 8 cases in which data are available either from echocardiogram or surgical resection.
[c]Electrocardiographic abnormalities on routine examination (3), aortic dissection, bicuspid aortic valve with coarctation, pneumonia and congenital syndrome, complex congenital heart disease.

219

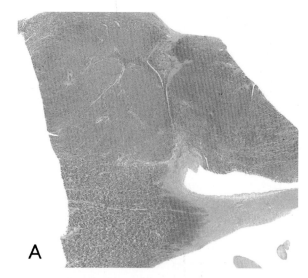

### Figure 13-1

**HAMARTOMA OF MATURE CARDIAC MYOCYTES**

A: A low-power view demonstrates no clear-cut lesion. A papillary muscle with chorda tendineae is at the bottom. The patient was a young boy who died suddenly. There were multiple firm nodules throughout the heart.

B: At higher magnification, the demarcation between the tumor (above) and the normal myocardium (below) is seen. The interface is marked with arrows.

C: Disordered myocytes and a thick-walled vessel are seen.

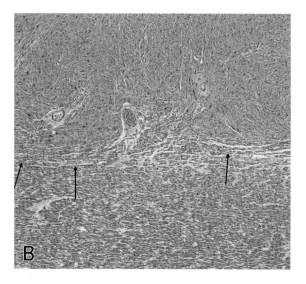

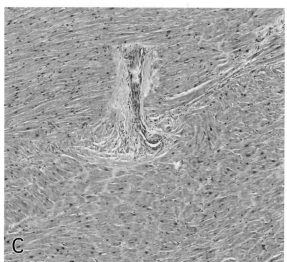

a congenital or acquired lesion, or if it is a heterogeneous entity.

Most reported cases are incidental findings. Manifestations, when present, include arrhythmias and sudden death (2,3). Hamartomas of mature cardiac myocytes may cause premature atrial and ventricular contractions, supraventricular tachycardia, and Wolff-Parkinson-White syndrome (1,2,5).

**Gross Findings.** At autopsy, the lesions are generally poorly circumscribed areas of fibrosis and firmness (2,3). Surgically, they may be difficult to distinguish from the surrounding myocardium, resulting in incomplete, or no attempt at, resection (2,6). In some cases, imaging studies show fairly circumscribed lesions (6,9).

**Microscopic Findings.** Histologically, hamartoma of mature cardiac myocytes is a poorly circumscribed area of enlarged, rounded or elongated myocytes, often with patterns of myofiber disarray (figs. 13-1–13-5) (2,3). Although arterial thickening is common, there are no areas of branching, thickened vessels as seen in hemangioma. Interstitial fibrosis is common, but is relatively minimal compared to the muscular hypertrophy. Fat infiltration is also common, but is a minor part of the tumor (Table 13-1). When present, myocyte vacuolization is limited to a small proportion of cells, in contrast to rhabdomyoma.

**Differential Diagnosis.** The differential diagnosis of hamartoma of mature cardiac myocytes

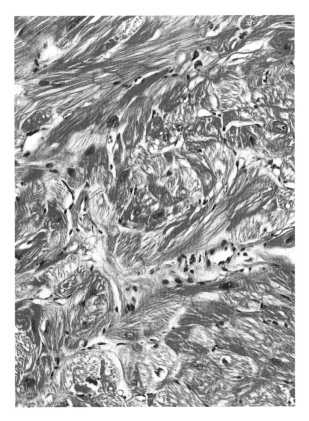

**Figure 13-2**

**HAMARTOMA OF MATURE CARDIAC MYOCYTES**

There are large, disorganized cardiomyocytes with marked hypertrophy and abundant cytoplasm. There is little interstitial fibrosis or myocyte vacuolization.

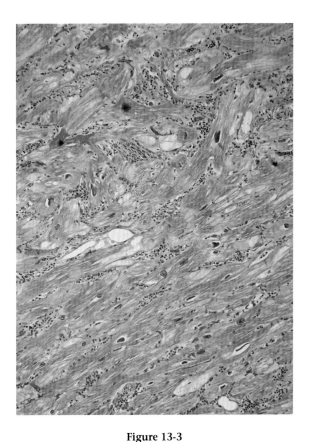

**Figure 13-3**

**HAMARTOMA OF MATURE CARDIAC MYOCYTES**

There is significant myocyte disorganization, but typical myofiber disarray, with branching or whorled muscle bundles, is absent.

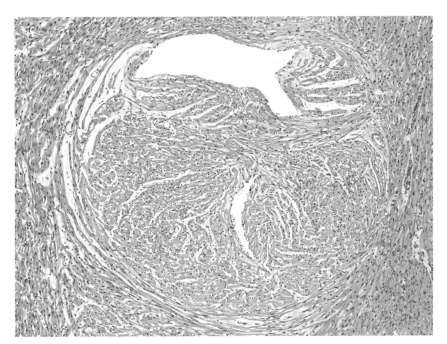

**Figure 13-4**

**HAMARTOMA OF MATURE CARDIAC MYOCYTES**

The border of the lesion is typically indistinct. There is a circular area of disorganized myocytes that extends from the central mass.

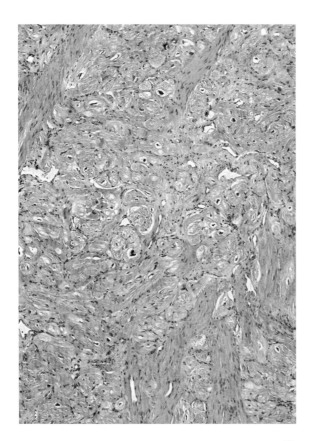
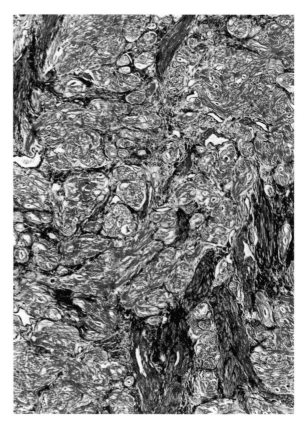

**Figure 13-5**

**HAMARTOMA OF MATURE CARDIAC MYOCYTES: INTERSTITIAL FIBROSIS**

Left: The fibrosis is mild on routine staining.
Right: A trichrome stain demonstrates extensive interstitial collagen. Nevertheless, most of the lesion is composed of cardiac muscle cells arranged in a haphazard fashion.

includes miscellaneous hamartomatous lesions that may be only partially sampled and difficult to classify, rhabdomyoma, and hypertrophic cardiomyopathy. Rhabdomyoma occurs exclusively in infants and children; in that age group, the distinction from hamartoma of mature cardiomyocytes rests on the presence of diffuse vacuolization, rounded cells, intracytoplasmic glycogen, and lack of enlarged, disorganized myocytes with abundant cytoplasm and interstitial fibrosis. The distinction from hypertrophic cardiomyopathy rests on the presence of a discrete mass and lack of clinical features. In some cases, this distinction is problematic, since hamartoma has been described in the ventricular septum, a site of predilection for hypertrophic cardiomyopathy, and clinical symptoms may overlap (10). In such cases, the imaging finding of a discrete, vascular mass favors hamartoma over cardiomyopathy.

**Miscellaneous Cardiac Hamartomas.** There have been several reports of cardiac hamartomas of mature cardiac myocytes that are composed primarily of proliferating vessels, with various amounts of fat, fibrous tissue, and interspersed myocytes; these tumors are probably best considered *intramuscular hemangiomas* (5,7,11). Other tumors designated "hamartomas" form a spectrum of non-neoplastic masses of disordered vessels, myocytes, and fat (4,8). A group of fibrofatty tumors with a variable vascular component has been described on the cardiac valves, with the term *fibromatous hamartoma* or *fibrolipoma of cardiac valves* (12,13). Zhang et al. (14) reported a giant cyst of the right ventricle containing myocytes, appropriately designated *giant atrial cystic hamartoma.*

**Treatment and Prognosis.** In those patients who present during life, the tumors are often difficult to resect, resulting in only partial excision in many cases (1,3,6,10,15). In some patients, patch repair or postoperative pacemaker insertion is necessary (2). No deaths have been reported in patients diagnosed at surgery, although follow-up is limited. One patient with a giant cardiac hamartoma was treated with heart transplant because of the size of the tumor (8). This case, however, is referred to only by subsequent reviews as a hamartoma of mature cardiac myocytes; the histologic illustration of proliferating vessels and fat composing most of the lesion suggests a diagnosis of intramuscular hemangioma (8).

## ADULT CELLULAR RHABDOMYOMA

**Definition.** *Adult cellular rhabdomyomas* of the heart are benign neoplasms that are histologically identical to the soft tissue adult rhabdomyomas that occur in the head, neck, and mediastinum. Rarely, this type occurs in the heart, and is also termed *cardiac extracardiac rhabdomyoma* (16).

**General Features.** Adult cellular rhabdomyomas of the heart are histologically distinct from congenital cardiac rhabdomyomas, but are histologically identical to so-called extracardiac rhabdomyomas, a term that distinguishes benign soft neoplasms from the hamartomatous rhabdomyomas of the heart associated with tuberous sclerosis (see chapter 8). Extracardiac rhabdomyomas of soft tissue are separated into three groups. The genital type consists of polyps, usually in the external genitalia of women, composed of large rhabdomyoblasts in a myxoid matrix; the adult and fetal types are solitary masses, usually in the head and neck region.

The adult rhabdomyoma is histologically composed of tightly packed, round to polygonal cells with eosinophilic, finely granular cytoplasm and occasional vacuoles and spider cells; unlike cardiac rhabdomyoma, there is abundant eosinophilic cytoplasm.

The first adult cellular rhabdomyoma was reported in a 42-year-old woman who presented with palpitations and a right atrial mass (17). Because of the patient's age and histologic features, this tumor was classified as a cardiac rhabdomyoma resembling an extracardiac rhabdomyoma. Subsequently, there were three cases reported, two in the atria and one in the

right ventricle (16). There have been no subsequent cases.

**Gross and Microscopic Findings.** Adult cellular rhabdomyoma is a well-demarcated lesion both by imaging and gross appearance (fig. 13-6). The cellular neoplasm is composed of striated muscle cells that have rounded or spindled shapes (figs. 13-7–13-10). There is little or no background fibrosis or other tissue elements. Vacuolization is minimal, and proliferation markers show scattered positive cells. Mitotic figures are rare.

**Differential Diagnosis.** Unlike congenital rhabdomyoma, adult cellular rhabdomyomas are tumors of adults, histologically resemble rhabdomyomas of the head and neck soft tissue, and show evidence of cellular proliferation. Spider cells are infrequent or absent. Many reported congenital rhabdomyomas occurring in adults are diagnosed based only on imaging and a patient or family history suggestive of tuberous sclerosis (18,19).

In contrast to hamartoma of mature cardiac myocytes, there is no cellular enlargement or disarray, and, again, there is evidence of cellular proliferation. There are no immunohistochemical studies that distinguish these three tumors, as all are tumors of striated muscle.

## GRANULAR CELL TUMOR

**Definition.** *Granular cell tumors* of the heart are benign epicardial neoplasms composed of cells with a characteristic granular cytoplasm and evidence of neural differentiation. They are histologically identical to granular cell tumors of extracardiac sites.

**General Features.** Granular cell tumors are often found in proximity to nerves, are diffusely positive for S-100 protein, and ultrastructurally often demonstrate myelinated and nonmyelinated axon-like structures.

There are few reported granular cell tumors of the heart: to date, approximately 10 cases have been reported in the English language literature, almost half of which were part of systemic involvement (20–27). Extracardiac involvement may occur as long as 20 years prior to cardiac involvement, and occurs in the skin, oropharynx, esophagus, stomach, and intestine (25,26). It is likely that many cases are not diagnosed because they are generally incidental epicardial nodules that are easily overlooked.

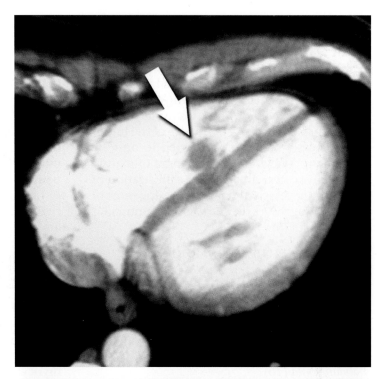

**Figure 13-6**

**ADULT CELLULAR RHABDOMYOMA**

Top: Contrast-enhanced axial computerized tomography (CT) in a 36-year-old male with dysrhythmias demonstrates a homogeneously enhancing 2-cm ovoid mass (arrow) attached to the interventricular septum and protruding into the right ventricular chamber.

Bottom: The resected bivalved specimen was a smooth-surfaced rhabdomyoma which measured 2 x 2 cm.

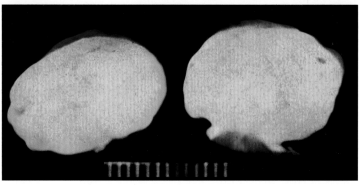

Patients are adults aged 24 to 55 years. Granular cell tumors are usually incidental autopsy findings or incidental findings during surgery for unrelated conditions (22). They are located on the ventricular or atrial epicardial surfaces close to the base of the heart, where nervous tissue is abundant.

**Gross Findings.** Cardiac granular cell tumors are circumscribed, gray or tan, and firm (figs. 13-11, 13-12). Despite their presumed neural origin, only one granular cell tumor of the heart has been shown to have direct continuity with nervous tissue (23). This tumor was in direct contact with the sinus node and perinodal tissue.

**Microscopic Findings.** Microscopically, the tumor cells merge with the surrounding cardiac tissue, and scattered normal myocytes are found entrapped within the tumor mass. The tumor histologically is identical to an extracardiac granular cell tumor (figs. 13-13–13-15). The tumor cells are round to elongated, and are filled with granular cytoplasm that stains weakly with the periodic acid–Schiff reagent after diastase pretreatment. Glycogen is absent. Tumor cells express S-100 protein, neuron-specific enolase, and various myelin proteins; they are negative for neurofilaments and glial fibrillary acidic protein. Electron microscopy shows the intracellular granules to consist of membrane bound, autophagic vacuoles containing cellular debris of mitochondria, rough endoplasmic reticulum, and myelinated and non-myelinated structures resembling axons.

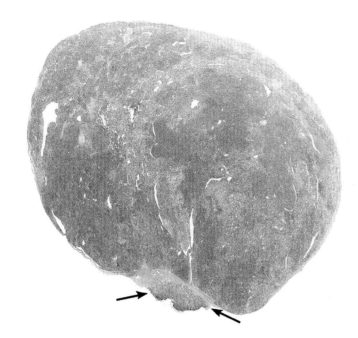

**Figure 13-7**

**ADULT CELLULAR RHABDOMYOMA**

At low magnification, a small amount of endocardium and normal myocardium (arrows) and a large, lobulated tumor are seen.

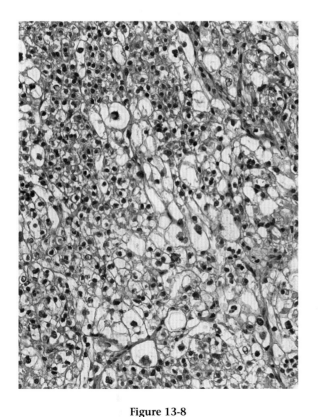

**Figure 13-8**

**ADULT CELLULAR RHABDOMYOMA**

Some cells show abundant eosinophilic cytoplasm, almost resembling rhabdomyoblasts. In contrast to rhabdomyosarcoma, there is little atypia or mitotic activity, and necrosis is absent.

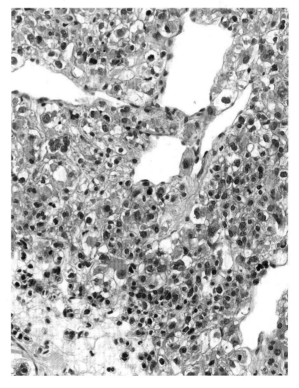

**Figure 13-9**

**ADULT CELLULAR RHABDOMYOMA**

The tumor is cellular, with a tumor-like vascular pattern of staghorn vessels. The paucity of cytoplasm and overall cellularity separate this lesion from hamartoma of mature cardiac myocytes.

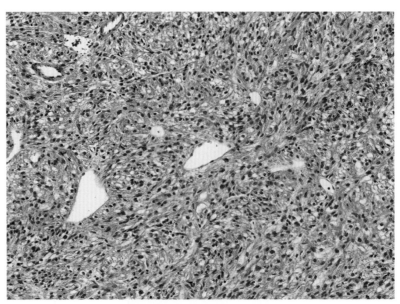

**Figure 13-10**

**ADULT CELLULAR RHABDOMYOMA**

The tumor cells are more elongated and spindled, typical of adult rhabdomyoma seen in the soft tissue of the head and neck.

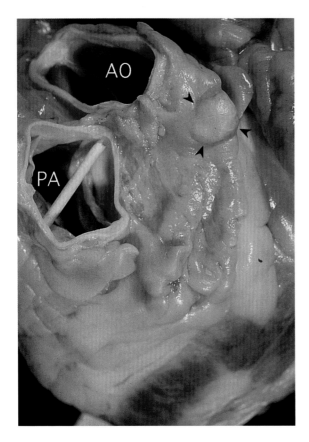

**Figure 13-11**

**GRANULAR CELL TUMOR**

Localized epicardial tumor (arrowheads) overlying the left main coronary artery close to its takeoff. The aorta (AO) is anterior to the pulmonary artery (PA).

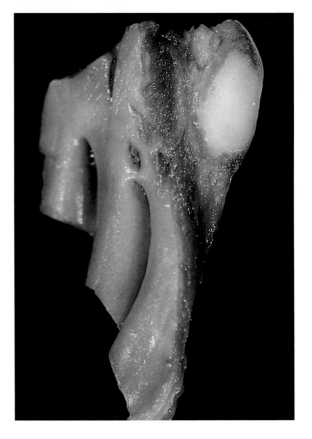

**Figure 13-12**

**GRANULAR CELL TUMOR**

The cut surface of a circumscribed white tumor on the epicardial surface. Underlying right ventricular trabeculations are seen.

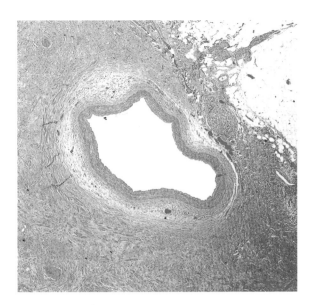
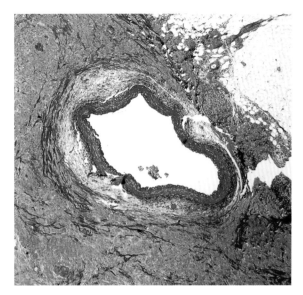

**Figure 13-13**

**GRANULAR CELL TUMOR**

Left: Low magnification demonstrates a cellular process around an epicardial coronary artery.
Right: A Masson trichrome stain shows the tumor (red) within a fibrous background (blue).

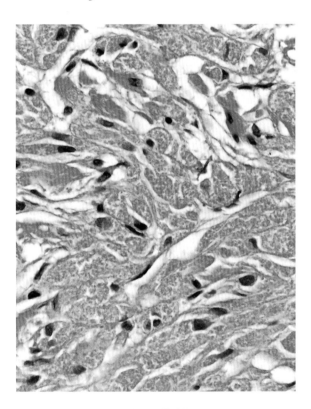
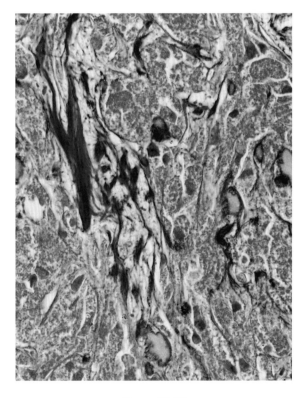

**Figure 13-14**

**GRANULAR CELL TUMOR**

High magnification shows the typical finely granular cells with a small, compressed eccentric nucleus.

**Figure 13-15**

**GRANULAR CELL TUMOR**

A Masson trichrome stain highlights the cytoplasmic granules and interstitial fibrosis.

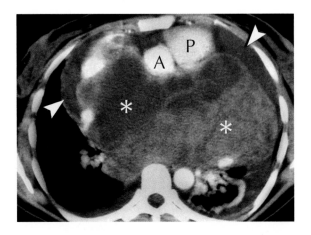 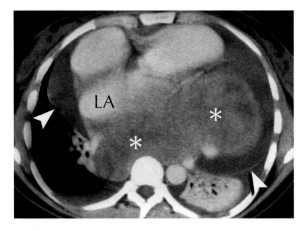

**Figure 13-16**

**INTRAPERICARDIAL SCHWANNOMA**

Left: Contrast-enhanced axial CT image at the level of the origin of the aorta (A) and main pulmonary artery (P) shows a large, partly cystic, partly heterogeneously enhancing mass (asterisks) associated with a pericardial effusion (arrowheads).

Right: Contrast-enhanced axial CT image at the level of the left atrium (LA) shows contiguous components of the heterogeneous mass clearly contained within the pericardial sac (arrowheads).

**Prognosis.** Malignant granular cell tumors constitute fewer than 2 percent of all granular cell tumors, and have not been reported in the myocardium except as metastatic deposits (21,28) or as part of disseminated congenital granular cell tumor (25).

## SCHWANNOMA

*Benign peripheral nerve sheath tumors* are classified as *neurofibromas* or *schwannomas*. Virtually all cardiac cases are schwannomas (or *neurilemoma* in the older literature). Malignant schwannomas of the heart are rare, and considered in chapter 16. Cardiac schwannomas are, by definition, intrapericardial, in contrast to the more common mediastinal soft tissue tumors. *Plexiform neurofibromas* may occur in the pericardium as part of systemic disease, in patients with neurofibromatosis (29).

Only 10 or so cases of primary cardiac schwannoma have been reported (30–39). Mediastinal schwannomas are common, especially in the posterior mediastinum, and may cause cardiac symptoms, especially by effusions and tamponade (40,41). Most cardiac schwannomas occur in the atria, especially the right (Table 13-2), or at the base of the heart near the origin of the great arteries. Patients may be asymptomatic and the tumors found as imaging findings (fig. 13-16) (30,39), incidental findings at autopsy

| Table 13-2 | |
|---|---|
| **CARDIAC SCHWANNOMAS**[a] | |
| Male:female ratio | 3:7 |
| Age, mean (range) | 52 years (30-70) |
| Symptoms (number) | |
| None (incidental) | 4 |
| Shortness of breath with pericardial effusion | 3 |
| Atrial fibrillation | 2 |
| Chest pain | |
| Site in heart | |
| RA[b]  6 | |
| LA   3 | |
| RVOT | |
| Size, cm, mean (range) | 7.1 (1.5-12) |
| Diagnostic procedure | |
| Surgical resection | 8 |
| Autopsy | 2 |

[a]Review of 10 reported cases from references 30–39.
[b]RA = right atrium; LA = left atrium; RVOT = right ventricular outflow tract.

(36,38,39), or as the cause of pericardial effusions (33,34,37). Some patients present with new-onset atrial fibrillation (31,35).

Cardiac schwannomas are firm well-circumscribed homogeneous masses that are often cystic (fig. 13-17, above). Histologically, they resemble schwannomas of soft tissue (fig. 13-17, right). Immunohistochemical (31,33) and ultrastructural analyses (36) confirm nerve sheath origin.

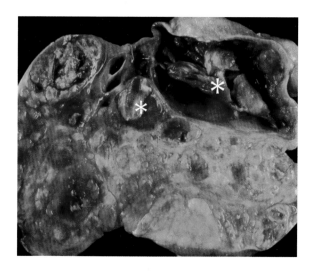

**Figure 13-17**

**INTRAPERICARDIAL SCHWANNOMA**

Above: The encapsulated gross specimen (17 x 16 x 6 cm) was fully resected from the transverse pericardial sinus, centered between the roof of the left atrium and inferior surface of the pulmonary artery. The cut surface shows macronodularity with foci of central hemorrhage, as well as multiple cysts containing gelatinous material (asterisks).

Right: There are pleomorphic and spindled cells with vague Antoni A and B areas in a neurofibrillary background. There were inflammatory and degenerative changes (so-called ancient schwannoma).

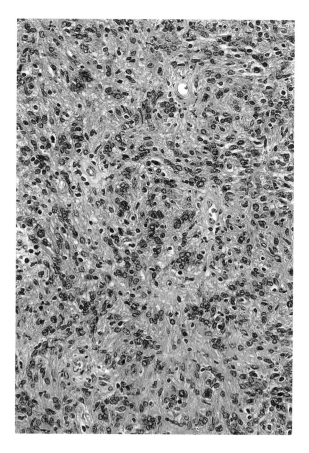

Surgical resection is curative. Pericardial patch reconstruction may be necessary for larger tumors (35).

## LEIOMYOMA AND LEIOMYOMATOSIS

**Definition.** *Primary leiomyomas* are benign soft tissue neoplasms with the histologic and immunohistochemical features of smooth muscle cells. *Intravenous leiomyomatosis* is the extension of a leiomyoma (usually from the myometrium) through venous channels; when extending into the heart, the term *intracardiac leiomyomatosis* is used. *Benign metastasizing leiomyoma* is a histologically benign leiomyoma that occurs in a woman with a prior hysterectomy for fibroids, generally in the lung, but also in the heart.

**General Features.** Primary leiomyomas of the heart are extremely rare. Two recently reported tumors (42,43) were not reliably distinguished from cardiac fibromas, since the diagnosis was based on immunohistochemical staining for actin, which is nonspecific and is expressed in fibromas (see chapter 7). A leiomyoma was re-cently reported as one of a series of heart tumors, without histologic documentation (44). The authors have seen a single cases arising in the right atrium of a middle-aged woman (fig. 13-18).

Benign smooth muscle tumors of extracardiac sites may extend into the right atrium, generally via the inferior vena cava. Such tumors may initially present with cardiac symptoms, and have been termed *intracardiac involvement by intravenous leiomyomatosis*. Leiomyomatosis accounts for a small number of surgical resections in published series of heart tumors (45).

There are two theories of pathogenesis of intravenous leiomyomatosis: that they arise in the vein wall or that they extend into the vein from the myometrial tumor. Most intravenous leiomatoses arise within a uterine leiomyoma, but the site of invasion is often not identified, and the intravenous component is usually diagnosed subsequent to hysterectomy. In total, about 10 percent of intravascular leiomyomas extend beyond the pelvic veins and reach the heart (46). There are over 100 reports of

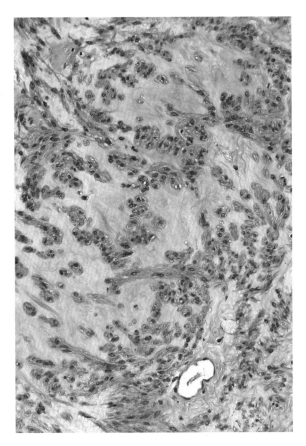

**Figure 13-18**

**CARDIAC LEIOMYOMA**

The tumor, which arose in the right atrium, is composed of bland spindled and rounded cells with the appearance of smooth muscle.

intravascular leiomyomatosis extending into the right atrium (45,46) including several in the last 5 years with surgical resection (47–52). All patients were female, most of child-bearing age.

For intravenous leiomyomatosis in general (including patients with cardiac involvement), the median age is 44 years, with a range of 23 to 80 years (53); there is a 4-year median interval from hysterectomy (54), although the tumors may present decades after the initial hysterectomy with the presumed invasive leiomyoma (46). Recently, an 81-year-old woman with intracardiac leiomyomatosis was reported (55). Although most patients are multigravida, an intracardiac leiomyoma has been reported in a nulliparous woman (56).

The symptoms related to intracardiac extension include syncope, congestive heart failure,

arrhythmias, and pulmonary embolism (46). The patients may present with symptoms related to tricuspid insufficiency, and the diagnosis of an atrial tumor is made without thought of a remote hysterectomy (46). Patients also present with what is believed to be multiple thromboemboli, with the initiation of anticoagulation and lack of regression of the tumor (56). The diagnosis is often not made before surgical resection, and imaging may initially suggest a thrombus (56). Other diagnostic possibilities include sarcoma, hepatocellular carcinoma, or renal cell carcinoma. Sudden death is a rare complication of intravenous leiomyomatosis, resulting from an arrhythmia secondary to right ventricular extension (57).

Benign metastasizing leiomyoma is a somewhat controversial entity that suggests that implants of benign myometrial tumors grow in distant sites after embolization. A few have been excised from the right atrium and ventricle (58,59). It is not clear whether some reported lesions, which are far more commonly reported in the lung than in the heart, are not low-grade leiomyosarcomas (60). One theory is that uterine leiomyoma with vascular invasion is the precursor to both benign metastasizing leiomyoma and intravascular leiomyomatosis (61). In support of this theory is a report of a benign metastasizing leiomyoma of the lung occurring years after resection of a uterine leiomyoma with extensive intravenous invasion (62).

**Gross Findings.** The diagnosis of intravascular leiomyoma involving the heart is often made at surgery or prior imaging by the identification of a continuity of the atrial mass with the uterus, extension along the inferior vena cava, and sometimes along hepatic, iliac, gonadal, and renal veins. Grossly, the tumors are described as "worm-like" (61). Although usually free floating without an attachment site in the heart or vena cava, there may be extensive adherence to the intima (63).

**Microscopic Findings.** Histologically, intravascular leiomyomatosis resembles leiomyoma of the uterine myometrium. Often, there is increased vascularity and collagen, and there may also be adipose tissue. The histologic features of intravenous leiomyomatosis in general, including those limited to the pelvis, demonstrate a wide range of changes, including epithelioid and symplastic types of leiomyoma (64).

**Differential Diagnosis.** The main entity in the differential diagnosis is leiomyosarcoma, which may clinically mimic intravenous leiomyomatosis (65). In contrast to sarcoma, there are no mitotic figures, nuclear atypia, or necrosis, and cellularity is low. In general, the histologic criteria separating intravenous leiomyomatosis from leiomyosarcomas of the inferior vena cava are the same as those for intrauterine smooth muscle tumors (60). In addition, leiomyosarcomas of the inferior vena cava are rarely exclusively intraluminal (see chapter 19).

**Treatment.** Surgery is the treatment of choice for intracardiac extension of intravenous leiomyomatosis, and may be performed as a one-stage or two-stage operation (first for the cardiac mass then for the infradiaphragmatic intravenous tumor) (55,66). Surgery may be complicated by serpiginous extension in multiple venous channels or by adherence of the tumor to the lumen wall. In the atypical case in which the patient has not had a prior hysterectomy, there are two surgeries, with extraction of the tumor by pulling it through the gonadal or iliac vein, followed by radical hysterectomy some time later (56,67). There is no need for postoperative filter placement in the inferior vena cava (46). Estrogen therapy is used as an adjunct to surgery since intravenous leiomyomas generally express estrogen receptors and are hormonally responsive (68).

## SOLITARY FIBROUS TUMOR

**Definition.** *Solitary fibrous tumors* are neoplasms of fibroblasts with a characteristic histologic and immunohistochemical profile, which may be benign or malignant. Synonyms include *localized fibrous tumor* and *hemangiopericytoma*.

**General Features.** Most solitary fibrous tumors occur in the pleura (approximately 80 percent); the remainder occur in a wide range of soft tissue sites. The anterior mediastinum is a common site for these tumors, which may be associated with the thymus gland (71,72). Of those that occur in the mediastinum, the minority are intrapericardial (73–76). Rarely, intrapericardial solitary fibrous tumors are intracardiac (77–79). In one series of 29 surgically resected cardiac tumors, 1 was a solitary fibrous tumor (80).

**Clinical Features.** Pericardial solitary fibrous tumors cause symptoms of pericarditis and pericardial effusion, and are tumors of adults of any age. Rare intracardiac tumors lead to heart failure, arrhythmias, tamponade, and embolism (79).

**Gross Findings.** Grossly, localized fibrous tumors are white and firm, with a whorled appearance on cut section. Most are attached to the pericardial surface either by a broad or narrow pedicle. There is typically no intracardiac extension, and there may be a pedunculated attachment site to the parietal or visceral pericardium. Rare intracardiac tumors are circumscribed homogeneous white-tan masses.

**Microscopic Findings.** Histologically, the tumor consists of spindle cells with interspersed hyalinized collagen, which is focally arranged in bundles of fibers, often with alternating cellular and acellular areas (figs. 13-19, 13-20). Small foci of calcification may be present, similar to cardiac fibroma. Myxoid areas and a hemangiopericytoma-like vascular pattern are common. Ultrastructural studies demonstrate spindle cells poor in organelles, with occasional strands of rough endoplasmic reticulum (76). Immunohistochemically, the cells express STAT6 and CD34 in the majority of cases, and frequently bcl-2 and CD99 (fig. 13-21) (81).

Mitotic figures, necrosis, and cellular atypia are generally absent; however, in 8 of 14 solitary fibrous tumors of the mediastinum reported by Witkin and Rosai (41), cellular areas with mitoses and necrosis were described. Malignant features include areas of de-differentiation with pleomorphism and necrosis, and a mitotic count exceeding 4 mitotic figures per 10 high-power fields (82).

**Differential Diagnosis.** Pericardial leiomyomas and neural tumors are rare, and may be excluded by immunohistochemical methods. Cardiac fibroma is histologically similar, but is an intracavitary tumor that lacks STAT6 and CD34 expression and typically lacks the hemangiopericytoma-like vascular pattern. Synovial sarcomas of the pericardium are generally more cellular, lack fibrous background, may show epithelial differentiation (epithelial membrane antigen or pancytokeratin positivity), and show typical translocation findings by cytogenetics or fluorescence in situ hybridization.

**Prognosis.** Reported solitary fibrous tumors of the pericardium and heart are benign,

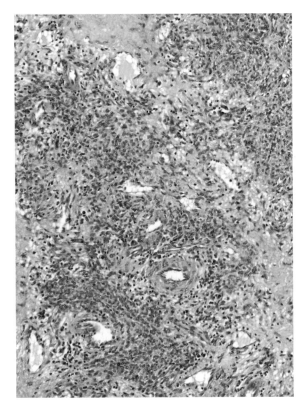

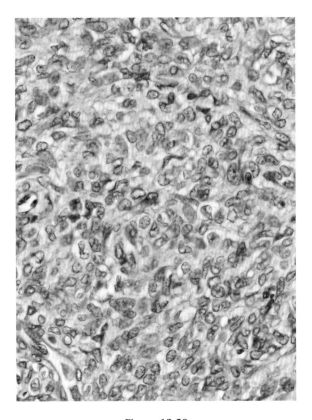

**Figure 13-19**

**SOLITARY FIBROUS TUMOR**

This tumor was resected from the cavity of the left atrium in a pregnant woman. On low magnification, there is a spindle cell proliferation with cellular and paucicellular areas. There is a prominent vascular pattern with scattered dilated vessels.

**Figure 13-20**

**SOLITARY FIBROUS TUMOR**

The cells are bland, with a fine collagenous background and lack of atypia.

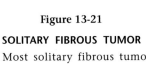

**Figure 13-21**

**SOLITARY FIBROUS TUMOR**

Most solitary fibrous tumors are CD34 positive (shown); other markers include bcl-2, STAT6, and CD99.

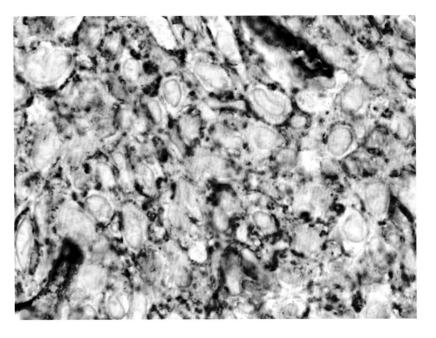

although malignant pleural tumors can spread and metastasize to the heart (81). Zhao et al. (79) did not document mitotic activity in a malignant solitary fibrous tumor of the heart, and follow-up was unavailable because the patient died postoperatively.

## INFLAMMATORY MYOFIBROBLASTIC TUMOR

**Definition.** *Inflammatory myofibroblastic tumors* are benign neoplasms of mesenchymal cells with smooth muscle and fibrocytic (myofibroblastic) differentiation. Synonyms include *inflammatory pseudotumor, pseudosarcomatous myofibroblastic proliferation,* and *myofibroblastic inflammatory tumor.*

**General Features.** Historically, inflammatory tumor-like masses with prominent spindle cells were designated inflammatory pseudotumors, which occurred most frequently in the lung. These were subsequently separated into two groups: inflammatory myofibroblastic tumor and plasma cell granuloma, depending on the predominant histologic features. Inflammatory myofibroblastic proliferations that mimic sarcomas are particularly frequent in the urinary tract, and occur in a minority of cases after instrumentation (83).

It is generally accepted that these lesions are neoplasms, and may even have a malignant counterpart (83). In the heart, there have been scattered older reports of "inflammatory pseudotumors" that are probably a heterogeneous group of non-neoplastic and neoplastic conditions. Only a single, more recent case of inflammatory myofibroblastic tumor of the heart occurred after surgical intervention (84). On the malignant end, there are intimal sarcomas with inflammation that may resemble inflammatory myofibroblastic tumors. The term "inflammatory myofibroblastic tumor," when applied to cardiac lesions, should probably be restricted to a histologically uniform set of tumors that arise from the endocardium, and hence are likely of intimal origin.

**Clinical Features.** Inflammatory myofibroblastic tumors of the heart are rare: fewer than 40 cases with histologic confirmation have been reported (Table 13-3). Several have been reported as sarcomas in children with long-term survival (85–89a).

The mean age at presentation is 16 years (median, 5.5 years). The earliest reported age is in a 5-week-old infant (90); the oldest in a 75-year-old man (91). There is slight female predominance. Most patients present with cardiac manifestations, including heart failure, cyanosis, peripheral edema, dyspnea, and syncope. Because cardiac inflammatory myofibroblastic tumors are endocardial-based lesions, pericardial effusions are uncommon (92). The second most frequent presentation involves systemic embolization, to the brain or lower extremities (86,87,90). Prolapse into the coronary arteries by lesions on the mitral or aortic valve can result in ischemia, myocardial infarction, and sudden death (88,93,94). A few patients present with inflammatory symptoms: fever, malaise, and elevated serum acute phase reactants (92,95,96). A single patient who had a family history of generalized myofibromatosis has been reported with an inflammatory myofibroblastic tumor on the mitral valve (97).

**Gross Findings.** Cardiac inflammatory myofibroblastic tumors are endocardial-based tumors that often have a stalk (fig. 13-22). Typically, they are multilobulated, often with a "grape-like" or clustered appearance (87,88,90,98). They may have a glistening, mucoid appearance that grossly mimics cardiac myxoma (99). About half are on the right side, the rest on the left (Table 13-3). The most frequent site is the right ventricle, followed by the valves and the atria. Most tumors are single, although they may be multicentric (97). When occurring on the right side, the tumors may prolapse through the pulmonary or tricuspid valves (96,100). More catastrophically, these tumors may embolize into the coronary ostia, resulting in acute myocardial infarction and sudden death (88,90,93,94). There is rarely deep involvement of myocardial tissue.

**Microscopic Findings.** Cardiac inflammatory myofibroblastic tumors are polypoid lesions, often with surface fibrin (figs. 13-23–13-26) (90,101). They may form filiform projections that protrude into the coronary artery. Histologically, they resemble their extracardiac counterparts (83). The spindle cells resemble myofibroblasts, with abundant cytoplasm and open, vesicular nuclei. Mitotic figures are infrequent, and are generally fewer than 2 per 10 high-power fields

| Table 13-3 | |
|---|---|
| **CARDIAC INFLAMMATORY MYOFIBROBLASTIC TUMORS**[a] | |
| Male:female:gender not stated | 16:21:1 |
| Age, mean (range) | 5.5 years (5 weeks-75 years) |
| Diagnostic designation (number) | |
| Inflammatory myofibroblastic tumor | 23 |
| Undifferentiated sarcoma[b] | 5 |
| Myofibroblastic inflammatory tumor | 2 |
| Inflammatory pseudotumor | 2 |
| Myofibroblastic tumor | 1 |
| Leiomyosarcoma[b] | 1 |
| Myxoma[b] | 1 |
| Rhabdomyoma[b] | 1 |
| Pseudosarcomatous proliferation | 1 |
| Myofibroma in congenital myofibromatosis | 1 |
| Site (number) | |
| Mitral valve | 9 |
| Right atrium | 7 |
| Right ventricle | 6 |
| Right ventricular outflow tract | 6 |
| Aortic valve | 3 |
| Left atrium | 3 |
| Left ventricle | 3 |
| Interventricular septum | 1 |
| Size (mean ± S.D.) | 3.5 ± 1.5 cm (maximum 6 cm) |
| Manifestations, symptoms[c] | |
| Cardiac related | 16 |
| Embolic (central nervous system) | 4 |
| Embolic (coronary artery) | 3 |
| Embolic (coronary artery and brain) | 1 |
| Embolic (lower extremities) | 1 |
| Inflammatory systemic | 3 |
| Incidental | 5 |
| Procedure | |
| Complete resection | 24 |
| Resection, coronary embolectomy, followed by OHT[d] | 1 |
| Autopsy | 4 |
| Resection with valve repair (2 PV, 1 MV) | 3 |
| Resection with aortic valve replacement | 2 |
| Resection with atrial reconstruction | 2 |
| Biopsy with referral for OHT | 1 |
| OHT | 1 |

[a]38 reported cases, primarily with adequate descriptions or illustrations, from references 84–96, 98–106, and 108–113.
[b]A diagnosis of inflammatory myofibroblastic tumor is favored for four reported undifferentiated sarcomas (86–89), one leiomyosarcoma (85), one myxoma (93), and one rhabdomyoma (108) based on histologic illustrations and benign follow-up in the case of the sarcomas.
[c]In 5 cases, not stated.
[d]OHT = orthotopic heart transplant; PV = pulmonary valve; MV = mitral valve.

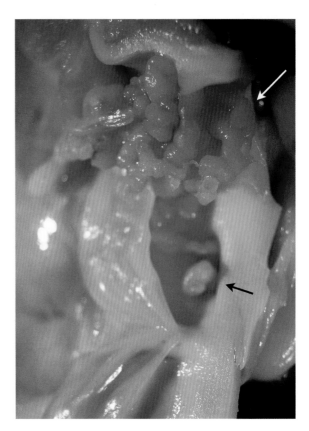

**Figure 13-22**

**INFLAMMATORY MYOFIBROBLASTIC TUMOR**

The tumor was polypoid, with grape-like clusters (white arrow). In contrast to papillary fibroelastoma, the papillary structures do not collapse and are clearly visible without immersion in water. In this case, the attachment to the aortic sinus was multifocal, with another tumor frond (black arrow) that prolapsed into the coronary ostium resulting in sudden death.

(90). Atypical mitotic figures are absent. There is variable inflammation, but lymphoid aggregates or germinal centers are rare. A myxoid background is frequent, but not consistently found.

**Immunohistochemical Findings.** All reported cases with immunohistochemical findings have been smooth muscle actin positive. Only one reported case expressed desmin (96). No case of cardiac inflammatory myofibroblastic tumor has shown immunohistochemical evidence of anaplastic lymphoma kinase (ALK-1) expression, with the exception of one weakly positive case (90). One tumor was tested for the *ALK-1* gene rearrangement, which was negative (91). Tumors show a low proliferative index by immunohistochemical staining with Ki-67 (102).

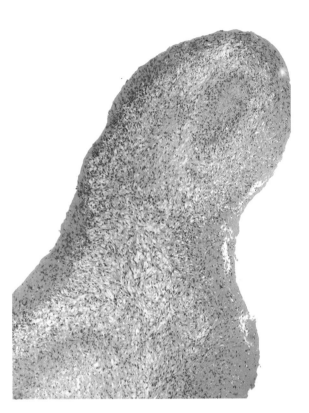

**Figure 13-23**

**INFLAMMATORY MYOFIBROBLASTIC TUMOR**

On low magnification, the papillary projections show central cellularity with a mild myxoid background.

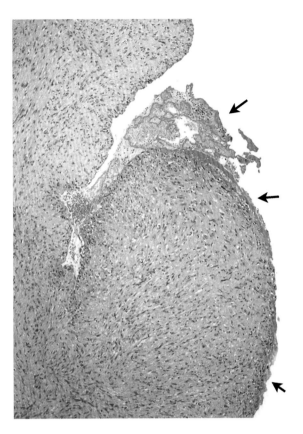

**Figure 13-24**

**INFLAMMATORY MYOFIBROBLASTIC TUMOR**

The surface typically shows fibrin (arrows).

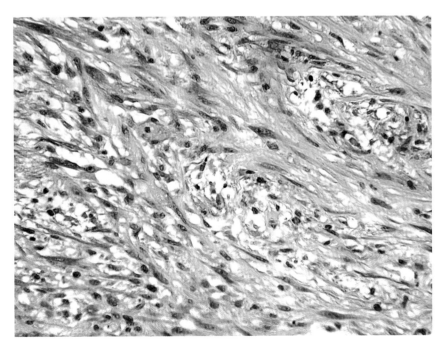

**Figure 13-25**

**INFLAMMATORY MYOFIBROBLASTIC TUMOR**

There is a proliferation of myofibroblasts with abundant collagen and scattered mononuclear inflammatory cells.

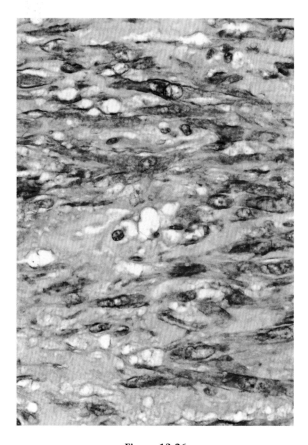

**Figure 13-26**

**INFLAMMATORY MYOFIBROBLASTIC TUMOR**

The neoplastic cells always express smooth muscle actin (antiactin immunohistochemical stain).

**Differential Diagnosis.** The differential diagnosis of cardiac inflammatory myofibroblastic tumor includes other endocardial-based lesions, such as myxoma and intimal sarcoma. Cardiac myxoma is distinguished by the presence of calretinin-positive tumor cells that are arranged in concentric vasoformative structures and cords. Cardiac fibromas are readily distinguished by their intramural location, presence of dense collagen, and lack of diffuse inflammation (101). Papillary fibroelastoma may also be confused with inflammatory myofibroblastic tumor by its location on the valve surface; however, the lack of cellularity and the presence of branch-ing frond-like excrescences distinguish papillary fibroelastoma.

The most difficult entity in the differential is intimal sarcoma, which may be relatively paucicellular and have a variable inflammatory background. In contrast to inflammatory myofibroblastic tumor, most intimal sarcomas occur in adults, and in the left atrium. Histologically, there are usually areas with increased mitotic activity and a high proliferative index. They generally deeply invade the atrial wall, an unusual occurrence with inflammatory myofibroblastic tumors. There are some cases, however, that are difficult to distinguish with certainty; only a long benign follow-up course will establish the diagnosis of inflammatory myofibroblastic tumor (103). Overexpression of MDM2 by immunohistochemistry or in-situ hybridization may prove relatively specific for cardiac "intimal" sarcoma (103a).

**Treatment and Prognosis.** Because of their endocardial location, cardiac inflammatory myofibroblastic tumors are generally resected completely. Valve tumors may necessitate repair or replacement of the valves (95,98,100,101,104). Large atrial tumors may require reconstruction of the atrium with a pericardial or xenograft patch (105). Very large tumors in infants, or tumors that result in infarcts by prolapsing into coronary arteries may necessitate orthotopic heart transplantation (88,90,92).

There has been one reported recurrence of cardiac inflammatory myofibroblastic tumor, resulting in the death of the patient (106). Generally, survival is excellent in patients with resected tumors, with one late death reported with unknown cause (90). Two children died 1 day after medical evaluation, one for symptoms of infarction (94) and the other for routine evaluation (93). One infant died suddenly at home, with a tumor on the mitral valve obstructing the orifice of the left main coronary artery (88). One child with "myxofibrosarcoma of the mitral valve" was successfully treated by heart transplantation, after presenting with myocardial infarction due to prolapse into the coronary artery (89a).

## REFERENCES

1. Sturtz CL, Abt AB, Leuenberger UA, Damiano R. Hamartoma of mature cardiac myocytes: a case report. Mod Pathol 1998;11:496-469.
2. Burke AP, Ribe JK, Bajaj AK, Edwards WD, Farb A, Virmani R. Hamartoma of mature cardiac myocytes. Hum Pathol 1998;29:904-909.
3. Fealey ME, Edwards WD, Miller DV, Menon SC, Dearani JA. Hamartomas of mature cardiac myocytes: report of 7 new cases and review of literature. Hum Pathol 2008;39:1064-1071.
4. Tanimura A, Kato M, Morimatsu M. Cardiac hamartoma. A case report. Acta Pathol Jpn 1988; 38:1481-1484.
5. Martinez Quesada M, Trujillo Berraquero F, Almendro Delia M, Hidalgo Urbano R, Cruz Fernández JM. [Cardiac hamartoma. Case report and literature review.] Rev Esp Cardiol 2005;58: 450-452. [Spanish]
6. Menon SC, Miller DV, Cabalka AK, Hagler DJ. Hamartomas of mature cardiac myocytes. Eur J Echocardiogr 2008;9:835-839.
7. Galeone A, Validire P, Gayet JB, Laborde F. Hamartoma of mature cardiac myocytes of the pulmonary infundibulum. Interact Cardiovasc Thorac Surg 2009;9:1029-1031.
8. Hsu PS, Chen JL, Hong GJ, Tsai YT, Tsai CS. Heart transplantation for ventricular arrhythmia caused by a rare hamartoma. J Heart Lung Transplant 2009;28:1114-1115.
9. Chu PH, Yeh HI, Jung SM, et al. Irregular connexin43 expressed in a rare cardiac hamartoma containing adipose tissue in the crista terminalis. Virchows Arch 2004;444:383-386.
10. Gilman G, Wright RS, Glockner JF, et al. Ventricular septal hamartoma mimicking hypertrophic cardiomyopathy in a 41-year-old woman presenting with paroxysmal supraventricular tachycardia. J Am Soc Echocardiogr 2005;18:272-274.
11. Movahedi N, Boroumand MA, Sotoudeh Anvari M, Yazdanifard P. Mature cardiac myocyte hamartoma in the right atrium. Asian Cardiovasc Thorac Ann 2008;16:e47-48.
12. Barberger-Gateau P, Paquet M, Desaulniers D, Chenard J. Fibrolipoma of the mitral valve in a child. Clinical and echocardiographic features. Circulation 1978;58:955-958.
13. Crotty TB, Edwards WD, Oh JK, Rodeheffer RJ. Lipomatous hamartoma of the tricuspid valve: echocardiographic-pathologic correlations. Clin Cardiol 1991;14:262-266.
14. Zhang F, Yin N, Yin B, Xu S, Yang Y. Giant right atrial cystic hamartoma: a case report and literature review. BMJ Case Rep 2009;2009:1587.
15. Dell'Amore A, Lanzanova G, Silenzi A, Lamarra M. Hamartoma of mature cardiac myocytes: case report and review of the literature. Heart Lung Circ 2011;20:336-340.
16. Burke AP, Gatto-Weis C, Griego JE, Ellington KS, Virmani R. Adult cellular rhabdomyoma of the heart: a report of 3 cases. Hum Pathol 2002; 33:1092-1097.
17. Yu GH, Kussmaul WG, DiSesa VJ, Lodato RF, Brooks JS. Adult intracardiac rhabdomyoma resembling the extracardiac variant. Hum Pathol 1993;24:448-451.
18. Eberle MC, Boudousq V, Becassis P, Mariano-Goulart D. Cardiac rhabdomyoma in an adult: an aspect of Tc-99m sestamibi myocardial perfusion. J Nucl Cardiol 2002;9:131-132.
19. Wage R, Kafka H, Prasad S. Images in cardiovascular medicine. Cardiac rhabdomyoma in an adult with a previous presumptive diagnosis of septal hypertrophy. Circulation 2008;117:e469-470.
20. Qi J, Yu J, Zhang M, et al. Multicentric granular cell tumors with heart involvement: a case report. J Clin Oncol 2012;30:e79-82.
21. Gualis J, Carrascal Y, de la Fuente L, Echevarría JR. Heart transplantation treatment for a malignant cardiac granular cell tumor: 33 months of survival. Interact Cardiovasc Thorac Surg 2007; 6:679-681.
22. Fujise K, Sacchi TJ, Williams RJ, DiCostanzo DP, Tranbaugh RF. Multicentric granular cell tumor of the heart presenting with aortic dissection. Ann Thorac Surg 1994;57:1653-1655.
23. Wang J, Kragel AH, Friedlander ER, Cheng JT. Granular cell tumor of the sinus node. Am J Cardiol 1993;71:490-1492.
24. Fujise K. Granular cell tumor with symptomatic cardiac involvement can be malignant or benign. Am J Cardiol 1993;72:862-863.
25. Park SH, Kim TJ, Chi JG. Congenital granular cell tumor with systemic involvement. Immunohistochemical and ultrastructural study. Arch Pathol Lab Med 1991;115:934-938.
26. Fenoglio JJ, McAllister HA. Granular cell tumors of the heart. Arch Pathol Lab Med 1976;100:276-8.
27. Roth D, Spain DM. Granular-cell myoblastoma of the myocardium; case report. Cancer 1952;5:302-306.
28. Kubac G, Doris I, Ondro M, Davey PW. Malignant granular cell myoblastoma with metastatic cardiac involvement: Case report and echocardiogram. Am Heart J 1980;100:227-229.
29. Ralis Z, Emery JL. Congenital plexiform neurofibroma of the vagus with cardiac, pulmonary and visceral involvement. J Pathol 1972;107:55-57.
30. Early SA, McGuinness J, Galvin J, Kennedy M, Hurley J. Asymptomatic schwannoma of the heart. J Cardiothorac Surg 2007;2:1.

31. Sirlak M, Uymaz OK, Tasoz R, Erden E, Ozyurda U, Akalin H. Primary benign schwannoma of the heart. Cardiovasc Pathol 2003;12:290-292.

32. Jassal DS, Légaré JF, Cummings B, et al., Primary cardiac ancient schwannoma. J Thorac Cardiovasc Surg 2003;125:733-735.

33. Hashimoto T, Eguchi S, Nakayama T, Ohzeki H, Hayashi J. Successful removal of massive cardiac neurilemoma with cardiopulmonary bypass. Ann Thorac Surg 1998;66:553-555.

34. Kodama M, Aoki M, Sakai K. Images in cardiovascular medicine. Primary cardiac neurilemoma. Circulation 1995;92:274-275.

35. Forbes AD, Schmidt RA, Wood DE, Cochran RP, Munkenbeck F, Verrier ED. Schwannoma of the left atrium: diagnostic evaluation and surgical resection. Ann Thorac Surg 1994;57:743-746.

36. Monroe B, Federman M, Balogh K. Cardiac neurilemoma. Report of a case with electron microscopic examination. Arch Pathol Lab Med 1984;108:300-304.

37. Betancourt B, Defendini EA, Johnson C, et al. Severe right ventricular outflow tract obstruction caused by an intracavitary cardiac neurilemoma: succesful surgical removal and postoperative diagnosis. Chest 1979;75:522-524.

38. Factor S, Turi G, Biempica L. Primary cardiac neurilemoma. Cancer 1976;37:883-890.

39. Gleason TH, Dillard DH, Gould VE. Cardiac neurilemoma. N Y State J Med 1972;72:2435-2436.

40. Kato M, Shiota S, Shiga K, et al. Benign giant mediastinal schwannoma presenting as cardiac tamponade in a woman: a case report. J Med Case Rep 2011;5:61.

41. Rausche T, El-Mokthari NE, Krüger D, et al. Benign mediastinal schwannoma: cardiac considerations—case report and a short review of the literature. Clin Res Cardiol 2006;95:422-424.

42. Melo IS, Belo F, Gouveia R, Anjos R. Primary cardiac leiomyoma of the ventricular septum: a rare form of pediatric intracardiac tumor. Pediatr Cardiol 2012;33:649-651.

43. Qin C, Chen L, Xiao YB, Chen BC. Giant primary leiomyoma of the right ventricle. J Card Surg 2010;25:169-171.

44. Strecker T, Rösch J, Weyand M, Strecker T. Primary and metastatic cardiac tumors: imaging characteristics, surgical treatment, and histopathological spectrum: a 10-year-experience at a German heart center. Cardiovasc Pathol 2012;21:436-443.

45. Matebele MP, Peters P, Mundy J, Shah P. Cardiac tumors in adults: surgical management and follow-up of 19 patients in an Australian tertiary hospital. Interact Cardiovasc Thorac Surg 2010; 10:892-895.

46. Castelli P, Caronno R, Piffaretti G, Tozzi M. Intravenous uterine leiomyomatosis with right heart extension: successful two-stage surgical removal. Ann Vasc Surg 2006;20:405-407.

47. Zhang Y, Zhu J, Wang C, Tu R, Jiang J, Lu W. Multimodality treatment of two cases of intracardiac leiomyomatosis with enormous mass in the abdominopelvic cavity. Expert Rev Anticancer Ther 2013;13:137-141.

48. Vaideeswar P, Kulkarni DV, Karunamurthy A, Hira P. Intracardiac leiomyomatosis: report of two cases. Indian J Pathol Microbiol 2011;54:158-160.

49. Song BG, Park YH, Kang GH, Chun WJ, Oh JH. Intravenous leiomyomatosis with intracardiac extension. Asian Cardiovasc Thorac Ann 2011;19:179.

50. Okamura H, Yamaguchi A, Kimura N, Adachi K, Adachi H. Partial resection of intravenous leiomyomatosis with cardiac extension. Gen Thorac Cardiovasc Surg 2011;59:38-41.

51. Lou YF, Shi XP, Song ZZ. Intravenous leiomyomatosis of the uterus with extension to the right heart. Cardiovasc Ultrasound 2011;9:25.

52. Senay S, Kaya U, Cagil H, Demirkiran F, Alhan C. Surgical management of intravenous leiomyoma with cardiac extension. Do we need total circulatory arrest? Thorac Cardiovasc Surg 2007;55:322-323.

53. Clement PB. Intravenous leiomyomatosis of the uterus. Pathol Annu 1988;23(Pt 2):153-183.

54. Kuenen BC, Slee PH, Seldenrijk CA, Wagenaar SS. Intravenous leiomyomatosis complicated by Budd-Chiari syndrome. Postgrad Med J 1996; 72:686-688.

55. Okada M, Miyoshi Y, Kato G, Ochi Y, Shimizu S, Nakai M. Successful one-stage surgical removal of intravenous leiomyomatosis with cardiac extension in an elderly patient. Gen Thorac Cardiovasc Surg 2012;60:153-156.

56. Matsuo K, Fleischman F, Ghattas CS, et al. Successful extraction of cardiac-extending intravenous leiomyomatosis through gonadal vein. Fertil Steril 2012;98:1341-1345 e1.

57. Roman DA, Mirchandani H. Intravenous leiomyoma with intracardiac extension causing sudden death. Arch Pathol Lab Med 1987;111:1176-1178.

58. Galvin SD, Wademan B, Chu J, Bunton RW. Benign metastasizing leiomyoma: a rare metastatic lesion in the right ventricle. Ann Thorac Surg 2010;89:279-281.

59. Takemura G, Takatsu Y, Kaitani K, et al. Metastasizing uterine leiomyoma. A case with cardiac and pulmonary metastasis. Pathol Res Pract 1996;192:622-629; discussion 630-633.

60. Anderson MC, Robboy SJ, Russell P. Uterine smooth muscle tumors. In: Robboy SJ, Anderson MC, Russell P, eds. Pathology of the female reproductive tract. Philadelphia: Churchill Livingstone; 2002:389-414.

61. Canzonieri V, D'Amore ES, Bartoloni G, Piazza M, Blandamura S, Carbone A. Leiomyomatosis with vascular invasion. A unified pathogenesis regarding leiomyoma with vascular microinvasion, benign metastasizing leiomyoma and intravenous leiomyomatosis. Virchows Arch 1994;425:541-545.

62. Mulvany NJ, Slavin JL, Ostör AG, Fortune DW. Intravenous leiomyomatosis of the uterus: a clinicopathologic study of 22 cases. Int J Gynecol Pathol 1994;13:1-9.

63. Nam MS, Jeon MJ, Kim YT, Kim JW, Park KH, Hong YS. Pelvic leiomyomatosis with intracaval and intracardiac extension: a case report and review of the literature. Gynecol Oncol 2003;89:175-180.

64. Clement PB, Young RH, Scully RE. Intravenous leiomyomatosis of the uterus. A clinicopathological analysis of 16 cases with unusual histologic features. Am J Surg Pathol 1988;12:932-945.

65. Peh WC, Cheung DL, Ngan H. Smooth muscle tumors of the inferior vena cava and right heart. Clin Imaging 1993;17:117-123.

66. Topcuoglu MS, Yaliniz H, Poyrazoglu H, et al. Intravenous leiomyomatosis extending into the right ventricle after subtotal hysterectomy. Ann Thorac Surg 2004;78:330-332.

67. Gehr NR, Lund O, Alstrup P, Nielsen JS, Villadsen AB, Bartholdy NJ. Recurrence of uterine intravenous leiomyomatosis with intracardiac extension. Diagnostic considerations and surgical removal. Scand Cardiovasc J 1999;33:312-314.

68. Mitsuhashi A, Nagai Y, Sugita M, Nakajima N, Sekiya S. GnRH agonist for intravenous leiomyomatosis with cardiac extension. A case report. J Reprod Med 1999;44:883-886.

69. Sinzelle E, Duong Van Huyen JP, Breiteneder-Geleff S, et al. Intrapericardial lymphangioma with podoplanin immunohistochemical characterization of lymphatic endothelial cells. Histopathology 2000;37:93-94.

70. Daubeney PE, Ogilvie BC, Moore IE, Webber SA. Intrapericardial lymphangioma presenting as neonatal cardiac tamponade. Pediatr Cardiol 1996;17:129-131.

71. Witkin GB, Rosai J. Solitary fibrous tumor of the mediastinum. A report of 14 cases. Am J Surg Pathol 1989;13:547-557.

72. Iwata T, Nishiyama N, Izumi N, Tsukioka T, Suehiro S. Solitary fibrous tumor of the thymus with local invasiveness and pleural dissemination: report of a case. Ann Thorac Cardiovasc Surg 2007;13:198-202.

73. Corgnati G, Drago S, Bonamini R, Trevi GP, Carra R, Di Summa M. Solitary fibrous tumor of the pericardium presenting itself as a pericardial effusion and right ventricular obstruction. J Cardiovasc Surg (Torino) 2004;45:393-394.

74. Segawa D, Yoshizu H, Haga Y, Hatori N, Tanaka S, Aida S. Successful operation for solitary fibrous tumor of the epicardium. J Thorac Cardiovasc Surg 1995;109:1246-1248.

75. Weidner N. Solitary fibrous tumor of the mediastinum. Ultrastruct Pathol 1991;15:489-492.

76. el-Naggar AK, Ro JY, Ayala AG, Ward R, Ordóñez NG. Localized fibrous tumor of the serosal cavities. Immunohistochemical, electron-microscopic, and flow-cytometric DNA study. Am J Clin Pathol 1989;92:561-565.

77. Bothe W, Goebel H, Kunze M, Beyersdorf F. Right atrial solitary fibrous tumor—a new cardiac neoplasm? Interact Cardiovasc Thorac Surg 2005;4:396-397.

78. Croti UA, Braile DM, Moscardini AC, Cury PM. [Solitary fibrous tumor in a child's heart.] Rev Bras Cir Cardiovasc 2008;23:139-141. [Portuguese]

79. Zhao XG, Wang H, Wang YL, Chen G, Jiang GN. Malignant solitary fibrous tumor of the right atrium. Am J Med Sci 2012;344:422-425.

80. Odim J, Reehal V, Laks H, Mehta U, Fishbein MC. Surgical pathology of cardiac tumors. Two decades at an urban institution. Cardiovasc Pathol 2003;12:267-270.

81. Cuadrado M, García-Camarero T, Expósito V, Val-Bernal JF, Gómez-Román JJ, Garijo MF. Cardiac intracavitary metastasis of a malignant solitary fibrous tumor: case report and review of the literature on sarcomas with left intracavitary extension. Cardiovasc Pathol 2007;16:241-247.

82. England DM, Hochholzer L, McCarthy MJ. Localized benign and malignant fibrous tumors of the pleura. A clinicopathologic review of 223 cases. Am J Surg Pathol 1989;13:640-658.

83. Montgomery EA, Shuster DD, Burkart AL, et al. Inflammatory myofibroblastic tumors of the urinary tract: a clinicopathologic study of 46 cases, including a malignant example inflammatory fibrosarcoma and a subset associated with high-grade urothelial carcinoma. Am J Surg Pathol 2006;30:1502-1512.

84. de Winkel N, Becker K, Vogt M. Echogenic mass in the right atrium after surgical ventricular septal defect closure: thrombus or tumour? Cardiol Young 2010;20:86-88.

85. Han P, Drachtman RA, Amenta P, Ettinger LJ. Successful treatment of a primary cardiac leiomyosarcoma with ifosfamide and etoposide. J Pediatr Hematol Oncol 1996;18:314-317.

86. Itoh K, Matsumura T, Egawa Y, et al. Primary mitral valve sarcoma in infancy. Pediatr Cardiol 1998;19:174-177.

87. Lee JR, Chang JM, Lee C, Kim CJ. Undifferentiated sarcoma of the mitral valve with unique clinicopathologic presentation. J Cardiovasc Surg (Torino) 2003;44:621-623.

88. McElhinney DB, Carpentieri DF, Bridges ND, Clark BJ, Gaynor JW, Spray TL. Sarcoma of the mitral valve causing coronary arterial occlusion in children. Cardiol Young 2001;11:539-542.

89. Takach TJ, Reul GJ, Ott DA, Cooley DA. Primary cardiac tumors in infants and children: immediate and long-term operative results. Ann Thorac Surg 1996;62:559-564.

89a. Zhang PJ, Brooks JS, Goldblum JR, et al., Primary cardiac sarcomas: a clinicopathologic analysis of a series with follow-up information in 17 patients and emphasis on long-term survival. Hum Pathol 2008;39:1385-1395.

90. Burke A, Li L, Kling E, Kutys R, Virmani R, Miettinen M. Cardiac inflammatory myofibroblastic tumor: a "benign" neoplasm that may result in syncope, myocardial infarction, and sudden death. Am J Surg Pathol 2007;31:1115-1122.

91. Nemolato S, Dettori T, Caria P, Frau DV, Faa G, Vanni R. Would a morphomolecular approach help in defining pseudosarcomatous myofibroblastic proliferations? A study of a heart polypoid lesion. J Clin Pathol 2009;62:377-379.

92. Di Maria MV, Campbell DN, Mitchell MB, Lovell MA, Pietra BA, Miyamoto SD. Successful orthotopic heart transplant in an infant with an inflammatory myofibroblastic tumor of the left ventricle. J Heart Lung Transplant 2008;27:792-796.

93. Kure K, Lingamfelter D, Taboada E. Large multifocal cardiac myxoma causing the sudden unexpected death of a 2-month-old infant—a rapidly growing, acquired lesion versus a congenital process?: a case report. Am J Forensic Med Pathol 2011;32:166-168.

94. Li L, Burke A, He J, Chang L, Zielke HR, Fowler DR. Sudden unexpected death due to inflammatory myofibroblastic tumor of the heart: a case report and review of the literature. Int J Legal Med 2011;125:81-85.

95. Anvari MS, Soleimani A, Abbasi A, et al. Inflammatory myofibroblastic tumor of the right ventricle causing tricuspid valve regurgitation. Tex Heart Inst J 2009;36:164-167.

96. Elkiran O, Karakurt C, Erdil N, Disli OM, Dagli AF. An unexpected cause of respiratory distress and cyanosis: cardiac inflammatory myofibroblastic tumor. Congenit Heart Dis 2013;8:E174-177.

97. de Montpreville VT, Zemoura L, Vaksmann G, Lecourt-Tierny G, Planché C, Dulmet E. Endocardial location of familial myofibromatosis revealed by cerebral embolization: cardiac counterpart of the frequent intravascular growth of the disease? Virchows Arch 2004;444:300-303.

98. Krishna L, Ng WL, Chachlani N. Inflammatory pseudotumor of the heart causing aortic regurgitation. Ann Thorac Surg 2001;71:1361-1363.

99. Li L, Cerilli LA, Wick MR. Inflammatory pseudotumor (myofibroblastic tumor) of the heart. Ann Diagn Pathol 2002;6:116-121.

100. Shamszad P, Morales DL, Slesnick TC. Right ventricular inflammatory myofibroblastic tumor characterization by cardiovascular magnetic resonance. J Am Coll Cardiol 2011;57:e205.

101. de Montpreville VT, Serraf A, Aznag H, Nashashibi N, Planché C, Dulmet E. Fibroma and inflammatory myofibroblastic tumor of the heart. Ann Diagn Pathol 2001;5:335-342.

102. Obikane H, Ariizumi K, Yutani C, Mitsumata M. Inflammatory pseudotumor (inflammatory myofibroblastic tumor) of the mitral valve of the heart. Pathol Int 2010;60:533-537.

103. Kelly SJ, Lambie NK, Singh HP. Inflammatory myofibroblastic tumor of the left ventricle in an older adult. Ann Thorac Surg 2003;75:1971-1973.

103a. Neuville A, Collin F, Bruneval P, et al. Intimal sarcoma is the most frequent primary cardiac sarcoma: clinicopathologic and molecular retrospective analysis of 100 primary cardiac sarcomas. Am J Surg Pathol 2014;38:461-469.

104. Rao N, Gajjar T, Ghosal N, Desai N. Inflammatory pseudotumor arising from the right ventricular outflow tract causing pulmonary stenosis. J Card Surg 2012;27:696-698.

105. Das Narla L, Siddiqi NH, Hingsbergen EA. Inflammatory pseudotumor of the right atrium. Pediatr Radiol 2001;31:351-353.

106. Yang X, Xiao C, Liu M, Wang Y. Cardiac inflammatory myofibroblastic tumor: does it recur after complete surgical resection in an adult? J Cardiothorac Surg 2012;7:44.

107. Raffa GM, Tarelli G, Balzarini L, Torta D, Monti L. Hamartoma of mature cardiac myocytes in adults and young: case report and literature review. Int J Cardiol 2013;163:e28-30.

108. Aktoz M, Tatli E, Ege T, et al. Cardiac rhabdomyoma in an adult patient presenting with right ventricular outflow tract obstruction. Int J Cardiol 2008;130:e105-107.

109. Gandy KL, Burtelow MA, Reddy VM, Silverman NH. Myofibroblastic tumor of the heart: a rare intracardiac tumor. J Thorac Cardiovasc Surg 2005;130:888-889.

110. Hoey ET, Ganesh V, Gopalan D, Screaton NJ. Cardiac inflammatory myofibroblastic tumor: evaluation with dual-source CT. J Cardiovasc Comput Tomogr 2009;3:114-116.

111. Jha NK, Trudel M, Eising GP, et al. Inflammatory myofibroblastic tumor of the right atrium. Case Rep Med, 2010;2010.

112. Thomas-de-Montpreville V, Nottin R, Dulmet E, Serraf A. Heart tumors in children and adults: clinicopathological study of 59 patients from a surgical center. Cardiovasc Pathol 2007;16:22-28.

113. Zhao D, Wang C. Guo C. An unusual case of severe aortic valve stenosis in an adult caused by aortic valve inflammatory myofibroblastic tumor. J Thorac Cardiovasc Surg 2013;146:479-480.

# HETEROTOPIAS AND GERM CELL TUMORS

## BRONCHOGENIC CYST

**Definition.** *Bronchogenic cysts* are congenital endodermal rests lined by columnar or cuboidal epithelium, usually with a muscular wall. They are located in the mediastinum, neck, lung, and rarely, within the pericardium (1). They contain elements derived from only two germ layers, mesoderm and endoderm. Synonyms include *inclusion cyst, epithelial cyst, entodermal cyst, heterotopic cyst, gastroenterogenous cyst,* and *enteric cyst.*

**General Features.** During embryogenesis, bronchogenic cysts arise from abnormal budding in the distal tracheobronchial tree. Resulting structures may migrate to subpleural, pericardial, myocardial, paravertebral, and cervical locations when embryologic connections with the parent bronchus are lost. The cysts arise from the migration of sequestered cells, with subsequent cyst formation, or the cyst may be preformed and subsequently migrates (1).

In a minority of cases, the cysts more closely resemble primitive gut than bronchus because of a lack of cartilage in the wall and a lack of mucin-producing cells. These cysts are designated "gastroenterogenous" or "enteric" cysts. Rarely, associated sequestered lung tissue is present within the cyst (2,3).

Bronchogenic or enteric cysts located within the pericardium are extremely rare, as most bronchogenic cysts occur in the mediastinum near but outside the pericardium (1). Four intrapericardial cysts, which were likely bronchogenic or enteric cysts, were compiled from the literature by Gould et al. in 1960 (4). Three of these were located on papillary muscles, and one was intramural in the left ventricle. The term "epithelial" cyst was used for these lesions; two other cases in this review are better classified as cystic tumors of the atrioventricular node because of their location in the atrial septum.

In 1974, a literature review found 21 cases of intrapericardial bronchogenic cysts (5).

Seven intrapericardial bronchogenic cysts were reported by McAllister and Fenoglio in 1978 (6). Since then there have been fewer than 15 reported cases (3,7–17).

**Clinical Features.** There is an approximate 2 to 1 female predominance for bronchogenic cysts that occur within the pericardium (5). Bronchogenic cysts in infants are often symptomatic. Manifestations include chest pain, shortness of breath (16), and arrhythmias, and vary according to the location of the cyst, its size, and the degree of compression of the heart and vessels. At presentation, approximately one third of patients are infants, half are over the age of 15 years, and most of the rest are children (5,11). Adults may present with heart block (10) or shortness of breath (16); generally, however, the cyst is an incidental finding (12,13). CA19-9 levels in adults may be increased (18).

There may be an association between intrapericardial bronchogenic cyst and multiple gestation (5), as well as between bronchogenic cyst and congenital heart disease, especially atrial septal defects (7,9,10,13). An epithelial cyst in an infant with esophageal atresia has been reported (19).

Generally, bronchogenic cysts are located on the epicardial surface of the right side of the heart, such as the right atrium (3,11), with the blood supply derived from the root of the ascending aorta (6). Symptoms usually result from compression of nearby heart structures. Rarely, cysts lie within heart muscle, such as the right ventricle (14) or atrial septum (12). In the latter case, heart block may result, as is the case with atrioventricular nodal tumors.

A surgically excised inclusion cyst overlying the septal leaflet of the tricuspid valve in a 5 1/5-year-old boy has recently been described (7), but this may represent a cystic tumor of the atrioventricular node. A histologically documented bronchogenic cyst with ciliated epithelium and underlying smooth muscle was

241

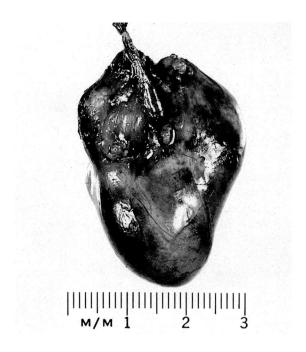

**Figure 14-1**

**BRONCHOGENIC CYST**

This example was removed from the epicardial surface of a 13-year-old boy.

surgically excised from the atrial septum near the atrioventricular node; the tumor caused heart block (10).

Bronchogenic cysts are generally detected by echocardiography; computed tomography (CT) and magnetic resonance imaging (MRI) may assist in delineating the size, extent, and involvement of adjacent structures (16,17).

**Gross Findings.** Intrapericardial bronchogenic cysts are usually located on the epicardial surface. The cysts are usually 1 to 3 cm in diameter, but may be up to 5 cm (fig. 14-1) (11).

**Microscopic Findings.** Histologically, the cyst lining is ciliated columnar or cuboidal epithelium, often resembling ciliated respiratory epithelium (fig. 14-2). There may be degenerative changes and areas of the cyst lining replaced by pseudocyst (fig. 14-2, right). Occasionally, pulmonary parenchyma reminiscent of extralobar sequestration accompanies the cyst (3). Both goblet cells and squamous epithelium may be present, especially if the cyst wall is inflamed.

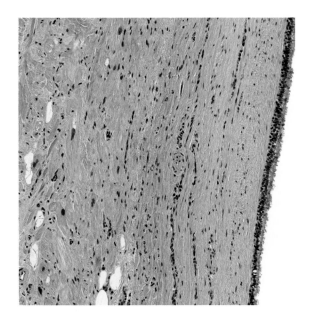

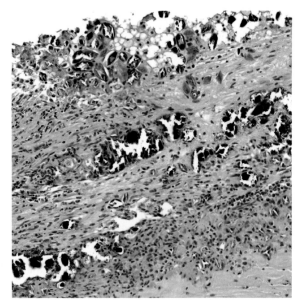

**Figure 14-2**

**BRONCHOGENIC CYST**

Left: The lining cells are cuboidal ciliated cells (right). There is a compact fibrous layer separating the cyst lining from atrial myocytes (left). The tumor arose in the interatrial septum of a young adult and was surgically excised. The diagnosis of probable bronchogenic cyst was made by imaging.

Right: Another area shows a pseudocyst with a calcified inflammatory lining, a nondiagnostic finding. The diagnosis of bronchogenic cyst was not made pathologically until the entire specimen was submitted for histologic evaluation.

The wall of the cyst generally contains smooth muscle that is often concentric, cartilage, lymphoid cells, lymphoid nodules, and seromucinous glands. In the absence of cartilage, the cyst is referred to as an *undifferentiated foregut cyst*, as this feature is necessary for the diagnosis of a bronchogenic cyst. When other types of ectodermal or endodermal tissue are present (such as gastric or pancreatic tissue), either the designation of "cystic teratoma" or, generically, "foregut cyst," is appropriate (5).

**Treatment and Prognosis.** With current surgical techniques, bronchogenic cysts are successfully excised with little morbidity. Even in the past, in a series of 25 cases surgically excised in the late 1960s and early 1970s, 20 patients survived the procedure (5). With involvement of the heart muscle, excision of the atrial wall may be necessary (11).

## CYSTIC TUMOR OF THE ATRIOVENTRICULAR NODE

**Definition.** *Cystic tumor of the atrioventricular (AV) node* is a benign, congenital, cystic mass located at the base of the atrial septum in the region of the AV node. Obsolete terms include *lymphangioendothelioma, mesothelioma*, and *inclusion cyst*. The designation *endodermal heterotopia* has been used for these lesions. Unlike bronchogenic cysts, the cysts are usually microscopic and multiple, and a muscular wall is absent.

**General Features.** The existence and clinical significance of cystic tumors of the AV node have been known since early the 20th century (20). However, divergent opinions regarding the histogenesis have resulted in numerous terms for these rare tumors (21). Although once considered of mesothelial or endothelial origin, these curious inclusions have been conclusively identified as of endodermal derivation. There is some evidence that they represent a form of ultimobranchial heterotopia (22). Immunohistochemical studies confirm that they are endodermal remnants and not mesothelial rests (23–27). The evidence for a mesothelial origin was based on ultrastructural data that was not entirely specific (28). For these reasons, we, as well as most recent authors, have abandoned the term "mesothelioma of the AV node" and prefer the term "cystic tumor of the AV node."

Six of 66 reported cases of AV nodal tumors (23) arose in patients with other midline defects, suggesting that these lesions represent misplaced embryologic tissue. They are located in the AV nodal region because this is an area of embryologic fusion (25,29), and therefore prone to abnormal incorporation of developing embryologic structures. The precise embryologic pathway from the primitive foregut to the atrial septum that allows for the existence of these inclusions is unknown. Travers (30) reviewed the embryologic data that may explain the origin of tumors of the AV nodal region. Fifty years ago it was argued that such cysts arise from sequestration or heterotopia during the period when the heart and foregut are in close approximation (31). Other authorities argued that the separation of the heart and foregut is too complete in man to allow for such a migration (32). They hypothesized that a form of metaplasia of mesodermal elements results in cystic tumors of the AV node and intrapericardial bronchogenic rests. There have been no recent studies regarding the pathogenesis of these rare lesions.

Cystic tumors of the AV node are rare: there have been fewer than 70 reports in the literature to date, approximately twice the number of intrapericardial bronchogenic cysts. The true incidence may be higher than the literature suggests because cases may be overlooked at autopsy.

**Clinical Features.** Most tumors are diagnosed at autopsy, although these lesions should be considered in the differential diagnosis of congenital heart block, especially in young women. Fewer than 10 cases have been diagnosed antemortem (33,34). Death is usually sudden and unexpected, but occasional patients have coexisting dilated cardiomyopathy (33,35). Ventricular arrhythmias are more frequent in patients with heart block, from any cause, than in patients without heart disease.

The mean age of presentation or of sudden death is 38 years, although there is a wide range, from birth to the eighth decade (23,36–38). The female to male ratio is approximately 3 to 1. Most patients with cystic tumors of the AV node present with complete heart block (33); in the remainder, patients die suddenly, presumably as a result of ventricular arrhythmias, without a history of heart problems. An incidental AV

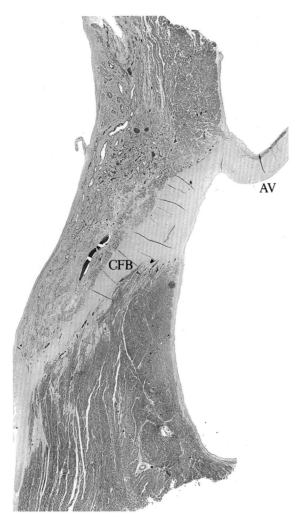

**Figure 14-3**

**CYSTIC TUMOR OF THE ATRIOVENTRICULAR NODE**

A glandular proliferation is replacing normal tissue at the atrioventricular (AV) node. The patient was a 20-year-old woman with a several-year history of first and second degree heart block treated intermittently by pacing. Structural heart disease had been ruled out. She presented with complete heart block during delivery of a healthy baby, and was given temporary pacing while hospitalized. She died suddenly several days postpartum while carrying her infant. The central fibrous body (CFB) contains the downward growth of the tumor. The aortic valve (AV) is at the top.

nodal tumor in an elderly man who had a normal electrocardiogram has been reported (40).

The diagnosis of heart block in patients with AV nodal tumors may occur at birth or as late as the ninth decade of life. Because of a female predominance, it has been suggested that the diagnosis be considered in teenage girls with

complete heart block (29,41). Rarely, patients become symptomatic during pregnancy (42). The clinical differential diagnosis of congenital heart block includes maternal lupus erythematosus, which can result in intrauterine destruction of nodal pathways, presumably by an autoimmune mechanism (41).

There have been at least five reports of successfully resected AV nodal tumors (39,40,43–46). One cystic tumor of the AV node was found in a cardiac explant after the patient underwent cardiac transplantation for presumed peripartum cardiomyopathy (33). One case was detected by MRI and surgically resected (45).

The majority of tumors of the AV node are sporadic. In these patients, however, there is an increased incidence of other midline defects, such as atrial septal defect (45), ventricular septal defect (23,47), nasal septal defect (48), encephalocele (48), thinning of the corpus callosum (49), absent septum pellucidum (49), and thyroglossal duct cyst (40). A familial history of sudden unexplained death and heart block has been reported (23,30,35).

**Gross Findings.** These tumors are located, by definition, in the region of the AV node. They appear in the region of the membranous septum as a cyst-like structure or as an area of thickening with small, fluid-filled cysts that are barely perceptible to the naked eye. At autopsy, they range in size from 2 to 20 mm. Often the cysts are first recognized at the time of microscopic examination of the conduction system. The gross examination of the heart is normal in 60 percent of patients (33), irregular cysts are seen in the area of the AV node in 20 percent, and a single dominant cyst in 10 percent (40). Surgically excised tumors are generally large, measuring several centimeters, and grossly multicystic, reflecting their ability to be detected by imaging (39,43–46).

**Microscopic Findings.** Histologically, the tumor is located in the inferior interatrial septum in the region of the AV node and proximal to the His bundles. It respects the boundary of the central fibrous body without extending into ventricular myocardium or valvular tissues (figs. 14-3–14-6). There are nests of cells that often form cysts of variable sizes (figs. 14-7–14-10). The cell nests can replace myocytes within the septum, and are composed of cuboidal, transitional, or squamous cells. Sebaceous cells

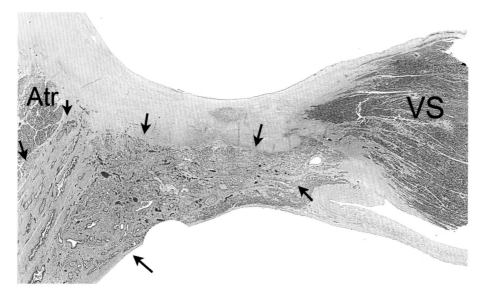

**Figure 14-4**

**CYSTIC TUMOR OF THE ATRIOVENTRICULAR NODE**

A tumor from a young man dying suddenly shows the proximal AV nodal area. The right atrial cavity is below, the tricuspid valve at the lower right, and the atrial septum (Atr) at the left. Above the tricuspid valve is the ventricular septum (VS).

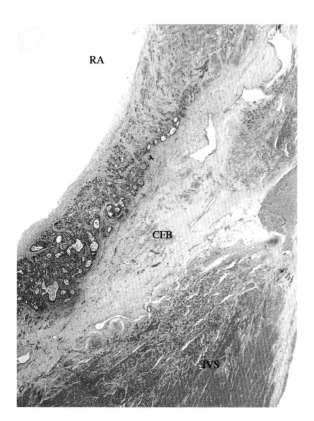

**Figure 14-5**

**CYSTIC TUMOR OF THE ATRIOVENTRICULAR NODE**

The typical location for this lesion is posterior to the position of the AV node. The central fibrous body (CFB) is at the top toward the interatrial septum, and the right atrial cavity (RA) at the top left. There is no evidence of residual nodal tissue. The interventricular septum is toward the bottom right.

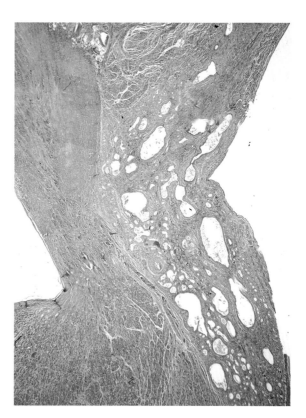

**Figure 14-6**

**CYSTIC TUMOR OF THE ATRIOVENTRICULAR NODE**

A different tumor, showing a similar distribution at a higher magnification. Multiple levels revealed no evidence of the atrioventricular node or the branching bundle, indicating the absence of these structures as a cause of congenital heart block.

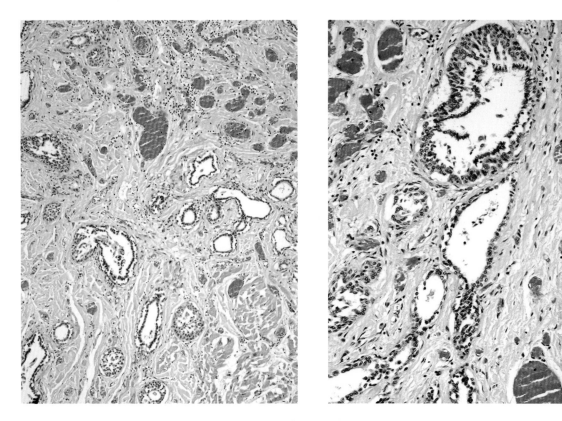

**Figure 14-7**

**CYSTIC TUMOR OF THE ATRIOVENTRICULAR NODE**

Left: There is a loose collection of small, open glands with a cuboidal, stratified and transitional type lining.

Right: At higher magnification, the typical glandular structures are seen, some compressed and some with lumens, with a basaloid or transitional histologic appearance.

**Figure 14-8**

**CYSTIC TUMOR OF THE ATRIOVENTRICULAR NODE**

Most of the epithelial rests are dilated and somewhat crowded, mimicking metastatic adenocarcinoma.

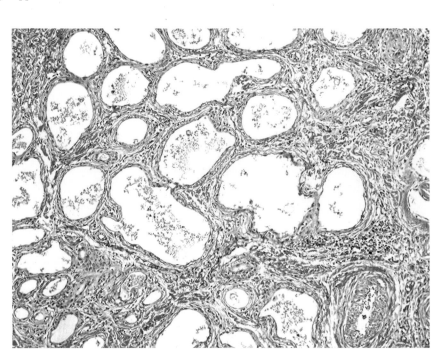

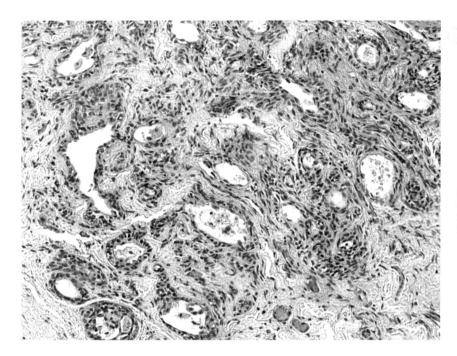

**Figure 14-9**

**CYSTIC TUMOR OF THE ATRIOVENTRICULAR NODE**

The haphazardly positioned glandular structures mimic metastatic adenocarcinoma. There is focal squamous differentiation in this case.

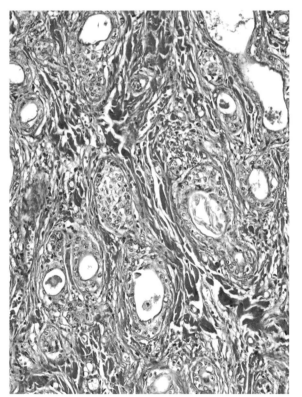
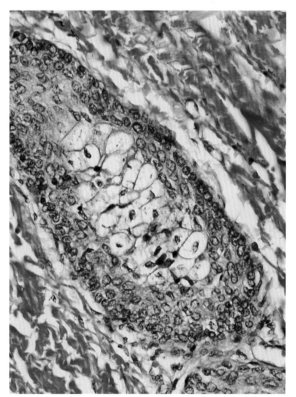

**Figure 14-10**

**CYSTIC TUMOR OF THE ATRIOVENTRICULAR NODE**

Left: There is sebaceous differentiation in this case, suggesting the diagnosis of teratoma. However, ectoderm and mesodermal structures are absent, and there is no single dominant cyst.

Right: The sebaceous-like differentiation at higher magnification.

may be interspersed among cuboidal cells, forming a two-cell population (fig. 14-10).

The lumens of the cysts contain periodic acid–Schiff (PAS)-positive, diastase-resistant material (33), which occasionally calcifies. The cysts often form two cell layers, a luminal, cuboidal, single cell layer overlying transitional cells. The epithelium can flatten, and the cysts can assume tortuous shapes, which may explain why early observers mistook them for endothelial cells. Often, there is dense fibrosis surrounding the cysts or cell nests, with a lymphocytic reaction. Cilia are sometimes visible on light microscopy. Endocrine granules have been reported in scattered epithelial cells of tumors of the AV nodal region, and these neuroendocrine cells may be detected immunohistochemically (see below).

**Immunohistochemical Findings.** The immunohistochemical profile of the lining cells indicates an epithelial origin, because they strongly express cytokeratin and epithelial membrane antigen. Immunohistochemical markers to distinguish mesothelial from endodermal tissues favor an endodermal derivation for these cells. Most cases are strongly positive for carcinoembryonic antigen as well as B72.3 antigen, epithelial membrane antigen, and CA19-9 (23,24,26,42,50). These four antigens are commonly found in embryonic or neoplastic glandular epithelium, and are generally absent in mesothelial cells.

As indicated above, there has been a report of endocrine cells interspersed among the lining cells of tumors of the AV node (25). These cells have exhibited reactivity with antibodies directed against calcitonin and serotonin. The presence of endocrine cells in these lesions further supports an endodermal, rather than mesothelial, origin.

**Differential Diagnosis.** The differential diagnosis of cystic tumor of the AV node is limited, because of its unique location. Bronchogenic cysts are larger, usually single cysts, that tend to occur on the epicardial surface, remote from the atrial septum, although this location has been reported (10). Teratomas may occur in a similar location, and are distinguished by the presence of neural and other ectodermal structures. An early example of an AV nodal tumor, originally misdiagnosed as metastatic clear cell carcinoma, was subsequently reported as a cystic tumor of the AV node (29). There has been a report of an AV nodal tumor that recurred as multiple nodules with the histologic features of a mature teratoma (51). Unlike metastatic carcinoma, cystic tumors of the AV node lack mitotic figures and cellular pleomorphism. Although the cysts of AV nodal tumors occasionally contain mucin, the myxoid background and extensive intracavitary growth of myxoma are absent. The tumors can be overlooked on gross inspection, necessitating histologic examination of the conduction system in all patients with sudden death, especially those with a history of arrhythmia or heart block.

**Treatment.** The treatment of congenital heart block consists of pacemaker implantation to prevent Stokes-Adams attacks (24), and antiarrhythmic drugs to suppress ventricular tachycardias. Nevertheless, treatment with pacemakers does not always prevent terminal arrhythmias in patients with AV nodal tumors. It has even been suggested that electrical pacing can precipitate arrhythmias in these patients (29). Surgical treatment is recommended for tumors that are diagnosed during life in patients with heart block (39,40,43–46). Postoperatively, patients require permanent pacing, however.

## CARDIAC GERM CELL TUMORS

A *germ cell tumor* is a neoplasm of germ cell origin that is classified by histologic type into *seminoma (dysgerminoma), embryonal carcinoma, yolk sac tumor (endodermal sinus tumor), choriocarcinoma, teratoma*, and *mixed type*. The majority of cardiac germ cell tumors are teratomas; the least common are nonseminomatous yolk sac tumors. Cardiac germ cell tumors, by definition, occur within the pericardium, mostly on the epicardial surface, with a minority present within heart muscle.

According to the germ cell theory, the cell of origin of extragonadal teratoma, including cardiac teratoma, is the primordial germ cell. Although normal germ cells migrate from the yolk sac to the gonad, it is hypothesized that they may lodge, early in embryogenesis, in midline structures such as the mediastinum and central nervous system. These ectopic germ cells give rise to germ cell tumors indistinguishable from those that occur in the testes and ovaries.

The mediastinum is the second most common location for germ cell tumors after the gonads. Only a small proportion occur within the pericardium, however; in one series, only 2 of 38 mediastinal germ cell tumors were intrapericardial (52). Rarely, intrapericardial germ cell tumors coexist with mediastinal germ cell tumors outside of the pericardium (53).

Intrapericardial cardiac germ cell tumors are rare. The first case of an intrapericardial teratoma was reported in 1890 (54). In 1983, 57 cases were collected in a review of the literature, 10 of which involved the myocardium (54). Since then, at least 50 have been reported in the literature (55–74).

### Cardiac Teratoma

**General and Clinical Features.** In the pediatric population, a female predilection of about 2 to 1 is seen, while in adults, mediastinal germ cell tumors are more frequent among men (5). In McAllister and Fenoglio's series of 14 patients with intrapericardial teratoma (6), the patient ages ranged from 1 day to 42 years. The majority of patients are infants, and over 75 percent of cardiac teratomas occur in children under age 15 years.

The symptoms depend on the location of the mass. Because most are on the epicardial or aortic surface, symptoms are typically related to effusions or recurrent tamponade (66); effusions may appear purulent due to rupture of cystic structures (75). In contrast, entirely intramyocardial teratomas may result in heart block or sudden death due to their typical location in the interventricular or interatrial septum (97). Fewer than 10 intramyocardial teratomas have been reported (6,40).

In newborns, the diagnosis of intrapericardial teratoma is typically made in utero (72,76,77), by sonographic detection of pericardial effusions and masses, often with ascites or hydrops (78). After delivery, there may be massive pericardial effusion, cardiac compression, and severe cardiorespiratory distress (79). Compression of the trachea results in life-threatening respiratory compromise (65,80,81). Infants may present after several months of life, with voluminous pericardial effusions (64) or cardiac tamponade; CT identifies a cardiac mass as the cause of the effusion, and a cystic appearance is typical of teratoma (62). Serum alpha fetoprotein (AFP) may be elevated, and does not necessarily indicate the presence of a yolk sac tumor (57). The presence of liver tissue within the teratoma has been reported as a source of the elevated AFP (60,82,83).

There were 46 cases of intrapericardial teratoma diagnosed prenatally from 1983 to 2005 (76). The clinicopathologic features of fetal and perinatal cardiac teratoma have been recently reviewed (84). Table 14-1 contains detailed clinical data on 56 selected cases reported to date. In utero diagnosis occurs as early as 19 weeks of gestation (73,85) with the identification of pericardial effusions and hydrops (60,68,83,86). There appears to be an increased incidence with twin gestation (68,87–90). If there is no treatment to prevent hydrops, intrauterine death may occur (61,63,91). After delivery, cardiac imaging, including 3D echocardiography, facilitates surgery by delineating the mass (56). The diagnosis of intrapericardial teratoma may be first diagnosed at autopsy in cases of hydrops (92), although with ultrasound screening most cases are identified prior to intrauterine death.

In adults, pericardial teratomas are often discovered as an incidental radiographic finding (fig. 14-11A), by the presence of cystic masses typically attached to the ascending aorta (59,70). Patients present as late as the sixth decade. Occasionally, there may be tamponade with circulatory compromise (93), or fever, tachycardia, and chest pain (94,95). Chest pain and friction rubs may be the result of hemorrhage within the tumor (96). Pericardial effusion is usually present and is serous, yellow, and clear. The cystic nature of the tumors and precise intrapericardial localization is readily visualized by cardiac CT and MRI (fig. 14-11B,C).

**Gross Findings.** Teratomas typically occur as a single, large, polycystic mass, in contact with the base of the heart and accompanied by pericardial effusion (figs. 14-12–14-14) (71,98). Intrapericardial teratoma can weigh up to 530 g (94) and measure from 2 to 15 cm (96,99). The large size may explain the high rate of hydrops and cardiac tamponade in fetuses and newborns (76). Teratomas are frequently attached to the ascending aorta, sometimes by a pedicle, with an arterial supply directly from the aorta (59,80). They can displace the heart and rotate it along

Table 14-1

CLINICAL FINDINGS OF 56 REPORTED INTRAPERICARDIAL TERATOMAS[a]

| | In Utero Diagnosis | Present After Birth (– 1 Year) | 1 to 15 Years | Adults (> 15 Years) |
|---|---|---|---|---|
| Number | 22 | 13 | 8 | 13 |
| % female | 33 | 30 | 86 | 31 |
| Multiple gestation | 2: twin | 1: triplet | 0 | 0 |
| Location in pericardialcavity | 12: attached to ascending aorta, by narrow or broad stalk, sometimes with feeder vessel 5: right-sided masses, with variable attachment, compressing RA, RV, IVC[b]; 5: intrapericardial, NOS | attached to ascending aorta, by narrow or broad stalk, sometimes with feeder vessel 3: attached to right atrial or ventricular epicardium; 5: intrapericardial, NOS | 2: attached to ascending aorta by distinct pedicle; 1: attached to adventitia of pulmonary trunk 3: intrapericardial, NOS | 7: intrapericardial, NOS 5: attached to ascending aorta; 2: with multiple pericardial attachments; 1: large tumor in the arch, extending on both sides of pericardium |
| Intramyocardial location | 0 | 0 | 2: interventricular septum | 1: interatrial |
| Diagnostic procedure | 17: complete resection 1: resection after intrauterine laser abalation 1: incomplete resection, with preservation of coronary artery 3: autopsy | 9: complete resection 4: autopsy | 4: complete resection 1: attempted surgical resection with postoperative death 3: autopsy | 13: surgical resection |
| Serum AFP elevation | 4 | 0 | 0 | 0 |
| Follow-up | 18: successful resection 2: died of massive tumor, one after attempted surgery 2: no data | 1: recurred with postexcision death (highgrade teratoma) 3: death due to massive tumor; 5: successful resection; 4: no data | 3: successful excision 3: died of massive tumor; 1: intraoperative death; 1: recurred with successful re-excision | 10: no recurrence after surgery; 3: no data |

[a]Data from references 51, 54, 57, 58, 60, 62, 63, 65, 66, 68–70, 72, 75, 76, 82, 83, 93–97, 99–102, and 148–167; some references cite several tumors.
[b]RA = right atrium; RV = right ventricle; IVC = inferior vena cava; NOS = not otherwise specified; AFP = alpha-fetoprotein.

its longitudinal axis. Intrapericardial teratomas are usually located on the right side of the heart, whereas intracardiac teratomas are almost always located in the ventricular septum (fig. 14-15).

The surface of teratomas is typically smooth and lobulated. On cut surface, the tumor is multicystic with intervening solid areas.

**Microscopic Findings.** Cardiac teratomas resemble teratomas of the testis or ovary: they contain cartilage, bone, respiratory epithelium, and squamous- and mucus-lined cysts (figs. 14-16, 14-17). Many reports of intrapericardial teratoma describe the presence of only one or two germ cell layers, and are therefore possibly cases of bronchogenic cyst, with which there is some overlap (5). There is also histologic overlap with cystic tumor of the AV node, as one tera-

toma has been reported to arise and recur after excision of an AV nodal tumor (51).

As in the testis, there is no prognostic difference between mature versus immature teratoma, since the lesions are essentially benign, in the absence of somatic malignancy. In contrast to teratomas of the testis, nonseminomatous elements rarely occur, and the lesions resemble ovarian desmoid tumors in adults. There has been some use of a grading system, as in immature teratoma of the ovary (82), but most are grade I lesions (53). There have been occasional reports of grade II tumors (83,100), one which recurred with areas of somatic malignancy (101). The lesion often exhibits more immature elements in infants (64,82), and more mature tissues in adults (70) and children. Occasionally there

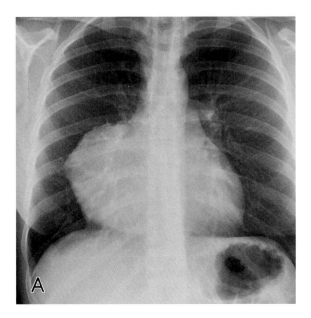

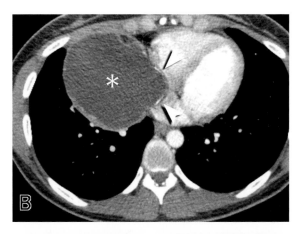

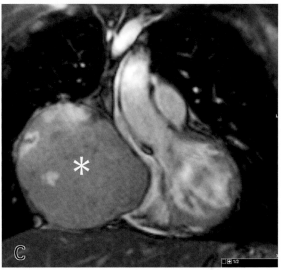

**Figure 14-11**

**PERICARDIAL TERATOMA**

A: Frontal chest radiograph demonstrates a large mass silhouetting the right cardiac border.

B: Contrast-enhanced computerized tomography (CT) shows a well-encapsulated, partly cystic 10-cm mass (asterisk) containing internal components of fluid, soft tissue, and focal fat with peripheral wall calcifications (arrowheads). The lesion exerts a mass effect upon the free right atrial wall.

C: Coronal steady-state free precession (SSFP) magnetic resonance image (MRI) shows a sharply circumscribed mass (asterisk) of heterogeneous internal signal compressing the right atrium.

is pancreatic tissue with endocrine function (102) or overgrown islets (51). The presence of hepatoid tissue is associated with elevated serum AFP levels (57,60,82,83).

In addition to squamous- or mucous-lined cysts, there may be cartilage, calcified neuroglial tissue, smooth muscle, mucous glands, intestinal tissue, pancreatic tissue, respiratory mucosa, ependyma, and bone. A myxoid stroma is often present.

The major entity in the differential diagnosis is bronchogenic cyst. The presence of elements of ectodermal origin, such as hair, teeth, or neurogenic elements, favors the diagnosis of teratoma.

McAllister and Fenoglio (6) reported four malignant pericardial germ cell tumors; the malignant foci were histologically composed of either embryonal carcinoma, squamous cell carcinoma arising in a teratoma, or choriocar-

cinoma. Three of these tumors metastasized to the lungs, and one was locally infiltrative. Since their report, no other primary malignant teratomas have been reported within the pericardium. Metastatic germ cell tumors may occur within the pericardium (101), occasionally as the presenting clinical event (102).

**Treatment and Prognosis.** Surgical excision is the only effective treatment for cardiac teratoma, and may necessitate full cardiopulmonary bypass (77). The timing of surgery for tumors diagnosed in utero has not been standardized, and evidence indicates that delayed surgery with stabilization is beneficial (103). Pericardiocentesis may be necessary prior to surgical excision (69). Since the blood supply is usually from the root of the ascending aorta, the surgeon must perform a careful dissection and ligation of

251

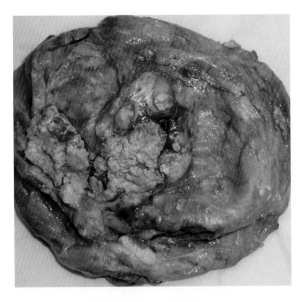

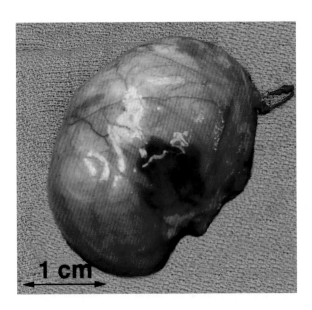

**Figure 14-12**

**PERICARDIAL TERATOMA**

Resected intrapericardial mature cystic teratoma contains proteinaceous fluid debris with elements of skin, sebaceous glands, hair follicles, smooth muscle, fat, cartilage, and respiratory epithelium.

**Figure 14-13**

**PERICARDIAL TERATOMA**

This intact cyst could represent a benign pericardial cyst or bronchogenic cyst. On sectioning, there was a single dominant cyst (not shown). The tumor was present entirely within the pericardium, and the surface is smooth and mesothelial-lined.

**Figure 14-14**

**TERATOMA AND YOLK SAC TUMOR**

Top: The tumor surface is smooth. Bottom: The cut surface demonstrates both solid and cystic areas. Histologically, the tumor was combined yolk sac tumor and teratoma.

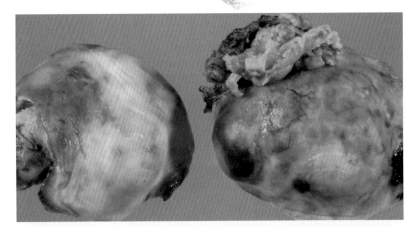

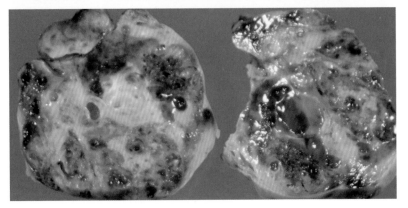

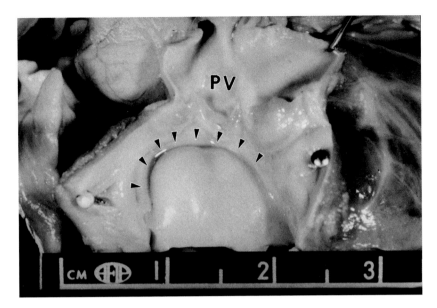

**Figure 14-15**

**INTRACARDIAC TERATOMA**

A bulging mass is in the right ventricular outflow tract (arrowheads). (PV = pulmonary valve.) The patient died minutes after birth at 37 weeks of gestation.

**Figure 14-16**

**BENIGN CYSTIC PERICARDIAL TERATOMA,**

A: A histologic section of the tumor illustrated in figure 14-12 shows a fluid-filled cyst with a simple lining, with fibrous and cellular areas.

B: A cellular area shows glandular structures composed predominantly of ducts resembling gastrointestinal differentiation.

C: Higher magnification of a cellular area shows pancreatic acini.

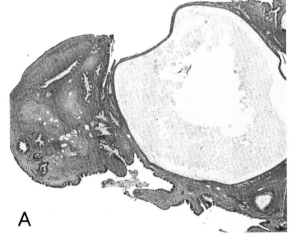

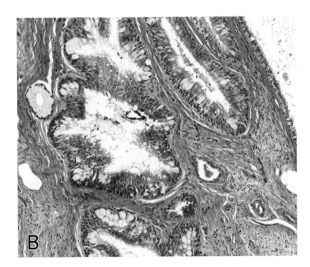

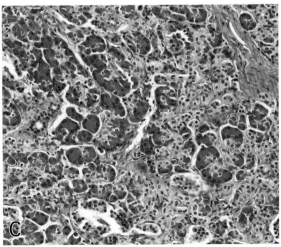

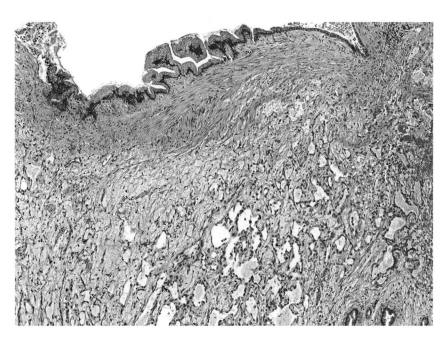

**Figure 14-17**

**TERATOMA AND YOLK SAC TUMOR**

A histologic section of the tumor illustrated in figure 14-14 shows a cyst at the top lined by mucus-secreting epithelium. The more cellular area below represents yolk sac tumor.

these vessels to prevent massive hemorrhage. Intracardiac teratomas, because of their location in the interventricular septum, are more difficult to remove than pericardial teratomas. However, even incomplete excision has been shown to be beneficial (96). Similar to the behavior of germ cell tumors in the gonads, pure teratomas are benign in the pediatric population. There is a report, however, of a histologically high-grade teratoma that recurred with areas of somatic adenocarcinoma, resulting in the child's death (101).

Teratomas occurring within the pericardium may be treated in utero by pregnancy termination (73,84), pericardioamniotic shunting (67, 74,84), prenatal pericardiocentesis (69,104, 105), and laser decompression (63). The treatment of twins with pericardial teratomas poses special problems in maintaining the viability of both fetuses (68,89). Surgical removal is accomplished soon after birth (60). Intrauterine fetal demise, however, often occurs before planned fetal surgery (91).

### Intrapericardial Yolk Sac Tumors

Similar to intrapericardial teratomas, most *yolk sac tumors* occur within the pericardial space. There are three reports of intramyocardial yolk sac tumor, occurring in the right atrium, right ventricle, and left ventricle, that resulted in heart block (106–108). Unlike with teratomas, the diagnosis is generally made after birth (Table

14-2). Patients are always infants or children, and usually girls; the serum AFP is invariably elevated (106–112). A report in a young man aged 17 shows that these tumors may occur late in adolescence (113). Yolk sac tumors associated with mature teratomas are rare and also occur in adolescents. The presenting symptoms are generally related to pericardial effusions (110). There was an association with myocarditis in a fatal case (112).

Histologically, yolk sac tumors of the pericardium resemble those of the testis (figs. 14-18, 14-19). There are a variety of histologic patterns, including reticular, microcystic, tubular, papillary, and solid (hepatoid).

Treatment includes chemotherapy, often including etoposide, ifosfamide, and carboplatin, which may result in long-term survival (115,116). There have been several deaths reported (109,113,114). One treated mediastinal yolk sac tumor that presented with metastatic disease to lungs, lymph nodes, and skeleton, recurred as a mature teratoma within the pericardial space (117).

### THYROID HETEROTOPIA

Ectopic thyroid tissue is usually found between the base of the tongue and the normal thyroid gland, and is a result of a migration failure along the pathway of the thyroglossal duct. *Heterotopic thyroid tissue* may be incidentally discovered in

**Table 14-2**

**NINE REPORTED INTRAPERICARDIAL YOLK SAC TUMORS[a]**

| | |
|---|---|
| Male:female | 2:7 |
| Age, range years (mean) | 1.2-17 (3.9) |
| Presenting manifestations | 3: Pericardial tamponade |
| | 1: Respiratory distress |
| | 1: Abdominal distension |
| | 1: Pulmonary metastasis |
| | 1: Fever, heart murmur |
| | 1: Heart block |
| | 1: Seizure, right ventricular outflow obstruction |
| Site | 5: Pericardial space, compressing right-sided structures, 1 with identified attachment site to ascending aorta |
| | 3: Intramyocardial, 2 right atrial extending into right ventricle across tricuspid valve, with extension into pericardium; 1 interventricular septum involving aortic valve |
| | 1: Mediastinal, involving pericardium, recurred as teratoma within the pericardium after chemotherapy |
| Surgical procedure | 6: Complete resection |
| | 2: Resection with patch repair |
| | 1: Incomplete resection |
| Chemotherapy | 4: Chemotherapy, NOS[b] |
| | 1: Vindesine, bleomycin, cisplatin |
| | 1: Etoposide, ifosfamide, cisplatin |
| | 1: Bleomycin, cisplatin, etoposide |
| | 2: Not given |
| Follow-up | 4: Response to chemotherapy, alive last follow-up |
| | 3: Deaths due to local recurrence |
| | 2: Metastatic disease, with response to chemotherapy |
| Metastatic sites | Lungs, lymph nodes, bone |

[a]Data from references 108–111 and 113–117.
[b]NOS = not otherwise specified.

the parietal pericardium, and more rarely, in the myocardium. The mechanism for thyroid tissue migration inferior to the thyroid gland is unclear, but may be a result of excessive migration in combination with traction of hyperplastic tissues. Ectopic thyroid in the heart may be the consequence of the intimate relationship between the cephalic portion of the developing foregut, which contains the thyroid anlage in the foramen cecum of the tongue, and the cardiac primordia.

Ectopic thyroid gland in the myocardium is called *struma cordis* (115) and is rare. Approximately 15 cases of intracardiac ectopic thyroid have been published in the English literature (115–123). The right ventricular outflow tract is generally involved (124), although left ventricular involvement with left ventricular outflow tract obstruction has also occurred (117,125). The condition is believed to occur early in embryogenesis, when part or all of the functioning thyroid tissue becomes lodged in the ventricular outflow region.

Although pulmonary stenosis with right ventricular hypertrophy may occur, most patients are asymptomatic (124). Radioiodide imaging is diagnostic (126).

Grossly, the lesions resemble thyroid gland (fig. 14-20). Histologically, the lesions are those of unremarkable thyroid tissue, although there may be inflammation and nodularity suggestive of an adenoma (129). There are follicular structures containing colloid; if there is any difficulty in diagnosis, immunohistochemical stains for thyroglobulin may be performed.

The differential diagnosis includes metastatic carcinoma of various origins (see chapter 18), and metastatic thyroid carcinoma. The latter distinction may be difficult purely on histologic grounds, and is made clinically by the exclusion of a dominant mass in the thyroid gland. The

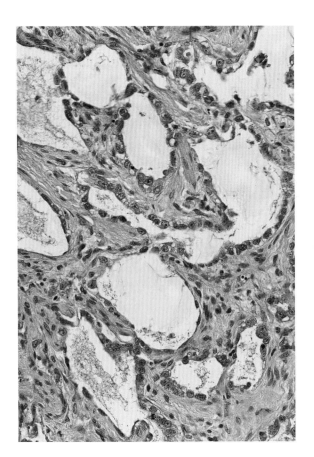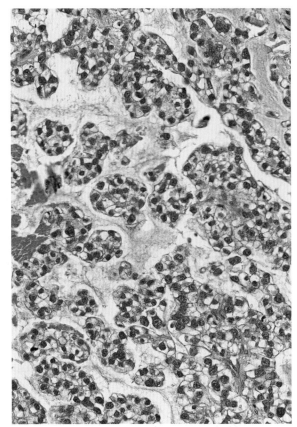

**Figure 14-18**

**INTRAPERICARDIAL YOLK SAC TUMOR**

Left: Higher magnification of the yolk sac element shown in figure 14-14 shows glandular structures lined by atypical cuboidal cells with inconspicuous nucleoli.

Right: In another area, the papillary configuration of the yolk sac tumor, with similar nuclear features, is seen.

**Figure 14-19**

**YOLK SAC TUMOR**

The characteristic pattern of glandular structures merging with more cord-like spindled cells in a myxoid matrix is seen in another area of the tumor in figure 14-18.

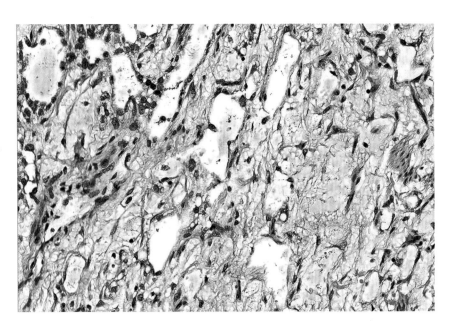

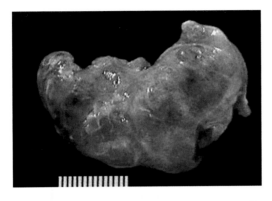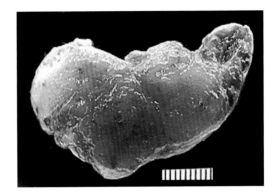

**Figure 14-20**

**MYOCARDIAL ECTOPIC THYROID TISSUE (STRUMA CORDIS)**

Left: This tumor was obstructing the right ventricular outflow tract in a young woman and was surgically excised. The tumor surface is shown.

Right: A cut section shows nodular lesions with abundant colloid-like material.

presence of papillary features indicates a metastasis from a thyroid primary. A case report of thyroid carcinoma of the heart, possibly arising in ectopic thyroid, has been reported (127).

Prior to the development of noninvasive technologies, cases of heterotopic cardiac thyroid tissue were discovered only at autopsy. Echocardiography has allowed the antemortem diagnosis of intracardiac thyroid tissue (128). In a middle-aged woman, a right ventricular mass, which may be obstructing the outflow tract causing a systolic murmur and right ventricular hypertrophy, should suggest the possibility of intracardiac thyroid tissue. Surgical removal is curative; however, care must be taken to initiate thyroid hormone replacement prior to surgery, because the ectopic tissue may be the only functioning thyroid tissue (116).

## PERICARDIAL THYMOMA AND ECTOPIC THYMIC TISSUE

*Thymomas* involving the heart are usually extensions of primary mediastinal tumors. Approximately 20 percent of thymomas are locally infiltrative (130), and pericardial involvement represents a late stage of tumor spread (see chapter 18) (131). Compression of the pulmonary trunk may occur (132), in addition to pericardial infiltration. Occasionally, mediastinal thymomas present as pericardial effusions (130), and the diagnosis is first made by examination of pericardial fluid or pericardial biopsy (130,133).

Rarely, thymomas are entirely intrapericardial; these tumors are believed to derive from pericardial thymic rests (6). Patients with pericardial thymomas are usually women (133,134). Intrapericardial thymic rests in children may be incidentally found during open heart surgery (138). Pericardial effusions lead to the symptoms of dyspnea or chest pain (135); other symptoms include dysphonia and myalgia (136).

Histologically, intrapericardial thymomas have not been extensively described (133,134), but are generally of epithelial type, with a background of lymphoid cells (figs. 14-21–14-23). An intrapericardial thymoma of World Health Organization (WHO) B2 type has been reported (136), as well as a thymoma arising in cardiac myxoma (139). Rare malignant thymomas occurring in the pericardium have been reported (137).

The treatment is generally surgical, although chemotherapy may result in tumor regression in inoperable cases (134).

## ECTOPIC LIVER

Most reported cases of *ectopic liver* occur within the abdominal cavity in the vicinity of the hepatic parenchyma, near or around the gallbladder. Fewer than 10 cases of intrathoracic ectopic liver have been reported (140–143). One case was in the right atrium, as an asymptomatic right atrial mass (fig. 14-24) (144).

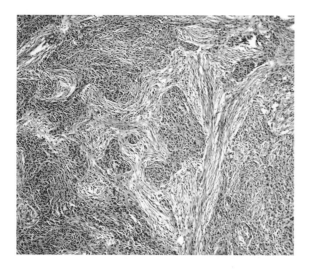

**Figure 14-21**

**INTRAPERICARDIAL THYMOMA**

There is an infiltrating epithelial tumor with a fibrous stroma.

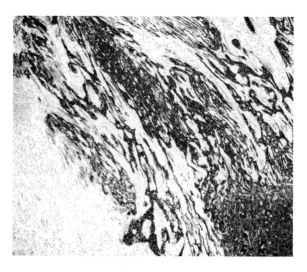

**Figure 14-22**

**INTRAPERICARDIAL THYMOMA**

An immunohistochemical stain (anticytokeratin 17) shows anastomosing cords of thymoma cells expressing low molecular weight cytokeratin.

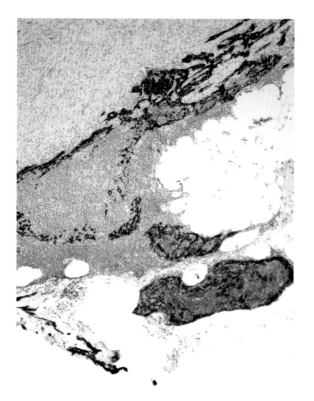

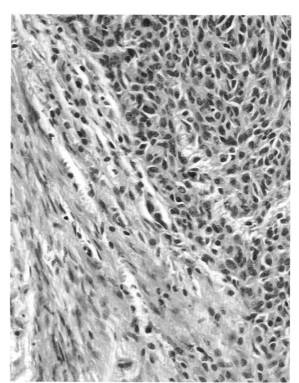

**Figure 14-23**

**RESIDUAL INTRAPERICARDIAL THYMUS, ADJACENT TO INTRAPERICARDIAL THYMOMA**

Left: An immunohistochemical stain (anticytokeratin 17) shows normal thymic tissue adjacent to the tumor illustrated in figure 14-22.

Right: At higher magnification, bland epithelial cells, without significant atypia or mitotic activity, are present, distinguishing this lesion from a thymic carcinoma.

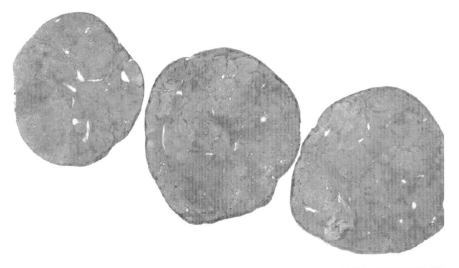

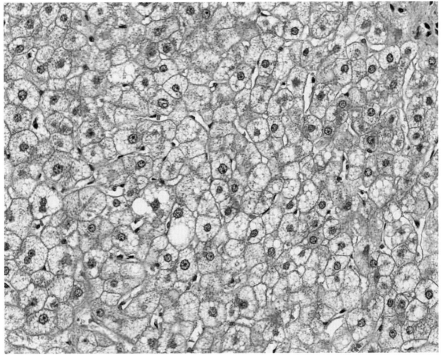

**Figure 14-24**

**ECTOPIC LIVER**

Top: A pedunculated nodule was excised from the right atrium in a woman without known liver disease. There was no communication with the liver.

Bottom: Higher magnification shows normal liver architecture, in contrast to metastatic hepatocellular carcinoma. There is mild fatty change.

**REFERENCES**

1. Di Lorenzo M, Collin PP, Vaillancourt R, Duranceau A. Bronchogenic cysts. J Pediatr Surg 1989; 24:988-991.
2. Wax JR, Pinette MG, Landes A, Blackstone J, Cartin A. Intrapericardial extralobar pulmonary sequestration-ultrasound and magnetic resonance prenatal diagnosis. Am J Obstet Gynecol 2002;187:1713-1714.
3. Hayashi AH, McLean DR, Peliowski A, Tierney AJ, Finer NN. A rare intrapericardial mass in a neonate. J Pediatr Surg 1992;27:1361-1363.
4. Gould SE. Cysts of the myocardium and heart valves, and diverticula. In: Gould SE, ed. Pathology of the heart, 2nd ed. Springfield, Ill: Thomas; 1960:883-886.

5. Deenadayalu RP, Tuuri D, Dewall RA, Johnson GF. Intrapericardial teratoma and bronchogenic cyst. Review of literature and report of successful surgery in infant with intrapericardial teratoma. J Thorac Cardiovasc Surg 1974;67:945-952.

6. McAllister HA, Fenoglio JJ Jr. Tumors of the cardiovascular system. Atlas of Tumor Pathology, 2nd Series, Fascicle 15. Washington DC: Armed Forces Institute of Pathology; 1978.

7. Machens G, Vahl CF, Hofmann R, Wolf D, Hagl S. Entodermal inclusion cyst of the tricuspid valve. Thorac Cardiovasc Surg 1991;39:296-298.

8. Shimizu M, Takeda R, Mifune J, Tanaka T. Echocardiographic features of intrapericardial bronchogenic cyst. Cardiology 1990;77:322-326.

9. Thomas R, Van Wesep R. Intracardiac epithelial cyst in association with an atrioventricular canal defect. Am J Cardiovasc Pathol 1990;3:325-328.

10. Martinez-Mateo V, Arias MA, Juarez-Tosina R, Rodriguez-Padial L. Permanent third-degree atrioventricular block as clinical presentation of an intracardiac bronchogenic cyst. Europace 2008;10:638-640.

11. Goksel OS, Sayin OA, Cinar T, Toker A, Tireli E, Dayioglu E. Bronchogenic cyst invading right atrium in a 5-year-old. Thorac Cardiovasc Surg 2008;56:435-436.

12. Chen CC. Bronchogenic cyst in the interatrial septum with a single persistent left superior vena cava. J Chin Med Assoc 2006;69:89-91.

13. Somwaru LL, Midgley FM, Di Russo GB. Intrapericardial bronchogenic cyst overriding the pulmonary artery. Pediatr Cardiol 2005;26:713-714.

14. Prates PR, Lovato L, Homsi-Neto A, et al. Right ventricular bronchogenic cyst. Tex Heart Inst J 2003;30:71-73.

15. Kobza R, Oechslin E, Jenni R. An intrapericardial bronchogenic cyst. Interact Cardiovasc Thorac Surg 2003;2:279-280.

16. Lugo-Olivieri CH, Schwartzman GJ, Beall DP, Lima JA, Fishman EK. Intrapericardial bronchogenic cyst: assessment with magnetic resonance imaging and transesophageal echocardiography. Clin Imaging 1999;23:81-84.

17. Padovani B, Hofman P, Chanalet S, Taillan B, Jourdan J, Serres JJ. Intrapericardial bronchogenic cyst: CT and MR demonstration. Eur J Radiol 1992;15:4-6.

18. Ferrari E, Taillan B, Jourdan J, Isetta C, Dujardin P, Morand P. Intrapericardial bronchogenic cyst: an unusual cause of CA 19-9 increase. Eur J Med 1992;1:122.

19. Scheimberg I, Rose S, Malone M. Intracardiac epithelial cyst associated with esophageal atresia. Pediatr Pathol Lab Med 1997;17:945-949.

20. Armstrong H, Monckeberg JG. Herzblock bedingt durch primaren herztumor, bei einem furf Jährigen Kinde. Deutsch Arch Klin Med 1911;102:144-166.

21. Veinot JP. Cardiac tumors of adipocytes and cystic tumor of the atrioventricular node. Semin Diagn Pathol 2008;25:29-38.

22. Cameselle-Teijeiro J, Abdulkader I, Soares P, Alfonsin-Barreiro N, Moldes-Boullosa J, Sobrinho-Simoes M. Cystic tumor of the atrioventricular node of the heart appears to be the heart equivalent of the solid cell nests (ultimobranchial rests) of the thyroid. Am J Clin Pathol 2005;123:369-375.

23. Burke AP, Anderson PG, Virmani R, James TN, Herrera GA, Ceballos R. Tumor of the atrioventricular nodal region. A clinical and immunohistochemical study. Arch Pathol Lab Med 1990; 114:1057-1062.

24. Duray PH, Mark EJ, Barwick KW, Madri JA, Strom RL. Congenital polycystic tumor of the atrioventricular node. Autopsy study with immunohistochemical findings suggesting endodermal derivation. Arch Pathol Lab Med 1985;109:30-34.

25. Fine G, Raju U. Congenital polycystic tumor of the atrioventricular node (endodermal heterotopia, mesothelioma): a histogenetic appraisal with evidence for its endodermal origin. Hum Pathol 1987;18:791-795.

26. Monma N, Satodate R, Tashiro A, Segawa I. Origin of so-called mesothelioma of the atrioventricular node. An immunohistochemical study. Arch Pathol Lab Med 1991;115:1026-1029.

27. Linder J, Shelburne JD, Sorge JP, Whalen RE, Hackel DB. Congenital endodermal heterotopia of the atrioventricular node: evidence for the endodermal origin of so-called mesotheliomas of the atrioventricular node. Hum Pathol 1984; 15:1093-1098.

28. Fenoglio J, Jacobs D, McAllister H. Ultrastructure of the mesothelioma of the atrioventricular node. Cancer 1977;40:721-727.

29. James TN, Galakhov I. De subitaneis mortibus. XXVI. Fatal electrical instabiltiy of the heart associated with benign congenital polycystic tumor of the atrioventricular node. Circulation 1977;56:667-678.

30. Travers H. Congenital polycystic tumor of the atrioventricular node. Arch Pathol Lab Med 1985; 109:704-706.

31. Sachs LJ, Angrist A. Congenital cyst of the myocardium. Am J Pathol 1945;21:187-193.

32. Prichard RW. Tumors of the heart; review of the subject and report of 150 cases. AMA Arch Pathol 1951;51:98-128.

33. Sharma G, Linden MD, Schultz DS, Inamdar KV. Cystic tumor of the atrioventricular node: An unexpected finding in an explanted heart. Cardiovasc Pathol 2010;19:e75-78.

34. Law KB, Feng T, Nair V, Cusimano RJ, Butany J. Cystic tumor of the atrioventricular node: Rare antemortem diagnosis. Cardiovasc Pathol 2012; 21:120-127.

35. Ford SE. Congenital cystic tumors of the atrioventricular node: Successful demonstration by an abbreviated dissection of the conduction system. Cardiovasc Pathol 1999;8:233-237.

36. Pan Y, Chen JL, Li ZJ, et al. Cystic tumour of the atrioventricular node: A case report and review of the literature. Chin Med J (Engl) 2012;125:4514-4516.

37. Oost E, Vermeulen T. Cystic tumour of the atrioventricular node: a case report. Pathology 2012; 44:487-489.

38. Patel J, Sheppard MN. Cystic tumour of the atrioventricular node: three cases of sudden death. Int J Legal Med 2011;125:139-142.

39. Kaminishi Y, Watanabe Y, Nakata H, Shimokama T, Jikuya T. Cystic tumor of the atrioventricular nodal region. Jpn J Thorac Cardiovasc Surg 2002; 50:37-39.

40. Burke AP, Virmani R. Tumors of the heart and great vessels. AFIP Atlas of Tumor Pathology, 3rd Series, Fascicle 16. Washington, DC: American Registry of Patholgy; 1996.

41. Subramanian R, Flygenring B. Mesothelioma of the atrioventricular node and congenital complete heart block. Clin Cardiol 1989;12:469-472.

42. Lewman LV, Demany MA, Zimmerman HA. Congenital tumor of atrioventricular node with complete heart block and sudden death. Mesothelioma or lymphangio-endothelioma of atrioventricular node. Am J Cardiol 1972;29:554-557.

43. Balasundaram S, Halees SA, Duran C. Mesothelioma of the atrioventricular node: first successful follow-up after excision. Eur Heart J 1992;13:718-719.

44. Saito S, Kobayashi J, Tagusari O, et al. Successful excision of a cystic tumor of the atrioventricular nodal region. Circ J 2005;69:1293-1294.

45. Tran TT, Starnes V, Wang X, Getzen J, Ross BD. Cardiovascular magnetics resonance diagnosis of cystic tumor of the atrioventricular node. J Cardiovasc Magn Reson 2009;11:13.

46. Guo J, Zuo S, Lin C, Ji Y. Surgical treatment of a giant cystic tumor of the atrioventricular nodal region. Interact Cardiovasc Thorac Surg 2009;8: 592-593.

47. Leighton J, Hurst JW, Crawford JD. Squamous epithelial cysts in the heart of an infant, with coincident cystic changes in the ovaries and breasts. AMA Arch Pathol 1950;50:632-643.

48. de Chatel A. Kongenitale epidermoid cyste des herzens. Frank Z Pathol 1932-33;44:426-429.

49. Morris AW, Johnson IM. Epithelial inclusion cysts of the heart. A case report and review of the literature. Arch Pathol 1964;77:36-40.

50. Arai T, Kurashima C, Wada S, Chida K, Ohkawa S. Histological evidence for cell proliferation activity in cystic tumor (endodermal heterotopia) of the atrioventricular node. Pathol Int 1998;48:917-923.

51. Ali SZ, Susin M, Kahn E, Hajdu SI. Intracardiac teratoma in a child simulating an atrioventricular nodal tumor. Pediatr Pathol 1994;14:913-917.

52. Billmire D, Vinocur C, Rescorla F, et al. Malignant mediastinal germ cell tumors: An intergroup study. J Pediatr Surg 2001;36:18-24.

53. Tollens T, Casselman F, Devlieger H, et al. Fetal cardiac tamponade due to an intrapericardial teratoma. Ann Thorac Surg 1998;66:559-560.

54. Cox JN, Friedli B, Mechmeche R, Ismail MB, Oberhaensli I, Faidutti B. Teratoma of the heart. A case report and review of the literature. Virchows Arch A Pathol Anat Histopathol 1983;402:163-174.

55. Ribeiro PJ, Amaral FT, Evora PR, Vicente WV. [Intrapericardial teratoma. A case report and a literature review.] Arq Bras Cardiol 1996;66:361-364. [Portuguese]

56. Herberg U, Berg C, Knopfle G, et al. Intrapericardial teratoma in the newborn—3D-echocardiography and course of disease. Ultraschall Med 2006; 27:577-581.

57. Meuris B, Gewillig M, Meyns B. Extreme levels of alpha-fetoprotein in a newborn with a benign intrapericardial teratoma. Cardiol Young 2006; 16:76-77.

58. Singh J, Sandeep Singh R. Some more about intrapericardial teratomas in perinatal period. J Pediatr Surg 2006;41:877-878; author reply 878.

59. Chataigner O, Mussot S, Fadel E, Dartevelle PG. Two cases of intra-pericardial tumors arising from the ascending aorta in adults. Eur J Cardiothorac Surg 2007;32:174-175.

60. Gobbi D, Rubino M, Chiandetti L, Zanon GF, Cecchetto G. Neonatal intrapericardial teratoma: a challenge for the pediatric surgeon. J Pediatr Surg 2007;42:E3-6.

61. Pachy F, Raiffort C, Mechler C, Zilberman S, Mandelbrot L. Intrapericardial teratoma with hydrops leading to in utero demise. Prenat Diagn 2007;27:970-972.

62. Taori K, Jawale R, Sanyal R, Sheorain VS, Chandanshive S. Intrapericardial teratoma diagnosed on CT. J Thorac Imaging 2007;22:185-187.

63. Liddle AD, Anderson DR, Mishra PK. Intrapericardial teratoma presenting in fetal life: intrauterine diagnosis and neonatal management. Congenit Heart Dis 2008;3:449-451.

64. Mirzaaghayan MR, Shabanian R. A huge intrapericardial teratoma in an infant. Pediatr Cardiol 2008;29:1122-1123.

65. Kumar IH, Shrote V, Kumar H. Anaesthetic management of a child presenting with intrapericardial teratoma compressing the airway and the heart. Ann Card Anaesth 2009;12:63-66.

66. Singh J, Rana SS, Kaur A, Srivastava V, Singh H, Sharma R. Intrapericardial teratoma presenting as recurrent pericardial tamponade: Report of a case. Surg Today 2009;39:700-704.

67. Steffensen TS, Quintero RA, Kontopoulos EV, Gilbert-Barness E. Massive pericardial effusion treated with in utero pericardioamniotic shunt in a fetus with intrapericardial teratoma. Fetal Pediatr Pathol 2009;28:216-231.

68. Fagiana AM, Barnett S, Reddy VS, Milhoan KA. Management of a fetal intrapericardial teratoma: a case report and review of the literature. Congenit Heart Dis 2010;5:51-55.

69. Goldberg SP, Boston US, Turpin DA, et al. Surgical management of intrapericardial teratoma in the fetus. J Pediatr 2010;156:848-849, 849 e841.

70. Gonzalez M, Krueger T, Schaefer SC, Ris HB, Perentes JY. Asymptomatic intrapericardial mature teratoma. Ann Thorac Surg 2010;89:e46-47.

71. Kalavrouziotis G, Konstantopoulou G, Stefanaki K, Eleftherakis N, Paphitis C, Azariades P. Intrapericardial teratoma in a premature neonate: Pre-delivery diagnosis and successful surgical removal. Hellenic J Cardiol 2010;51:278-280.

72. Shrestha GK, Mora B, Agarwala B. Intrapericardial teratoma in a newborn. Pediatr Cardiol 2010; 31:157-158.

73. Soor GS, Chakrabarti MO, Luk A, Abraham JR, Phillips K, Butany J. Prenatal intrapericardial teratomas: Diagnosis and management. Cardiovasc Pathol 2010;19:e1-4.

74. Tomek V, Vlk R, Tlaskal T, Skovranek J. Successful pericardio-amniotic shunting for fetal intrapericardial teratoma. Pediatr Cardiol 2010;31:1236-1238.

75. Dewan RK, Gupta K, Meena BK, Aggarwal M. Intrapericardial benign teratoma with unusual presentation. Indian J Chest Dis Allied Sci 1998; 40:287-290.

76. MacKenzie S, Loken S, Kalia N, et al. Intrapericardial teratoma in the perinatal period. Case report and review of the literature. J Pediatr Surg 2005;40:e13-18.

77. Pratt JW, Cohen DM, Mutabagani KH, Davis JT, Wheller JJ. Neonatal intrapericardial teratomas: clinical and surgical considerations. Cardiol Young 2000;10:27-31.

78. Milovanovic V, Lukac M, Krstic Z. Intrapericardial immature teratoma in a newborn: a case report. Cardiol Young 2013(Feb 6):1-3.

79. Ragupathy R, Nemeth L, Kumaran V, Rajamani G, Krishnamoothy P. Successful surgical management of a prenatally diagnosed intrapericardial teratoma. Pediatr Surg Int 2003;19:737-739.

80. Vaideeswar P, Deshpande JR, Sivaraman A. Intrapericardial teratoma—a report of two cases. Indian J Pathol Microbiol 2000;43:351-352.

81. Sievers RF, Tang AT, Haw MP. Complete surgical resection of intrapericardial teratoma in a neonate with compression of the central airways. Cardiol Young 2000;10:64-66.

82. Roy N, Blurton DJ, Azakie A, Karl TR. Immature intrapericardial teratoma in a newborn with elevated alpha-fetoprotein. Ann Thorac Surg 2004;78:e6-8.

83. Isaacs H Jr. Fetal and neonatal cardiac tumors. Pediatr Cardiol 2004;25:252-273.

84. Bader R, Hornberger LK, Nijmeh LJ, et al. Fetal pericardial teratoma: presentation of two cases and review of literature. Am J Perinatol 2006;23: 53-58.

85. Czernik C, Stiller B, Hubler M, Hagen A, Henrich W. Hydrops fetalis caused by a large intrapericardial teratoma. Ultrasound Obstet Gynecol 2006; 28:973-976.

86. Iacona GM, Barber MA, Medina M, Abella R. Intrapericardial teratoma in a low birth weight preterm infant: A successful multidisciplinary approach. Interact Cardiovasc Thorac Surg 2011; 12:287-289.

87. Levin SE, Harrisberg JR, Govendrageloo K. Intrapericardial teratoma in a twin with severe failure to thrive. Cardiovasc J S Afr 2002;13:237-240.

88. Valioulis I, Aubert D, Lassauge F, Slimane MA. Intrapericardial teratoma diagnosed prenatally in a twin fetus. Pediatr Surg Int 1999;15:284-286.

89. Sklansky M, Greenberg M, Lucas V, Gruslin-Giroux A. Intrapericardial teratoma in a twin fetus: diagnosis and management. Obstet Gynecol 1997;89:807-809.

90. Paw PT, Jamieson SW. Surgical management of intrapericardial teratoma diagnosed in utero. Ann Thorac Surg 1997;64:552-554.

91. Riskin-Mashiah S, Moise KJ Jr, Wilkins I, Ayres NA, Fraser CD Jr. In utero diagnosis of intrapericardial teratoma: A case for in utero open fetal surgery. Prenat Diagn 1998;18:1328-1330.

92. Perez-Aytes A, Sanchis N, Barbal A, et al. Non-immunological hydrops fetalis and intrapericardial teratoma: Case report and review. Prenat Diagn 1995;15:859-863.

93. Brown KM, Banerjee S, Kane PA, Marrinan MT. Intrapericardial teratoma presenting with circulatory compromise. Ann Thorac Surg 2006;81: 374.

94. Bitar FF, el-Zein C, Tawil A, Gharzuddine W, Obeid M. Intrapericardial teratoma in an adult: a rare presentation. Med Pediatr Oncol 1998;30: 249-251.

95. Cohen R, Mirrer B, Loarte P, Navarro V. Intrapericardial mature cystic teratoma in an adult: case presentation. Clin Cardiol 2013;36:6-9.

96. Garcia Cors M, Mulet J, Caralps J, Oller G. Fast-growing pericardial mass as first manifestation of intrapericardial teratoma in a young man. Am J Med 1990;89:818-820.

97. Swalwell CI. Benign intracardiac teratoma. A case of sudden death. Arch Pathol Lab Med 1993;117:739-742.

98. Marianeschi SM, Seddio F, Abella RF, Colagrande L, Iorio FS, Marcelletti CF. Intrapericardial teratoma in a newborn: a case report. J Card Surg 1999;14:169-171.

99. Rasmussen SL, Hwang WS, Harder J, Nicholson S, Davies D, Nimrod CA. Intrapericardial teratoma. Ultrasonic and pathological features. J Ultrasound Med 1987;6:159-162.

100. Ertugrul T, Dindar A, Elmaci TT, Onursal E, Kilicaslan I. An intrapericardial teratoma with endocrine function. J Cardiovasc Surg (Torino) 2001;42:781-783.

101. Pickuth D, Eeles R, Mason M, Pumphrey C, Goldstraw P, Horwich A. Intracardiac metastases from germ cell tumours—an unusual but important site of metastasis. Br J Radiol 1992; 65:672-673.

102. Chandrashekar G. Choriocarcinoma presenting as intracardiac (intracavitary) tumour. Int J Cardiol 1995;50:197.

103. Mitanchez D, Grebille AG, Parat S, et al. Delayed surgery in pericardial teratoma with neonatal hydrops. Eur J Pediatr Surg 2005;15:431-433.

104. Laquay N, Ghazouani S, Vaccaroni L, Vouhe P. Intrapericardial teratoma in newborn babies. Eur J Cardiothorac Surg 2003;23:642-644.

105. Fujimori K, Honda S, Akutsu H, et al. Prenatal diagnosis of intrapericardial teratoma: a case report. J Obstet Gynaecol Res 1999;25:133-136.

106. Morin MJ, Hopkins RA, Ferguson WS, Ziegler JW. Intracardiac yolk sac tumor and dysrhythmia as an etiology of pediatric syncope. Pediatrics 2004;113:e374-376.

107. Chintala K, Bloom DA, Walters HL 3rd, Pettersen MD. Images in cardiology: pericardial yolk sac tumor presenting as cardiac tamponade in a 21-month-old child. Clin Cardiol 2004; 27:411.

108. Graf M, Blaeker H, Schnabel P, Serpi M, Ulmer HE, Otto HF. Intracardiac yolk sac tumor in an infant girl. Pathol Res Pract 1999;195:193-197.

109. Parvathy U, Balakrishnan KR, Ranjit MS, Kuruvilla S, Rao KR. Primary intracardiac yolk sac tumor. Pediatr Cardiol 1998;19:495-497.

110. Skillington PD, Brawn WJ, Edis BD, et al. Surgical excision of primary cardiac tumours in infancy. Aust N Z J Surg 1987;57:599-604.

111. Nelson E, Stenzel P. Intrapericardial yolk sac tumor in an infant girl. Cancer 1987;60:1567-1569.

112. Sicari MC, Fyfe B, Parness I, Rossi A, Unger P. Intrapericardial yolk sac tumor associated with acute myocarditis. Arch Pathol Lab Med 1999;123:241-243.

113. Liang TC, Lu MY, Chen SJ, Lu FL, Lin KH. Cardiac tamponade caused by intrapericardial yolk sac tumor in a boy. J Formos Med Assoc 2002; 101:355-358.

114. Bath LE, Walayat M, Mankad P, Godman MJ, Wallace WH. Stage IV malignant intrapericardial germ cell tumor: a case report. Pediatr Hematol Oncol 1997;14:451-455.

115. Pollice L, Caruso G. Struma cordis. Ectopic thyroid goiter in the right ventricle. Arch Pathol Lab Med 1986;110:452-453.

116. Ansani L, Percoco G, Zanardi F, Peranzoni P, Gamba G, Antonioli G. Intracardiac thyroid heterotopia. Am Heart J 1993;125:1797-1801.

117. Kon ND, Headley RN, Cordell AR. Successful operative management of struma cordis obstructing the left ventricular outflow tract. Ann Thorac Surg 1988;46:244-245.

118. Polvani GL, Antona C, Porqueddu M, et al. Intracardiac ectopic thyroid: Conservative surgical treatment. Ann Thorac Surg 1993;55:1249-1251.

119. Richmond I, Whittaker JS, Deiraniya AK, Hassan R. Intracardiac ectopic thyroid: a case report and review of published cases. Thorax 1990;45:293-294.

120. Scrofani R, Rossi RS, Antona C. Ectopic thyroid in the right ventricle. J Cardiovasc Med (Hagerstown) 2011;12:689-691.

121. Irvine RW, Ramphal PS, Hall C, Char G. Struma cordis in a Jamaican woman. Interact Cardiovasc Thorac Surg 2005;4:83-84.

122. Carson W. Intracardiac thyroid. Am Heart J 1988;116:1650-1651.

123. Greco-Lucchina P, Ottino GM, Avonto L, Carini G, Pozzi R, Emanuelli G. Ectopic thyroid remnants within the myocardium: an unusual case of right ventricular mass. Am Heart J 1988;115:195-198.

124. Chosia M, Waligorski S, Listewnik MH, Wiechowski S. Ectopic thyroid tissue as a tumour of the heart—case report and review of the literature. Pol J Pathol 2002;53:173-175.

125. Baykut D, Fiegen U, Krian A, Thiel A. Ectopic thyroid tissue in the left ventricular outflow tract. Ann Thorac Surg 2000;69:620-621.

126. Rieser GD, Ober KP, Cowan RJ, Cordell AR. Radioiodide imaging of struma cordis. Clin Nucl Med 1988;13:421-422.

127. Hirnle T, Szymczak J, Ziolkowski P, Lenartowska L. Ectopic thyroid malignancy in the right ventricle of the heart. Eur J Cardiothorac Surg 1997;12:147-149.

128. Comajuan SM, Ayerbe JL, Ferrer BR, et al. An intracardiac ectopic thyroid mass. Eur J Echocardiogr 2009;10:704-706.

129. Wu Z, Zhou Q, Wang DJ. An intracardiac ectopic thyroid adenoma. Interact Cardiovasc Thorac Surg 2009;8:587-588.

130. Venegas RJ, Sun NC. Cardiac tamponade as a presentation of malignant thymoma. Acta Cytol 1988;32:257-261.

131. Masaoka A, Monden Y, Nakahara K, Tanioka T. Follow up study of thymomas with special reference to their clinical stages. Cancer 1981;48:2485-2492.

132. Nishimura T, Kondo M, Miyazaki S, Mochizuki T, Umadome H, Shimono Y. Two dimensional echocardiographic findings of cardiovascular involvement by invasive thymoma. Chest 1982;81:752-754.

133. Eglen DE. Pericardial based thymoma: diagnosis by fine needle aspiration. Indiana Med 1986; 79:526-528.

134. Ileceto S, Quagliara D, Calabrese P, Rizzon P. Visualization of pericardial thymoma and evaluation of chemotherapy by two dimensional echocardiography. Am Heart J 1984;107:605-606.

135. Sumner TE, Crowe JE, Klein A, McKone RC, Weaver RL. Intrapericardial teratoma in infancy. Pediatr Radiol 1980;10:51-53.

136. Azoulay S, Adem C, Gatineau M, et al. Pericardial ectopic thymoma. Virchows Arch 2005; 446:185-188.

137. Calderon AM, Merchan JA, Rozo JC, et al. Intrapericardial primary thymic carcinoma in a 73-year-old man. Tex Heart Inst J 2008;35:458-461.

138. Karolczak MA, Bec L, Madry W. Intrapericardial ectopic thymic tissue. Interact Cardiovasc Thorac Surg 2004;3:300-301.

139. Miller DV, Tazelaar HD, Handy JR, Young DA, Hernandez JC. Thymoma arising within cardiac myxoma. Am J Surg Pathol 2005;29:1208-1213.

140. Chen F, Heller DS, Bethel C, Faye-Petersen O. Intrathoracic ectopic lobe of liver presenting as pulmonary sequestration. Fetal Pediatr Pathol 2005;24:155-159.

141. Leone N, De Paolis P, Carrera M, et al. Ectopic liver and hepatocarcinogenesis: Report of three cases with four years' follow-up. Eur J Gastroenterol Hepatol 2004;16:731-735.

142. Luoma R, Raboei E. Supradiaphragmatic accessory liver: a rare cause of respiratory distress in a neonate. J Pediatr Surg 2003;38:1413-1414.

143. Yoshino I, Yamaguchi M, Kameyama T, et al. Extension of liver tissue into the thorax following a right extrapleural pneumonectomy for malignant pleural mesothelioma. Ann Thorac Cardiovasc Surg 2006;12:355-357.

144. Xu L, Jeudy J, Burke AP. Ectopic hepatic tissue presenting as right atrial mass. Hum Pathol 2012;43:958-960.

# 15 CARDIAC ANGIOSARCOMA AND EPITHELIOID HEMANGIOENDOTHELIOMA

## CARDIAC ANGIOSARCOMA

**Definition.** *Angiosarcoma* is an aggressive, malignant mesenchymal neoplasm demonstrating endothelial differentiation. Endothelial differentiation manifests morphologically by vascular channels lined by atypical endothelial cells and immunohistochemically by the expression of endothelial antigens. Angiosarcomas may have epithelioid features, with abundant cytoplasm and expression of epithelial antigens; in this case the term *epithelioid angiosarcoma* may be used. In contrast, *epithelioid hemangioendothelioma* is a distinctive low-grade sarcoma with endothelial differentiation that also occurs in the heart, although at a far lower frequency. It is defined by its histologic features, as well as immunohistochemical confirmation of coexpression of endothelial and epithelial markers.

**General Features.** Angiosarcomas are the most common primary cardiac malignancies with specific differentiation, accounting for approximately 40 percent of cardiac sarcomas (1–9). There have been approximately 200 cases reported (10,11). They account for a small fraction of primary cardiac tumors, estimated at 0.021 percent in a compilation of autopsy studies (12,13). In series of biopsy-proven cardiac tumors, they represent up to 10 percent, but are fewer in series of resected tumors because they are often infiltrative and not amenable to surgical excision (Table 15-1).

Epithelioid hemangioendothelioma is rarer in the heart. In several recent series of cardiac tumors that included angiosarcoma, 2 of 77 malignant vascular tumors were epithelioid hemangioendotheliomas (Table 15-1).

**Clinical Features.** There have been several reviews of cardiac angiosarcoma outlining the clinical features (14–21). Cardiac angiosarcomas occur over a wide age range (childhood to over 80 years), with a peak incidence in the fourth to fifth decade (Table 15-1) (2,12,15,22). Cardiac angiosarcoma occurs with equal frequency in men and women in most series, although there may be a male predilection (2,18). Familial angiosarcoma has been reported (23–26). It most often arises in the right atrium near the atrioventricular groove (80 percent), but is also reported in the other three chambers as well as in the pericardium (21,27–30). The pericardium is often involved as extension from the atrium, and rarely is the dominant site of tumor.

The clinical features are related to the location, size, and extent of regional involvement, as well as to the presence or absence of metastases (21). The most common presenting symptoms are chest pain (31–33), dyspnea related to pericardial and pleural effusions (34–39), recurrent pericarditis (36,40), and supraventricular arrhythmias (21). Presenting clinical symptoms may also be related to obstruction of right ventricular blood flow, superior vena cava syndrome (41), recurrent pulmonary embolism (42), and right heart failure (43,44), and include seizures (45), hemothorax (46), and hemoptysis (47,48). When the tumor has a significant intracavitary component, it may obstruct a valve orifice, simulating a stenotic lesion, usually on the right side, and precipitating syncope related to the patient's body position (17). In about 1 of 10 patients there is a long history related to constitutional symptoms and pericarditis, resulting in delayed diagnosis, ineffective treatment, and advanced stage at diagnosis (40,49,50). Pericardial involvement can lead to a diagnosis of mycobacterial infection in countries endemic for tuberculosis (51). In some cases, the diagnosis is made first at autopsy after a period of clinical investigation for pericardial disease (34,52). The first clinical manifestations may relate to metastatic disease, where the initial tissue diagnosis is made (8).

An unusual presentation is cardiac rupture, either of the atrium or aortic root (53–57). We have seen one case that ruptured during mediastinoscopic biopsy, causing fatal

**Table 15-1**

**CARDIAC SARCOMAS WITH ENDOTHELIAL DIFFERENTIATION**[a]

| | |
|---|---|
| % of all tumors, surgical series of heart tumors | 0-10%, mean 2.6%[b] |
| % of sarcomas, surgical series of heart tumors | 0-100%, mean 31%[b] |
| Number of epithelioid hemangioendotheliomas (EHEs) | 2[b] |
| Age, years at presentation, range[c] | 39, 14-80 |
| % men | 66% |
| Size, mean, range | 6.6 cm, 1.5-11 cm |
| Site[d] | |
|    Right atrium | 81% |
|    Pericardium | 10% |
|    Left atrium | 6% |
|    Right ventricle | 4% |
|    Left ventricle | 4% |
| Surgical procedure | |
|    Resection, incomplete or positive margins (R1) | 46% |
|    Complete resection (R0) | 16% |
|    Debulking, no attempt at complete resection (R2) | 11% |
|    Resection with atrial reconstruction | 8% |
|    Biopsy only | 18% |
| Metastasis at time of surgery or within 6 months | 53% |
|    Lung | 51% |
|    Bone | 5% |
|    Brain | 7% |
|    Liver | 2% |
| Median survival (data for 75 patients) | 5–17 months |
| Died of sarcoma during follow-up period | 95%, range 1 day–75 months |
| Alive without evidence of disease at follow-up | 0 |
| Alive with evidence of disease | n=4: 20, 42, 60, 64 months |
| Chemotherapy treatment given, % patients | Approximately 75% |
|    Drugs | Vincristine |
| | Ifosfamide |
| | Actinomycin drugs |
| | Cyclophosphamide |
| | Cisplatin |
| | Anthracyclines |
| | Imatinib (Glivec)[e] |
| | Herceptin[e] |

[a]79 resected or biopsied tumors with histologic confirmation. Data from references 6, 8, 10, 11, 16, 17, 40, 97, 113–115, and 146–148.

[b]The proportion of angiosarcomas is higher in series that include biopsies, because most are not completely resectable at the time of diagnosis and are generally less resectable than other types of heart sarcomas. The two EHEs were in two separate series (8,97). One was an incidental finding at explant, and one caused embolic symptoms. Both occurred in the atria. Neither caused the death of the patient, although one died of complications of transplant and the other was followed only 7 months. The data in the table otherwise refer only to angiosarcomas.

[c]One tumor in an infant was excluded based on lack of histologic confirmation and atypical benign course (6).

[d]Three tumors were in more than one chamber, total exceeds 100%.

[e]Occasionally, clinicians will request her2neu or CD117 staining on tumors for directed chemotherapy (16).

hemopericardium. Paraneoplastic syndromes related to cardiac angiosarcoma are rare, but there was a report of membranoproliferative glomerulonephritis diagnosed before the cardiac tumor (58). One patient presenting with seizure has been reported (45) as well as a case found incidentally (59).

Because of the propensity for pericardial involvement, cardiac tamponade occurs more frequently than with other types of cardiac sarcomas (50,54,60–65). In a series of 37 cases, tamponade occurred in 4 patients (12 percent) (2). Involvement of the coronary arteries is uncommon (66,67).

A single cardiac angiosarcoma of the right atrium has been reported to occur years after ascending aortic repair (68). Because of the proximity of the tumor to the graft, a causative association between the foreign material (Dacron) and the tumor was suggested.

Echocardiographically, angiosarcomas are echogenic, nodular or lobulated masses in the right atrium (59). Pericardial effusions with direct pericardial extension are frequently seen. Transesophageal echocardiography may be used to delineate the tumor (69).

On magnetic resonance imaging (MRI), angiosarcoma usually appears as a heterogeneous, nodular mass in the right atrium (70–73). MRI sequences are sensitive for hemorrhage and may show areas of nodularity on T1-weighted imaging (70,74,75). After the administration of intravenous contrast (gadolinium-DTPA), enhancement along vascular lakes may be seen (described as a "sunray" appearance) (76). Similar to echocardiography, MRI also shows pericardial effusion or direct pericardial invasion (37), although MRI is more sensitive for distinguishing between pericardial fluid and pericardial tumor (71,73,77).

Similar to MRI, computerized tomography (CT) usually shows a heterogeneous, nodular mass in the right atrium, with effusion or invasion into the pericardium, and variable attenuation (low attenuation due to necrosis but high attenuation due to hemorrhage). With MRI or CT, the presence of a hemorrhagic, irregular right atrial mass is very suggestive of angiosarcoma, especially if accompanied by a pericardial effusion (70). Multimodality cardiac imaging is useful to further characterize the mass and may help guide a diagnostic biopsy (78,79). However, CT and MRI may underestimate the extent of tumor because of its infiltrative nature.

A preoperative positron emission tomography (PET) scan may help evaluate cardiac angiosarcoma and the presence of metastatic disease (81–84) and may detect early recurrence and pulmonary metastasis (85). A right atrial angiosarcoma evaluated by real-time 3-dimensional echocardiography has been reported

(31). Intracardiac echocardiography may aid in catheter-based tissue sampling (78).

Angiography often demonstrates the vascular supply of the tumor and typically shows a blush at the tumor site (86,87). The tumor may erode the right coronary artery and result in fistulas within the atrium (88) mimicking ruptured sinus or Valsalva aneurysm (56), or resulting in coronary pseudoaneurysm (67).

**Gross Findings.** Angiosarcoma is typically a large, multilobular mass replacing the right atrial wall and either protruding into or filling the chamber (figs. 15-1, 15-2). The pericardium is typically involved, and may be the primary site. The third most common location is the left atrium, occurring in about 6 percent of patients (Table 15-1) (27). The mass (or masses) is typically dark brown or black. Invasion of the vena cava and tricuspid valve is common, but the atrial septum and pulmonary artery are usually spared. The pericardium is frequently involved, and is sometimes diffusely infiltrated. Rarely, it is the only site of tumor without myocardial infiltration (15,89). Angiosarcoma has been reported to infiltrate a coronary artery, resulting in pseudoaneurysm formation and rupture (67,90,91).

Cardiac angiosarcomas range from 2 to 10 cm (Table 15-1; figs. 15-3–15-8). The masses are typically dark gray-brown to black; spindled tumors appear firm and yellow-white and lack the classic hemorrhagic appearance.

**Tissue Sampling.** Cardiac angiosarcoma is diagnosed by open biopsy, mediastinoscopy (37), echocardiogram-guided fine-needle aspiration biopsy (92), and pericardiotomy (57). Often, the pericardial cytology is negative prior to biopsy or resection, despite bloody pericardial fluid (36). Intracardiac echocardiography is currently used for the precise localization of the tumor (78). Cytologic examination of the pericardial effusion has not proven sensitive (17,34,58,93), although fine-needle aspiration may establish the diagnosis in some cases (92). The predominant right-sided location allows for the diagnosis by endomyocardial biopsy; all other sarcoma types have a predilection for the left atrium. Transvenous endomyocardial biopsy guided by transesophageal echocardiography is a less invasive mode of diagnosis compared with thoracotomy (94).

**Microscopic Findings.** Angiosarcoma is an infiltrating mass that typically invades muscle,

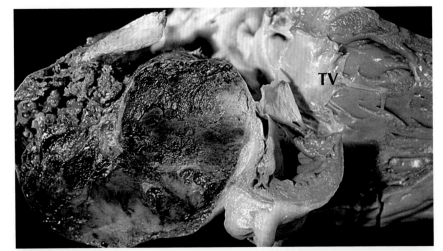

**Figure 15-1**

**ANGIOSARCOMA: AUTOPSY**

Top: This hemorrhagic mass fills the right atrium. The right ventricle is at the right (TV = tricuspid valve).

Bottom: A different level through the tumor shows the 6-cm mass with a variegated cut surface filling the right atrium and respecting the border of the atrioventricular sulcus (RCA = right coronary artery).

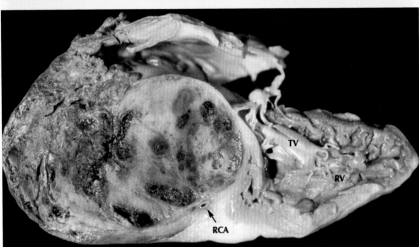

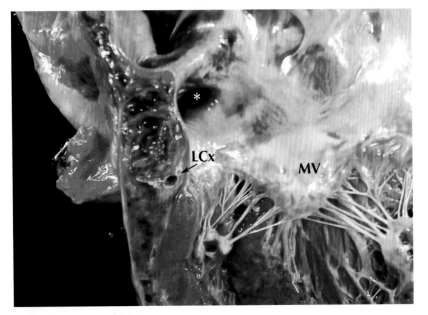

**Figure 15-2**

**ANGIOSARCOMA: AUTOPSY**

The main mass was in the right atrium, and spread along the pericardium from the interatrial septum to the left side of the heart. The tumor is seen in the wall of the left atrium and in the epicardium above the left circumflex artery (LCx). MV = mitral valve. The asterisk shows the orifice of the left atrial appendage, to the left of the interatrial septum, as seen from the left atrium.

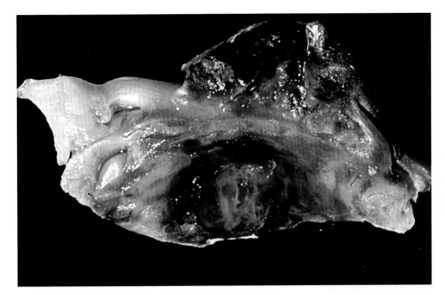

**Figure 15-3**

**ANGIOSARCOMA: RIGHT ATRIUM**

There is a hemorrhagic tumor on the luminal aspect (below) and epicardial surface of the right atrium (above). A right atrial reconstruction with pericardial patch procedure was required.

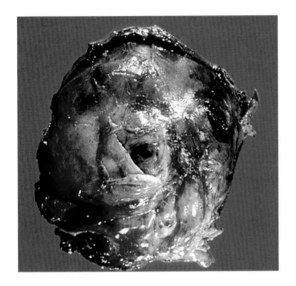

**Figure 15-4**

**ANGIOSARCOMA: RIGHT ATRIUM**

The tumor is dark, with surface adhesions of pericardium.

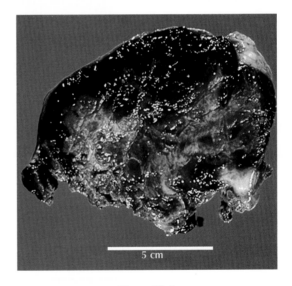

**Figure 15-5**

**ANGIOSARCOMA: RIGHT ATRIUM**

The typical variegated hemorrhagic appearance is seen on cut surface.

and may form polypoid projections into the atrial lumen (figs. 15-9–15-11). Approximately two thirds of cardiac angiosarcomas are fairly differentiated, composed of malignant endothelial cells that form papillary structures or vascular channels. The vascular channels are irregular, anastomosing, and sinusoidal (figs. 15-12–15-18). The lining cells are usually pleomorphic and atypical. They may form cord-like structures in which the lumens are difficult to demonstrate. Mitoses are usually present. The remaining third are poorly differentiated and composed predominantly of anaplastic spindle cells (figs. 15-19–15-26).

In angiosarcomas with a focal or dominant spindle cell pattern, poorly formed vascular channels and extravascular red blood cells are usually identified. In these cases, the identification of vacuoles containing red blood cells helps in the diagnosis, and extensive sampling of the tumor usually reveals diagnostic areas.

Metastatic as opposed to primary lesions often show areas of better differentiation. Metastatic deposits are often more vasoformative than the primary lesions (15), and occasionally, the histologic appearance of metastases is more diagnostic than the primary tumor.

The *epithelioid variant of angiosarcoma* is unusual in the heart, in contrast to the aortic intima (95). In the soft tissue, epithelioid angiosarcomas are described as possessing "solid sheets of highly atypical, mitotically active, epithelioid endothelial cells. Necrosis is common, and vascular differentiation is expressed primarily by the formation of irregular sinusoidal vascular channels" (96). Although the tumor cells have eosinophilic cytoplasm with occasional cytoplasmic vacuoles, they are distinct from epithelioid hemangioendothelioma (8,16,97,98). The nuclei in this variant are usually large and hyperchromatic, and have prominent eosinophilic nucleoli. The stroma may be abundant and hyalinized; these tumors often co-express epithelial and endothelial markers.

A specific subtype of angiosarcoma is the *serosal angiosarcoma*, which is reported in the pleura and pericardium (129). Serosal angiosarcoma may mimic mesothelioma, and demonstrate diffuse sheet-like and clustered patterns of growth, with only subtle evidence of vascular differentiation. A tubulopapillary growth pattern, often seen in mesothelioma, may be seen, as well as spindle cell areas imparting a biphasic growth pattern, further suggesting mesothelioma. Most serosal angiosarcomas do not show strong cytokeratin or calretinin staining, however, and express endothelial markers (see below) by immunohistochemistry.

**Grading.** Angiosarcomas of soft tissue are typically not graded, either by the National Cancer Institute (NCI) guidelines or those of the FNLCC (Fédération Nationale des Centres de Lutte Contre le Cancer) (see chapter 16), because they are considered high grade regardless of the histologic features. However, the presence of epithelioid morphology and necrosis may indicate a poor prognosis (100,101). Some reports of cardiac

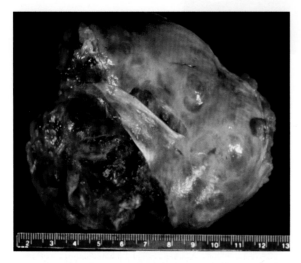

Figure 15-6

**ANGIOSARCOMA: RIGHT ATRIUM**

The necrotic hemorrhagic tumor is partly invested with pericardium.

Figure 15-7

**ANGIOSARCOMA: RIGHT ATRIUM**

The typical variegated, hemorrhagic appearance, with some more solid firm white areas (right), is seen.

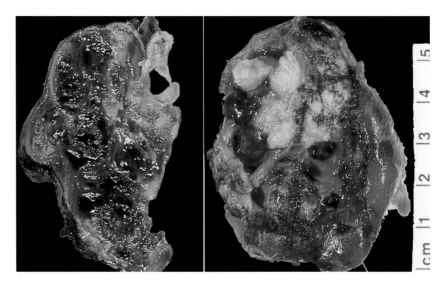

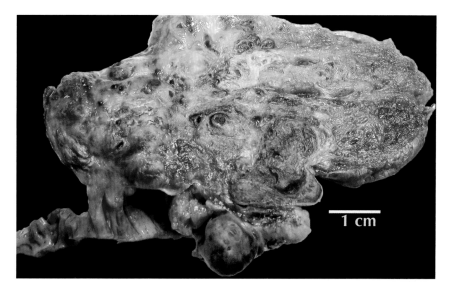

**Figure 15-8**

**ANGIOSARCOMA:
RIGHT ATRIUM**

This tumor is firm and fleshy, and is more typical of the solid spindle type of angiosarcoma. A portion of the right atrium with pectinate muscles is seen at the bottom left.

**Figure 15-9**

**ANGIOSARCOMA:
RIGHT ATRIUM**

The tumor, which is fairly well differentiated, is filling the right atrial invaginations with a polypoid pattern that grows into the trabeculae. At this magnification, the tumor is difficult to differentiate from atrial pectinate muscle.

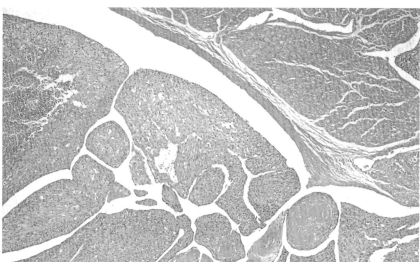

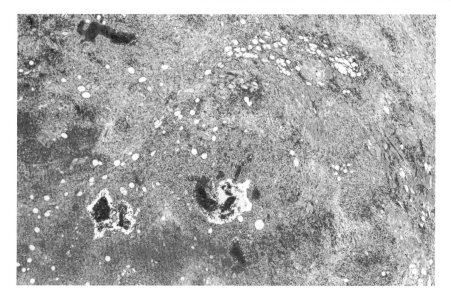

**Figure 15-10**

**ANGIOSARCOMA:
RIGHT ATRIUM**

At low magnification, the tumor is hemorrhagic and infiltrates the atrial wall and atrial fat.

**Figure 15-11**

**ANGIOSARCOMA: RIGHT ATRIUM**

A: At low magnification, there is patchy infiltration of the atrial muscle by a cellular tumor.

B: At higher magnification, a cellular vasoformative neoplasm (above) infiltrates the myocardium (below).

C: The interface between the angiosarcoma, on the right, and the atrial muscle at top left, is seen. The neoplasm has a spindled component, with poorly formed vascular structures.

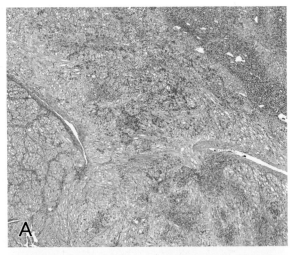

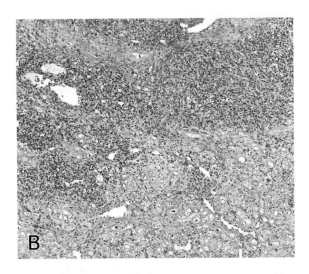

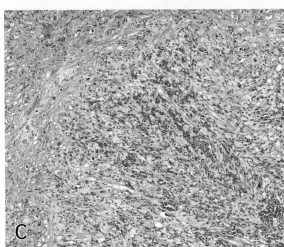

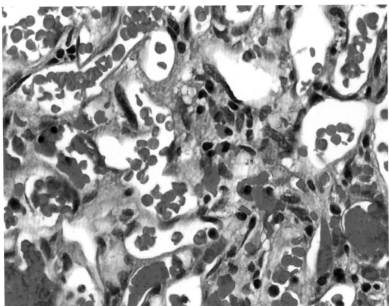

**Figure 15-12**

**ANGIOSARCOMA**

In well-differentiated areas, vascular structures are easily identified. Typically, there are anastomosing channels lined by markedly atypical cells.

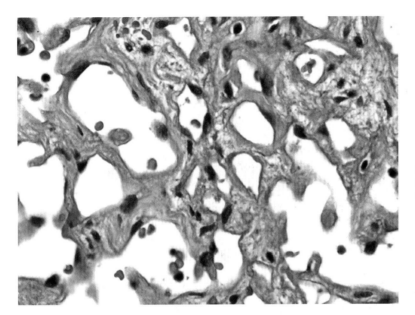

**Figure 15-13**

**ANGIOSARCOMA**

Irregular channels are lined by atypical endothelial cells that vary in size and shape. Large numbers of red blood cells are lacking.

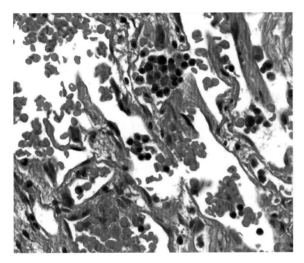

**Figure 15-14**

**ANGIOSARCOMA**

Occasionally, nests of extramedullary hematopoiesis are present, as here.

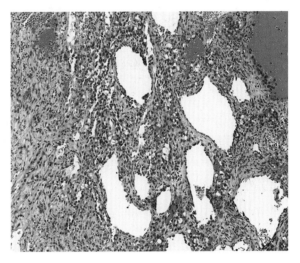

**Figure 15-15**

**ANGIOSARCOMA: DILATED CHANNELS**

This angiosarcoma is composed of cellular spindled areas surrounding larger channels that are lined by atypical endothelial cells.

angiosarcoma grade the tumors on a three-point scale without specifying a specific system (11).

Because there are too few primary cardiac angiosarcomas reported, it is not known whether the histologic features affect prognosis, because the completeness of excision and stage at time of presentation are far more important factors. In those series reported, cardiac angiosarcomas had high mitotic rates (often over 10 mitoses per 10 high-power fields) with necrosis present in at least 50 percent, but in only a few cases with histologic data (11).

The type of specimen (biopsy versus resection) affects sampling and the ability to evaluate these grading features. In the 10 cardiac angiosarcomas reported by Kim et al. (6), the mean mitotic rate was 3 per 10 high-power fields, with a range of 1 to 8, which is much lower than in the series of Look-Hong et al. (11). A review of cardiac angiosarcomas does

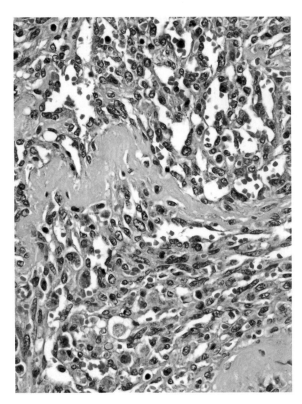
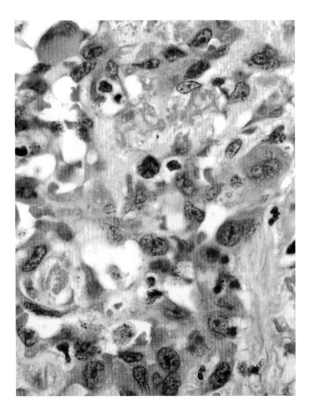

**Figure 15-16**

**ANGIOSARCOMA**

Left: Most typically, the vascular channels are irregular, with small, compressed lumens. Highly atypical tumor cells infiltrate into the stromal background.

Right: At higher magnification, compressed, irregular vascular channels are lined by highly atypical endothelial cells.

not mention that histologic parameters affect survival (17). In the authors' experience with 36 cardiac angiosarcomas with adequate sampling, the mean mitotic rate was 40 per 10 high-power fields, higher than any other histologic subtype other than embryonal rhabdomyosarcoma. One third of these angiosarcomas have a mitotic rate of above 50 per 10 high-power fields, and over one third had fewer than 5 per 10 high-power fields, indicating a wide range in the proliferative rate. In these same tumors, in the authors' files, angiosarcoma had the highest average necrosis score among all cardiac sarcomas, with one third demonstrating zonal necrosis (areas over 5 mm), half with microscopic areas of necrosis, and the remainder without necrosis.

**Immunohistochemical Findings.** Immunohistochemical staining for CD31 has shown great diagnostic sensitivity in soft tissue angiosarcomas, and is positive in about 90 percent of

cases (figs. 15-27–15-30). CD34 is not a specific marker for endothelial cells, but is consistently detected in cardiac angiosarcoma (fig. 15-31) (130). Factor VIII-related antigen has low diagnostic sensitivity (fig. 15-32). Herrmann et al. (18) noted staining for this antigen in only 1 of 6 cases, and Tazelaar et al. (102) in 1 of 2 cases. Newer immunohistochemical markers for angiosarcoma with high sensitivity and specificity include the nuclear factors ERG transcription factor (103) and Fli-1 (104).

Serosal angiosarcomas consistently express at least two of four endothelial markers (CD31, CD34, von Willebrand factor, and Ulex europaeus agglutinin-I). Weibel-Palade bodies, which are specific for endothelial differentiation, are unfortunately not always present by ultrastructural evaluation. Vascular channels may be highlighted by the use of laminin and type IV collagen (99).

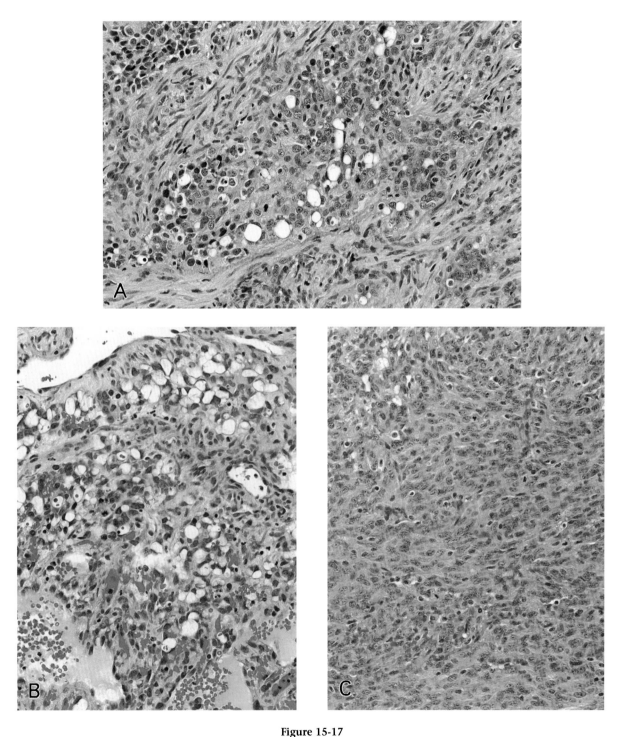

**Figure 15-17**

**ANGIOSARCOMA**

A: This tumor, also illustrated in figures 15-15 and 15-22, demonstrates the variety of patterns represented in an angiosarcoma. This area has a vaguely epithelioid appearance, but the amount of cytoplasm is not enough to be designated as the epithelioid variant. There may be a subset of cells with prominent vacuoles (a nonspecific feature).

B: A different area shows vacuoles with an almost adenomatoid appearance.

C: In this area, there is a prominent spindle cell component, and the vascular nature of the tumor is inconspicuous. The diagnosis is confirmed by the presence of better-differentiated areas (see A and B) or immunohistochemical methods.

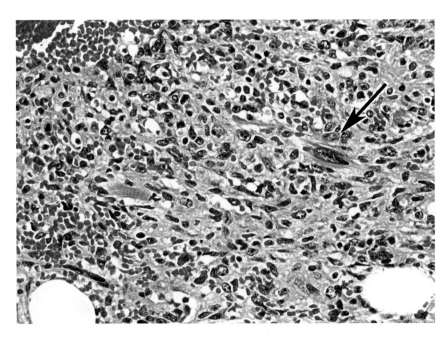

**Figure 15-18**

**ANGIOSARCOMA**

The vascular nature of the tumor is inconspicuous. There are rare entrapped cardiac myocytes (arrow).

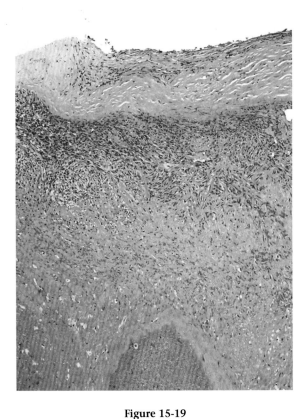

**Figure 15-19**

**ANGIOSARCOMA: PREDOMINANTLY SPINDLED TYPE**

The tumor is largely hemorrhagic and necrotic (bottom), and is spindled in the area adjacent to the fibrous pericardium (top).

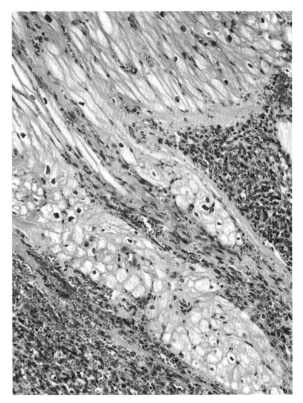

**Figure 15-20**

**ANGIOSARCOMA: INFILTRATING ATRIAL MUSCLE**

The spindle cell neoplasm infiltrates atrial myocytes, which are prominently vacuolated, possibly due to chronic ischemia. There are numerous red blood cells within the tumor, giving a clue to the diagnosis.

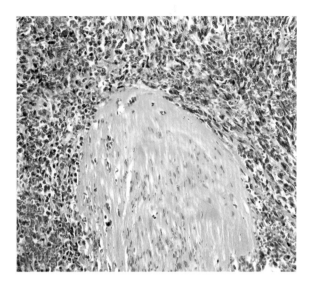

**Figure 15-21**

**ANGIOSARCOMA: INFILTRATING
NECROTIC CARDIAC MUSCLE**

This hemorrhagic spindle cell tumor, histologically compatible with angiosarcoma, infiltrates around atrial muscle.

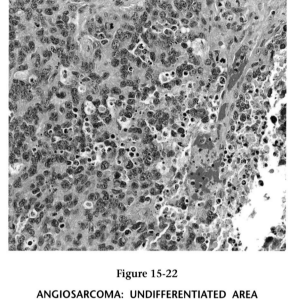

**Figure 15-22**

**ANGIOSARCOMA: UNDIFFERENTIATED AREA**

Angiosarcoma, in addition to the spindling, can be difficult to diagnose because of small undifferentiated round cells. Other areas of the tumor were diagnostic (see figs. 15-15, 15-17A).

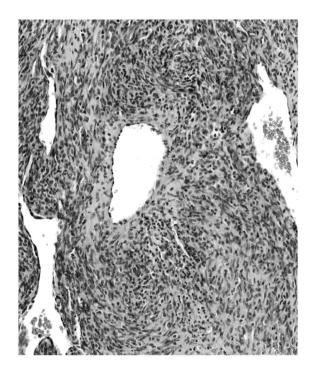

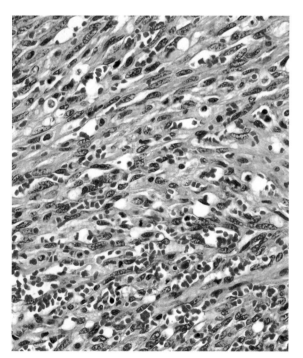

**Figure 15-23**

**ANGIOSARCOMA: WITH DILATED VASCULAR SPACES**

Left: Occasionally, there are dilated irregular vascular channels within the tumor, mimicking a hemangiopericytoma-like pattern.

Right: At higher magnification, the typical spindled pattern with compressed vascular channels containing red blood cells is seen.

277

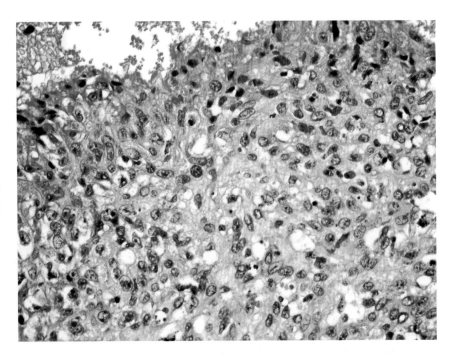

**Figure 15-24**

**ANGIOSARCOMA: EPITHELIOID PATTERN**

In some cases, there is abundant cytoplasm, a more solid pattern of growth, and absent vascular channels and erythrocytes.

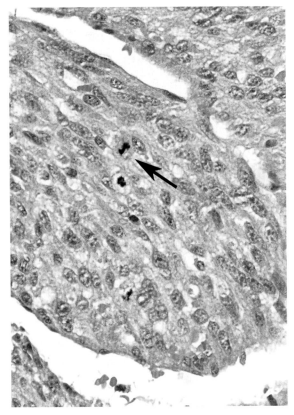
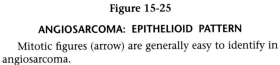

**Figure 15-25**

**ANGIOSARCOMA: EPITHELIOID PATTERN**

Mitotic figures (arrow) are generally easy to identify in angiosarcoma.

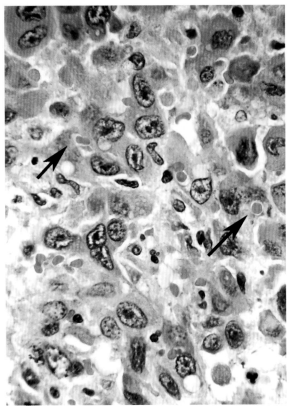

**Figure 15-26**

**ANGIOSARCOMA: EPITHELIOID PATTERN**

The arrow shows a tumor cell with a capillary-like intracytoplasmic lumen containing a red blood cell.

Cytokeratin and epithelial membrane antigen may be focally positive in conventional angiosarcomas and diffusely positive in epithelioid angiosarcomas (figs. 15-33, 15-34). There is one report of an epithelioid angiosarcoma expressing CD117 and HER2/neu (16).

**Molecular Findings.** There is no known etiology for cardiac angiosarcoma. A single case was associated with prior mediastinal radiation for Hodgkin lymphoma (105), and one related to the ascending aortic Dacron graft (68). Rare familial cases, including primary cardiac angiosarcomas in identical twins (23–26), suggest the possibility of a genetic basis. Although cytogenetic analyses of cardiac angiosarcomas show no consistent chromosomal abnormality, a case of right atrial angiosarcoma demonstrated hyperdiploid clonal populations with changes in chromosome number as follows: 55, XY, +der(1;17)(q10:q10), +2, +7, +8, +19, +20, +21, +22, as well as polysomy of chromosome 8 (106). Other chromosomal changes reported are gains of 5pter-p11, 8p12-qter, 2opter-q12 and losses of 4p, 7p15-pter-y, and abnormalities involving 22q (107). Genetic alterations of *TP53* and *KRAS* have also been documented in cardiac angiosarcomas in humans as well as animal models (108–110).

**Differential Diagnosis.** The spindle cell areas of angiosarcoma may be difficult, if not impossible, to distinguish from unclassifiable spindle cell sarcomas, fibrosarcomas, or pleomorphic

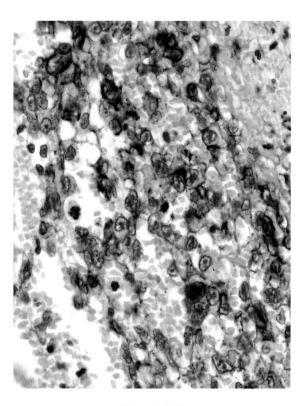

**Figure 15-27**

**ANGIOSARCOMA: CD31 IMMUNOHISTOCHEMICAL STAIN**

In tumors without obvious endothelial differentiation, endothelial expression is demonstrated by immunohistochemistry. The tumor is diffusely positive for endothelial markers, and care must be taken to avoid misinterpreting intratumoral vessels.

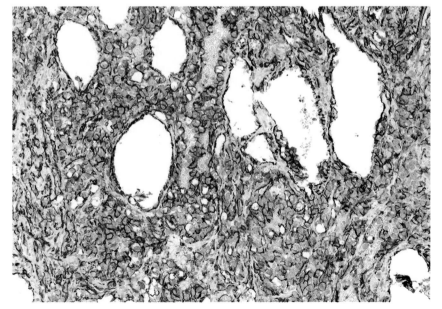

**Figure 15-28**

**ANGIOSARCOMA: CD31 IMMUNOHISTOCHEMICAL STAIN**

The cells lining dilated channels and more solid areas are positive for CD31. The tumor cells must be differentiated from normal vessels, as capillaries are numerous in neoplasms of all types. A background of capillaries is usually not prominent or evident in angiosarcoma.

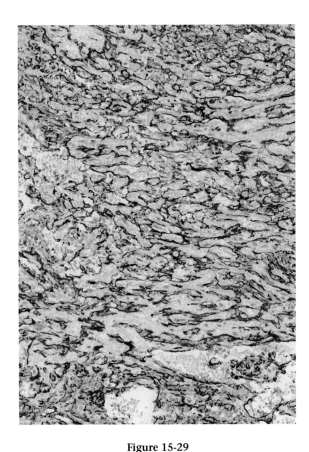

**Figure 15-29**

**ANGIOSARCOMA: CD31
IMMUNOHISTOCHEMICAL STAIN**

Endothelial differentiation is obvious in this fairly spindled tumor. On routine staining, such a tumor may mimic a different type of sarcoma.

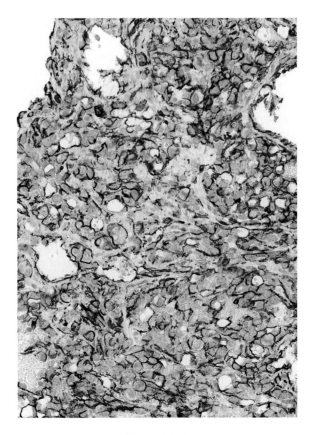

**Figure 15-30**

**ANGIOSARCOMA: CD31
IMMUNOHISTOCHEMICAL STAIN**

In this more epithelioid tumor there is prominent cytoplasmic staining.

undifferentiated sarcomas. In such tumors, extensive sampling is important to detect endothelial vacuoles or diagnostic papillary structures. Endothelial differentiation is assessed by immunohistochemical staining for CD31, CD24, factor VIII-related antigen, and erythroblast transformation specific gene (ERG) protein (18,103).

Angiosarcomas of the pericardium can be quite difficult to diagnose in pericardial biopsies and can be mistaken for mesotheliomas, and nests of reactive mesothelial cells may be trapped in areas of an angiosarcoma. The tumor cells may be difficult to detect in pericardial biopsies, leading to the mistaken impression of reactive mesothelium, and delay in diagnosis (111). Nests of reactive mesothelial cells may become incorporated into the sarcoma and be mistaken for malignant cells. Immuno-

histochemical stains for calretinin, WT1, and cytokeratin 5/6 (mesothelial markers) help to differentiate mesothelial cells from endothelial cells (CD31, CD34, and others).

Papillary endothelial hyperplasia (Masson tumor) may be present in cardiac hemangiomas, and superficially resemble the papillary growths of angiosarcoma. Unlike angiosarcoma, however, marked cellular atypia and mitoses are absent, and unequivocally benign structures of hemangioma are present elsewhere within the tumor.

**Treatment and Prognosis.** Cardiac angiosarcoma is generally treated by a combination of surgery, radiation, and sarcoma-type chemotherapy (6,11,97,112–115). Resection is impossible in almost one fifth of tumors, and biopsy is the only tissue sampling performed (Table 15-1). Complete surgical excision cannot be achieved in most cases

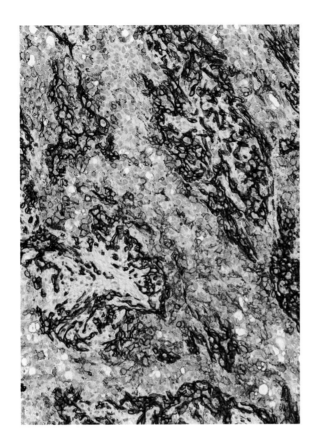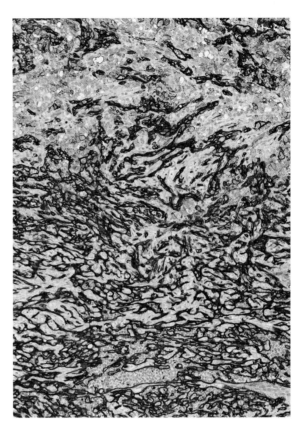

**Figure 15-31**

**ANGIOSARCOMA, CD34 IMMUNOHISTOCHEMICAL STAIN**

Left: In this example, not all the cells express endothelial markers, but there is intense staining of the anastomosing channels.

Right: Another area highlights the growth pattern, which is more vascular at the top and spindled in the center.

due to the lack of a dissection plane and myocardial encroachment of tumor tissue. Reconstructive techniques with atrial repair using pericardial patching (112,116,117) and valve replacement or repair (118) may be necessary. Coronary bypass grafting of the right coronary artery may be necessary for infiltrative or especially large right atrial tumors (119). Heart transplantation has been used to treat cardiac angiosarcoma, but without long-term survival (121–126).

The ability of postoperative chemotherapy to extend survival has been questioned (17), although there are anecdotal reports of remissions (20,35,127). Short-term responses with sarcoma treatments (e.g., cisplatin, epirubicin, and ifosfamide) in combination with herceptin and imatinib (Glivec) have been reported (16,57,120), but the benefit of chemotherapy has not been substantiated. Paclitaxel and docetaxel have also

been used as chemotherapy for cardiac angiosarcoma (49,83,128,129). Radiation therapy may be sensitized by razoxane (130).

The survival of patients with angiosarcoma of the heart is poor, with many patients dying in the postoperative period (41,55), or dying from metastatic, inoperable disease (18). In series from the 1990s, combined data from seven institutions demonstrated a mean survival period in 17 patients of 6.6 months until death, with 1 living survivor at 16 months (12). Herrmann et al. (18) found a mean survival period of 6 months in 6 patients, and somewhat longer (10 months) in 2 patients with surgical resection (18). Blondeau et al. (131) reported a mean survival period of 2.14 years in 11 French patients; the reason for this disparity in mean survival is unclear.

In this century, survival has not increased considerably. In the largest series of 18 patients

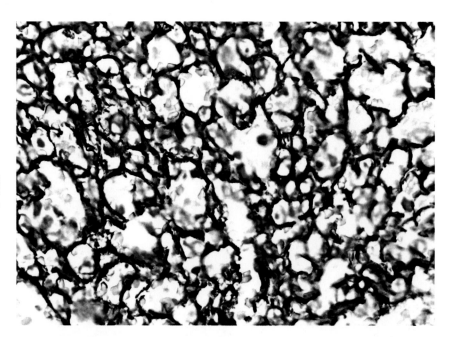

**Figure 15-32**

**ANGIOSARCOMA: FACTOR VIII-RELATED ANTIGEN**

There is diffuse tumor staining for factor VIII. The tumor had a somewhat epithelioid morphology.

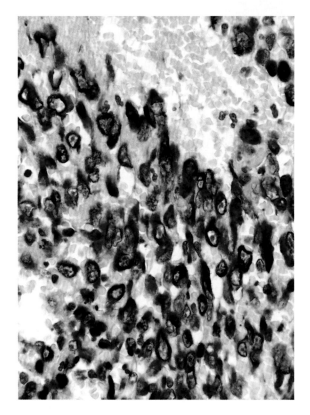

**Figure 15-33**

**ANGIOSARCOMA: PANCYTOKERATIN**

Cytokeratins may be coexpressed in angiosarcoma, but in order to exclude an epithelial neoplasm, diffuse staining for an endothelial marker is required.

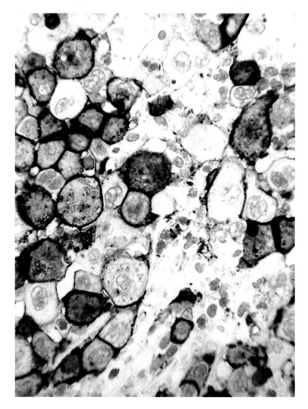

**Figure 15-34**

**ANGIOSARCOMA: EPITHELIOID TYPE, CD31 IMMUNOSTAINING**

In this tumor with obvious epithelioid characteristics, diffuse CD31 staining confirmed the diagnosis of angiosarcoma.

with cardiac angiosarcomas, the median survival period was 13 months, with better survival among patients with localized disease (11). In this series, 15 of 17 patients with follow-up died of disease (1 to 84 months), and 2 were alive with disease. In the 10 patients reported by Kim et al. (6), the median survival period was 10 months: 8 patients died of disease and 2 were alive with disease, 1 at 64 months. In the 10 patients reported by Simpson et al. (115), the median survival period was only 5 months, worse than for other histologic sarcoma subtypes, although one patient was alive at 42 months. In most of these series, factors related to longer survival were absence of metastasis at the time of diagnosis and completeness of excision.

In general, necrosis and mitotic activity are negative prognostic signs in cardiac sarcomas, but these are findings typical of angiosarcoma and do not predict outcome in this subset of high-grade sarcomas (2). One angiosarcoma patient with a long-term cure was reported, but occurred in an infant and was described as well-differentiated (8). Because angiosarcomas are by definition high grade, and because the illustrated lesion suggested a form of hemangioma, it is uncertain whether this lesion should be considered a true angiosarcoma.

In soft tissue (extracardiac) angiosarcomas, the morphologic features that are statistically correlated with poor outcome include age, large tumor size, and high MIB-1 (Ki-67) index (29). No significant correlation has been reported between DNA ploidy patterns and clinical outcome in these angiosarcomas (22).

Patients with cardiac angiosarcomas have an especially poor prognosis because they typically present with metastasis, often in multiple sites (132). Metastases occur in 66 to 89 percent of patients, most often to the lungs (11,48,133), frequently at the time of presentation (10,17). Other sites of metastases include bone (11,16, 112,117), liver (11,15), adrenal gland (28), spleen (11,16,134), brain (11,61,135,136), retroperitoneum (112), and breast (137).

## EPITHELIOID HEMANGIOENDOTHELIOMA

*Epithelioid hemangioendothelioma* is a low-grade angiosarcoma composed of epithelioid cells that form short strands or solid nests. The endothelial cells form small intracellular lumens and infil-

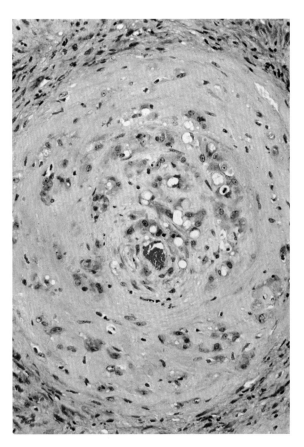

**Figure 15-35**

**EPITHELIOID HEMANGIOENDOTHELIOMA**

The tumor cells show minimal atypia and form linear cohesive nests.

trate the muscular walls of vessels (figs. 15-35, 15-36). About 12 cases have been reported in the heart (8,95,97,138–143), 1 in association with myelodysplastic syndrome (95). The intracellular lumens of epithelioid hemangioendothelioma may mimic the vacuoles of adenocarcinoma, which may be initially considered in the microscopic differential diagnosis. Immunohistochemical stains for factor VIII-related antigen, CD31, or CD34 identify the cells as endothelial in origin (fig. 15-37).

Approximately 10 percent of extracardiac hemangioendotheliomas result in metastases, and up to one third recur or metastasize (144). The biologic behavior of epithelioid hemangioendotheliomas of the heart, however, is unknown. These tumors should be considered potentially malignant, based on available data

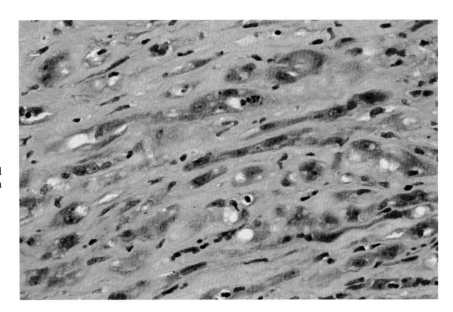

**Figure 15-36**

**EPITHELIOID HEMANGIOENDOTHELIOMA**

Cytoplasmic vacuoles and circumferential growth around a vessel are typical of this tumor.

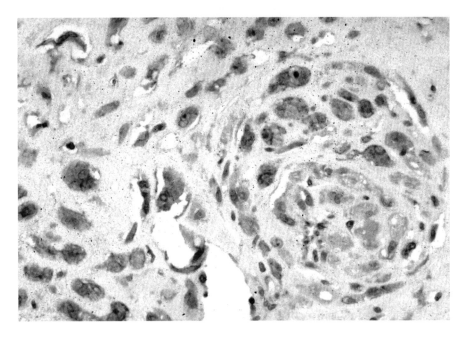

**Figure 15-37**

**EPITHELIOID HEMANGIOENDOTHELIOMA**

Immunohistochemical stains show coexpression of endothelial and epithelial markers. This tumor is diffusely positive for CD34.

on histologically similar extracardiac tumors, and one tumor developed distant metastases (143).

Epithelioid hemangioendothelioma should not be confused with the epithelioid variant of angiosarcoma or epithelioid hemangioma. The latter, which has been reported in the heart (145), is also called angiolymphoid hyperplasia with eosinophilia. It is probably a reactive condition characterized by a proliferation of epithelioid endothelial cells, reactive lymphoid aggregates, and tissue eosinophilia, typically occurring near an artery in the subcutaneous tissues of the head and neck (see chapter 10).

## REFERENCES

1. Bear P, Moodie D. Malignant primary cardiac tumors. The Cleveland Clinic experience, 1956 to 1986. Chest 1987;92:860-862.
2. Burke AP, Cowan D, Virmani R. Primary sarcomas of the heart. Cancer 1992;69:387-395.
3. Murphy MC, Sweeney MS, Putnam JB Jr, et al. Surgical treatment of cardiac tumors: A 25 year experience. Ann Thorac Surg 1990;49:612-617.
4. Putnam JB Jr, Sweeney MS, Colon R, Lanza LA, Frazier OH, Cooley DA. Primary cardiac sarcomas. Ann Thorac Surg 1991;51:906-910.
5. Donsbeck AV, Ranchere D, Coindre JM, Le Gall F, Cordier JF, Loire R. Primary cardiac sarcomas: an immunohistochemical and grading study with long-term follow-up of 24 cases. Histopathology 1999;34:295-304.
6. Kim CH, Dancer JY, Coffey D, et al. Clinicopathologic study of 24 patients with primary cardiac sarcomas: a 10-year single institution experience. Hum Pathol 2008;39:933-938.
7. Llombart-Cussac A, Pivot X, Contesso G, et al. Adjuvant chemotherapy for primary cardiac sarcomas: the IGR experience. Br J Cancer 1998;78:1624-1628.
8. Zhang PJ, Brooks JS, Goldblum JR, et al. Primary cardiac sarcomas: a clinicopathologic analysis of a series with follow-up information in 17 patients and emphasis on long-term survival. Hum Pathol 2008;39:1385-1395.
9. Raaf HN, Raaf JH. Sarcomas related to the heart and vasculature. Semin Surg Oncol 1994;10:374-382.
10. Fatima J, Duncan AA, Maleszewski JJ, et al. Primary angiosarcoma of the aorta, great vessels, and the heart. J Vasc Surg 2013;57:756-764.
11. Look-Hong NJ, Pandalai PK, Hornick JL, et al. Cardiac angiosarcoma management and outcomes: 20-year single-institution experience. Ann Surg Oncol 2012;19:2707-2715.
12. Burke A, Virmani R. Tumors of the heart and great vessels. AFIP Atlas of tumor pathology, 3rd Series, Fascicle 16. Washington, DC: American Registry of Pathology; 1996.
13. Burke A. Primary malignant cardiac tumors. Semin Diagn Pathol 2008;25:39-46.
14. Glancy D, Morales J, Roberts W. Angiosarcoma of the heart. Cancer 1968;21:413-418.
15. Janigan D, Husain A, Robinson N. Cardiac angiosarcomas. A review and a case report. Cancer 1986;57:852-859.
16. Batzios S, Michalopoulos A, Kaklamanis L, et al. Angiosarcoma of the heart: case report and review of the literature. Anticancer Res 2006;26:4837-4842.
17. Brandt RR, Arnold R, Bohle RM, Dill T, Hamm CW. Cardiac angiosarcoma: case report and review of the literature. Z Kardiol 2005;94:824-828.
18. Herrmann MA, Shankerman RA, Edwards WD, Shub C, Schaff HV. Primary cardiac angiosarcoma: a clinicopathologic study of six cases. J Thorac Cardiovasc Surg 1992;103:655-664.
19. Makhoul N, Bode FR. Angiosarcoma of the heart: review of the literature and report of two cases that illustrate the broad spectrum of the disease. Can J Cardiol 1995;11:423-428.
20. Luk A, Nwachukwu H, Lim KD, Cusimano RJ, Butany J. Cardiac angiosarcoma: a case report and review of the literature. Cardiovasc Pathol 2010;19:e69-74.
21. Butany J, Yu W. Cardiac angiosarcoma: two cases and a review of the literature. Can J Cardiol 2000;16:197-205.
22. Burke AP, Tazelaar H, Butany JW, et al. Cardiac sarcomas. In: Travis WD, Brambilla E, Müller-Hermelink HK, Harris CC, eds. Pathology and genetics of tumours of the lung, pleura, thymus, and heart. Lyon: IARC Press; 2004:273-281.
23. Hu R, Polga JP, McCann JC. Primary angiosarcoma of the heart in identical twins. J Comput Assist Tomogr 1999;23:963-965.
24. Lundkvist L, Erntell H. [A case report of two siblings. Cardiac angiosarcoma—rare tumor with non-specific symptoms and poor prognosis.] Lakartidningen 2002;99:4165-4167. [Swedish]
25. Casha AR, Davidson LA, Roberts P, Nair RU. Familial angiosarcoma of the heart. J Thorac Cardiovasc Surg 2002;124:392-394.
26. Keeling IM, Ploner F, Rigler B. Familial cardiac angiosarcoma. Ann Thorac Surg 2006;82:1576.
27. Ho CK, Wang E, Au WK, Cheng LC. Primary cardiac angiosarcoma of left atrium. J Card Surg 2009;24:524-525.
28. Kuwabara F, Hirate Y, Sugiura T, et al. [Primary cardiac angiosarcoma in the left atrium with adrenal metastasis; report of a case.] Kyobu Geka 2005;58:396-398. [Japanese]
29. Dennig K, Lehmann G, Richter T. An angiosarcoma in the left atrium. N Engl J Med 2000;342:443-444.
30. Montiel J, Ruyra X, Carreras F, Caralps JM, Aris A, Padro JM. [A report of a rare case of primary angiosarcoma of left atrium and a review of the literature.] Rev Esp Cardiol 1994;47:768-770. [Spanish]

31. Yang HS, Sengupta S, Umland MM, Chandrasekaran K, Mookadam F. Primary cardiac angiosarcoma evaluated with contrast two-dimensional and real-time three-dimensional echocardiography. Eur J Echocardiogr 2008;9:733-738.

32. Baeza-Roman A, Latour-Perez J, Alzamora DR, et al. Prinzmetal's angina in a patient with angiosarcoma of the right cardiac chambers. Heart Lung 2011;40:346-348.

33. Duyuler S, Demirkan B, Guray Y, Demir C, Guray U. Echocardiography in differential diagnosis of chest pain and elevated cardiac biomarkers: a case of cardiac angiosarcoma. Eur J Echocardiogr 2011;12:406-407.

34. Riles E, Gupta S, Wang DD, Tobin K. Primary cardiac angiosarcoma: A diagnostic challenge in a young man with recurrent pericardial effusions. Exp Clin Cardiol 2012;17:39-42.

35. Afonso PV, Antunes MJ. Primary cardiac angiosarcoma. Extended resection of the right atrial wall. Case report. Rev Port Cardiol 2007;26:1189-1194.

36. Kontogiorgi M, Exarchos D, Charitos C, et al. Primary right atrium angiosarcoma mimicking pericarditis. World J Surg Oncol 2007;5:120.

37. Valeviciene N, Mataciunas M, Tamosiunas A, Petrulioniene Z, Briediene R. Primary heart angiosarcoma detected by magnetic resonance imaging. Acta Radiol 2006;47:675-679.

38. Chenier M, Johnson D, Ohman M, Pavlisko E. Cardiac angiosarcoma presenting as progressive dyspnea on exertion. J Cardiovasc Med (Hagerstown) 2011;12:904-907.

39. Demirkan B, Ozen A, Turhan N, Guray Y, Birincioglu L. Fever, dyspnea and chest pain with pericardial effusion. Primary cardiac angiosarcoma. Anadolu Kardiyol Derg 2012;12:525, 533.

40. Kurian KC, Weisshaar D, Parekh H, Berry GJ, Reitz B. Primary cardiac angiosarcoma: case report and review of the literature. Cardiovasc Pathol 2006; 15:110-112.

41. Murinello A, Mendonca P, Abreu A, et al. Cardiac angiosarcoma—a review. Rev Port Cardiol 2007;26:577-584.

42. O'Callaghan DS, Breen DP, Young V. Angiosarcoma of the right atrium masquerading as recurrent pulmonary embolism. Thorac Cardiovasc Surg 2008;56:488-490.

43. Bahammam A. Cardiac angiosarcoma presenting as right heart failure secondary to pulmonary vascular carcinomatosis. Ann Saudi Med 1999;19:42-44.

44. Sidhu MS, Singh HP, Chopra AK, Kapila D, Chopra S, Anand M. Primary right atrial angiosarcoma: atypical presentation and echocardiographicassessment of right atrial mass. Echocardiography 2009;26:1276-1277.

45. Navarro Calzada J, Sierra Bergua B. [Epileptic seizure as a first sign of a cardiac angiosarcoma.] Neurologia 2010;25:198-199. [Spanish]

46. Lafçı G, Caglı K, Tok D, Yalçınkaya A. An unusual cause of spontaneous hemothorax: cardiac angiosarcoma. Turk Kardiyol Dern Ars 2013;41:526-528.

47. Mahdhaoui A, Bouraoui H, Cheniour M, et al. [Right atrium angiosarcoma disclosed by alveolar hemorrhage.] Rev Med Suisse Romande 2004; 124:115-116. [French]

48. Amonkar GP, Deshpande JR. Cardiac angiosarcoma. Cardiovasc Pathol 2006;15:57-58.

49. Castilla E, Pascual I, Roncales F, Aguirre E, Del Rio A. Transient response of cardiac angiosarcoma to paclitaxel. Eur J Cancer Care (Engl) 2010;19:699-700.

50. El-Osta HE, Yammine YS, Chehab BM, Fields AS, Moore DF Jr, Mattar BI. Unexplained hemopericardium as a presenting feature of primary cardiac angiosarcoma: a case report and a review of the diagnostic dilemma. J Thorac Oncol 2008;3: 800-802.

51. Jain G, Mukhopadhyay S, Kurien S, Yusuf J, Tyagi S, Jain R. Ruptured cardiac angiosarcoma with pulmonary metastases: a rare disease with a common (mis)diagnosis! Indian Heart J 2012;64:603-606.

52. Uto T, Bando M, Yamauchi H, et al. Primary cardiac angiosarcoma of the right auricle with difficult-to-treat bilateral pleural effusion. Intern Med 2011;50:2371-2374.

53. Bertoli F, Remon Valera JA, Arrocha R. [Angiosarcoma of the heart and its spontaneous rupture. A rare cause of effusive-constrictive pericarditis. A case report and review of the literature.] Rev Med Panama 1995;20:84-91. [Spanish]

54. Corso RB, Kraychete N, Nardeli S, et al. Spontaneous rupture of a right atrial angiosarcoma and cardiac tamponade. Arq Bras Cardiol 2003;81: 611-613, 608-610.

55. Sakaguchi M, Minato N, Katayama Y, Nakashima A. Cardiac angiosarcoma with right atrial perforation and cardiac tamponade. Ann Thorac Cardiovasc Surg 2006;12:145-148.

56. Yoshitake I, Hata M, Sezai A, et al. Cardiac angiosarcoma with cardiac tamponade diagnosed as a ruptured aneurysm of the sinus valsalva. Jpn J Clin Oncol 2009;39:612-615.

57. Antonuzzo L, Rotella V, Mazzoni F, et al. Primary cardiac angiosarcoma: a fatal disease. Case Rep Med 2009;2009:591512.

58. Shahani L, Beckmann M, Vallurupalli S. Cardiac angiosarcoma-associated membranoproliferative glomerulonephropathy. Case Report Med 2011; 2011:956089.

59. Pourmand A, Boniface K. Incidental identification of right atrial mass using bedside ultrasound: cardiac angiosarcoma. West J Emerg Med 2011; 12:478-480.

60. Holtan SG, Allen RD, Henkel DM, et al. Angiosarcoma of the pericardium presenting as hemorrhagic pleuropericarditis, cardiac tamponade, and thromboembolic phenomena. Int J Cardiol 2007;115:e8-9.

61. Ikeya E, Taguchi J, Yamaguchi M, Shibuya M, Kanabuchi K. Primary cardiac angiosarcoma: presenting with cardiac tamponade followed by cerebral hemorrhage with brain metastases. Jpn J Thorac Cardiovasc Surg 2006;54:528-531.

62. Kim DM, Hong JH, Kim SY, et al. Primary cardiac angiosarcoma presenting with cardiac tamponade. Korean Circ J 2010;40:86-89.

63. Sosnik K, Lewczuk J, Ludwik B, et al. [Cardiac tamponade due to angiosarcoma--was surgical treatment necessary? A case report.] Kardiol Pol 2006;64:1426-1427. [Polish]

64. Chalhoub E, Mattar BI, Shaheen W, Schulz TK. Cardiac angiosarcoma presenting with tamponade. Intern Med 2012;51:2905-2907.

65. van der Lee C, Klootwijk PJ, van Geuns RJ, Maat LP, den Bakker MA. Angiosarcoma of the right atrium presenting as collapse. Int J Cardiol 2009; 132:e17-19.

66. Gualis J, Castano M, Gomez-Plana J, Mencia P, Alonso D. Palliative surgical treatment of primary cardiac angiosarcoma complicated with recurrent tamponade. J Surg Oncol 2009;100:744.

67. Chaturvedi A, Vummidi D, Shuman WP, Dubinsky TJ, Maki JH. Cardiac angiosarcoma: an unusual cause of coronary artery pseudoaneurysm. J Thorac Imaging 2012;27:W8-9.

68. Almeida NJ, Hoang P, Biddle P, Arouni A, Esterbrooks D. Primary cardiac angiosarcoma: in a patient with a dacron aortic prosthesis. Tex Heart Inst J 2011;38:61-65; discussion 65.

69. Jaafari A, Benyoussef S, Boukhriss B, Zakhama L, Thameur M, Boussabah E. [Angiosarcoma of the right atrium detected by transesophageal echocardiography. A case report.] Tunis Med 2003;81(Suppl 8):680-684. [French]

70. Araoz PA, Eklund HE, Welch TJ, Breen JF. CT and MR imaging of primary cardiac malignancies. Radiographics 1999;19:1421-1434.

71. Deetjen AG, Conradi G, Mollmann S, Hamm CW, Dill T. Cardiac angiosarcoma diagnosed and characterized by cardiac magnetic resonance imaging. Cardiol Rev 2006;14:101-103.

72. Vogt FM, Hunold P, Ruehm SG. Images in vascular medicine. Angiosarcoma of superior vena cava with extension into right atrium assessed by MD-CT and MRI. Vasc Med 2003;8:283-284.

73. Keenan N, Davies S, Sheppard MN, Maceira A, Serino W, Mohiaddin RH. Angiosarcoma of the right atrium: a diagnostic dilemma. Int J Cardiol 2006;113:425-426.

74. Mader MT, Poulton TB, White RD. Malignant tumors of the heart and great vessels: MR imaging appearance. Radiographics 1997;17:145-153.

75. Restrepo CS, Largoza A, Lemos DF, et al. CT and MR imaging findings of malignant cardiac tumors. Curr Probl Diagn Radiol 2005;34:1-11.

76. Yahata S, Endo T, Honma H, et al. Sunray appearance on enhanced magnetic resonance image of cardiac angiosarcoma with pericardial obliteration. Am Heart J 1994;127:468-471.

77. Chryssogonidis IA, Vorkas GA, Papadopoulos XA, Dimitriadis AS. Angiosarcoma of right cardiac atrium. JBR-BTR 2006;89:118-119.

78. Kuppahally SS, Litwin SE, Michaels AD. Endomyocardial biopsy of right atrial angiosarcoma guided by intracardiac echocardiography. Cardiol Res Pract 2010;2010:681726.

79. Vaidya OU, Dobson JR 3rd, Wible BC, Main ML. Usefulness of multimodality cardiac imaging in the diagnosis of a right atrial angiosarcoma. J Am Soc Echocardiogr 2010;23:792.e3-4.

80. Park WK, Jung SH, Lim JY. Cardiac angiosarcoma on the right atrium: two cases. Korean J Thorac Cardiovasc Surg 2012;45:120-123.

81. Higashiyama S, Kawabe J, Hayashi T, et al. Effectiveness of preoperative PET examination of huge angiosarcoma of the heart. Clin Nucl Med 2009;34:99-102.

82. Bilski M, Kaminski G, Dziuk M. Metabolic activity assessment of cardiac angiosarcoma by 18FDG PET-CT. Nucl Med Rev Cent East Eur 2012;15:83-84.

83. Nakamura-Horigome M, Koyama J, Eizawa T, et al. Successful treatment of primary cardiac angiosarcoma with docetaxel and radiotherapy. Angiology 2008;59:368-371.

84. Tan H1, Jiang L, Gao Y, Zeng Z, Shi H. 18F-FDG PET/CT imaging in primary cardiac angiosarcoma: diagnosis and follow-up. Clin Nucl Med 2013;38:1002-1005.

85. Juergens KU, Hoffmeier A, Riemann B, Maintz D. Early detection of local tumour recurrence and pulmonary metastasis in cardiac angiosarcoma with PET-CT and MRI. Eur Heart J 2007;28:663.

86. Malani AK, Hindupur M, Gupta C. Vascular tumour blush of cardiac angiosarcoma on coronary angiography. Heart 2007;93:1237.

87. Khanji M, Lee E, Ionescu A. Blushing primary cardiac angiosarcoma. Heart 2014;100:266.

88. Yildiz A, Yakut N, Kurtoglu T, Okcun B, Kupelioglu A. Primary cardiac angiosarcoma with right coronary-to-right atrium fistula. Cardiovasc J Afr 2008;19:26-27.

89. Poole-Wilson PA, Farnsworth A, Braimbridge MV, Pambakian H. Angiosarcoma of pericardium. Problems in diagnosis and management. Br Heart J 1976;38:240-243.

90. Berry MF, Williams M, Welsby I, Lin S. Cardiac angiosarcoma presenting with right coronary artery pseudoaneurysm. J Cardiothorac Vasc Anesth 2010;24:633-635.

91. Tang K, Shang QL, Zhou QC, Zhou JW, She XL, Zhang M. Primary cardiac angiosarcoma with spontaneous ruptures of the right atrium and right coronary artery. Echocardiography 2013; 30:E156-160.

92. Bhalla R, Nassar A. Cardiac angiosarcoma: report of a case diagnosed by echocardiographic-guided fine-needle aspiration. Diagn Cytopathol 2007;35:164-166.

93. Iwa N, Masuda K, Yutani C, Kobayashi TK. Imprint cytology of primary cardiac sarcomas: A report of 3 cases. Ann Diagn Pathol 2009;13:239-245.

94. Savoia MT, Liguori C, Nahar T, et al. Transesophageal echocardiography-guided transvenous biopsy of a cardiac sarcoma. J Am Soc Echocardiogr 1997;10:752-755.

95. Agaimy A, Kaiser A, Wunsch PH. [Epithelioid hemangioendothelioma of the heart in association with myelodysplastic syndrome.] Z Kardiol 2002;91:352-356. [German]

96. Goldblum JR, Folpe AL, Weiss SW. Enzinger and Weiss's soft tissue tumors, 6th ed. Philadelphia: Saunders/Elsevier; 2014.

97. Thomas-de-Montpreville V, Nottin R, Dulmet E, Serraf A. Heart tumors in children and adults: clinicopathological study of 59 patients from a surgical center. Cardiovasc Pathol 2007;16:22-28.

98. Matzke LA, Knowling MA, Grant D, et al. A rare cardiac neoplasm: case report of cardiac epithelioid angiosarcoma. Cardiovasc Pathol 2011;20:e197-201.

99. Lin BT, Colby T, Gown AM, et al. Malignant vascular tumors of the serous membranes mimicking mesothelioma. A report of 14 cases. Am J Surg Pathol 1996;20:1431-1439.

100. Deyrup AT, McKenney JK, Tighiouart M, Folpe AL, Weiss SW. Sporadic cutaneous angiosarcomas: a proposal for risk stratification based on 69 cases. Am J Surg Pathol 2008;32:72-77.

101. Deyrup AT, Miettinen M, North PE, et al. Angiosarcomas arising in the viscera and soft tissue of children and young adults: a clinicopathologic study of 15 cases. Am J Surg Pathol 2009;33:264-269.

102. Tazelaar HD, Locke TJ, McGregor CG. Pathology of surgically excised primary cardiac tumors. Mayo Clin Proc 1992;67:957-965.

103. Miettinen M, Wang ZF, Paetau A, et al. ERG transcription factor as an immunohistochemical marker for vascular endothelial tumors and prostatic carcinoma. Am J Surg Pathol 2011;35: 432-441.

104. Folpe AL, Chand EM, Goldblum JR, Weiss SW. Expression of Fli-1, a nuclear transcription factor, distinguishes vascular neoplasms from potential mimics. Am J Surg Pathol 2001;25:1061-1066.

105. Killion MJ, Brodovsky HS, Schwarting R. Pericardial angiosarcoma after mediastinal irradiation for seminoma. A case report and a review of the literature. Cancer 1996;78:912-917.

106. Zu Y, Perle MA, Yan Z, Liu J, Kumar A, Waisman J. Chromosomal abnormalities and p53 gene mutation in a cardiac angiosarcoma. Appl Immunohistochem Molecul Morphol 2001;9:24-28.

107. Schuborg C, Mertens F, Rydholm A, et al. Cytogenetic analysis of four angiosarcomas from deep and superficial soft tissue. Cancer Genet Cytogenet 1998;100:52-56.

108. Garcia JM, Gonzalez R, Silva JM, et al. Mutational status of K-ras and TP53 genes in primary sarcomas of the heart. Br J Cancer 2000;82: 1183-1185.

109. Naka N, Tomita Y, Nakanishi H, et al. Mutations of p53 tumor-suppressor gene in angiosarcoma. Int J Cancer 1997;71:952-955.

110. Hong HH, Devereux TR, Melnick RL, Moomaw CR, Boorman GA, Sills RC. Mutations of ras protooncogenes and p53 tumor suppressor gene in cardiac hemangiosarcomas from B6C3F1 mice exposed to 1,3-butadiene for 2 years. Toxicol Pathol 2000;28:529-534.

111. Wong CW, El-Jack S, Edwards C, Patel H. Primary cardiac angiosarcoma: morphologically deceptive benign appearance and potential pitfalls in diagnosis. Heart Lung Circ 2010;19:473-475.

112. Slepicka C, Durci M. Cardiac angiosarcoma treated with resection and adjuvant radiation therapy. J La State Med Soc 2012;164:92-93.

113. Elbardissi AW, Dearani JA, Daly RC, et al. Survival after resection of primary cardiac tumors: a 48-year experience. Circulation 2008;118:S7-15.

114. Kamiya H, Yasuda T, Nagamine H, et al. Surgical treatment of primary cardiac tumors: 28 years' experience in kanazawa university hospital. Jpn Circ J 2001;65:315-319.

115. Simpson L, Kumar SK, Okuno SH, et al. Malignant primary cardiac tumors: review of a single institution experience. Cancer 2008;112:2440-2446.

116. Pigott C, Welker M, Khosla P, Higgins RS. Improved outcome with multimodality therapy in primary cardiac angiosarcoma. Nat Clin Pract Oncol 2008;5:112-115.

117. Benassi F, Maiorana A, Melandri F, Stefanelli G. A case of primary cardiac angiosarcoma: extensive right atrial wall reconstruction with autologous pericardium. J Card Surg 2010;25: 282-284.

118. Nath MP, Dhawan N, Chauhan S, Kiran U. A large angiosarcoma of the right atrium involving tricuspid valve and right ventricle. Ann Card Anaesth 2010;13:165-166.

119. Liu XR, Miao Q, Zhang CJ, Guo QB, Di Y. Successful resection of cardiac angiosarcoma combined with right coronary artery bypass grafting. Chin Med Sci J 2007;22:66-68.

120. Sanli M, Tuncozgur B, Sevinc A, Daglar B, Bakir K, Elbeyli L. Surgical treatment of a giant primary cardiac angiosarcoma. Acta Medica (Hradec Kralove) 2008;51:237-239.

121. Aoka Y, Kamada T, Kawana M, et al. Primary cardiac angiosarcoma treated with carbon-ion radiotherapy. Lancet Oncol 2004;5:636-638.

122. Frota Filho JD, Lucchese FA, Leaes P, Valente LA, Vieira MS, Blacher C. Primary cardiac angiosarcoma. A therapeutical dilemma. Arq Bras Cardiol 2002;78:586-591.

123. Hoffmeier A, Scheld HH, Tjan TD, et al. Ex situ resection of primary cardiac tumors. Thorac Cardiovasc Surg 2003;51:99-101.

124. Sinatra R, Brancaccio G, di Gioia CR, De Santis M, Sbraga F, Gallo P. Integrated approach for cardiac angiosarcoma. Int J Cardiol 2003;88:301-304.

125. Stein M, Deitling F, Cantor A, Perner Y, Bezwoda W. Primary cardiac angiosarcoma: a case report and review of therapeutic options. Med Pediatr Oncol 1994;23:149-152

126. Uberfuhr P, Meiser B, Fuchs A, et al. Heart transplantation: an approach to treating primary cardiac sarcoma? J Heart Lung Transplant 2002;21:1135-1139.

127. Kodali D, Seetharaman K. Primary cardiac angiosarcoma. Sarcoma 2006;2006:39130.

128. Ram Prabu MP, Thulkar S, Ray R, Bakhshi S. Primary cardiac angiosarcoma with good response to Paclitaxel. J Thorac Oncol 2011;6:1778-1779.

129. Suderman D, Cooke A, Wong R, Klein J. Treatment of cardiac angiosarcoma with radiation and docetaxel: A case report with partial response and prolonged stable disease. J Thorac Oncol 2011;6:834-835.

130. Rhomberg W, Grass M. [Angiosarcoma of the right atrium: Local control via low radiation doses and razoxane. A case report.] Strahlenther Onkol 1999;175:102-104. [German]

131. Blondeau P. Primary cardiac tumors. French studies of 533 cases. Thorac Cardiovasc Surg 1990;38:192-195.

132. Erpolat OP, Icli F, Dogan OV, et al. Primary cardiac angiosarcoma: a case report. Tumori 2008;94:892-897.

133. Herr W, Schwarting A, Wittig B, et al. Enormous hemangiosarcoma of the heart. Clin Investig 1994;72:372-376.

134. Val-Bernal JF, Figols J, Arce FP, Sanz-Ortiz J. Cardiac epithelioid angiosarcoma presenting as cutaneous metastases. J Cutan Pathol 2001; 28:265-270.

135. Liassides C, Katsamaga M, Deretzi G, Koutsimanis V, Zacharakis G. Cerebral metastasis from heart angiosarcoma presenting as multiple hematomas. J Neuroimaging 2004;14:71-73.

136. Jung SH, Jung TY, Joo SP, Kim HS. Rapid clinical course of cerebral metastatic angiosarcoma from the heart. J Korean Neurosurg Soc 2012;51:47-50.

137. Kim EK, Park IS, Sohn BS, et al. Angiosarcomas of the bilateral breast and heart: which one is the primary site? Korean J Intern Med 2012;27:224-228.

138. Messias P, Bernardo J, Antunes MJ. Primary left atrial haemangioendothelioma. Interact Cardiovasc Thorac Surg 2008;7:945-946.

139. Safirstein J, Aksenov S, Smith F. Cardiac epithelioid hemangioendothelioma with 8-year follow-up. Cardiovasc Pathol 2007;16:183-186.

140. Lisy M, Beierlein W, Muller H, Bultmann B, Ziemer G. Left atrial epithelioid hemangioendothelioma. J Thorac Cardiovasc Surg 2007; 133:803-804.

141. Moulai N, Chavanon O, Guillou L, et al. Atypical primary epithelioid hemangioendothelioma of the heart. J Thorac Oncol 2006;1:188-189.

142. Guray Y, Demirkan B, Guray U, Boyaci A. Right atrial hemangioendothelioma: a three-dimensional echocardiographic evaluation. Anadolu Kardiyol Derg 2010;10:E7-8.

143. Marchiano D, Fisher F, Hofstetter S. Epithelioid hemangioendothelioma of the heart with distant metastases. A case report and literature review. J Cardiovasc Surg (Torino) 1993;34:529-533.

144. Makhlouf HR, Ishak KG, Goodman ZD. Epithelioid hemangioendothelioma of the liver: a clinicopathologic study of 137 cases. Cancer 1999;85:562-582.

145. de Nictolis M, Brancorsini D, Goteri G, Prat J. Epithelioid haemangioma of the heart. Virchows Arch 1996;428:119-123.

146. Bossert T, Gummert JF, Battellini R, et al. Surgical experience with 77 primary cardiac tumors. Interact Cardiovasc Thorac Surg 2005;4:311-315.

147. Endo A, Ohtahara A, Kinugawa T, et al. Characteristics of 161 patients with cardiac tumors diagnosed during 1993 and 1994 in Japan. Am J Cardiol 1997;79:1708-1711.

148. Matebele MP, Peters P, Mundy J, Shah P. Cardiac tumors in adults: surgical management and follow-up of 19 patients in an australian tertiary hospital. Interact Cardiovasc Thorac Surg 2010;10:892-895.

# 16 PRIMARY CARDIAC SARCOMAS, OTHER THAN ANGIOSARCOMA

## GENERAL FEATURES

*Primary cardiac sarcomas* are malignant mesenchymal tumors that arise in the heart. In addition to those with endothelial differentiation (angiosarcoma, see chapter 15), they represent a wide range of histologic types. The classification of soft tissue sarcoma is based on the differentiation of tumor cells to a specific cell type (Table 16-1). Cardiac sarcomas presumably arise from stromal stem cells that occur anywhere in the heart, which may differentiate into virtually any soft tissue. Tumor classification is facilitated in some instances by cytogenetic alterations that identify a certain tumor type and may impact prognosis and treatment.

In series of primary cardiac malignancies, most are sarcomas, about a third of which are angiosarcomas (Table 16-2) (1). The second most common subtype are those with fibrous or myofibroblastic differentiation, sometimes with heterologous matrix-forming sarcoma, which include a range of overlapping growth patterns. These include well-differentiated sarcomas (usually with prominent collagen or myxoid matrix, sometimes referred to as myxofibrosarcoma); undifferentiated sarcoma with pleomorphic spindle cells (also known as malignant fibrous histiocytoma, or MFH); and undifferentiated sarcomas without significant spindling. The World Health Organization (WHO) has recently classified undifferentiated sarcomas into round cell, spindle cell, pleomorphic, and "not otherwise specified" groups (2). Unfortunately, there is no universally accepted nomenclature for these types of sarcoma in the heart. The third largest group of cardiac sarcomas includes specific subtypes with corresponding soft tissue counterparts, including leiomyosarcoma, synovial sarcoma, rhabdomyosarcoma, and liposarcoma.

For the purpose of this chapter, cardiac sarcomas that typically form intracavitary, endocardial-based tumors are grouped into 5 headings. *Myxofibrosarcoma* has no specific soft tissue counterpart, and includes the previously termed myxoid MFH, and possibly undifferentiated spindle cell sarcoma according to the recent WHO classification (2), and is relatively well-differentiated. *Undifferentiated pleomorphic sarcomas* are tumors that were previously called MFH, and are high-grade tumors with some evidence of fibroblastic or myofibroblastic differentiation and a disorganized spindled "storiform" pattern. *Undifferentiated sarcomas* (not otherwise specified) are composed of discohesive rounded or epithelioid cells and correspond to round cell and epithelioid types of undifferentiated sarcoma of soft tissue (2). *Osteosarcoma* is the term for any of the above growth patterns (most frequently pleomorphic undifferentiated) with osteosarcoma or chondrosarcoma. *Leiomyosarcoma* is used for low- or high-grade sarcomas with uniform fascicular or epithelioid patterns and expression of smooth muscle-specific antigens, especially desmin; they conceptually arise either from precursor spindle cells of the atrial endocardium or adjacent veins, especially pulmonary veins. The term *undifferentiated spindle cell sarcoma* will be used for MFH, unless citing a specific reference using the term, in which case it will be designated in quotation marks. The first four groups often show overlapping patterns.

Although there is no consensus regarding how to classify tumors with heterogenous histologic features, it seems appropriate to classify them by defining areas, even in a minority of the tumor. In other words, tumors with any osteosarcoma or chondrosarcoma, significant myxoid areas, and pleomorphic storiform growth pattern, would exclude the designation undifferentiated sarcoma, and would be designated based on the feature in the order listed.

The subclassification of cardiac sarcomas in published series varies widely, especially because of the lack of reproducibility in certain categories, such as the divisions among undifferentiated pleomorphic sarcomas, "MFH," and myxofibrosarcoma.

**Table 16-1**

**CLASSIFICATION OF CARDIAC SARCOMAS, INCLUDING ANGIOSARCOMA**

| Cellular Differentiation | Diagnostic Designation | Comments |
|---|---|---|
| Endothelial differentiation | Angiosarcoma[a] | High-grade tumor composed of anastomosing channels, spindled cells, or epithelioid cells with endothelial differentiation; epithelioid type may express cytokeratins |
| | Epithelioid hemangioendothelioma | Low-grade tumor with characteristic cord-like growth of bland occasionally vacuolated cells that express endothelial and epithelial markers |
| "Intimal" origin with myofibroblastic differentiation | Myxofibrosarcoma | Spindle cell tumor with variably fibrous and/or myxoid background, without significant pleomorphism, cellularity, or necrosis; lacks "storiform" pattern; has variety of synonyms (fibrosarcoma, myxosarcoma, fibromyxosarcomas); usually smooth muscle actin positive |
| | Pleomorphic spindle cell sarcoma | Similar to myxofibrosarcoma (which is often present), with storiform pattern, necrosis, or dense cellularity; smooth muscle actin often negative; the term "malignant fibrous histiocytoma" is gradually being phased out for soft tissue counterparts |
| | Leiomyosarcoma | Similar to leiomyosarcomas of soft tissue, may be low- or high grade, may have epithelioid features; expresses desmin (at least focally) in addition to actin; typical histologic features |
| | Osteosarcoma (matrix-forming sarcomas) | Areas of osteosarcoma, malignant giant cell tumor, or chondrosarcoma; usually with areas of myxofibrosarcoma or pleomorphic spindle cell sarcoma |
| | Undifferentiated sarcoma | Sheets of polygonal or small cells, without significant fibrous or myxoid matrix; negative markers/genetics for synovial sarcoma, rhabdomyosarcoma, MPNST[b], or primitive neuroectodermal tumor (CD99); increased frequency of diagnosis with limited sampling |
| Striated muscle differentiation | Rhabdomyosarcoma | Far less frequent than angiosarcoma or myofibrointimal sarcomas; most common in children and young adults |
| Miscellaneous differentiation (all identical to those in soft tissue) | Synovial sarcoma | The most common cardiac sarcoma after those of endothelial or myofibrointimal differentiation; biphasic growth (EMA, pancytokeratin positive areas) in over half; X;18 translocation positive by FISH or PCR |
| | Liposarcoma | Rare in the myocardium or pericardium |
| | Malignant solitary fibrous tumor | Overlap with malignant hemangiopericytoma; usually in the pericardium |
| | Malignant peripheral nerve sheath tumor | "Triton" tumor if there is rhabdomyosarcoma |
| | Malignant mesenchymoma | Combination of two types of specific differentiation, other than myofibroblastic types (e.g., chondrosarcoma and angiosarcoma) |

[a]May have epithelioid features but differs from epithelioid hemangioepithelioma, a low-grade neoplasm.
[b]MPNST = malignant peripheral nerve sheath tumor; EMA = epithelial membrane antigen; FISH = fluoresence in situ hybridization; PCR = polymerase chain reaction.

In older series, there was an over-representation of rhabdomyosarcoma, which was diagnosed in the absence of confirmatory immunohistochemical staining. In recent series, the largest group is undifferentiated sarcoma, followed by angiosarcoma. Other relatively common types include leiomyosarcomas, synovial sarcoma (3), and undifferentiated sarcomas with matrix formation (osteosarcoma and chondrosarcoma).

The most common site for spindle cell sarcomas of various types, including matrix-forming tumors, is the left atrium (4), in contrast to angiosarcoma, with its predilection for the right atrium (see chapter 15) (5). Of 110 primary heart tumors excised at Mayo Clinic, 8 patients had primary cardiac sarcomas: angiosarcoma, leiomyosarcoma, and MFH in two patients each and undifferentiated and osteogenic sarcoma in

**Table 16-2**

**FREQUENCY OF HISTOLOGIC SUBTYPES OF CARDIAC SARCOMAS, INCLUDING ANGIOSARCOMA[a]**

| Type | Frequency (n,%) | Mean age, years ± S.D. | % Male |
|---|---|---|---|
| Pleomorphic spindle sarcoma | 50 (26%) | 48 ± 21 | 46% |
| Angiosarcoma | 47 (24%) | 40 ± 17 | 79% |
| Undifferentiated sarcoma | 20 (10%) | 51 ± 20 | 45% |
| Osteosarcoma (matrix-forming sarcoma) | 19 (10%) | 40 ± 18 | 37% |
| Fibromyxosarcoma | 18 (9%) | 42 ± 19 | 56% |
| Leiomyosarcoma | 14 (7%) | 27 ± 16 | 57% |
| Synovial sarcoma | 9 (5%) | 46 ± 13 | 89% |
| Rhabdomyosarcoma | 8 (4%) | 20 ± 16 | 25% |
| MPNST[b] | 2 (<1%) | 52 ± 5 | 100% |
| Liposarcoma | 2 (<1%) | 67 ± 4 | 50% |
| EHE, malignant SFT, malignant mesenchymoma | 1 each (1.5% total) | 71, 21, 46 | 0% |
| Total | 192 (100%) | 43 ± 20 | 56% |

[a]From a database of 192 tumors seen by one coauthor in consultation.
[b]MPNST = malignant peripheral nerve sheath tumor; EHE = epithelioid hemangioendothelioma; SFT= solitary fibrous tumor.

**Table 16-3**

**SITES OF MOST COMMON CARDIAC SARCOMA SUBTYPES (OTHER THAN ANGIOSARCOMA)[a]**

| Type (n) | LA[b] (n, %) | RA | Biatrial | RV | LV | Valve | Pericardium | Multiple Chambers |
|---|---|---|---|---|---|---|---|---|
| Pleomorphic spindle sarcoma (50) | 31 (62%) | 3 (6%) | 1 (2%) | 7 (14%) | 4 (8%) | 0 | 3 (6%) | 1 (2%) |
| Fibromyxosarcoma (18) | 9 (50%) | 4 (22%) | 0 | 2 (11%) | 3 (17%) | 0 | 0 | 0 |
| Undifferentiated sarcoma (20) | 12 (60%) | 4 (20%) | 0 | 3 (15%) | 1 (5%) | 0 | 0 | 0 |
| Matrix-forming sarcoma (19) | 15 (79%) | 0 | 0 | 2 (11%) | 1 (5%) | 1 (5%) | 0 | 0 |
| Leiomyosarcoma (16) | 9 (64%) | 2 (14%) | 0 | 0 | 1 (7%) | 1 (7%) | 1 (7%) | 0 |
| Synovial sarcoma | 1 (11%) | 2 (22%) | 0 | 2 (22%) | 2 (22%) | | 2 (22%) | 0 |
| Rhabdomyosarcoma | 1 (12.5%) | 1 (12.5%) | 0 | 1 (12.5%) | 4 (50%) | 0 | 1 (12.5%) | 0 |
| Total (including rare sarcomas) | 83 (43%) | 41 (21%) | 3 (2%) | 30 (15%) | 16 (8%) | 3 (2%) | 15 (8%) | 1 (<1%) |

[a]From database presented in Table 16-1.
[b]LA = left atrium; RA = right atrium; RV = right ventricle; LV = left ventricle.

one patient each (5). In a series of unresectable left atrial tumors, the majority were sarcomas, either undifferentiated sarcomas or "MFH" (7). In a compilation of recently published surgically excised heart tumors, the majority (26 percent) were designated by different terms for "MFH" (a term no longer used), followed by angiosarcoma, undifferentiated sarcoma, osteosarcoma, fibromyxosarcoma (under various designations), and a few others (Table 16-2). In recent series, undifferentiated spindle cell sarcomas with or without smooth muscle or osteochondrosarcomatous differentiation

(undifferentiated pleomorphic sarcoma, undifferentiated sarcoma, fibromyxosarcoma, leiomyosarcoma, osteosarcoma) were seen at least 50 percent of the time in the left atrium, usually as endoluminal growths (Table 16-3). Also, it is not unusual for the same left atrial sarcoma to show low-grade areas similar to fibrosarcoma, areas typical of "MFH," and undifferentiated areas with or without matrix formation.

The percentage of sarcomas (including angiosarcomas) among heart tumors in surgical resection series varies, but is approximately 10 percent (1,8–10). In a series from China, the rate

**Table 16-4**

**CHARACTERISTICS OF 106 REPORTED CARDIAC SARCOMAS (OTHER THAN ANGIOSARCOMAS)[a]**

| | |
|---|---|
| Histologic types (number) | Undifferentiated pleomorphic sarcoma[b], 23 |
| | Myxofibrosarcoma[c], 15 |
| | Undifferentiated[d], 20 |
| | Leiomyosarcoma, 19 |
| | Synovial sarcoma, 10 |
| | Rhabdomyosarcoma, 8 |
| | Extraskeletal osteosarcoma[e], 5 |
| | Malignant peripheral nerve sheath tumor, 3 |
| | Malignant SFT,[f] 1 |
| | Malignant mesenchymoma, 1 |
| | Liposarcoma, 1 |
| % male | 55% |
| Age in years (range)[g] | 42 (4–84) |
| Site in heart | |
| LA[h] | 40% |
| RV/PV | 28% |
| RA | 26% |
| LV | 5% |
| pericardium | 1% |
| Surgical procedure | Resection with positive margin, 18/53 |
| | Complete excision, 16/53 |
| | Excision after chemotherapy, 1/53 |
| | Partial resection/debulking, 4/53 |
| | Reresection, 3/53 |
| | Transplant, 2/53 |
| | Autotransplant, 4/53 |
| | Biopsy, 5/53 |
| Chemotherapy | 75%, often only if positive margins or metastatic disease |
| Prognosis | Post-op deaths, 5 |
| | Dead of disease, 26 (1 month–131 months) |
| | 7 NED[i]: 13, 18, 22, 60, 34, 36, and 78 months |
| | Median survival: 17 months[j] |
| Features associated with poor prognosis | High grade (Zhan et al., p=.05) |
| | Incomplete excision (p=.01), metastases at the time of diagnosis (Simpson et al., p = .05) |

[a]Data from references 3, 14, 17, 20, 57, 58, 74–76, 211, and 212. Some tumors were excluded based on benign clinical course and lack of histologic documentation. Many tumors were not documented immunohistochemically. Rhabdomyosarcomas are often over-represented in surgical series not documented immunohistochemically.

[b]Variably designated malignant fibrous histiocytoma, undifferentiated pleomorphic.

[c]Variably designated fibrosarcoma, myxoid fibrosarcoma, myxoid sarcoma.

[d]Often designated unclassified in series with others designated as malignant fibrous histiocytoma (MFH) or pleomorphic sarcoma; the nine unclassified in Kim et al.'s series (74a) are placed in this group as there were none in the pleomorphic category and based on histologic illustration.

[e]Designated osteosarcoma, chondrosarcoma.

[f]SFT = solitary fibrous tumor.

[g]Two sarcomas in infants were not included, as they had an excellent prognosis and were not histologically documented, and possibly represented inflammatory myofibroblastic tumors.

[h]Two designated as pedunculated.

[i]No evidence of disorder.

[j]Versus 5 months for angiosarcoma (Simpson et al. (200), p=.04).

was somewhat higher, close to 20 percent (11), a rate similar to that reported in an older series from Stanford (12). Overall, the rate ranges from 6 percent (13,14) to anywhere between 8 and 40 percent (15–21). In a compilation of recent series (13,14,20–23), however, the overall estimate of primary cardiac sarcomas, as a proportion of surgically resected heart tumors, was 10 percent (4 percent angiosarcoma, 6 percent other sarcomas) (1).

**Table 16-5**

**THE NATIONAL CANCER INSTITUTE (NCI) GRADING SYSTEM FOR SOFT TISSUE SARCOMAS**

| Grade 1 | Grade 2 | Grade 3 |
|---|---|---|
| [Well differentiated and myxoid liposarcoma][a] Epithelioid hemangioendothelioma | [Pleomorphic liposarcoma] Fibrosarcoma[b] Malignant fibrous histiocytoma[d] Synovial sarcoma Leiomyosarcoma [Neurofibrosarcoma] | Alveolar rhabdomyosarcoma Osteosarcoma[c] PNET (primitive neuroectodermal tumor) Alveolar soft part sarcoma Chondrosarcoma[b] |
| No tumor necrosis | Or necrosis, < 15% | Or necrosis, >15% |

[a]Tumors in brackets occur rarely, if ever, in the heart.
[b]To include myxofibrosarcoma in current classification.
[c]Mesenchymal or extraskeletal, by definition if applied to cardiac tumors.
[d]Pleomorphic undifferentiated sarcoma with storiform features.

**Table 16-6**

**THE FÉDÉRATION NATIONALE DES CENTRES DE LUTTE CONTRE LE CANCER (FNCLCC) GRADING SYSTEM FOR SOFT TISSUE SARCOMAS**

| Numeric Score | Differentiation Score | Mitotic Score Per 10 High-Power Fields | Necrosis | Overall Grade |
|---|---|---|---|---|
| 0 | N/A | N/A | None | Grade I: sum of scores = 2-3 |
| 1 | Resembling adult mesenchymal tissue[a] | 0-9 | < 50% | Grade II: sum of scores = 4-5 |
| 2 | Certain histotype[b] | 10-19 | > 50% | Grade III: sum of scores = 6-8 |
| 3 | Embryonal/undifferentiated or uncertain differentiation[c] | 20 or more | N/A | |

[a]Includes well-differentiated leiomyosarcoma, fibrosarcoma, and liposarcoma; only the first has been reported in the heart.
[b]Includes myxoid liposarcoma, fibrosarcoma, myxofibrosarcoma, pleomorphic undifferentiated sarcoma with storiform pattern (MFH), leiomyosarcoma, well-differentiated angiosarcoma.
[c]Including *synovial sarcomas*, epithelioid sarcomas, *osteosarcomas*, embryonal sarcomas, round cell liposarcoma, *pleomorphic liposarcoma*, poorly differentiated fibrosarcoma, *pleomorphic undifferentiated sarcoma* (without storiform pattern), *poorly differentiated or epithelioid leiomyosarcoma, rhabdomyosarcoma, chondrosarcoma, primitive neuroectodermal tumor, poorly differentiated or epithelioid angiosarcoma*, epithelioid sarcoma, and clear cell sarcoma; those in italics have been described in the heart.

If all the subtypes of cardiac sarcoma (other than angiosarcoma) are taken together, there is a slight male predominance, with a mean age of 42 years at surgery. Only one third are resectable without residual tumor (Table 16-4).

There is no known cause for cardiac sarcoma. One "MFH" of the mitral valve was reported years after mitral valve replacement, obstructing the mitral valve orifice and presenting as a cerebral embolism, diagnosed at autopsy (24).

## GRADING

There is no single established grading scheme for soft tissue sarcomas, and none has been modified for cardiac sarcomas. Several recent reviews address the complexities of grading schemes, which generally involve the histo-pathologic type, mitotic activity, and presence of necrosis (25–28). The major schemes include that of the National Cancer Institute (NCI), which is now over 25 years old (Table 16-5) (29) and the more recent Fédération Nationale des Centres de Lutte Contre le Cancer (FNCLCC) grading system (Table 16-6) (25,26).

The differences between the NCI and FNCLCC grading systems include the absence of a mitotic rate in the NCI system, lesser amount of tumor necrosis in the NCI scheme as a cut-off (15 percent versus 50 percent), and the different placement of some tumor types (for example, synovial sarcoma).

The difficulties in the application of a grading system include the quantification of necrosis, the changing classifications of low-grade tumors

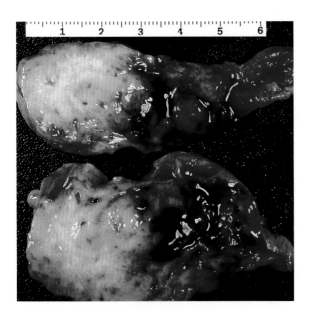

**Figure 16-1**

**LEFT ATRIAL SARCOMA**

A 70-year-old man presented with dyspnea; an echocardiogram demonstrated a left atrial mass. Histologically, the tumor had pleomorphic undifferentiated areas, as well as areas of malignant fibrous histiocytoma (MFH). The cut surface is variegated, with solid hemorrhagic and necrotic areas.

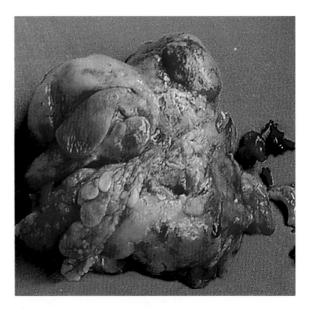

**Figure 16-2**

**LEFT ATRIAL SARCOMA**

A 20-year-old man presented with dyspnea. An echocardiogram demonstrated a left atrial tumor, histologically a leiomyosarcoma. Better-differentiated low-grade sarcomas lack the gross features of necrosis, and are relatively homogeneous on cut section, as here.

such as myxofibrosarcoma, and the confusion about the distinction between undifferentiated pleomorphic sarcoma and "MFH." Furthermore, angiosarcoma, one of the more common heart sarcomas, is not included in a grading system but considered high-grade regardless of the histologic features. It has been recommended that the MIB-1 (Ki-67) proliferative index be substituted for the mitotic count to improve reproducibility (30–32). In this scheme, a proliferative index of 0 to 9 percent is substituted for a mitotic rate of 0 to 9 mitoses per 10 high-power fields; 10 to 29 percent is substituted for a mitotic rate of 10 to 19 mitoses per 10 high-power fields; and 30 percent or more is substituted for a mitotic rate of over 20 mitoses per 10 high-power fields.

## CLINICAL AND RADIOLOGIC FEATURES

The initial clinical symptoms that result from cardiac tumors are generally related to the size and site of the mass, and not the histologic type of tumor. In general, symptoms are caused either by obstruction of blood flow, which may result in heart failure or pulmonary hypertension, with dyspnea and cough (33); superior

vena cava obstruction (34); embolic phenomena (24); ischemia or pericardial abnormalities causing chest pain (35); growth into airways with hemoptysis (36); or pericardial constriction due to effusions. Rarely, tumor infiltration results in ventricular arrhythmias and sudden death (37). Systemic symptoms such as weight loss are common, as with any malignancy (33).

Echocardiography establishes the presence of a cardiac tumor in most cases. Computed tomography (CT) and magnetic resonance imaging (MRI) provide additional information, owing to their superior resolution. Calcification and fat are detected with CT, and better characterization of the heart, pericardium, mediastinum, and lungs is done with MRI. The addition of contrast helps distinguish the neoplasm from myocardium, thrombus, and blood flow artifact.

MRI best facilitates surgical planning and post-treatment follow-up with its superior resolution (38). Three-dimensional echocardiography with MRI has been used to delineate the extent of invasion preoperatively (39). Features that indicate malignancy with MRI include

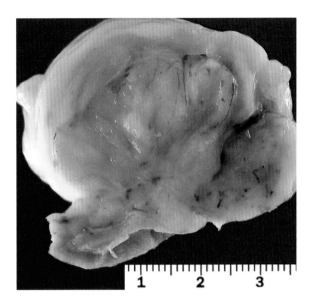

**Figure 16-3**

**LEFT ATRIAL SARCOMA**

A 30-year-old man had a left atrial mass surgically removed, requiring atrial reconstruction. The tumor was a well-differentiated myxofibrosarcoma histologically, reflected in the homogeneous gross appearance of this low-grade sarcoma.

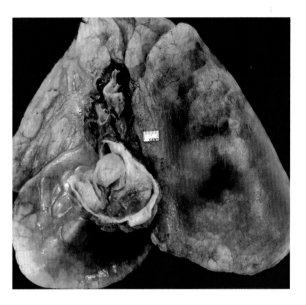

**Figure 16-4**

**LEFT ATRIAL SARCOMA**

A 50-year-old female presented with shortness of breath. Open heart surgery demonstrated an osteosarcoma of the left atrium, which was growing into the right pulmonary veins, necessitating right pneumonectomy (see fig. 3-30).

wide point of attachment to the endocardium; large size with near complete occupation of the cardiac chamber; involvement of more than one cardiac chamber or great vessel; pericardial or extracardiac extension; and the identification of necrosis (40,41). Features on MRI have been reported as useful in a variety of cases of primary cardiac sarcoma (42–45). When the sarcoma arises in the left atrium, cardiac sarcoma can mimic cardiac myxoma (46).

## TISSUE SAMPLING AND GROSS SPECIMEN HANDLING

Most cardiac tumors are sampled as open surgical resections, after the diagnosis is made by imaging (Table 16-4). When frozen section is requested, a diagnosis of malignancy should be considered if the typical features of myxoma are not present, if there is infiltration of the atrial wall, or if the tumor does not arise from the atrial septum, as is typical of myxoma. The resection margin should be noted (and inked if possible), as well as involvement of tumor margins, on the final diagnostic report. Occasionally, the diagnosis is made by biopsy (Table 16-4) or fine-needle aspiration (47).

Most cardiac sarcomas are bulky, infiltrating, nodular masses with irregular margins (figs. 16-1–16-4). Occasionally, sarcomas are discrete masses that are pedunculated and mimic myxomas. Although typically firm and white, areas of hemorrhage or calcification can impart a variegated and gritty surface. Most sarcomas of the heart, other than angiosarcomas (see chapter 15), occur in the left atrium, although any site may be involved, including the ventricle (48,49).

## SARCOMA VARIANTS

### Cardiac Sarcomas of "Intimal" Origin

The term *"intimal" sarcoma* denotes the site of origin rather than the tumor cell differentiation. It is generally used for sarcomas of the great vessels (50), although the term is also applied to sarcomas in the left atrium (51–53). The reason for using the term "intimal" is that sarcomas of left atrial origin are often exophytic intraluminal masses, which may have a narrow stalk or base of attachment, similar to cardiac myxoma. Therefore, the site of origin of these tumors is considered to be the intimal myofibroblasts, a concept that is strengthened based on the finding

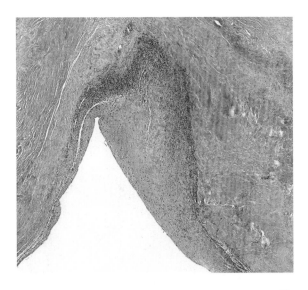 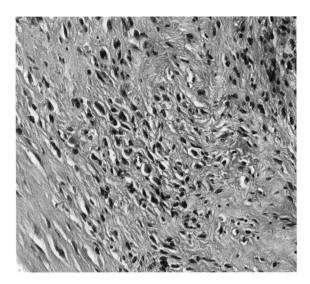

**Figure 16-5**

**CARDIAC OSTEOSARCOMA: INTIMAL SPREAD**

Left: Left atrial sarcomas can grow laterally along the endocardium, giving credence to the concept of an intimal origin.
Right: At higher magnification, the intimal growth is deceptively bland. This tumor was at the edge of the sarcoma with the osteosarcomatous differentiation illustrated in figure 16-33.

of intimal atypia (in situ sarcoma) (8) adjacent to some left atrial tumors (fig. 16-5), as well as the preponderance of tumors with fibroblastic or smooth muscle cell differentiation in this location. Recently, the finding of MDM2 nuclear expression in pleomorphic sarcomas of the left atrium has enforced the concept of "intimal cardiac sarcoma" because intimal sarcomas of the pulmonary artery also demonstrate amplification of the *MDM2* gene (53a).

### Undifferentiated Cardiac Sarcomas

After angiosarcoma, *undifferentiated sarcoma* is the most common sarcoma subtype to occur as a primary lesion in the heart (7,11). There is an overlap between the designation "pleomorphic undifferentiated sarcoma" and simply "undifferentiated sarcoma"; if there are areas of storiform growth, then it is best to use the designation pleomorphic undifferentiated sarcoma.

In the soft tissue, undifferentiated sarcomas include undifferentiated round cell, undifferentiated epithelioid, and undifferentiated spindle cell types (2); these terms have not been applied to cardiac sarcomas to this date, however.

In a series of cardiac sarcomas with detailed pathologic study, the largest group was the undifferentiated category (3), constituting 8

of 22 intracardiac tumors (2). Of these, 4 were in men of a mean age of 49 years (range, 27 to 77 years); 6 were in the left atrium; and 1 each was in the right ventricle and atrium. The most common manifestation was dyspnea, with others including weight loss, fever, chest pain, palpitations, anasarca, hemoptysis, and congestive heart failure. In the previous Atlas of Tumor Pathology on heart lesions (8), unclassified sarcomas constituted 24 percent of tumors, with a mean patient age of 45 years, a slight male predominance, and a mostly left atrium location (49 percent). In the above study, most patients died within months, although two survived for 1 year or more. Undifferentiated sarcomas of the heart are associated with an especially poor prognosis (54,55) and have been reported during pregnancy (56).

Histologically, undifferentiated cardiac sarcomas show polygonal or rounded discohesive cells, without significant spindling (figs. 16-6–16-10). There may be a focally myxoid or collagenous background. The differential diagnosis includes metastatic sarcoma (for right-sided tumors), metastatic carcinoma, and lymphoma. The histologic grade of undifferentiated sarcomas is generally high grade, whether the FNCLCC or NCI system is used (57,58).

Immunohistochemically, undifferentiated sarcomas typically express vimentin. They are negative for smooth muscle markers, including actin and desmin; S-100 protein; endothelial markers, including CD34 and CD31; and lymphoid markers.

### Undifferentiated Pleomorphic Sarcoma

*Undifferentiated pleomorphic sarcoma* was previously called "MFH" in the heart (59–70), and still currently is in some cases (71,72). The term "pleomorphic" denotes the distinctive spindle cell differentiation with a classic "storiform" pattern, which is lacking in undifferentiated sarcomas. If undifferentiated and pleomorphic sarcomas are combined into one group, they account for approximately 40 percent of heart sarcomas, about the frequency of angiosarcomas.

Cardiac undifferentiated pleomorphic sarcomas are typically located in the left atrium, and have prominent luminal growth, which occurs before extensive infiltration into the

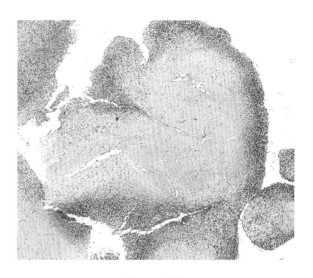

**Figure 16-6**

**UNDIFFERENTIATED SARCOMA**

A 73-year-old female had a polypoid left atrial mass. As often occurs with sarcomas of putative intimal origin, the tumor area toward the luminal surface is more cellular, with a more fibrous center. In some foci, the tumor showed typical storiform features (not shown).

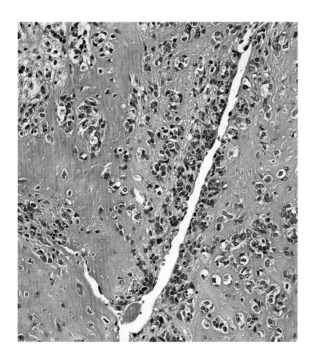

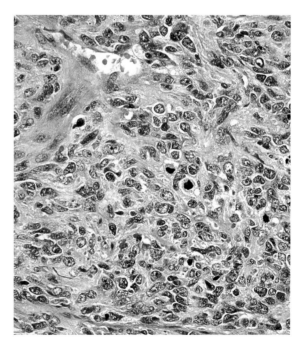

**Figure 16-7**

**UNDIFFERENTIATED CARDIAC SARCOMA**

Left: There are large, pleomorphic cells with epithelioid features. Although the background is collagenized, there were no areas of spindling. In the absence of spindling or a storiform pattern, with predominantly epithelioid features, this tumor was classified as undifferentiated pleomorphic sarcoma. There is extensive fibrosis underlying the more cellular surface of the tumor.

Right: At higher magnification, there are large pleomorphic tumor cells, with minimal spindling. The differential diagnosis includes large cell undifferentiated neoplasms, including lymphoma.

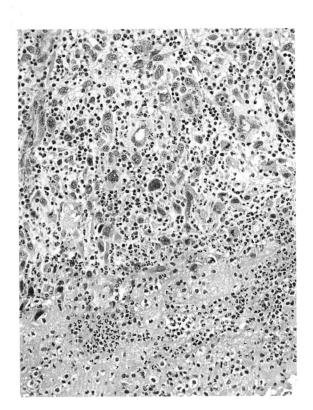
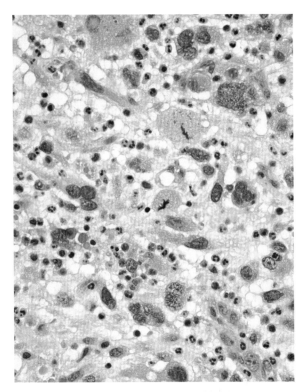

**Figure 16-8**

**UNDIFFERENTIATED SARCOMA**

This undifferentiated malignant neoplasm with markedly pleomorphic, noncohesive cells has an inflammatory background. There is no spindling. The tumor elsewhere showed fibromyxosarcoma (see fig. 16-28). A large number of left atrial sarcomas show three patterns of growth: undifferentiated, MFH-like, and myxofibrosarcoma-like. There is no precise designation of these tumors, although a term such as "pleomorphic undifferentiated sarcoma, with areas of storiform and myxofibrosarcoma growth patterns" is a possibility.

Right: At higher magnification, numerous mitotic figures are seen. There is also acute and chronic inflammation (inflammatory type of MFH, previous designation).

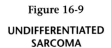

**Figure 16-9**

**UNDIFFERENTIATED SARCOMA**

An 82-year-old man underwent resection of a left ventricle tumor, which histologically was an undifferentiated pleomorphic sarcoma with epithelioid features. The arrow points to a mitotic figure.

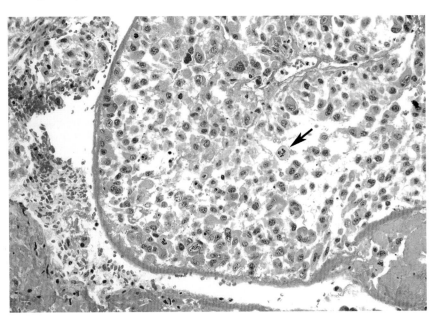

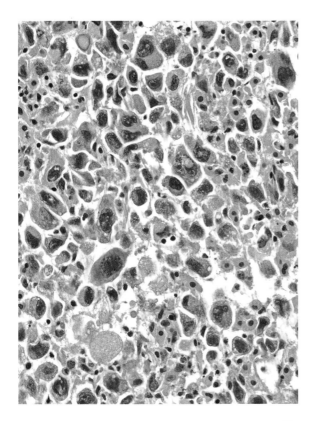 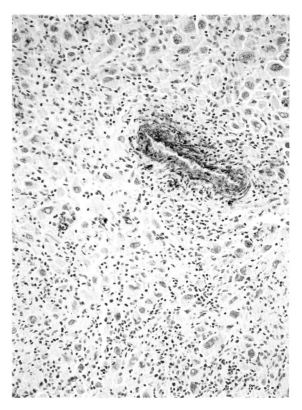

**Figure 16-10**

**UNDIFFERENTIATED SARCOMA**

Left: A 74-year-old man had a left atrial mass, metastatic at the time of surgery to the left femur. The tumor was undifferentiated, with pleomorphic epithelioid features. Because the left atrium is a rare site of distant metastasis, a large endoluminal sarcoma is considered primary, if there are tumor deposits in locations that are prone to delayed metastasis, such as long bones.

Right: An immunohistochemical stain for smooth muscle actin is negative.

myocardium and pericardium (7,10). There is no gender predilection and the mean patient age is around 45 years (64). The site of attachment is commonly the posterior wall or interatrial septum. In a recent review, 81 percent of 47 cases were located in the left atrium (64). The other reported locations included the pericardial space, right ventricular outflow tract and pulmonary valve, right atrium, (73), and left ventricle.

Because of the typical location in the left atrium, signs and symptoms are related to pulmonary hypertension, mitral stenosis and pulmonary vein obstruction. Tumors may also present with metastases, and the lungs, lymph nodes, kidney, and skin are common sites. Rarely, tumors present with embolism, such as retinal occlusion mimicking giant cell arteritis (24).

The histologic appearance of undifferentiated pleomorphic sarcoma ranges from the typical features of "MFH," with a storiform appearance, to epithelioid undifferentiated areas (figs. 16-11–16-19). By definition, there is cellular pleomorphism, which separates these tumors from myxofibrosarcoma. Necrosis is variable, as is the degree of collagenization. Occasionally, there is a prominent vascular background that has been associated with myxoid "MFH." The surface of the tumor projecting into the atrial lumen is often denuded and covered by fibrin.

Pleomorphic sarcomas with giant cells have been described in the heart. Formerly designated "giant cell MFH," these tumors are characterized by numerous giant cells resembling giant cell tumor of bone (3).

Most undifferentiated pleomorphic sarcomas of the heart are high grade, either by FNCLCC or NCI criteria (57,74). The majority of tumors have necrosis. The mean mitotic activity is 9

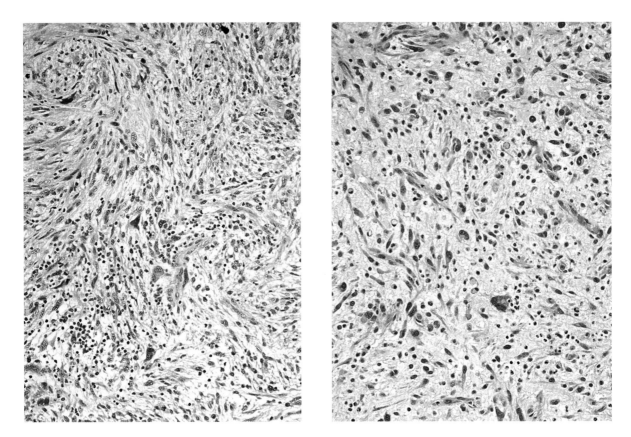

**Figure 16-11**

**UNDIFFERENTIATED PLEOMORPHIC SARCOMA**

Left: If there are areas with pleomorphic spindle cells in a "storiform" pattern, the term MFH or pleomorphic sarcoma with storiform growth pattern is used. The tumor was excised from a 23-year-old man with a left atrial mass who presented with cerebral embolism.

Right: In this field, the storiform growth pattern, inflammation, and scattered tumor giant cells are seen.

mitoses per 10 high-power fields, with a range of 1 to 22 mitoses (74).

Immunohistochemically, undifferentiated pleomorphic sarcoma is positive for vimentin, and negative for other markers, with the exception of smooth muscle actin, which is focally expressed in the majority of tumors (74).

Unusual sites of cardiac pleomorphic undifferentiated sarcoma include the left ventricle (62) and right ventricle (68). Tumors may metastasize to a variety of locations, including the brain (63). There may be metastatic disease at the time of diagnosis of the primary heart tumor (70). After surgical resection, the tumor may recur outside the heart (64–66).

There are few follow-up reports for undifferentiated pleomorphic sarcoma, because of variation in classification and terminology. In Kim et al.'s series (74a) of 6 patients with "unclassified" cardiac sarcomas with a microscopic description consistent with undifferentiated pleomorphic sarcoma, 3 were dead of disease at 3 to 68 months, and 3 were alive, up to 78 months. The four "malignant fibrous histiocytomas" in two other series of heart tumors resulted in the death of the patients from 1 month to 6 years (57,75). Series of surgically resected malignant cardiac tumors frequently include few undifferentiated pleomorphic sarcomas and so there is little histologic data (76).

### Cardiac Myxofibrosarcoma

*Myxofibrosarcoma* has been used as a replacement term for "myxoid MFH" (see Table 16-5). If there is 25 percent myxoid background in a tumor that otherwise resembles undifferentiated

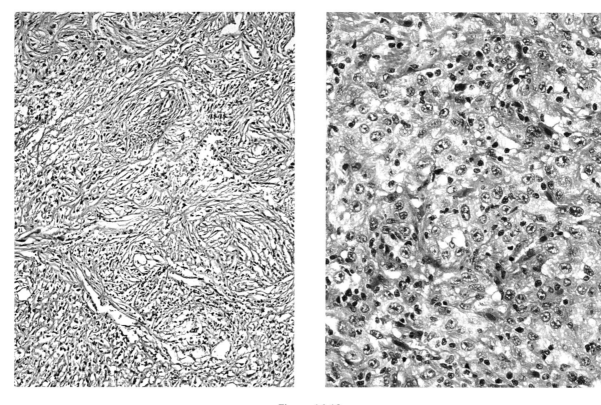

**Figure 16-12**

**UNDIFFERENTIATED PLEOMORPHIC SARCOMA**

Left: A 54-year-old female with a left atrial tumor presented with a cerebrovascular accident. In this field, there is the typical storiform area of so-called MFH.

Right: In another area, undifferentiated large, pleomorphic, epithelioid tumor cells are seen.

pleomorphic sarcoma, then the term myxofibrosarcoma is appropriate. It must be remembered, however, that a myxoid background is common in heart tumors, ranging from benign (myxoma and inflammatory myofibroblastic tumor, the latter occurring primarily in children) to malignant neoplasms, including leiomyosarcoma. If there are areas of matrix formation (osteoid or cartilage), then the tumor is considered high grade and classified based on the presence of these elements.

The term *fibrosarcoma* is used rarely in current terminology, especially in the heart, and is generally restricted to the specific subtypes of sarcoma that occur in the extremities. The term still persists for isolated case reports of cardiac tumors, but must be distinguished from pleomorphic sarcoma or myxofibrosarcoma in the presence of significant cellular atypia, and fibroma, especially in children, in whom fibromas may be deceptively cellular.

Cardiac myxofibrosarcomas have been described most frequently in the left atrium (77), typically causing obstruction and symptoms of mitral stenosis (78,79). From several series of heart tumors, using variable terminology, 6 of 8 primary cardiac sarcomas with myxoid features were in the left atrium (57,58,74). Less common sites include the right atrium (80), right ventricle (81), and ventricular septum (82).

Histologically, myxofibrosarcomas demonstrate spindle cells within a fibrous matrix, without significant pleomorphism or a storiform pattern, or rounded cells in a myxoid matrix without marked atypia (figs. 16-20–16-28). Although there is a continuum with undifferentiated pleomorphic sarcoma, there is no storiform pattern or marked pleomorphism. There are many tumors that show a variety of patterns, including fibromyxosarcoma, undifferentiated pleomorphic sarcoma, and undifferentiated sarcoma. Of those reported with histologic data,

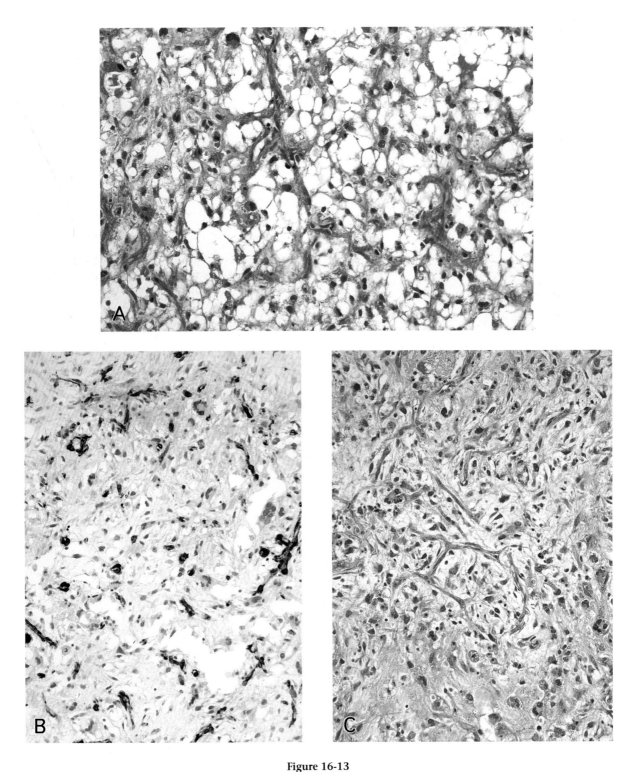

**Figure 16-13**

**UNDIFFERENTIATED PLEOMORPHIC SARCOMA**

A: A 45-year-old woman with a left atrial mass presented with heart failure. The tumor showed the typical vascular pattern of myxoid MFH.

B: As is frequently the case, actin is generally negative in these tumors (smooth muscle actin stain).

C: Areas have a typical storiform pattern.

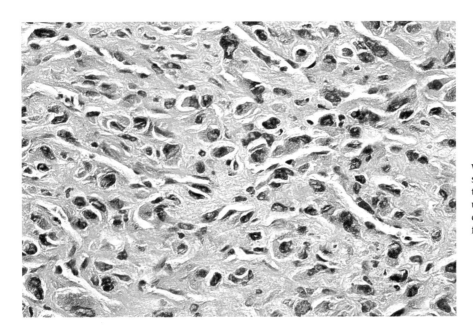

**Figure 16-14**

**UNDIFFERENTIATED PLEOMORPHIC SARCOMA**

An 82-year-old woman with a left atrial mass presented with pulmonary symptoms. The tumor is largely undifferentiated, but the cells are focally spindled in a fibrous stroma.

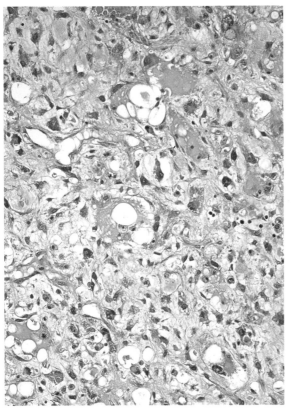

**Figure 16-15**

**UNDIFFERENTIATED PLEOMORPHIC SARCOMA**

An undifferentiated area has pleomorphic large cells, with the appearance of histiocytes, which led to the origin of the term MFH. These cells are known now to lack histiocytic markers. (Same case as fig. 16-13.)

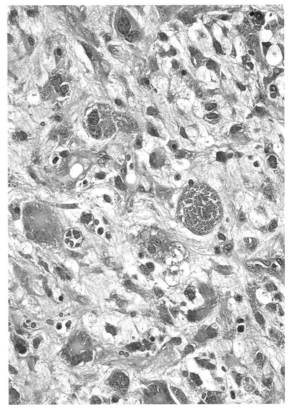

**Figure 16-16**

**UNDIFFERENTIATED PLEOMORPHIC SARCOMA**

Some of the histiocyte-like large undifferentiated tumor cells have small eosinophilic inclusions. (Same case as fig. 16-13.)

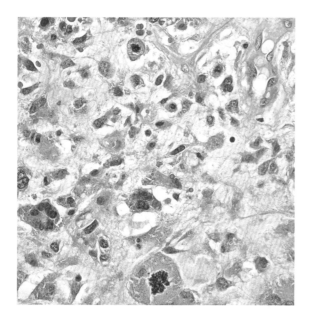

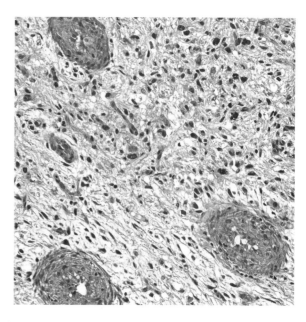

**Figure 16-17**

**UNDIFFERENTIATED PLEOMORPHIC SARCOMA**

Histiocyte-like giant cells are present in an undifferentiated area with mitotic figures. (Same case as fig. 16-13.)

**Figure 16-18**

**UNDIFFERENTIATED PLEOMORPHIC SARCOMA**

There may be a thick smooth muscle cell proliferation around tumor vessels. This change is present in other sarcomas as well. (Same case as fig. 16-13.)

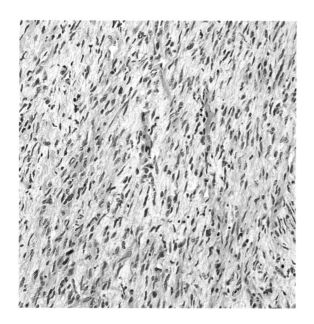

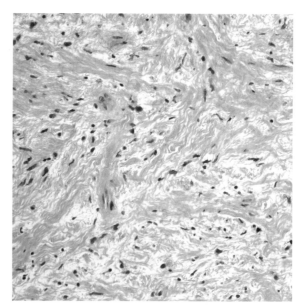

**Figure 16-19**

**FIBROMYXOSARCOMA**

Left: A different area of the tumor shown in figure 16-14 demonstrates areas with features of fibrosarcoma or myxofibrosarcoma.

Right: In another area, the bland features of fibromyxosarcoma are seen. Although in the soft tissue there is evidence that better-differentiated areas of myxofibrosarcoma impart a better prognosis than a tumor that is entirely pleomorphic, there is no such data in the heart; overall tumor grading is likely important, as is a description of the sarcoma growth patterns.

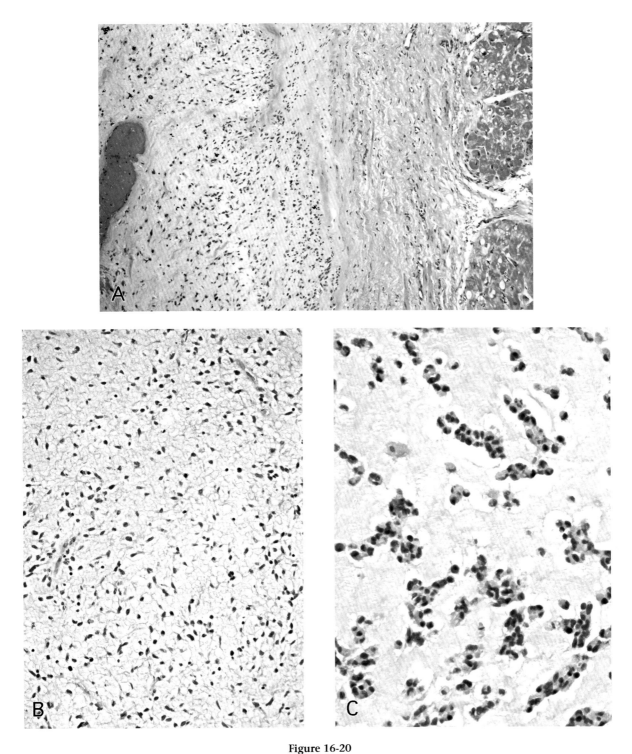

**Figure 16-20**

**CARDIAC MYXOFIBROSARCOMA**

A: A 36-year-old female with shortness of breath had a tumor in the left atrium that infiltrated the pulmonary veins. The junction of atrial wall (right) and tumor (left) is seen.

B: The tumor has bland areas, mimicking myxoma of soft tissue. However, there is no resemblance to cardiac myxoma, as the tumor lacks myxomatous structures.

C: Some areas show epithelioid features.

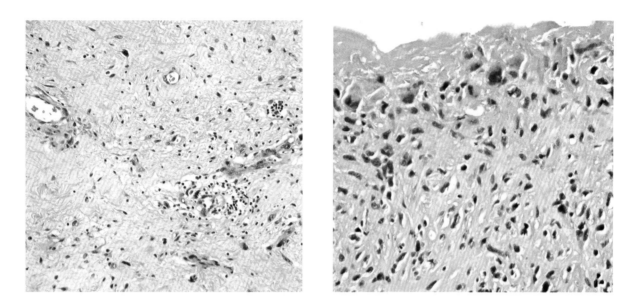

**Figure 16-21**

**CARDIAC MYXOFIBROSARCOMA**

Left: Some areas of the tumor seen in figure 16-20 are deceptively bland. Exhaustive sampling of left atrial sarcomas may be necessary to confirm the diagnosis of malignancy, especially of necrotic, hemorrhagic, and variegated tumor foci.

Right: With adequate sampling, areas of atypia that are absent in benign tumors are identified. Typically, there is fibrin on the endoluminal surface.

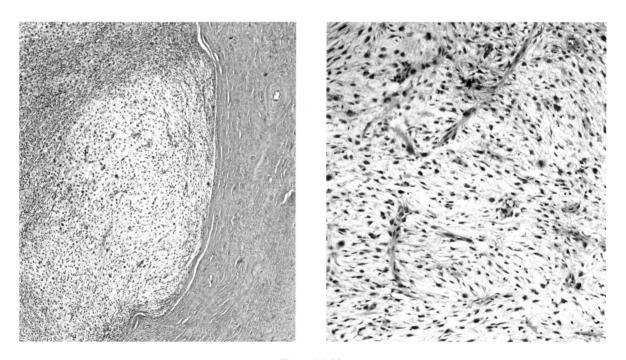

**Figure 16-22**

**CARDIAC MYXOFIBROSARCOMA**

Left: A 66-year-old woman had a recurrent "myxoma" of the left atrium. The initial tumor, upon review, was also a myxofibrosarcoma. The tumor is well differentiated but heterogeneous, with a bland fibrous area (top), a more cellular area (bottom), and a clearly myxoid focus (center).

Right: The typical myxoid MFH vascular pattern is seen in this field.

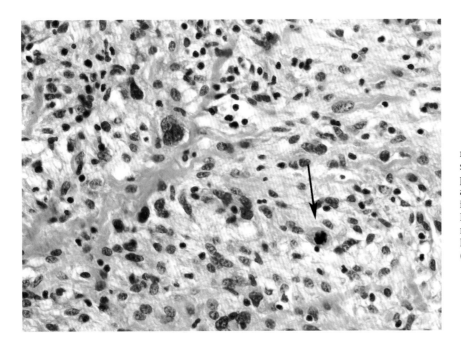

**Figure 16-23**

**CARDIAC MYXOFIBROSARCOMA**

As is the case with the fibro-myxosarcoma/pleomorphic spindle cell/undifferentiated pleomorphic sarcoma spectrum, all three growth types often coexist in left atrial cardiac sarcomas. Here, a pleomorphic area with mitotic figures (arrow) and large histiocyte-like giant cells is seen. (Same case as fig. 16-22.)

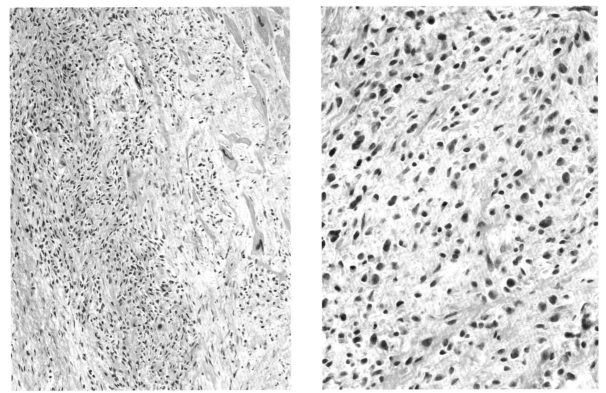

**Figure 16-24**

**CARDIAC MYXOFIBROSARCOMA**

Left: A 19-year-old woman had a right ventricular mass surgically excised. Several features of inflammatory myofibroblastic tumor (IMFT) were seen, especially because of the lack of significant atypia. This tumor infiltrates cardiac muscle (above), unusual for IMFT. Although the young age is characteristic of IMFT, cardiac sarcomas of higher grade also occur at this age range.

Right: In other areas, the tumor is more cellular, consistent with a low-grade sarcoma with fibrous differentiation.

**Figure 16-25**

**CARDIAC MYXOFIBROSARCOMA: MITRAL VALVE**

A: A young man with shortness of breath presented with a left atrial mass and liver metastasis. The primary tumor occurred mostly on the mitral valve and extended onto the left atrial wall. At low magnification, the tumor resembles IMFT (see chapter 13).

B: The pleomorphism in this area exceeds that seen in IMFT.

C: On the surface, there was fibrin with a cellular area underneath.

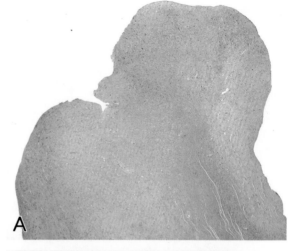

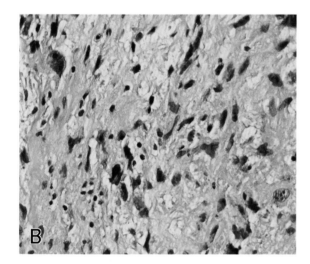

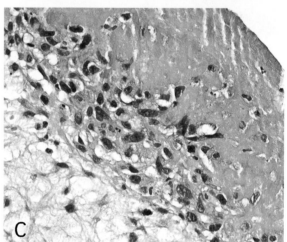

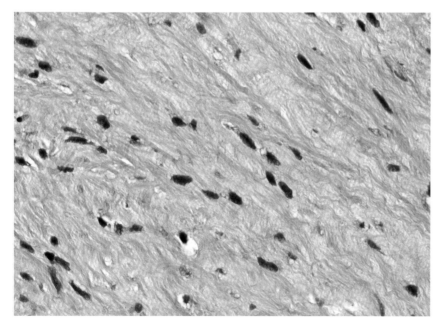

**Figure 16-26**

**CARDIAC MYXOFIBROSARCOMA**

Often in left atrial sarcomas, there are very bland fibrous areas. This field is from the tumor illustrated in figure 16-25. The malignant nature of the tumor was evident in histologic findings in other areas, and in the metastatic spread.

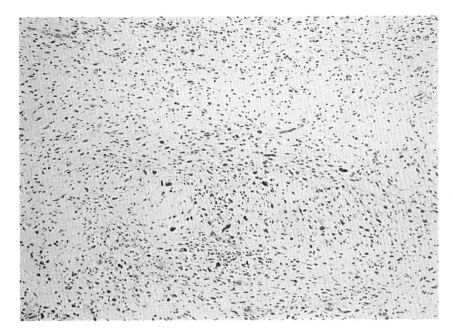

**Figure 16-27**

**CARDIAC
MYXOFIBROSARCOMA**

This is a bland low-grade tumor, mostly fibrous, with scattered larger cells in a myxoid background. Elsewhere there were high-grade areas (not shown). The differential diagnosis of low-grade left atrial sarcoma is myxoma, but there are no myxoma structures present. (Same case as fig. 16-11.)

**Figure 16-28**

**CARDIAC MYXOFIBROSARCOMA**

A: This tumor presented as a metastatic lesion to the vertebra. The primary tumor had areas that looked completely bland and benign, almost like a fibroma; unlike fibroma, the tumor arose from the lining of the left atrium, and was predominantly endoluminal.

B: The atypical areas are predominantly perivascular.

C: The perivascular cells show the clear-cut pleomorphism indicative of malignancy.

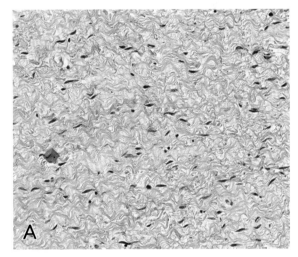

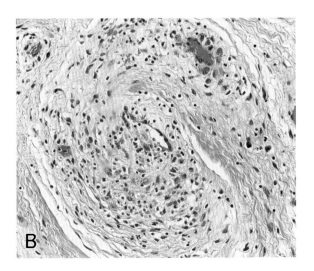

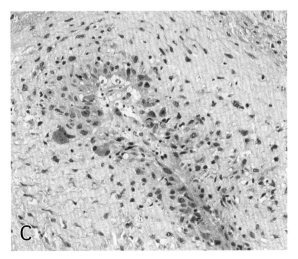

there was a spectrum of low-, intermediate-, and high-grade tumors (57,58,74). Mitotic figures and tumor necrosis are generally present (74). In the authors' experience with 15 myxofibrosarcomas, 7 had a mitotic rate of 0-1 mitosis per 10 high-power fields, 5 had a mitotic rate of 1-10 mitoses per 10 high-power fields, and 3 had greater than 10 per 10 high-power fields. Tumor necrosis was present in two thirds of these tumors.

The prognosis of patients with cardiac myxofibrosarcoma is probably better than for other cardiac sarcomas, as they include low-grade tumors, although data is scarce. Of six patients with cardiac myxofibrosarcoma from three series (57,58,74), three patients were alive without disease at 12,19, and 60 months; two were alive with disease at 33 and 37 months; and one died soon after surgical excision.

## Leiomyosarcoma

*Leiomyosarcoma* is one of the more common differentiated forms of primary cardiac sarcoma. There is usually expression of smooth muscle–specific markers, such as desmin. Alternatively, the diagnosis is used if there are the typical histologic features of fascicular tumor bundles, which often are organized at right angles to one another; blunt-ended nuclei and often perinuclear vacuoles; and actin expression in the absence of more specific smooth muscle markers. Actin positivity is, in itself, not specific for smooth muscle differentiation, and may be present in myofibroblastic lesions and undifferentiated pleomorphic sarcoma.

Cardiac leiomyosarcoma represents approximately 6 percent of cardiac sarcomas. In one series, it represented over one in four cardiac sarcomas, with a mean patient age of 47 years (range, 31 to 69 years) (3). Most cardiac leiomyosarcomas are located in the left atrium (posterior wall) and involve the pulmonary veins or mitral valve. There is no sex predilection, and most occur in patients between 40 and 50 years of age. Dyspnea is the main clinical feature.

Although the left atrium is the most common site (83–85), with a possible origin from the pulmonary veins (86,87), cardiac leiomyosarcomas may arise in the right atrium (88–90); right ventricle, with or without outflow tract obstruction (45,91); or in the left ventricle with left ventricle outflow tract obstruction (92,93).

Leiomyomas and leiomyosarcomas occurring in the adrenal gland and soft tissues have been associated with Epstein-Barr virus (EBV) infection, in association with immunosuppression caused by human immunodeficiency virus (HIV) infection or allografts. A single leiomyosarcoma of the heart in a transplant patient has been described, but EBV infection was not documented in that case (94).

Histologically, leiomyosarcoma has the recognizable features of smooth muscle cells (fascicular growth, often at right angles, often with perinuclear vacuoles) (fig. 16-29, left). Expression of desmin by immunohistochemistry is sometimes considered a prerequisite for the diagnosis (fig. 16-29, right), and actin is also expressed. Cardiac leiomyosarcoma may be high grade, with a very high mitotic rate and abundant necrosis (58,74) or low grade (95). In the authors' experience, two thirds of cardiac leiomyosarcomas have fewer that 10 mitotic figures per 10 high-power fields, and one third have more than that, with necrosis typical. Epithelioid features and a myxoid background may occur (90,96). Unlike at other sites, the mitotic rate is not essential in the distinction between leiomyoma and leiomyosarcoma, as the former does not occur within the myocardium.

Treatment includes chemotherapy (97) in addition to attempted complete surgical excision.

## Rhabdomyosarcoma

*Rhabdomyosarcoma* was at one time considered a common type of cardiac sarcoma. With strict diagnostic criteria, however, including expression of desmin or myogenin, the incidence of cardiac rhabdomyosarcoma has decreased, and it is currently considered a rare cardiac tumor that occurs primarily in children (98). Most published reports are single cases with incomplete documentation of striated muscle differentiation (99–107). In a recent series of cardiac sarcomas, rhabdomyosarcomas constituted about 5 percent of all cases (108), although a large series reported none (3,58), emphasizing the rarity of this tumor. Nevertheless, cardiac rhabdomyosarcoma is the most common malignant heart tumor in children (98,109), in whom primary cardiac malignancies are exceptionally rare.

Cardiac rhabdomyosarcomas have been reported at all ages, but there is a predominance in

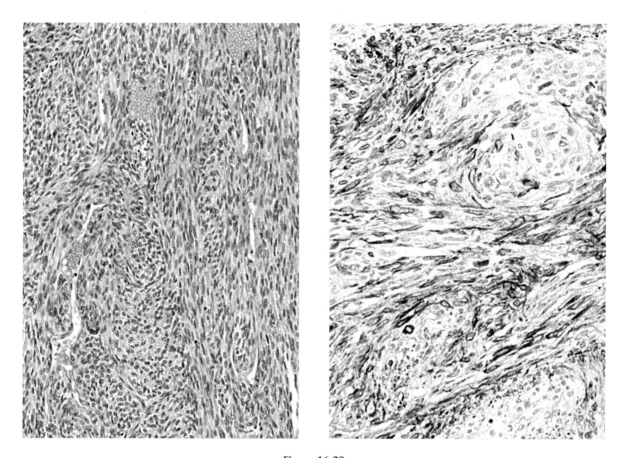

**Figure 16-29**

**CARDIAC LEIOMYOSARCOMA**

Left: Most well-differentiated smooth muscle sarcomas occur in the left atrium. Fascicles are oriented at right angles to one another.

Right: Desmin positivity is generally a prerequisite for the diagnosis of leiomyosarcoma.

childhood, and the tumor may occur in infants (42,106). The mean age at presentation is about 14 years, and survival is poor (8). The clinical symptoms are diverse, and depend on the site of the tumor within the heart. Those arising in the left atrium may present as severe mitral stenosis, similar to undifferentiated pleomorphic sarcomas (110). Embolization may result in stroke (111,112). In contrast to other cardiac sarcomas, most cardiac rhabdomyosarcomas arise in the ventricular walls (110,111), but they also occur in the atria (8,113).

Histologically, most cardiac rhabdomyosarcomas are of the embryonal type, although there are reports of alveolar cardiac rhabdomyosarcomas (figs. 16-30–16-32) (114). Occasional cardiac rhabdomyosarcomas with a botryoid endocardial growth pattern have been reported

(115,116); one was likely a metastasis from a prior chest wall tumor (105). A case of spindle cell embryonal type has been reported (117). Pleomorphic rhabdomyosarcomas are considered rare in any location, and it is possible that some reports have misidentified undifferentiated pleomorphic sarcoma (47,118).

Cardiac rhabdomyosarcomas typically have abundant mitotic figures (in the authors' experience, greater on average than all other types), dense cellularity, and invariable necrosis.

Most extracardiac alveolar rhabdomyosarcomas carry the specific *PAX3(7)/FKHR* translocation, corresponding cytogenetically to the t(2;13) or t(1;13) translocation. Chromosomal translocations are infrequently encountered in embryonal rhabdomyosarcoma; none has been reported to date in cardiac rhabdomyosarcoma.

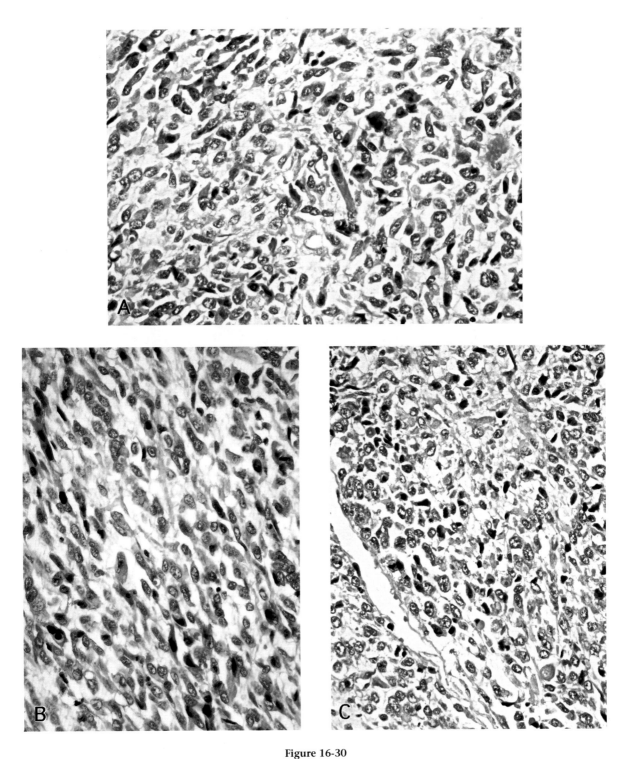

**Figure 16-30**

**CARDIAC RHABDOMYOSARCOMA**

A: A 49-year-old man died soon after the diagnosis of right ventricular outflow tract obstruction due to a bulky mass. Rhabdomyosarcomas of the heart are more common in the ventricle than are pleomorphic undifferentiated sarcomas. Occasional "strap" cells or rhabdomyoblasts are seen. Most cardiac rhabdomyosarcomas in heart are of the embryonal type.

B: A more primitive undifferentiated area is seen in this field.

C: In another field, the rhabdomyosarcoma resembles a small round cell tumor.

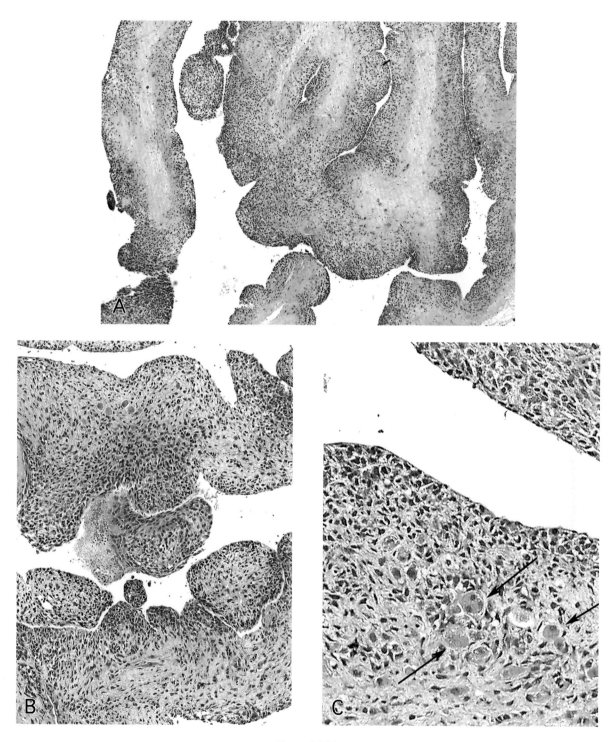

**Figure 16-31**

**CARDIAC RHABDOMYOSARCOMA**

A: A 39-year-old woman with a left atrial tumor presented with shortness of breath. Low magnification shows an endoluminal polypoid tumor.

B: Greater cellularity is seen toward the luminal surface, but no real cambium layer, as seen in botryoid sarcoma, an occasionally described tumor in the heart cavities, is present.

C: There are occasional rhabdomyoblasts (arrows).

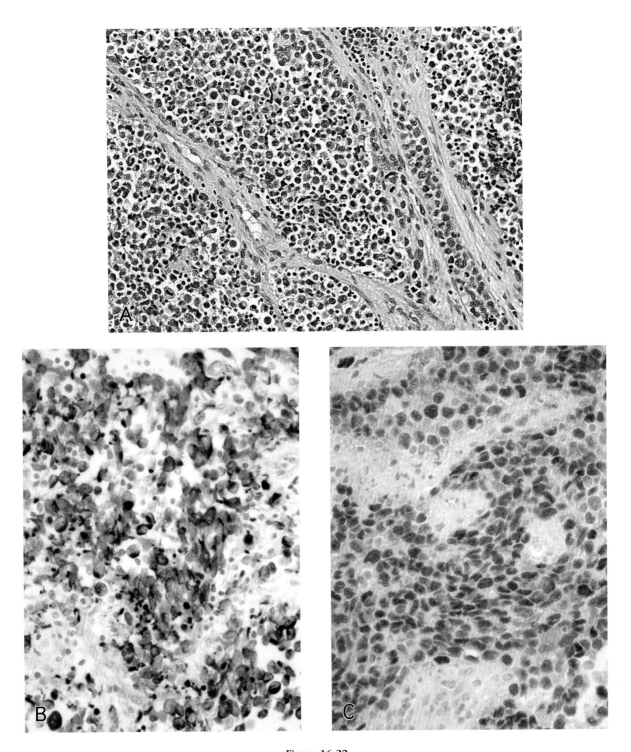

**Figure 16-32**

**CARDIAC RHABDOMYOSARCOMA**

A: A small round cell tumor in the heart elicits the same differential as elsewhere, including embryonal rhabdomyosarcoma and lymphoma (less likely, peripheral neuroendocrine tumor [PNET] and metastatic small cell carcinoma).

B: Rhabdomyosarcomas express muscle-specific antigens, including desmin and myogenin. The desmin positivity is cytoplasmic.

C: The myogenin positivity is nuclear.

The differential diagnosis of embryonal and alveolar rhabdomyosarcomas includes other small round cell sarcomas, which are exceptionally rare in the heart as primary tumors. There have been rare reports of cardiac primitive neuroectodermal tumors (PNET) arising in the heart (119). Immunohistochemically, rhabdomyosarcoma expresses desmin and myogenin, with more focal staining for myogenin in embryonal rhabdomyosarcoma as compared to the alveolar type. WT1 is also positive in rhabdomyosarcoma, in contrast to Ewing sarcoma and synovial sarcoma, which do not express these muscle markers. CD99 and synaptophysin are usually negative, but are not reliable in distinguishing alveolar rhabdomyosarcoma from synovial or Ewing family sarcomas.

There is no effective treatment for cardiac rhabdomyosarcoma. Attempts have been made at heart transplantation (113).

### Cardiac Osteosarcoma

Osteosarcomatous or chondrosarcomatous differentiation occurs in approximately 15 percent of undifferentiated cardiac sarcomas (120). Virtually all *osteosarcomas* of the heart arise in the left atrium, and may extend into the pulmonary veins (120–123). Men and women are equally affected. The mean patient age is 40 years, with a range of 14 to 70 years. These tumors appear to occur in slightly younger patients (124) than pleomorphic sarcomas, and have been reported in patients as young as 14 years of age (125).

Dyspnea is the most common presenting symptom, often related to mitral valve obstruction secondary to the left atrial cavitary location (124,126) or involvement of the mitral valve (127). Congestive heart failure may occur early in the course (128). Peripheral and cerebral embolisms have been reported as complications of left atrial osteosarcoma (129). Rarely, primary cardiac osteosarcomas occur in the right atrium, but in this location an extracardiac primary tumor must be excluded (125,128). One case was reported in a pregnant woman (127). Imaging does not always reveal calcification, as the tumors histologically may be composed primarily of osteoid (121).

Most primary cardiac sarcomas lack chromosomal recurrent translocations, with the exception of synovial sarcoma. Interestingly, the authors have noted one 70-year-old man

with a *JAZF1/PHF1* translocation in a primary ossifying cardiac sarcoma, a translocation previously only observed in endometrial stromal neoplasms (130).

Histologically, the osteosarcomatous component varies from well-differentiated trabecular patterns to high-grade tumors with a solid background of osteoid. Almost half of extracellular osteosarcomas in the heart possess areas of chondrosarcoma, with smaller foci of myxofibrosarcoma or undifferentiated pleomorphic sarcoma (figs. 16-33–16-38) (123). Chondrosarcomatous areas may be the only heterologous element (74,131). Osteoclastic giant cells may be a component of the tumor (120). Cardiac osteosarcoma may be intermediate or high grade, and mitotic figures are typically numerous (58).

The prognosis of patients with cardiac osteosarcoma is poor (128). Cardiac osteosarcoma has an aggressive course, with early metastases to sites including the lung, skin, skeleton (122), and thyroid gland. Patients may develop widespread metastases despite complete resection of the primary tumor and absence of metastatic disease at the time of surgery (134). Survival beyond 1 year is unusual (132), although there is one report of a patient living 7 years, with local recurrence and distant metastasis to the stomach (133).

Pure *cardiac chondrosarcoma* is rarer than primary osteosarcoma. In contrast to osteosarcoma, which occurs in the left atrium, cardiac chondrosarcoma has been described in various cardiac locations in addition to the left atrium (135), including the left ventricle and right atrium (131,136–138). A cardiac chondrosarcoma secreting parathyroid hormone (PTH)-like protein has been reported (135), as well as a patient surviving 20 months postoperatively (136). Extraskeletal (mesenchymal) chondrosarcoma is characterized by a proliferation of small cells in a chondroid background, and the translocation der(13;21)(q10;q10) (139). This particular combination has not yet been documented in a primary cardiac chondrosarcoma.

### Synovial Sarcoma

*Synovial sarcoma* represents 3 to 5 percent of primary heart sarcomas (3,9,21,140). The mean age at presentation is 41 years (141) and tumors have been described in children as young as 13 years (141,142). The atrium is the most common

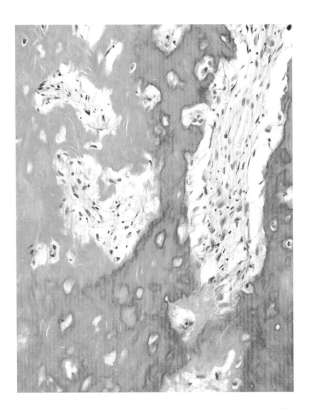
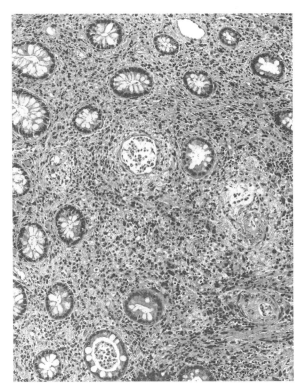

**Figure 16-33**

**CARDIAC OSTEOSARCOMA**

Left: A 48-year-old man had a left atrial mass; the tumor presented with small bowel metastases. Low magnification demonstrates areas of osteoid and chondroid matrix formation.

Right: The metastases were undifferentiated, whereas the primary tumor had areas of osteosarcoma, chondrosarcoma, and pleomorphic spindle cell sarcoma (MFH-like).

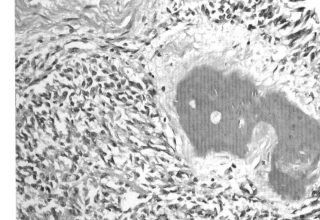

**Figure 16-34**

**CARDIAC OSTEOSARCOMA**

Osteoid within a high-grade spindle cell sarcoma.

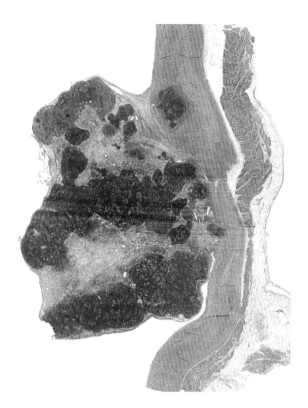 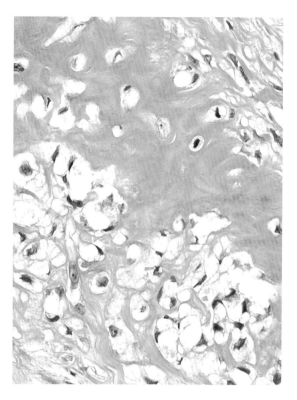

**Figure 16-35**

**CARDIAC OSTEOSARCOMA**

Left: A 26-year-old man had a left atrial mass with mitral obstruction. Low magnification shows an area of malignant osteoid.
Right: At higher magnification, malignant osteoid is clearly seen.

location of intracardiac synovial sarcomas, usually the left (143–150). Nevertheless, also reported have been biatrial synovial sarcomas (151), a synovial sarcoma isolated to the mitral valve (152), and an atrial synovial sarcoma extending through the mitral and aortic valve (153). There may be an extension of right atrial tumors onto the tricuspid valves (151,154,155). The left ventricular myocardium may be the primary site of tumor (156).

The presenting manifestations are typically dyspnea, as with other heart tumors (3), congestive heart failure (145), and rarely, cerebral ischemia due to embolism (144). There have been two reports in patients with asbestos exposure (157,158). Diagnosis by ultrasound-guided fine-needle aspiration has been reported (156).

Synovial sarcomas arising within the pericardium are more common than those arising within the myocardium (142–144,159–165). The symptoms are related to pericardial effusions, tamponade, and constrictive pericarditis.

Histologically, there are several patterns of synovial sarcoma of soft tissue, including most commonly three types: biphasic, monophasic (spindle) type, and poorly differentiated (round cell) types. The biphasic pattern is a mixture of glandular spaces and spindled areas, both readily seen on routine stains. The spindled component often resembles fibrosarcoma, with dense uniform cellularity, sometimes with a neural appearance. A hemangiopericytoma-like vascular pattern may be present. Monophasic spindle cell synovial sarcoma is probably the most common type to occur in the heart (figs. 16-39–16-49), all of which are high grade (58,74). Cardiac synovial sarcoma may also be of the undifferentiated type, with a round cell morphology and little cytologic spindling.

Immunohistochemically, synovial sarcomas are positive for vimentin in all cases, and frequently positive for epithelial membrane antigen (EMA) (up to 97 percent), and less frequently pan-cytokeratin, synaptophysin, and CD99.

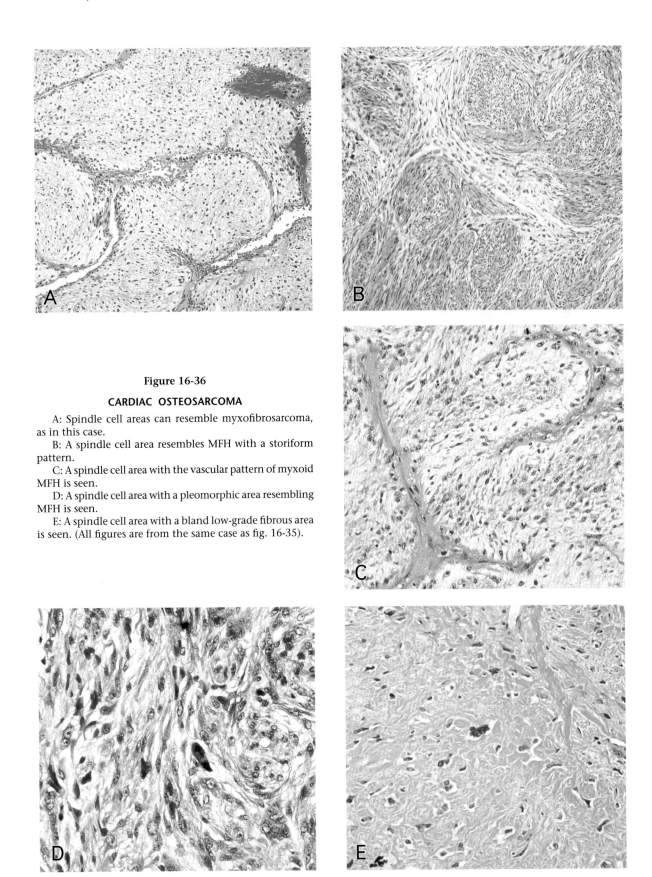

**Figure 16-36**

**CARDIAC OSTEOSARCOMA**

A: Spindle cell areas can resemble myxofibrosarcoma, as in this case.

B: A spindle cell area resembles MFH with a storiform pattern.

C: A spindle cell area with the vascular pattern of myxoid MFH is seen.

D: A spindle cell area with a pleomorphic area resembling MFH is seen.

E: A spindle cell area with a bland low-grade fibrous area is seen. (All figures are from the same case as fig. 16-35).

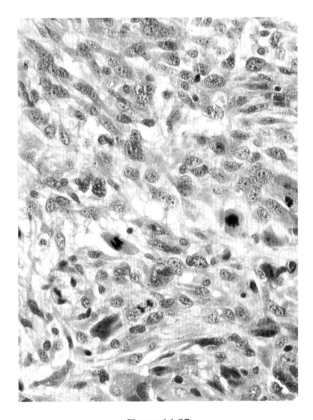

**Figure 16-37**

**CARDIAC OSTEOSARCOMA**

In the nonmatrix-producing regions of the tumor, the pleomorphic undifferentiated area with epithelioid features resembles pleomorphic left atrial sarcomas in general. Shown is a different area of the tumor illustrated in figure 16-35. The spindle cell component of cardiac osteosarcoma may resemble any or all of the spectrum of myxofibrosarcoma –undifferentiated pleomorphic sarcoma (MFH).

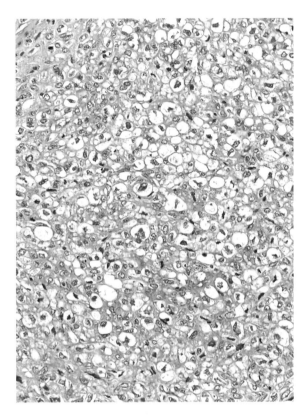

**Figure 16-38**

**CARDIAC CHONDROSARCOMA (EXTRASKELETAL CHONDROSARCOMA)**

A 70-year-old woman presented with shortness of breath related to a left atrial tumor. In this rare example, most of the tumor was chondrosarcoma, with only small spindle cell areas and essentially no osteosarcoma.

However, they may show little expression of antigens other than vimentin (74). EMA and cytokeratin are more diffusely expressed in the epithelial component. Because most cardiac synovial sarcomas are often of the monophasic spindle or undifferentiated types, epithelial differentiation may be difficult to identify on small biopsies or poorly sampled tumors.

Molecular studies confirm the diagnosis of cardiac synovial sarcoma, as in soft tissue locations. The *SYT-SSX* gene fusion product resulting from the X;18 translocation can be demonstrated by cytogenetics, reverse transcriptase-polymerase chain reaction (RT-PCR), and COBRA-fluorescence in situ hybridization (FISH), the latter two methods on paraffin sections (146,151,152,158, 162,164,166,167). Generally, only the *SYT-SSX1*

fusion has been demonstrated in the heart, in contrast to the less common *SYT-SSX2* fusion, which is associated with a better prognosis in patients with soft tissue synovial sarcomas.

The differential diagnosis of biphasic synovial sarcoma includes carcinosarcoma and mesothelioma. The former does not exist as a primary cardiac tumor, other than in a single case report, which likely demonstrates a variant of glandular malignant peripheral nerve sheath tumor (MPNST) with rhabdomyosarcomatous elements (168). Malignant mesothelioma is a consideration in the differential diagnosis of pericardial synovial sarcoma, if it is of the biphasic or sarcomatoid type, and can be differentiated based on the presence of pleomorphic spindle cells, tubulopapillary epithelial structures, expression of the mesothelial markers calretinin and WT1, and absence of t(X;18) translocation.

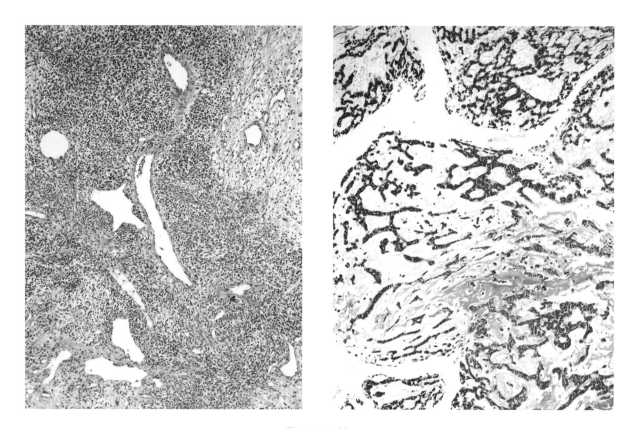

**Figure 16-39**

**CARDIAC SYNOVIAL SARCOMA**

Left: A 34-year-old man with a right atrial tumor and lung metastasis died 2 years after initial tumor resection. Low magnification shows a hemangiopericytoma-like vascular pattern and alternative cellular and more acellular areas.

Right: In a different area of the tumor there are epithelioid cells with myxoid background.

**Figure 16-40**

**CARDIAC SYNOVIAL SARCOMA**

There is condensation around vessels of a highly cellular monomorphic spindle cell tumor. (Same case as fig. 16-39.)

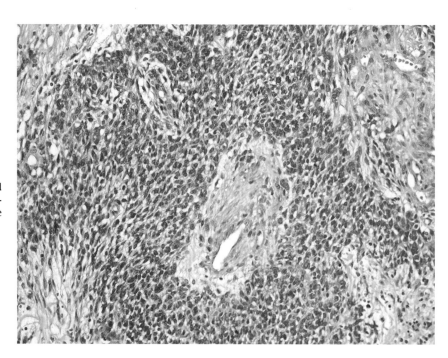

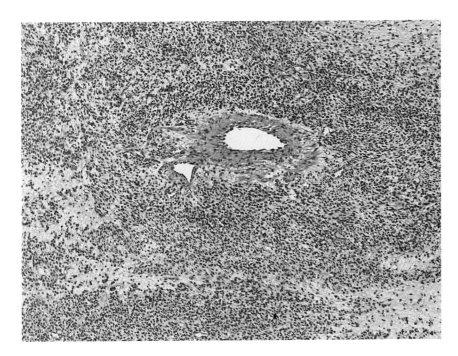

**Figure 16-41**

**CARDIAC
SYNOVIAL SARCOMA**

There are dense spindle cells, with a monomorphic cellular growth pattern and perivascular accentuation.

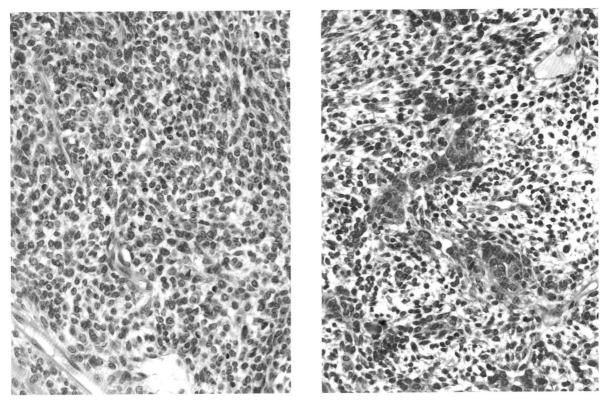

**Figure 16-42**

**CARDIAC SYNOVIAL SARCOMA**

Left: The appearance is of a small round sarcoma cell with a very monotonous growth pattern.

Right: A biphasic area of the tumor confirms the epithelial differentiation and suggests the diagnosis of synovial sarcoma. (Same case as fig. 16-41.)

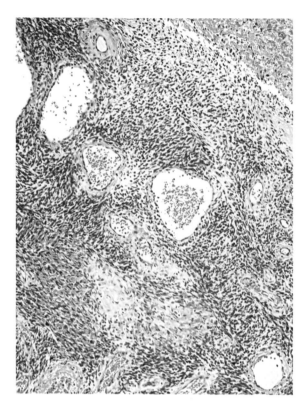 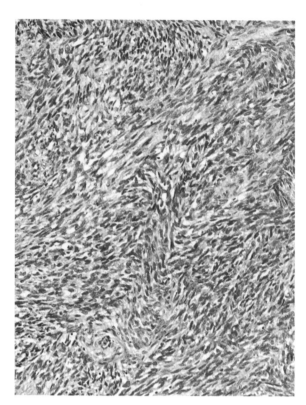

**Figure 16-43**

**CARDIAC SYNOVIAL SARCOMA**

Left: A 19-year-old-man had a right ventricular tumor. At low magnification, the differential diagnosis includes angiosarcoma, especially given the right-sided location. The cells are more uniform, however, than the typical angiosarcoma.

Right: There is a herringbone fibrosarcoma-like growth pattern. The diagnosis of monomorphic synovial sarcoma was confirmed by detection of a t(X;18) translocation by fluorescence in situ hybridization.

The differential diagnosis of monomorphic synovial sarcoma includes myxofibrosarcoma, MPNST, and solitary fibrous tumor (SFT). Myxofibrosarcoma generally demonstrates more pleomorphism and does not express epithelial antigens. SFT is a consideration in the pericardium, as it rarely occurs within the myocardium. The distinction of SFT from monophasic spindle synovial sarcoma of the pericardium may require an immunohistochemical panel that includes epithelial markers, which are generally negative in SFT, reliance on the histologic blandness of most SFTs, and confirmation of the diagnosis of synovial sarcoma by molecular studies. CD99 and BCL2 protein are often expressed in both synovial sarcoma and SFT.

Monophasic synovial sarcoma may also mimic MPNST, which is uncommon in the heart. In the absence of epithelial differentiation, MPNST is difficult to distinguish from synovial sarcoma, which may express S-100 protein. In such cases, the identification of epithelial differentiation with the use of CK7 or CK19 may be helpful, as well as the expression of TLE1, a novel marker that is specific for synovial sarcoma and rarely expressed in MPNST (169).

The differential diagnosis of undifferentiated synovial sarcoma includes embryonal rhabdomyosarcoma and Ewing sarcoma (primitive neuroectodermal tumor [PNET]). These three tumors are all exquisitely rare in an intracardiac location, and are most readily distinguished by the presence of muscle differentiation in the case of rhabdomyosarcoma, epithelial differentiation in the case of PNET, and genetic studies for confirmative diagnosis.

The prognosis of patients with cardiac synovial sarcoma is poor, but may be improving, as synovial sarcomas are very sensitive to chemotherapy. There have been reports of survival of over 1 year

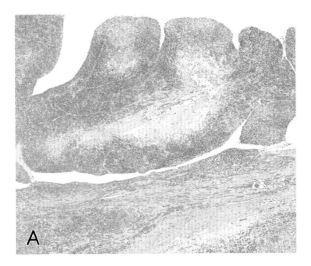

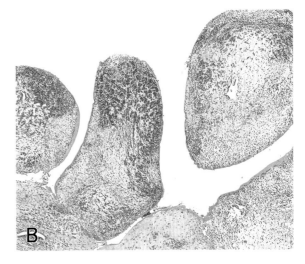

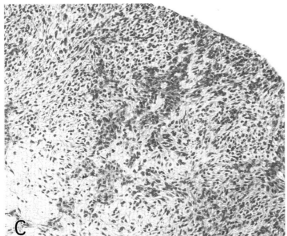

**Figure 16-44**

**CARDIAC SYNOVIAL SARCOMA**

A: A 72-year-old man had a tumor arising from the posteromedial papillary muscle of the left ventricle. There was a polypoid endoluminal configuration. The diagnosis was confirmed by detecting the t(X;18) translocation in tumor cells by polymerase chain reaction (PCR).

B: The typical biphasic area of synovial sarcoma is seen.

C: Higher magnification of a biphasic area.

**Figure 16-45**

**CARDIAC SYNOVIAL SARCOMA**

Surface fibrin is typical of endoluminal cardiac tumors of various histogenetic types.

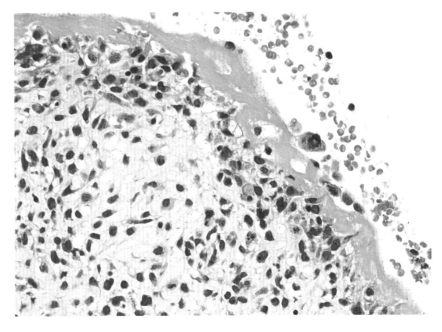

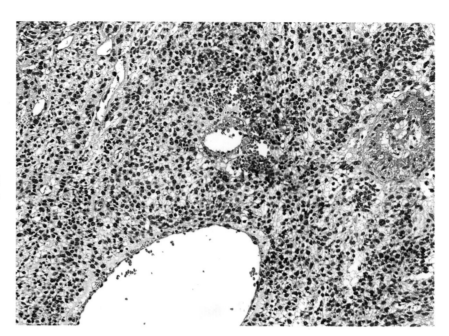

**Figure 16-46**

**CARDIAC
SYNOVIAL SARCOMA**

The monomorphic small cell area has prominent vascularity. (Same case as fig. 16-44.)

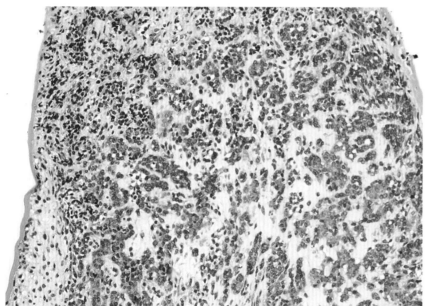

**Figure 16-47**

**CARDIAC
SYNOVIAL SARCOMA**

The growth pattern is predominantly epithelioid. (Same case as fig. 16-44.)

(8,154). Treatment includes chemotherapy and aggressive tumor resection (156). Although little data are available for cardiac synovial sarcoma, among four patients in recent series, two were alive with evidence of disease after treatment, at 13 and 34 months; the other two patients were dead of disease at 9 and 10 months. Prolonged survival of over 10 years has been reported with multimodality therapy in a patient with pericardial synovial sarcoma (142).

## Miscellaneous Cardiac Sarcomas

Sarcoma subtypes that have been anecdotally described in the heart include liposarcoma (8,170,171), Ewing sarcoma/PNET (119, 172,173), MPNST sarcomas with divergent differentiation (malignant mesenchymoma) (2,58,174), malignant rhabdoid tumor (175), and carcinosarcoma (168). The three MPNSTs described in the series of Zhang et al. (58) were diagnosed based solely on the focal expression

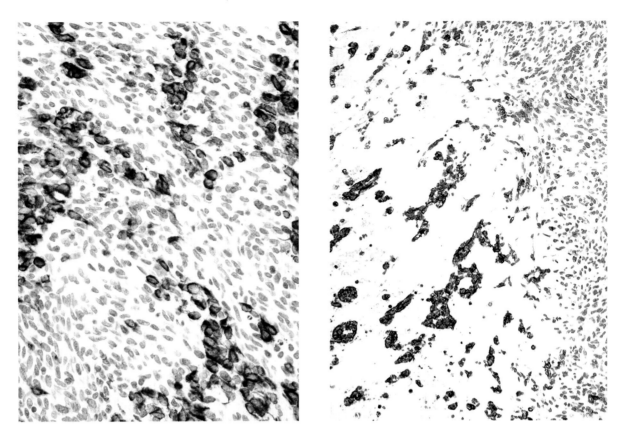

**Figure 16-48**

**CARDIAC SYNOVIAL SARCOMA**

Left: Epithelial areas express cytokeratin (immunohistochemical stain for pancytokeratin).
Right: The epithelial area is seen below with a myxoid background. (Same case as fig. 16-44.)

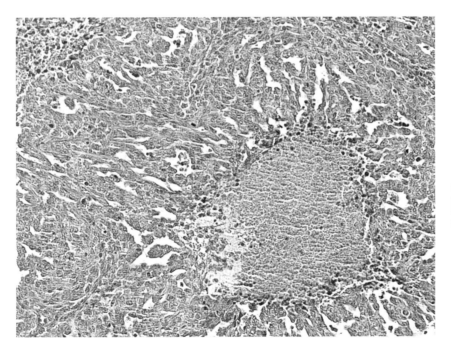

**Figure 16-49**

**CARDIAC
SYNOVIAL SARCOMA**

A 41-year-old male had a right atrial mass and multiple pulmonary nodules. This tumor was almost purely epithelioid. Central necrosis is present.

of S-100 protein, which can also occur in synovial sarcoma. A recent report described an intracardiac tumor with features of desmoplastic small round cell tumor (176).

### Sarcomas of Cardiac Valves

Valvular involvement by cardiac sarcoma is usually as an extension from atrial tumors, such as pleomorphic sarcomas, osteosarcomas, synovial sarcomas, and leiomyosarcomas. Pulmonary valve involvement may occur with sarcomas of the pulmonary artery (see chapter 19) (177,178). Pure valvular sarcomas are rare; lesions such as papillary fibroelastoma and inflammatory myofibroblastic tumor are much more common as primary valve lesions. Sarcoma subtypes that have been reported as primarily involving valves include rhabdomyosarcoma (115), undifferentiated sarcomas (179,180), and synovial sarcoma (152).

The differential diagnosis of valve sarcomas includes inflammatory myofibroblastic tumor, which occurs primarily in children (182) (see chapter 13), and papillary fibroelastoma, which is acellular and has a distinctive histologic appearance (see chapter 6). Treatment, in addition to chemotherapy, includes valve replacement, including homograft valve replacement (181).

### Sarcomas in Infants and Children

Malignant primary cardiac tumors are extremely rare in infants and children, and are generally the subject of case reports (37). In series of heart tumors in children, there is typically only one instance of sarcoma, such as rhabdomyosarcoma or PNET (109,172,183). Of 40 primary pediatric heart tumors, 3 were sarcomas, the highest proportion reported (classified as rhabdomyosarcoma, undifferentiated sarcoma, and fibrosarcoma, although without histologic or immunohistochemical descriptions) (184). One series of cardiac sarcomas reported one left-sided undifferentiated sarcoma arising in a 4-year-old that metastasized widely to the brain, kidney, adrenal glands, and bone (58). Several pediatric heart tumors, reported in the medical literature as sarcomas, are likely inflammatory myofibroblastic tumors, given the good prognosis, location on valves, and available histologic descriptions (58,97,180,185,186). One atrial leiomyosar-

coma in an infant was successfully resected with apparent cure at 96 months, although a histologic description is absent (58). A case of sarcoma of the ventricle may in fact represent fibroma (37).

In a series of 16 pediatric cardiac sarcomas (187), most patients were male. The clinical presentation was variable, including recurrent pericardial effusion, respiratory distress, pulmonary emboli, shortness of breath, arrhythmias, chest pain, and congestive heart failure. Heart failure may be the result of right ventricular outflow obstruction, and infants may present with failure to thrive, supraventricular arrhythmias (184), or sudden death (37).

Most lesions are single, and occur anywhere in the heart, but most frequently in the left atrium, and less commonly, the pericardium (188). The 10 lesions reported were undifferentiated sarcomas, with 3 angiosarcomas, 2 rhabdomyosarcomas, and 1 osteosarcoma. The tumors were uniformly fatal, with survival up to only 13 months (182). Death was related to recurrent disease or distant spread, including pulmonary (184) and cerebral metastases (118,189). One 3-month-old infant reportedly survived 10 years, but histologic confirmation of the sarcomatous nature of the tumor was lacking (184).

### Pericardial Sarcomas

Sarcomas limited to, or primarily involving, the pericardium are extremely rare, and are most typically synovial sarcomas (see above). Angiosarcomas with predominant pericardial involvement have also been reported, but generally infiltrate the myocardium (see chapter 15). Most reports of primary pericardial sarcomas are undifferentiated sarcomas or fibrosarcomas (190–195); one liposarcoma has been reported (196).

### DIFFERENTIAL DIAGNOSIS

The differential diagnosis of sarcoma includes reactive soft tissue lesions with a deceptively aggressive appearance. In the heart, however, few, if any, pseudosarcomatous lesions occur. One tumor that should be distinguished from primary cardiac sarcoma is inflammatory myofibroblastic tumor, which has not demonstrated the capacity for metastatic potential in the cardiac location (see chapter 13). These tumors have a characteristic appearance, and occur on the heart valves almost exclusively in children and adolescents.

Sarcomas of the left atrium are frequently myxofibrosarcomas, myxoid MFHs, or other myxoid sarcomas, such as leiomyosarcomas. Even though none of these tumors is significantly histologically similar to cardiac myxoma to cause confusion, myxoma is frequently in the differential diagnosis because it is more common and better recognized. The lack of myxomatous structures and myxoma cells in the variants of left atrial sarcoma should exclude myxoma from the differential diagnosis, especially in cases of well-differentiated myxofibrosarcoma.

Sarcomas of the heart can be metastatic lesions (96,186,187), therefore, the differential diagnosis of primary cardiac sarcoma includes a metastasis. However, metastatic sarcomas to the heart are invariably right sided, and not angiosarcomas. Any right-sided sarcoma that is not angiosarcoma should be considered a potential metastasis until a primary tumor of the soft tissue has been excluded.

## TREATMENT

Cardiac sarcomas are treated by multimodal therapy, including combined radiation and chemotherapy (201,202), in addition to resection of the mass (Table 16-4). Because of the frequent difficulty in complete excision because of adjacent vital structures, heart transplantation has been successfully performed in patients with primary cardiac sarcomas (113,203). In the largest series of four patients with transplantation, all tumors recurred, three with distant metastases, for a median patient survival period of 31 months, a better average survival period than for cardiac sarcomas treated conventionally (198). A patient has been reported to have lived over 7 years after transplantation for cardiac sarcoma (113). If the margins are negative at the anastomotic site between donor and recipient, the prognosis is improved, with up to 78 months survival (203). If there is local recurrence after transplant, resection with chemotherapy may extend survival time (56). The role of immunosuppression in tumor recurrence is unclear.

Short of orthotopic transplant, unresectable cardiac sarcomas may be surgically treated by radical resection with autotransplantation (7,33,44,204,205), atrial transplantation (206), and stereotactic radiosurgery (207).

## PROGNOSIS

The overall survival period for patients with cardiac sarcomas averages 11 to 16 months (3,9). The histologic type has not been shown to affect outcome, but necrosis, mitotic activity, and the presence of metastasis at the time of diagnosis negatively impact survival. Metastases are present in about 50 percent of patients at the time of diagnosis; almost all of the remainder develop metastases later. The metastatic sites are most frequently lungs (3,45), followed by long bones (47,197), adrenal gland (3,197), brain (197–199), pleura (3), liver (70), kidney (3), thyroid gland (120), soft tissue (3), skin (2,120), chest wall (3), stomach (133), and vertebra (3). Right-sided sarcomas are more likely to metastasize to lungs (45), which accounts for the high rate of metastatic angiosarcoma to the lungs (see chapter 15). In some patients, metastatic disease appears after complete excision of the primary tumor (197).

Patients die of metastatic disease or because local recurrence results in heart failure or sudden death (90). Local recurrence includes sites in the heart itself, especially the atria, or the pulmonary artery (199,200). Prolonged survival for years despite multiple recurrences has been reported in a patient with osteosarcoma (133). Survival of up to 131 months has been reported in a patient with primary cardiac osteosarcoma who had multiple recurrences and metastases (58).

## REFERENCES

1. Burke A. Primary malignant cardiac tumors. Semin Diagn Pathol 2008;25:39-46.
2. Fletcher CD, Chibon F, Mertens F. Undifferentiated/unclassified sarcomas, in WHO Classification of Tumours of Soft Tissue and Bone. In: Fletcher CD, et al., eds. Lyon: IARC Press; 2013: 236-238.
3. Donsbeck AV, Ranchere D, Coindre JM, Le Gall F, Cordier JF, Loire R. Primary cardiac sarcomas: an immunohistochemical and grading study with long-term follow-up of 24 cases. Histopathology 1999;34:295-304.
4. Bear PA, Moodie DS. Malignant primary cardiac tumors. The Cleveland Clinic experience, 1956 to 1986. Chest 1987;92:860-862.
4. Putnam JB Jr, Sweeney MS, Colon R, Lanza LA, Frazier OH, Cooley DA. Primary cardiac sarcomas. Ann Thorac Surg 1991;51:906-910.
5. Tazelaar HD, Locke TJ, McGregor CG. Pathology of surgically excised primary cardiac tumors. Mayo Clin Proc 1992;67:957-965.
6. Blackmon SH, Patel AR, Bruckner BA, et al. Cardiac autotransplantation for malignant or complex primary left-heart tumors. Tex Heart Inst J 2008;35:296-300.
7. Burke A, Virmani R. Primary cardiac sarcomas. AFIP Atlas of Tumor Pathology. Tumors of the heart and great vessels, 3rd Series, Fascicle 16. Washington, DC: American Registry of Pathology; 1996:127-170.
8. Burke AP, Cowan D, Virmani R. Primary sarcomas of the heart. Cancer 1992;69:387-395.
9. Burke AP, Tazelaar H, Butany JW, et al. Cardiac sarcomas. In: Travis WD, Brambilla E, Müller-Hermelink HK, Harris CC, eds. Pathology and genetics of tumours of the lung, pleura, thymus and heart. Lyon: ARC Press; 2004:273-281.
10. Meng Q, Lai H, Lima J, Tong W, Qian Y, Lai S. Echocardiographic and pathologic characteristics of primary cardiac tumors: a study of 149 cases. Int J Cardiol 2002;84:69-75.
11. Dein JR, Frist WH, Stinson EB, et al. Primary cardiac neoplasms. Early and late results of surgical treatment in 42 patients. J Thorac Cardiovasc Surg 1987;93:502-511.
12. Fernandes F, Soufen HN, Ianni BM, Arteaga E, Ramires FJ, Mady C. Primary neoplasms of the heart. Clinical and histological presentation of 50 cases. Arq Bras Cardiol 2001;76:231-237.
13. Kamiya H, Yasuda T, Nagamine H, et al. Surgical treatment of primary cardiac tumors: 28 years' experience in Kanazawa university hospital. Jpn Circ J 2001;65:315-319.
14. Jae-Kuo, Lai WY, Young MS, Ding YA. Primary malignant cardiac tumor: an analysis of seven cases. Zhonghua Yi Xue Za Zhi (Taipei) 1994;54:329-335.
15. Kosuga T, Fukunaga S, Kawara T, et al. Surgery for primary cardiac tumors. Clinical experience and surgical results in 60 patients. J Cardiovasc Surg (Torino) 2002;43:581-587.
16. Endo A, Ohtahara A, Kinugawa T, et al. Characteristics of 161 patients with cardiac tumors diagnosed during 1993 and 1994 in Japan. Am J Cardiol 1997;79:1708-1711.
17. Miralles A, Bracamonte L, Soncul H, et al. Cardiac tumors: clinical experience and surgical results in 74 patients. Ann Thorac Surg 1991; 52:886-895.
18. Murphy MC, Sweeney MS, Putnam JB Jr, et al. Surgical treatment of cardiac tumors: a 25-year experience. Ann Thorac Surg 1990;49:612-617; discussion 617-618.
19. Odim J, Reehal V, Laks H, Mehta U, Fishbein MC. Surgical pathology of cardiac tumors. Two decades at an urban institution. Cardiovasc Pathol 2003;12:267-270.
20. Piazza N, Chughtai T, Toledano K, Sampalis J, Liao C, Morin JF. Primary cardiac tumours: eighteen years of surgical experience on 21 patients. Can J Cardiol 2004;20:1443-1448.
21. Alfaro-Gomez F, Careaga-Reyna G, Valero-Elizondo G, Arguero-Sanchez R. [Tumors of the heart. 16 years experience in Hospital De Cardiologia, Del Centro Medico Nacional Siglo XXI in Mexico City. Cir Cir 2003;71:179-185. [Spanish]
22. Hoffmeier A, Schmid C, Deiters S, et al. Neoplastic heart disease—the Muenster experience with 108 patients. Thorac Cardiovasc Surg 2005;53:1-8.
23. Coindre JM. Grading of soft tissue sarcomas: review and update. Arch Pathol Lab Med 2006; 130:1448-1453.
24. Coindre JM, Trojani M, Contesso G, et al. Reproducibility of a histopathologic grading system for adult soft tissue sarcoma. Cancer 1986;58:306-309.
25. Deyrup AT, Weiss SW. Grading of soft tissue sarcomas: the challenge of providing precise information in an imprecise world. Histopathology 2006;48:42-50.
26. Guillou L, Coindre JM, Bonichon F, et al. Comparative study of the National Cancer Institute and French Federation of Cancer Centers Sarcoma Group grading systems in a population of 410 adult patients with soft tissue sarcoma. J Clin Oncol 1997;15:350-362.

27. Costa J, Wesley RA, Glatstein E, Rosenberg SA. The grading of soft tissue sarcomas. Results of a clinicohistopathologic correlation in a series of 163 cases. Cancer 1984;53:530-541.
28. Hasegawa T, Yamamoto S, Yokoyama R, Umeda T, Matsuno Y, Hirohashi S. Prognostic significance of grading and staging systems using MIB-1 score in adult patients with soft tissue sarcoma of the extremities and trunk. Cancer 2002;95:843-851.
29. Hasegawa T, Yokoyama R, Lee YH, Shimoda T, Beppu Y, Hirohashi S. Prognostic relevance of a histological grading system using MIB-1 for adult soft-tissue sarcoma. Oncology 2000;58:66-74.
30. Khoury JD, Coffin CM, Spunt SL, Anderson JR, Meyer WH, Parham DM. Grading of nonrhabdomyosarcoma soft tissue sarcoma in children and adolescents: a comparison of parameters used for the Federation Nationale des Centers De Lutte Contre le Cancer and Pediatric Oncology Group Systems. Cancer 2010;116:2266-2274.
31. Wu JT, Frazier OH, Nasser MM, Reul RM. A novel surgical approach to cardiac autotransplantation in complex cardiac sarcoma resection. Innovations (Phila) 2010;5:364-368.
32. Thakker M, Keteepe-Arachi T, Abbas A, et al. A primary cardiac sarcoma presenting with superior vena cava obstruction. Am J Emerg Med 2012;30:264 e263-265.
33. Vallakati A, Shetty V, Shani J. Acute myocardial infarction as a complication of cardiac sarcoma: a rare presentation. J Invasive Cardiol 2012;24:E209-211.
34. Solla-Ruiz I, Villanueva-Benito I, Iglesias-Rodriguez MB, Asorey-Veiga V, Yas SR, Pereira-Loureiro MA. Hemoptysis as the presenting symptom in cardiac sarcoma. Rev Port Cardiol 2012;31:463-464.
35. Cascini F, Longo F, Parenti D, Capelli A. A case of sudden infant death due to a primary cardiac sarcoma. J Forensic Sci 2012;57:1368-1371.
36. Restrepo CS, Largoza A, Lemos DF, et al. CT and MR imaging findings of malignant cardiac tumors. Curr Probl Diagn Radiol 2005;34:1-11.
37. Bhattacharyya S, Roussin I, Prasad S, et al. Characterization of cardiac sarcoma with 2- and 3-dimensional echocardiography, myocardial contrast echocardiography and cardiac magnetic resonance imaging. Circulation 2012;126:e298-300.
38. Siripornpitak S, Higgins CB. MRI of primary malignant cardiovascular tumors. J Comput Assist Tomogr 1997;21:462-466.
39. Mader MT, Poulton TB, White RD. Malignant tumors of the heart and great vessels: Mr imaging appearance. Radiographics 1997;17:145-153.
40. Villacampa VM, Villarreal M, Ros LH, Alvarez R, Cozar M, Fuertes MI. Cardiac rhabdomyosarcoma: diagnosis by MR imaging. Eur Radiol 1999;9:634-637.
41. Clarke NR, Mohiaddin RH, Westaby S, Banning AP. Multifocal cardiac leiomyosarcoma. Diagnosis and surveillance by transoesophageal echocardiography and contrast enhanced cardiovascular magnetic resonance. Postgrad Med J 2002;78:492-493.
42. Hoffmeier A, Deiters S, Schmidt C, et al. Radical resection of cardiac sarcoma. Thorac Cardiovasc Surg 2004;52:77-81.
43. Ishikawa K, Takanashi S, Mihara W, Fukui T, Hosoda Y. Surgical treatment for primary cardiac leiomyosarcoma causing right ventricular outflow obstruction. Circ J 2005;69:121-123.
44. Etschmann B, Krombach G, Boning A, Gattenlohner S. Pleomorphic high-grade sarcoma of the heart mimicking cardiac myxoma. BMJ Case Rep 2012;2012.
45. Ali SZ, Smilari TF, Teichberg S, Hajdu SI. Pleomorphic rhabdomyosarcoma of the heart metastatic to bone. Report of a case with fine needle aspiration biopsy findings. Acta Cytol 1995;39:555-558.
46. Aggeli C, Lampropoulos K, Kartalis A, et al. Primary left ventricular cardiac sarcoma. Cardiol J 2010;17:632-633.
47. Hirota M, Ishikawa N, Oi M, Tedoriya T. Large primary cardiac sarcoma on the left ventricular free wall: Is total excision contraindicated? Interact Cardiovasc Thorac Surg 2010;11:670-672.
48. Zhang H, Macdonald WD, Erickson-Johnson M, Wang X, Jenkins RB, Oliveira AM. Cytogenetic and molecular cytogenetic findings of intimal sarcoma. Cancer Genet Cytogenet 2007;179:146-149.
49. Li Z, Hsieh T, Salehi A. Recurrent cardiac intimal (spindle cell) sarcoma of the left atrium. J Cardiothorac Vasc Anesth 2013;27:103-107.
50. Colon G, Quint DJ, Blaivas M, McGillicuddy J. Cardiac sarcoma metastatic to the brain. AJNR Am J Neuroradiol 1995;16:1739-1741.
51. Domanski MJ, Delaney TF, Kleiner DE Jr, et al. Primary sarcoma of the heart causing mitral stenosis. Am J Cardiol 1990;66:893-895.
52. Son HS, Sun K, Jung JS, Park SM, Lee SH, Kim KT. Intimal cardiac sarcoma in a pregnant woman. Asian Cardiovasc Thorac Ann 2007;15:66-68.
53. Montalescot G, Chapelon C, Drobinski G, Thomas D, Godeau P, Grosgogeat Y. Diagnosis of primary cardiac sarcoma. Report of 4 cases and review of the literature. Int J Cardiol 1988;20:209-219.
53a. Neuville A, Collin F, Bruneval P, et al. Intimal sarcoma is the most frequent primary cardiac sarcoma: clinicopathologic and molecular retrospective analysis of 100 primary cardiac sarcomas. Am J Surg Pathol 2014;38:461-469.
54. Georghiou GP, Shapira Y, Tobar A, Vidne BA, Sahar G. Primary cardiac pleomorphic sarcoma: An aggressive tumor. Isr Med Assoc J 2005;7:470-471.

55. Cho GJ, Kim HJ, Kang JS. Primary cardiac sarcoma in pregnancy: a case report. J Korean Med Sci 2006;21:940-943.

56. Akhter SA, McGinty J, Konys JJ, Giesting RM, Merrill WH, Wagoner LE. Recurrent primary cardiac malignant fibrous histiocytoma following orthotopic heart transplantation. J Heart Lung Transplant 2004;23:1447-1450.

57. Dorobantu M, Fruntelata A, Constantinescu D, et al. Primary left heart malignant fibrous histiocytoma. Eur J Echocardiogr 2005;6:225-227.

58. Suh SH, Park TH, Yoo JN, et al. Primary undifferentiated pleomorphic sarcoma of the left atrium that presented as acute pulmonary edema. Yonsei Med J 2007;48:131-134.

59. Fang CY, Fu M, Chang JP, Eng HL, Hung JS. Malignant fibrous histiocytoma of the left ventricle: a case report. Changgeng Yi Xue Za Zhi 1996;19:187-190.

60. Maruki C, Suzukawa K, Koike J, Sato K. Cardiac malignant fibrous histiocytoma metastasizing to the brain: Development of multiple neoplastic cerebral aneurysms. Surg Neurol 1994;41:40-44.

61. Okamoto K, Kato S, Katsuki S, et al. Malignant fibrous histiocytoma of the heart: Case report and review of 46 cases in the literature. Intern Med 2001;40:1222-1226.

62. Okita Y, Miki S, Ueda Y, Tahata T, Sakai T, Matsuyama K. Recurrent malignant fibrous histiocytoma of the left atrium with extracardiac extension. Am Heart J 1994;127:1624-1628.

63. Ovcak Z, Masera A, Lamovec J. Malignant fibrous histiocytoma of the heart. Arch Pathol Lab Med 1992;116:872-874.

64. Pasquale M, Katz NM, Caruso AC, Bearb ME, Bitterman P. Myxoid variant of malignant fibrous histiocytoma of the heart. Am Heart J 1991; 122(Pt 1):248-250.

65. Teramoto N, Hayashi K, Miyatani K, et al. Malignant fibrous histiocytoma of the right ventricle of the heart. Pathol Int 1995;45:315-319.

66. Rashidi A, Silverberg ML, McCray RD. Malignant fibrous histiocytoma of the heart. Echocardiography 2011;28:E217-218.

67. Hsieh SC, Chen CY, Chan WP. Malignant fibrous histiocytoma of the heart: a case report. Acta Cardiol 2010;65:85-87.

68. Furukawa N, Gummert J, Borgermann J. Complete resection of undifferentiated cardiac sarcoma and reconstruction of the atria and the superior vena cava: case report. J Cardiothorac Surg 2012;7:96.

69. Lazaros GA, Matsakas EP, Madas JS, et al. Primary myxofibrosarcoma of the left atrium: case report and review of the literature. Angiology 2008;59: 632-635.

70. Heletz I, Abramson SV. Large obstructive cardiac myxofibrosarcoma is nearly invisible on transthoracic echocardiogram. Echocardiography 2009;26:847-851.

71. Knobel B, Rosman P, Kishon Y, Husar M. Intracardiac primary fibrosarcoma. Case report and literature review. Thorac Cardiovasc Surg 1992;40:227-230.

72. Basso C, Stefani A, Calabrese F, Fasoli G, Valente M. Primary right atrial fibrosarcoma diagnosed by endocardial biopsy. Am Heart J 1996;131:399-402.

73. Jyothirmayi R, Jacob R, Nair K, Rajan B. Primary fibrosarcoma of the right ventricle—a case report. Acta Oncol 1995;34:972-974.

74. Shih WJ, McCullough S, Smith M. Diagnostic imagings for primary cardiac fibrosarcoma. Int J Cardiol 1993;39:157-161.

74a. Kim CH, Dancer JY, Coffey D, et al. Clinicopathologic study of 24 patients with primary cardiac sarcomas: a 10-year single institution experience. Hum Pathol 2008;39:933-938.

75. Boey S, Tribouilloy C, Lesbre JP, et al. [Surgical treatment of leiomyosarcoma of the left atrium report of a case and review of the literature.] Arch Mal Coeur Vaiss 1994;87:291-294. [French]

76. Fyfe AI, Huckell VF, Burr LH, Stonier PM. Leiomyosarcoma of the left atrium: case report and review of the literature. Can J Cardiol 1991;7:193-196.

77. Stoian I, Piser IT, Kulcsar I, Chioncel O, Carp A, Macarie C. Rare tumors of the heart—angiosarcoma, pericardial lipoma, leiomyosarcoma. Three case reports. J Med Life 2010;3:178-182.

78. Gyhra AS, Santander CK, Alarcon EC, Mucientes FH, Carrillo H. Leiomyosarcoma of the pulmonary veins with extension to the left atrium. Ann Thorac Surg 1996;61:1840-1841.

79. Patel SM, Kadakia KC, Maleszewski JJ, Marks RS. Straight to the heart: pulmonary vein leiomyosarcoma. Am J Med 2013;126:117-119.

80. Gehrmann J, Kehl HG, Diallo R, Debus V, Vogt J. Cardiac leiomyosarcoma of the right atrium in a teenager: unusual manifestation with a lifetime history of atrial ectopic tachycardia. Pacing Clin Electrophysio. 2001;24:1161-1164.

81. Takamizawa S, Sugimoto K, Tanaka H, Sakai O, Arai T, Saitoh A. A case of primary leiomyosarcoma of the heart. Intern Med 1992;31:265-268.

82. Morin JE, Rahal DP, Huttner I. Myxoid leiomyosarcoma of the left atrium: a rare malignancy of the heart and its comparison with atrial myxoma. Can J Cardiol 2001;17:331-336.

83. Lee SH, Kim WH, Choi JB, et al. Huge primary pleomorphic leiomyosarcoma in the right ventricle with impending obstruction of both inflow and outflow tracts. Circ J 2009;73:779-782.

84. Fox JP, Freitas E, McGiffin DC, Firouz-Abadi AA, West MJ. Primary leiomyosarcoma of the heart: A rare cause of obstruction of the left ventricular outflow tract. Aust N Z J Med 1991;21:881-883.

85. Ogimoto A, Hamada M, Ohtsuka T, et al. Rapid progression of primary cardiac leiomyosarcoma with obstruction of the left ventricular outflow tract and mitral stenosis. Intern Med 2003; 42:827-830.

86. van Gelder T, Jonkman FA, Niesters HG, Vuzevski VD, Spillenaar Bilgen EJ, Weimar W. Absence of epstein-barr virus involvement in an adult heart transplant recipient with an epitheloid leiomyosarcoma. J Heart Lung Transplant 1996;15:650-651.

87. Pucci A, Gagliardotto P, Papandrea C, et al. An unusual myxoid leiomyosarcoma of the heart. Arch Pathol Lab Med 1996;120:583-586.

88. Han P, Drachtman RA, Amenta P, Ettinger LJ. Successful treatment of a primary cardiac leiomyosarcoma with ifosfamide and etoposide. J Pediatr Hematol Oncol 1996;18:314-317.

89. Ashraf T, Day TG, Marek J, Hughes M, Giardini A. A triad: cardiac rhabdomyosarcoma, stroke and tamponade. Pediatr Cardiol 2012;34:771-773.

90. Vujin B, Benc D, Srdic S, Bikicki M, Vuckovic D, Dodic S. Rhabdomyosarcoma of the heart. Herz 2006;31:798-800.

91. Damjanovic M, Djordjevic-Radojkovic D, Perisic Z, et al. Heart failure caused by cardiac rhabdomyosarcoma. Kardiol Pol 2008;66:1207-1209.

92. Sokullu O, Sanioglu S, Deniz H, Ayoglu U, Ozgen A, Bilgen F. Primary cardiac rhabdomyosarcoma of the right atrium: case report. Heart Surg Forum 2008;11:E117-119.

93. Skopin II, Serov RA, Makushin AA, Sazonenkov MA. Primary rhabdomyosarcoma of the right atrium. Interact Cardiovasc Thorac Surg 2003; 2:316-318.

94. Selvaraj T, Kapoor PM, Kiran U. Large rhabdomyosarcoma of the right ventricle obstructing tricuspid valve, pulmonary valve and left ventricular outflow tract. Ann Card Anaesth 2009; 12:81-82.

95. Fan HG, Meng J, Pan SW, Zheng Z, Hu SS. Diagnosis, operation, recurrence, metastasis, and death: a case of primary cardiac rhabdomyosarcoma. J Card Surg 2009;24:480-482.

96. Scott RS, Jagirdar J. Right atrial botryoid rhabdomyosarcoma in an adult patient with recurrent pleomorphic rhabdomyosarcomas following doxorubicin therapy. Ann Diagn Pathol 2007; 11:274-276.

97. Tutak E, Satar M, Ozbarlas N, et al. A newborn infant with intrapericardial rhabdomyosarcoma: a case report. Turk J Pediatr 2008;50:179-181.

98. Lima Rde C, Mendes A, Bezerra E, Oliveira W. Surgical treatment of primary cardiac rhabdomyosarcoma. Rev Bras Cir Cardiovasc 2009;24: 242-244.

99. Burke A, Virmani R. Tumors of the heart and great vessels. AFIP Atlas of Tumor Pathology, t3rd Series, Fascicle, 16. Washington, DC: American Registry of Pathology; 1996:1-12.

100. Chan HS, Sonley MJ, Moes CA, Daneman A, Smith CR, Martin DJ. Primary and secondary tumors of childhood involving the heart, pericardium, and great vessels. A report of 75 cases and review of the literature. Cancer 1985;56:825-836.

101. Castorino F, Masiello P, Quattrocchi E, Di Benedetto G. Primary cardiac rhabdomyosarcoma of the left atrium: an unusual presentation. Tex Heart Inst J 2000;27:206-208.

102. Attanasio A, Romitelli S, Mauriello A, Palmieri G, Stefani A, Pierangeli L. Cardiac rhabdomyosarcoma: a clinicopathologic and electron microscopy study. G Ital Cardiol 1998;28:383-386.

103. Awad M, Dunn B, al Halees Z, et al. Intracardiac rhabdomyosarcoma: transesophageal echocardiographic findings and diagnosis. J Am Soc Echocardiogr 1992;5:199-202.

104. Grandmougin D, Fayad G, Decoene C, Pol A, Warembourg H. Total orthotopic heart transplantation for primary cardiac rhabdomyosarcoma: factors influencing long-term survival. Ann Thorac Surg 2001;71:1438-1441.

105. Orsmond GS, Knight L, Dehner LP, Nicoloff DM, Nesbitt M, Bessinger FB Jr. Alveolar rhabdomyosarcoma involving the heart. An echocardiographic, angiographic and pathologic study. Circulation 1976;54:837-843.

106. Hajar R, Roberts WC, Folger GM Jr. Embryonal botryoid rhabdomyosarcoma of the mitral valve. Am J Cardiol 1986;57:376.

107. Hui KS, Green LK, Schmidt WA. Primary cardiac rhabdomyosarcoma: definition of a rare entity. Am J Cardiovasc Pathol 1988;2:19-29.

108. Fraternali Orcioni G, Ravetti JL, Gaggero G, Bocca B, Bisceglia M. Primary embryonal spindle cell cardiac rhabdomyosarcoma: case report. Pathol Res Pract 2010;206:325-330.

109. Altunbasak S, Demirtas M, Tunali N, Zorludemir S, Polat S. Primary rhabdomyosarcoma of the heart presenting with increased intracranial pressure. Pediatr Cardiol 1996;17:260-264.

110. Charney DA, Charney JM, Ghali VS, Teplitz C. Primitive neuroectodermal tumor of the myocardium: a case report, review of the literature, immunohistochemical, and ultrastructural study. Hum Pathol 1996;27:1365-1369.

111. Burke AP, Virmani R. Osteosarcomas of the heart. Am J Surg Pathol 1991;15:289-295.

112. Hashimoto W, Hashizume K, Ariyoshi T, et al. Primary cardiac osteosarcoma with imaging that revealed no calcification. Gen Thorac Cardiovasc Surg 2011;59:184-186.

113. Ahn S, Choi JA, Chung JH, et al. MR imaging findings of a primary cardiac osteosarcoma and its bone metastasis with histopathologic correlation. Korean J Radiol 2011;12:135-139.

114. Ye Z, Shi H, Peng T, Han A. Clinical and pathological features of high grade primary cardiac osteosarcoma. Interact Cardiovasc Thorac Surg 2011;12:94-95.

115. Takeuchi I, Kawaguchi T, Kimura Y, et al. Primary cardiac osteosarcoma in a young man with severe congestive heart failure. Intern Med 2007;46:649-651.

116. Lurito KJ, Martin T, Cordes T. Right atrial primary cardiac osteosarcoma. Pediatr Cardiol 2002;23:462-465.

117. Reynard JS Jr, Gregoratos G, Gordon MJ, Bloor CM. Primary osteosarcoma of the heart. Am Heart J 1985;109:598-600.

118. Kocak H, Karapolat S, Gundogdu C, Bozkurt E, Unlu Y. Primary cardiac osteosarcoma in a pregnant woman. Heart Vessels 2006;21:56-58.

119. Dohi T, Ohmura H, Daida H, Amano A. Primary right atrial cardiac osteosarcoma with congestive heart failure. Eur J Cardiothorac Surg 2009;35:544-546.

120. Jahns R, Kenn W, Stolte M, Inselmann G. A primary osteosarcoma of the heart as a cause of recurrent peripheral arterial emboli. Ann Oncol 1998;9:775-778.

121. Seidal T, Wandt B, Lundin SE. Primary chondroblastic osteogenic sarcoma of the left atrium. Case report. Scand J Thorac Cardiovasc Surg 1992;26:233-236.

122. Shuhaiber J, Cabrera J, Nemeh H. Treatment of a case of primary osteosarcoma of the left heart: a case report. Heart Surg Forum 2007;10:E30-32.

123. Parwani AV, Esposito N, Rao UN. Primary cardiac osteosarcoma with recurrent episodes and unusual patterns of metastatic spread. Cardiovasc Pathol 2008;17:413-417.

124. Lopez M, Pinto A, Moreno V, Diaz M, Gonzalez Baron M. Primary cardiac osteosarcoma. Clin Transl Oncol 2008;10:515-516.

125. Kase S, Nakamoto S, Miyasaka S, et al. Cardiac chondrosarcoma producing parathyroid hormone-related protein. Circ J 2004;68:715-718.

126. Jinno T, Morimoto T, Itoh A, Tago M. Primary cardiac chondrosarcoma with large cell pulmonary carcinoma. Jpn J Thorac Cardiovasc Surg 2006;54:228-231.

127. Miwa S, Konishi Y, Matsumoto M, Minakata K. Primary cardiac chondrosarcoma—a case report. Jpn Circ J 1997;61:795-797.

128. Ng SH, Ko SF, Yang TS, Wong HF, Wan YL, Ho YS. Primary cardiac chondrosarcoma. Am J Emerg Med 1996;14:285-287.

129. Naumann S, Krallman PA, Unni KK, Fidler ME, Neff JR, Bridge JA. Translocation der(13;21)(q10;q10) in skeletal and extraskeletal mesenchymal chondrosarcoma. Mod Pathol 2002;15:572-576.

130. Yokouchi Y, Hiruta N, Oharaseki T, et al. Primary cardiac synovial sarcoma: a case report and literature review. Pathol Int 2011;61:150-155.

131. Nicholson AG, Rigby M, Lincoln C, Meller S, Fisher C. Synovial sarcoma of the heart. Histopathology 1997;30:349-352.

132. Van der Mieren G, Willems S, Sciot R, et al. Pericardial synovial sarcoma: 14-year survival with multimodality therapy. Ann Thorac Surg 2004;78:e41-42.

133. Casselman FP, Gillinov AM, Kasirajan V, Ratliff NB, Cosgrove DM 3rd. Primary synovial sarcoma of the left heart. Ann Thorac Surg 1999;68:2329-2331.

134. Bittira B, Tsang J, Huynh T, Morin JF, Huttner I. Primary right atrial synovial sarcoma manifesting as transient ischemic attacks. Ann Thorac Surg 2000;69:1949-1951.

135. Hannachi Sassi S, Zargouni N, Saadi Dakhlia M, Mrad K, Cammoun M, Ben Romdhane K. Primary synovial sarcoma of the heart. A clinicopathologic study of one case and review of the literature. Pathologica 2004;96:29-34.

136. Hazelbag HM, Szuhai K, Tanke HJ, Rosenberg C, Hogendoorn PC. Primary synovial sarcoma of the heart: a cytogenetic and molecular genetic analysis combining RT-PCR and COBRA-FISH of a case with a complex karyotype. Mod Pathol 2004;17:1434-1439.

137. Varma T, Adegboyega P. Primary cardiac synovial sarcoma. Arch Pathol Lab Med 2012;136:454-458.

138. Mohamed AA, Al-Khaldi A, Omran AS. Primary cardiac synovial sarcoma demonstrated by 3D transesophageal echocardiogram. Eur J Echocardiogr 2011;12:409.

139. Talukder M, Joyce L, Marks R, Kaplan K. Primary cardiac synovial sarcoma. Interact Cardiovasc Thorac Surg 2010;11:490-492.

140. Lv X, Guo X, Chen X, et al. Primary cardiac synovial sarcoma. J Card Surg 2010;25:288-290.

141. Zhao Q, Geha AS, Devries SR, et al. Biatrial primary synovial sarcoma of the heart. J Am Soc Echocardiogr 2007;20:197 e191-194.

142. Miller DV, Deb A, Edwards WD, Zehr KJ, Oliveira AM. Primary synovial sarcoma of the mitral valve. Cardiovasc Pathol 2005;14:331-333.

143. Sakai M, Takami H, Joyama S, et al. Cardiac synovial sarcoma swinging through the aortic valve. Ann Thorac Surg 2011;92:1129.

144. Provenzano SC, Con R, Jones OD, Grant PW. Synovial sarcoma of the heart. Heart Lung Circ 2006;15:278-279.

145. White RW, Rushbrook J, Sivananthan MU, Mc-Goldrick JP. Primary cardiac synovial sarcoma with imminent tricuspid valve obstruction. Ann Thorac Surg 2009;87:322.

146. Policarpio-Nicolas ML, Alasadi R, Nayar R, De Frias DV. Synovial sarcoma of the heart: Report of a case with diagnosis by endoscopic ultrasound-guided fine needle aspiration biopsy. Acta Cytol 2006;50:683-686.

147. Le March'hadour F, Peoc'h M, Pasquier B, Leroux D. Cardiac synovial sarcoma with translocation (X;18) associated with asbestos exposure. Cancer 1994;74:986.

148. Karn CM, Socinski MA, Fletcher JA, Corson JM, Craighead JE. Cardiac synovial sarcoma with translocation (X;18) associated with asbestos exposure. Cancer 1994;73:74-78.

149. Kojima KY, Koslin DB, Primack SL, Kettler MD. Synovial sarcoma arising from the pericardium: radiographic and CT findings. AJR Am J Roentgenol 1999;173:246-247.

150. Anand AK, Khanna A, Sinha SK, Mukherjee U, Walia JS, Singh AN. Pericardial synovial sarcoma. Clin Oncol (R Coll Radiol) 2003;15:186-188.

151. Constantinou LL, Charitos CE, Lariou CM, et al. Primary synovial cardiac sarcoma: a rare cause of tamponade. Eur Heart J 1996;17:1766-1768.

152. Hing SN, Marshall L, Al-Saadi R, Hargrave D. Primary pericardial synovial sarcoma confirmed by molecular genetic studies: a case report. J Pediatr Hematol Oncol 2007;29:492-495.

153. Al-Rajhi N, Husain S, Coupland R, McNamee C, Jha N. Primary pericardial synovial sarcoma: a case report and literature review. J Surg Oncol 1999;70:194-198.

154. Oizumi S, Igarashi K, Takenaka T, et al. Primary pericardial synovial sarcoma with detection of the chimeric transcript SYT-SSX. Jpn Circ J 1999;63:330-332.

155. Schumann C, Kunze M, Kochs M, Hombach V, Rasche V. Pericardial synovial sarcoma mimicking pericarditis in findings of cardiac magnetic resonance imaging. Int J Cardiol 2007;118: e83-84.

156. Iyengar V, Lineberger AS, Kerman S, Burton NA. Synovial sarcoma of the heart. Correlation with cytogenetic findings. Arch Pathol Lab Med 1995;119:1080-1082.

157. Boulmay B, Cooper G, Reith JD, Marsh R. Primary cardiac synovial sarcoma: a case report and brief review of the literature. Sarcoma 2007; 2007:94797.

158. Paraf F, Bruneval P, Balaton A, et al. Primary liposarcoma of the heart. Am J Cardiovasc Pathol 1990;3:175-180.

159. Uemura S, Watanabe M, Iwama H, Saito Y. Extensive primary cardiac liposarcoma with multiple functional complications. Heart 2004;90:e48.

160. Higgins JC, Katzman PJ, Yeager SB, et al. Extraskeletal Ewing's sarcoma of primary cardiac origin. Pediatr Cardiol 1994;15:207-208.

161. Small EJ, Gordon GJ, Dahms BB. Malignant rhabdoid tumor of the heart in an infant. Cancer 1985;55:2850-2853.

162. Cho WC, Jung SH, Lee SH, Bang JH, Kim J, Lee JW. Malignant peripheral nerve sheath tumor arising from the left ventricle. J Card Surg 2012; 27:567-570.

163. Zhang PJ, Brooks JS, Goldblum JR, et al. Primary cardiac sarcomas: a clinicopathologic analysis of a series with follow-up information in 17 patients and emphasis on long-term survival. Hum Pathol 2008;39:1385-1395.

164. Ramnarine IR, Davidson L, van Doorn CA. Primary cardiac carcinosarcoma: a rare, aggressive tumor. Ann Thorac Surg 2001;72:927-929.

165. Romanos-Sirakis EC, Meyer DB, Chun A, Gardner S. A primary cardiac sarcoma with features of a desmoplastic small round cell tumor in an adolescent male. J Pediatr Hematol Oncol 2010; 32:236-239.

166. Bloomberg RD, Butany JW, Cusimano RJ, Leask RL. Primary cardiac sarcoma involving the pulmonary artery and valve. Can J Cardiol 2003;19:843-847.

167. Edwards FH, Hale D, Cohen A, Thompson L, Pezzella AT, Virmani R. Primary cardiac valve tumors. Ann Thorac Surg 1991;52:1127-1131.

168. Kalangos A, Sierra J, Hohn L, et al. Cardiac sarcoma originating from the tricuspid valve. J Card Surg 2001;16:173-175.

169. Lee JR, Chang JM, Lee C, Kim CJ. Undifferentiated sarcoma of the mitral valve with unique clinicopathologic presentation. J Cardiovasc Surg (Torino) 2003;44:621-623.

170. Zerkowski HR, Hofmann HS, Gybels I, Knolle J. Primary sarcoma of pulmonary artery and valve: Multimodality treatment by chemotherapy and homograft replacement. J Thorac Cardiovasc Surg 1996;112:1122-1124.

171. Burke A, Virmani R. Pediatric heart tumors. Cardiovasc Pathol 2008;17:193-198.

172. Sallee D, Spector ML, van Heeckeren DW, Patel CR. Primary pediatric cardiac tumors: a 17 year experience. Cardiol Young 1999;9:155-162.

173. Takach TJ, Reul GJ, Ott DA, Cooley DA. Primary cardiac tumors in infants and children: immediate and long-term operative results. Ann Thorac Surg 1996;62:559-564.

174. Itoh K, Matsumura T, Egawa Y, et al. Primary mitral valve sarcoma in infancy. Pediatr Cardiol 1998;19:174-177.

175. McElhinney DB, Carpentieri DF, Bridges ND, Clark BJ, Gaynor JW, Spray TL. Sarcoma of the mitral valve causing coronary arterial occlusion in children. Cardiol Young 2001;11:539-542.

176. Burke A, Tavora F, Ozbudak I, Franks T, Miettinen M. Pediatric cardiac sarcomas, a series of 16 new cases with literature review. Virchows Arch 2007; 451:489-490.

177. Lazarus KH, D'Orsogna DE, Bloom KR, Rouse RG. Primary pericardial sarcoma in a neonate. Am J Pediatr Hematol Oncol 1989;11:343-347.

178. Mahar LJ, Lie JT, Groover RV, Seward JB, Puga FJ, Feldt RH. Primary cardiac myxosarcoma in a child. Mayo Clin Proc 1979;54:261-266.

179. Koga S, Ikeda S, Urata J, et al. Primary high-grade myofibroblastic sarcoma arising from the pericardium. Circ J 2008;72:337-339.

180. Lajos P, Hasaniya N, Ehrman W, Razzouk A. Spindle cell sarcoma of the pericardium: a case report. J Card Surg 2004;19:139-141.

181. Rangasetty UC, Martinez JD, Ahmad M. Images in cardiovascular medicine. Contrast-enhanced echocardiography in spindle cell sarcoma of the pericardium. Circulation 2007;115:e329-331.

182. Calvert PA, Bell AD, Lynch M. Effusive constrictive pericarditis secondary to undifferentiated pericardial sarcoma. Heart 2006;92:1034.

183. Kim NH, Kweon KH, Oh SK, et al. A case of primary pericardial undifferentiated sarcoma. J Korean Med Sci 2003;18:742-745.

184. Zhengrong W, Yun Z, Fuchun Z. Primary malignant pericardial sarcoma. Int J Cardiol 2009; 136:96-99.

185. Kindl TF, Hassan AM, Booth RL, Jr., Durham SJ, Papadimos TJ. A primary high-grade pleomorphic pericardial liposarcoma presenting as syncope and angina. Anesth Analg 2006;102:1363-1364.

196. Kamlow FJ, Padaria SF, Wainwright RJ. Metastatic cardiac malignant fibrous histiocytoma presenting as right ventricular outflow tract obstruction. Clin Cardiol 1991;14:173-175.

197. Harting MT, Messner GN, Gregoric ID, Frazier OH. Sarcoma metastatic to the right ventricle: Surgical intervention followed by prolonged survival. Tex Heart Inst J 2004;31:93-95.

188. Lin MH, Yu HY, Wang SS. Haematogenous metastases after complete resection of primary cardiac sarcoma from the left atrium. Acta Cardiol 2011;66:395-397.

189. Talbot SM, Taub RN, Keohan ML, Edwards N, Galantowicz ME, Schulman LL. Combined heart and lung transplantation for unresectable primary cardiac sarcoma. J Thorac Cardiovasc Surg 2002;124:1145-1148.

190. Myruski KS, Manecke GR Jr, Kotzur A, Wahrenbrock EA, Jamieson SW. Late recurrence of cardiac sarcoma presenting as giant pulmonary artery aneurysm. J Heart Lung Transplant 2004; 23:1445-1446.

191. Uberfuhr P, Meiser B, Fuchs A, et al. Heart transplantation: an approach to treating primary cardiac sarcoma? J Heart Lung Transplant 2002;21:1135-1139.

192. Mery GM, Reardon MJ, Haas J, Lazar J, Hindenburg A. A combined modality approach to recurrent cardiac sarcoma resulting in a prolonged remission: a case report. Chest 2003; 123:1766-1768.

193. Movsas B, Teruya-Feldstein J, Smith J, Glatstein E, Epstein AH. Primary cardiac sarcoma: a novel treatment approach. Chest 1998;114:648-652.

194. Goldstein DJ, Oz MC, Rose EA, Fisher P, Michler RE. Experience with heart transplantation for cardiac tumors. J Heart Lung Transplant 1995; 14:382-386.

195. Hoffmeier A, Scheld HH, Tjan TD, et al. Ex situ resection of primary cardiac tumors. Thorac Cardiovasc Surg 2003;51:99-101.

196. Wippermann J, Albers JM, Brandes H, Wahlers T. Redo-extirpation of a cardiac leiomyosarcoma to avoid transplantation. Thorac Cardiovasc Surg 2002;50:62-63.

197. Stoica SC, Mitchell IM, Foreman J, Hunt CJ, Wallwork J, Large SR. Atrial transplantation for recurrent cardiac sarcoma. J Heart Lung Transplant 2001;20:1220-1223.

198. Soltys SG, Kalani MY, Cheshier SH, Szabo KA, Lo A, Chang SD. Stereotactic radiosurgery for a cardiac sarcoma: a case report. Technol Cancer Res Treat 2008;7:363-368.

199. Grande AM, Ragni T, Vigano M. Primary cardiac tumors. A clinical experience of 12 years. Tex Heart Inst J 1993;20:223-230.

200. Simpson L, Kumar SK, Okuno SH, et al. Malignant primary cardiac tumors: Review of a single institution experience. Cancer 2008;112:2440-2446.

201. Thomas-de-Montpreville V, Nottin R, Dulmet E, Serraf A. Heart tumors in children and adults: clinicopathological study of 59 patients from a surgical center. Cardiovasc Pathol 2007;16:22-28.

202. Bakaeen FG, Reardon MJ, Coselli JS, et al. Surgical outcome in 85 patients with primary cardiac tumors. Am J Surg 2003;186:641-647; discussion 647.

203. Strecker T, Rosch J, Weyand M, Agaimy A. Primary and metastatic cardiac tumors: imaging characteristics, surgical treatment, and histopathological spectrum: a 10-year-experience at a German heart center. Cardiovasc Pathol 2012;21:436-443.

204. Bossert T, Gummert JF, Battellini R, et al. Surgical experience with 77 primary cardiac tumors. Interact Cardiovasc Thorac Surg 2005;4:311-315.

# 17 HEMATOLOGIC TUMORS OF THE HEART AND PERICARDIUM

## CARDIAC LYMPHOMA

**Definition.** *Lymphoma* is a malignant proliferation of lymphoid cells that occasionally involves the heart and pericardium. Lymphoma is broadly categorized as of Hodgkin and non-Hodgkin types, although in general, only the latter occurs as a primary neoplasm in the heart, almost all of which are of B-cell origin.

The term *primary cardiac lymphoma* is used to indicate different situations. Some observers use it to denote cardiac symptoms at the onset of disease manifestation; others use it to indicate that the bulk of the tumor mass is present within the pericardium. The term is also used to describe a tumor confined to the myocardium as determined by multimodality imaging or at autopsy (1,2). It is reasonable to classify lymphomas that cause initial symptoms by their mass effect within the pericardium as primary cardiac lymphomas, especially if the bulk of tumor appears to be intrapericardial (3).

**General Features.** The precise location of the lymphoid cell at the time of incipient clonal expansion can never be stated with certainty (4). Because lymphocytes are not normal constituents of the myocardium, cardiac lymphomas, like those of soft tissue, have no known precursor cells. In contrast, extranodal lymphomas that occur in organs with a resident lymphoid tissue population arise from this tissue and have in the past been termed "MALToma," or "derived from mucosa-associated lymphoid tissue," as well as other designations.

Anatomic studies of cardiac lymphatic drainage in animals (5–7) demonstrate a network of lymphatic vessels in the epicardium, which connects to the sinoatrial and atrioventricular nodes. This may explain the predilection of cardiac lymphoma for the epicardium as well as the reported development of conduction abnormalities (6). The cardiac valves do not appear to contain lymphatics, which is consistent with the absence of valvular involvement in most patients with cardiac lymphoma (7–9).

Lymphatic obstruction by tumor may result in pericardial effusions (8,9).

A subset of cardiac B-cell lymphomas occurs in immunocompromised patients. About 80 percent of these tumors contain episomal Epstein-Barr virus (EBV) DNA (10) which is believed to be oncogenic. The resulting clonal expansion of B lymphocytes may progress through a polyclonal or oligoclonal initial phase. This spectrum of lesions has been termed "post-transplant lymphoproliferative disorder" in allograft recipients who are iatrogenically immunocompromised (see Cardiac Lymphoma in Immunocompromised Patients).

Cardiac involvement occurs in 25 percent of patients with disseminated lymphoma (11,12). Primary cardiac lymphoma is, however, rare, accounting for 1.3 percent of primary cardiac tumors and 0.5 percent of extranodal lymphomas (12). Most series of surgically excised cardiac tumors include few or no examples of lymphoma (13–27). In the authors' experience, however, cardiac lymphomas are becoming more frequent as surgical specimens, and are the fourth most common surgically excised cardiac mass (other than thrombi and vegetations) after papillary fibroelastoma, myxoma, and sarcoma.

Primary cardiac lymphomas were initially recognized as autopsy findings, as antemortem diagnosis was impossible prior to the era of open heart surgery (28,29). The autopsy incidence of primary cardiac lymphoma is unknown, but is estimated at 1 percent of .005 percent, a rough estimate of the incidence of primary heart tumors (30), or about 1 in 2 million patients. Most reports of primary cardiac lymphoma diagnosed during life are case reports or small series (1,2,31–66).

**Clinical Features.** Men are somewhat more likely than women to have cardiac lymphomas, with an overall male to female ratio of approximately 1.3 to 1.0. Cardiac lymphoma is a disease of adults of a mean age of approximately 60 years (range, 12 to 86 years) (3,35,67,50,67).

337

As is the case with heart tumors of any type, symptoms related to cardiac lymphomas depend on location, and whether there is obstruction of blood flow, interference with cardiac contractility, formation of pericardial effusions, and involvement of conduction pathways and nerves. The presenting symptoms are most commonly related to congestive heart failure, pericardial effusions, vena caval obstruction, and conduction system disturbances (1,29,33,42,44,50,53,56,67–72). Anginal pain indicates infiltration of a coronary artery (32). Conduction system disturbances caused by cardiac lymphoma include complete heart block (33,58,73,74), atrial fibrillation or flutter (52), and sudden cardiac death (41). There are reports of initial symptoms related to cardiac tamponade (75), tumor embolism to the pulmonary arteries (31), systemic embolic phenomena (stroke) (76,77), right heart obstruction (54), and valvular obstruction (42). Rarely, initial symptoms mimic viral myocarditis (60). Heart block may reverse after treatment (73).

**Radiologic Findings.** Localization of tumor and assessment of response to treatment is performed by imaging techniques, primarily transthoracic and transesophageal echocardiography (37,78), magnetic resonance imaging (MRI), and computed tomography (CT) (38,61). Both CT and MRI have significantly improved tissue and contrast resolution, allowing for the evaluation of tissue based on density or signal intensity (79–82). Because cardiac lymphomas may be ill-defined infiltrative masses, they are often best evaluated with MRI because of its superior soft tissue contrast (79). Lymphomas have variable signal intensity on MRI, may have similar or lower attenuation than the adjacent muscle on CT, and may show increased or decreased contrast enhancement with gadolinium (67,83). In some cases, pericardial effusion or pericardial thickening may be the only finding. Gallium-67 uptake is nonspecific, but is increased in lymphomatous deposits. Fluorine-18 fluorodeoxyglucose positron emission tomography (PET) may be useful for evaluating tumor location and chemotherapy response (67,83).

**Tissue Sampling.** The diagnosis of cardiac lymphoma is made by biopsy, open resection, or cytologic examination of pericardial fluid (32, 35,39). Tumor staging, including the detection of extracardiac tumor, includes bone marrow biopsies, mediastinal CT or MRI, and PET scanning. Mediastinal lymphadenopathy may, on histologic examination, represent reactive hyperplasia (28,42) and imaging does not always detect the presence of a mediastinal lymphoma (57).

When pericardial effusion is present, pericardiocentesis may have both palliative and diagnostic purposes. Lymphoma cells are detected in serous fluid in up to 88 percent of cases (84). When cytology is not available, the diagnosis of primary cardiac lymphoma is usually assessed by explorative thoracotomy and cardiac mass biopsy. Recently, less invasive procedures have been performed, such as transesophageal ultrasound-guided percutaneous intracardiac biopsy or transvenous endomyocardial biopsy (51,55).

**Gross Findings.** Primary cardiac lymphomas typically occur as multiple masses of firm, white, homogeneous nodules with a "fish flesh" consistency (figs. 17-1–17-6). The heart is usually enlarged; autopsy weights range from 410 to 1,570 g (31,42), with a mean weight of approximately 700 g in untreated cases (3). The gross appearance may suggest sarcoidosis; sarcoid granulomas, however, do not usually form large nodules that extend onto epicardium/pericardium, as is typical for lymphoma, and are generally more firm and fibrous. Grossly, lymphomas may be impossible to distinguish from sarcomas. The latter, however, are more likely to demonstrate hemorrhage and necrosis, and often extend into the ventricular or atrial cavities.

The sites of the heart most often affected by lymphoma are the right atrium, followed by the right ventricle, left ventricle, left atrium, atrial septum, and ventricular septum (fig. 17-1) (3,35,67,85,86). Extension of tumor onto valves is unusual, but extension onto the pericardial surface is typical. More than one cardiac chamber is involved in over 75 percent of cases, although tumors confined to the atria, pericardium (35), and coronary arteries (34) have been reported.

**Microscopic Findings.** Histologically, cardiac lymphomas span the spectrum of B-cell proliferations, and include *diffuse large B-cell lymphoma* (nearly 80 percent of published cases) (figs. 17-7–17-13) (3,46,50,56,88,89), *follicular lymphoma* (fig. 17-14), and *Burkitt lymphoma* (fig. 17-15). In a series of 40 primary cardiac lymphomas in immunocompetent patients, 37 were

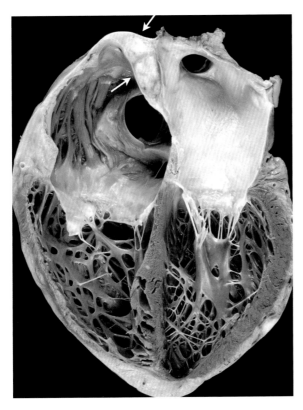

**Figure 17-1**

**CARDIAC LYMPHOMA**

A four-chamber view of a heart at autopsy shows white masses in the atrial septum (arrows). Histologically, this was an anaplastic large cell lymphoma.

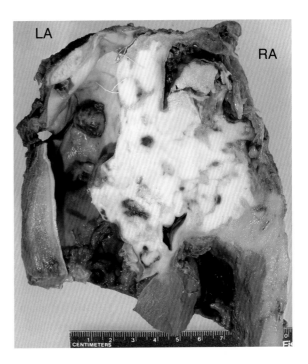

**Figure 17-2**

**CARDIAC LYMPHOMA**

There is massive involvement of the atrial septum and destruction of the basilar heart structures. The atrial septum and right atrium were extensively replaced by tumor, with polypoid subendocardial nodular projections into the left atrium. (LA = left atrium, RA = right atrium.)

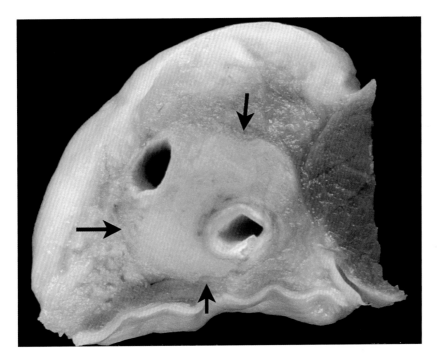

**Figure 17-3**

**CARDIAC LYMPHOMA**

The tumor forms a homogeneous, white fleshy mass nearly surrounding the left circumflex artery (lower right) and partly surrounding the great cardiac vein (upper left). The borders of the tumor are demarcated by arrows. At the bottom is atrial endocardium; on the right, left ventricular muscle.

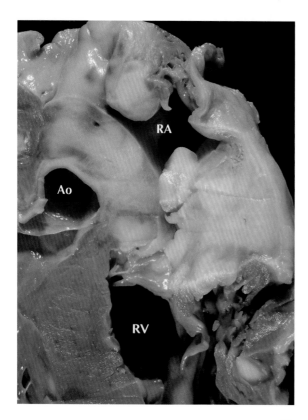 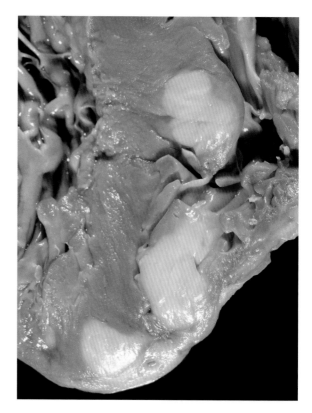

**Figure 17-4**

**CARDIAC LYMPHOMA: SECONDARY**

Left: This patient had a history of cutaneous T-cell lymphoma and presented with supraventricular arrhythmias late in the course of disease. There is extensive involvement of the right atrium (RA), with a homogeneous fleshy tumor extending into the wall of the ascending aorta (Ao). The heart is seen from the posterior aspect. (RV= right ventricle.)

Right: The right side of the ventricular apex has homogeneous fleshy masses without significant fibrosis, necrosis, or hemorrhage.

**Figure 17-5**

**CARDIAC LYMPHOMA: SECONDARY**

In patients with disseminated lymphoma, heart failure may ensue due to massive biventricular and biatrial involvement. The valves, however, are generally spared by lymphoma.

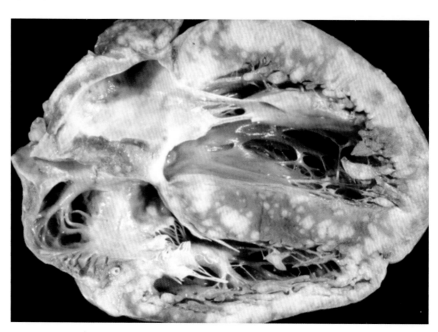

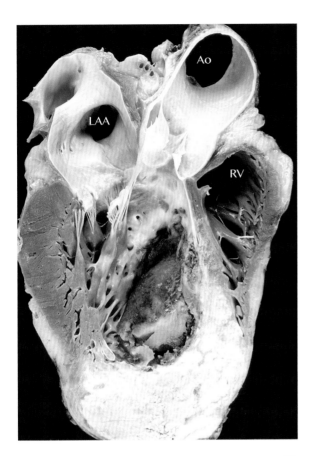
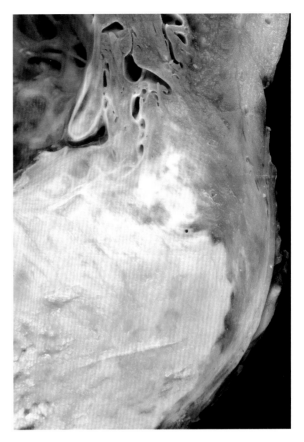

**Figure 17-6**

**CARDIAC T-CELL LYMPHOMA: APICAL VENTRICULAR INVOLVEMENT AND APICAL ANEURYSM**

Left: The left ventricular apex and a portion of the interventricular septum is replaced by fleshy tumor. The left ventricular cavity has a mural thrombus. The tumor typed as a T-cell lymphoma. (LAA = left atrial appendage; RV = right ventricle; Ao = ascending aorta.)

Right: At high magnification, there is marked thinning of the ventricular muscle with replacement by tumor.

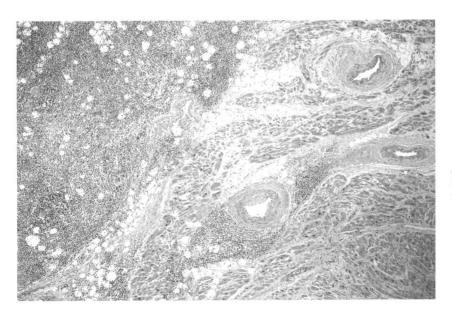

**Figure 17-7**

**CARDIAC LYMPHOMA**

The tumor invades the epicardial fat (left). An infiltrating margin is seen at the myocardial interface (right).

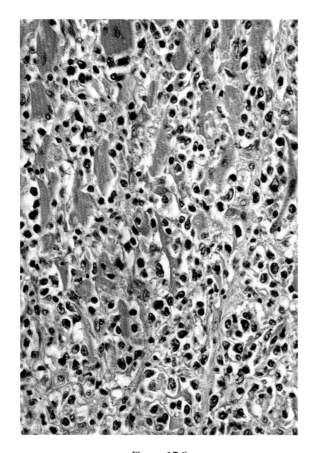

**Figure 17-8**

**CARDIAC LYMPHOMA**

Tumor cells infiltrate around and within myocytes, resulting in myocyte necrosis. The tumor typed as a diffuse large B-cell lymphoma, the most common subtype of primary cardiac lymphomas.

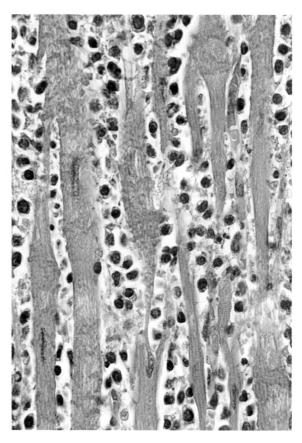

**Figure 17-9**

**CARDIAC LYMPHOMA: INTERSTITIAL GROWTH WITH MYOCYTE NECROSIS**

In some instances, there is contraction band necrosis resulting from infiltrating tumor cells. The tumor typed as a diffuse large B-cell lymphoma.

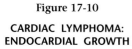

**Figure 17-10**

**CARDIAC LYMPHOMA: ENDOCARDIAL GROWTH**

Leukemic and lymphomatous involvement of the heart often has a predilection for the endocardial surface, similar to myocarditis. The thickness of the tumor infiltrate, formation of discrete masses, atypia of myocytes, and general typing as B cells distinguish myocarditis from lymphoma.

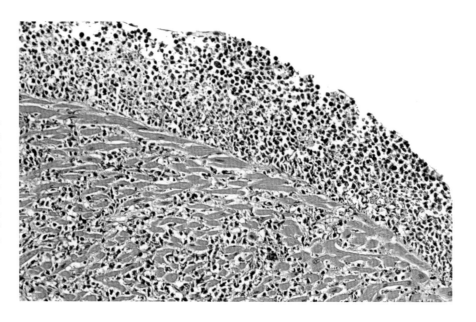

**Table 17-1**

**LYMPHOMA TYPES: PRIMARY VERSUS SECONDARY CARDIAC LYMPHOMAS[a]**

| | Primary (n=14) | Secondary (n=7) |
|---|---|---|
| Histologic type | | |
| Diffuse large B-cell lymphoma | 6 | 3 |
| Burkitt lymphoma | 4 | 0 |
| Follicular lymphoma | 1 | 1 |
| Primary effusion lymphoma | 2 | 0 |
| Peripheral T-cell lymphoma | 0 | 2 |
| Anaplastic large cell lymphoma | 1 | 1 |
| Primary site in heart | | |
| Right atrium | 5 | 2 |
| Right ventricle | 2 | 2 |
| Pericardium | 3 | 1 |
| Left ventricle | 2 | 1 |
| Biatrial/atrial septum | 1 | 1 |
| Left atrium | 1 | 0 |
| Diagnostic procedure | | |
| Open biopsy | 7 | 1 |
| Lymph node/liver biopsy | 0 | 4 |
| Endomyocardial biopsy | 1 | 1 |
| Pericardial cytology | 2 | 0 |
| Autopsy | 1 | 1 |
| Needle biopsy | 1 | 0 |
| Pleural cytology | 1 | 0 |

[a]21 patients with imaging and histopathologic data; adapted from reference 67.

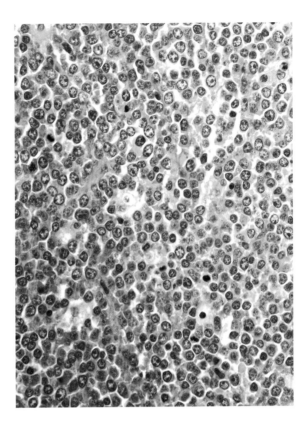

**Figure 17-11**

**CARDIAC LYMPHOMA: DIFFUSE LARGE CELL**

There is a monotonous population of large atypical lymphoid cells with a high mitotic rate and scattered macrophages.

of B-cell lineage, 2 were of T-cell lineage, and 1 was not determined (50). A more recent series of 14 primary cardiac lymphomas included 6 diffuse large B-cell lymphomas, 4 Burkitt lymphomas, 2 primary effusion lymphomas (seen in immunocompromised patients, discussed below), and 1 each of large cell anaplastic and follicular lymphomas (Table 17-1). In this series, the most common site was the right atrium. In a recent review of cardiac lymphomas (67), the most common type was diffuse large B-cell lymphoma, followed by Burkitt lymphoma, follicular lymphoma, effusion lymphoma, anaplastic large cell lymphoma, and peripheral T-cell lymphoma (Table 17-1).

Primary cardiac *T-cell lymphomas* are rare, and occur only in immunocompetent patients (figs. 17-16, 17-17) (87). Histologically, they are difficult to distinguish from large B-cell lymphomas without immunophenotyping (fig. 17-18). In patients with acquired immunodeficiency syndrome (AIDS), most lymphomas are of diffuse aggressive subtypes (85), including Burkitt-like and primary effusion lymphomas.

*Endemic-type Burkitt lymphoma* (occurring in children with EBV infection) has not been reported in the heart, but sporadic and immunodeficiency-related Burkitt lymphoma may occur within the pericardium. Burkitt lymphoma is defined by the morphologic features and expression of pan-B-cell antigens, including CD19, CD20, CD22, and CD79a, and coexpression of CD10, bcl-6, and CD43. The cells of classic Burkitt morphology are small, with multiple small chromocenters and dark blue cytoplasm (vacuolated on touch preparations); plasmacytoid features are common in immunodeficiency-related Burkitt lymphoma, and there can be moderate pleomorphism in atypical Burkitt lymphoma. Unlike follicular lymphomas, there is a lack of expression of CD5, CD23, and bcl-2. The proliferation fraction, as measured by

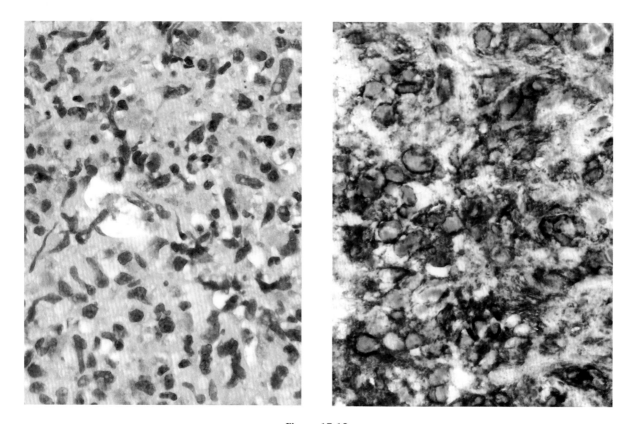

**Figure 17-12**

**CARDIAC LYMPHOMA: DIFFUSE LARGE B-CELL**

Left: In small samples, as in other sites, crush artifact may render a diagnosis difficult. There is an infiltrate of pleomorphic malignant cells of uncertain lineage on routine stains (transvenous biopsy).

Right: An immunohistochemical stain for CD20 shows that most of the atypical cells have a B-cell phenotype, consistent with B-cell lymphoma (transvenous biopsy).

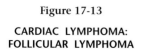

**Figure 17-13**

**CARDIAC LYMPHOMA: FOLLICULAR LYMPHOMA**

The epicardium and surface myocardium are infiltrated by tumor. It is typical of lymphomas to infiltrate the interface with cardiac muscle.

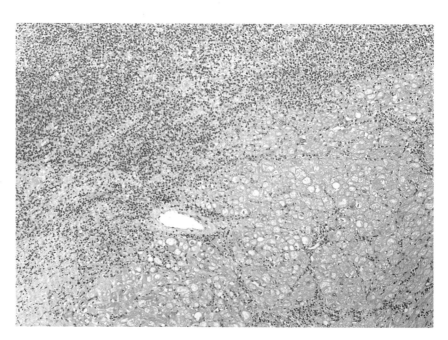

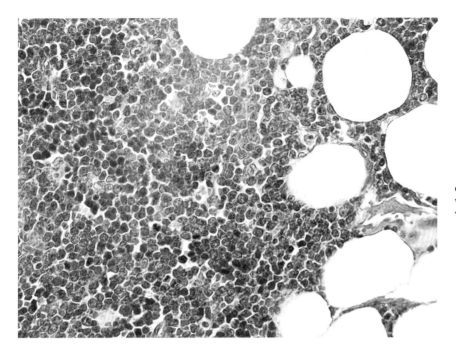

**Figure 17-14**

**FOLLICULAR LYMPHOMA**

The tumor is present within epicardial fat cells (right), with little infiltration of the ventricular myocardium (left).

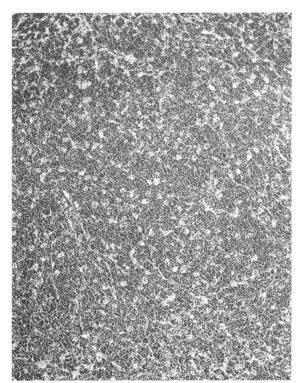

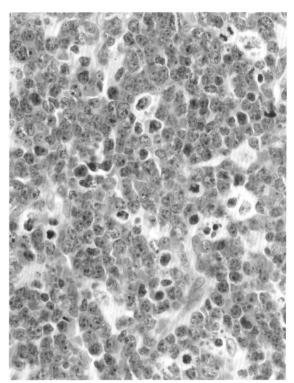

**Figure 17-15**

**BURKITT LYMPHOMA**

Left: On low magnification, the tumor is intensely blue, with a starry sky appearance.

Right: On higher magnification, the starry sky appearance is evident, caused by tingible body macrophages. The definitive diagnosis rests on characteristic phenotyping, high proliferative index documented by Ki-67 staining, and gene rearrangements.

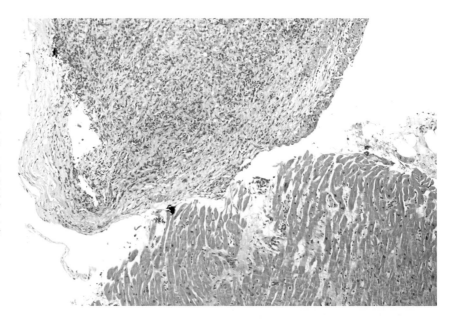

**Figure 17-16**

**T-CELL LYMPHOMA**

The patient had a history of disseminated T-cell lymphoma, which had infiltrated the superior vena cava, right atrium, and right ventricle. There are two fragments of tissue: one myocardial fragment uninvolved by tumor and one diffusely replaced by a malignant neoplasm. (Diagnosis by right ventricular endomyocardial biopsy.)

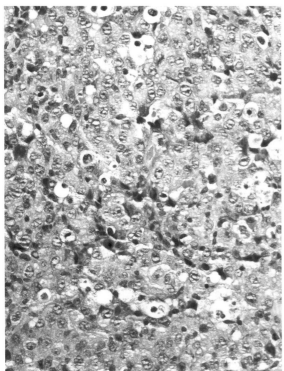

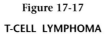

**Figure 17-17**

**T-CELL LYMPHOMA**

A higher magnification of the tumor in figure 17-16 shows a monomorphous tumor composed of round cells. The differential diagnosis includes lymphoma, undifferentiated carcinoma, melanoma, and sarcoma. Immunophenotyping confirmed lymphoma, consistent with the patient's prior T-cell lymphoma. (Diagnosis by right ventricular endomyocardial biopsy.)

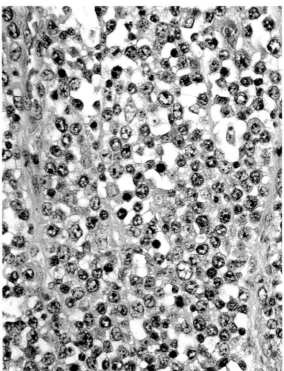

**Figure 17-18**

**T-CELL LYMPHOMA**

High magnification of the tumor illustrated grossly in figures 17-5 and 17-6 shows a large cell lymphoma, which by immunophenotyping was of T-cell derivation.

Ki-67 staining, approaches 100 percent. The diagnosis is often corroborated by characteristic gene translocations, specifically between the *c-myc* gene and the *IgH* gene (t(8;14)) or between *c-myc* and the gene for either the kappa or lambda light chain (t(2;8) or t(8;22), respectively).

**Differential Diagnosis.** The differential diagnosis of large cell lymphoma includes round cell sarcoma, undifferentiated carcinoma, malignant melanoma, and granulocytic sarcoma. In general, the distinction is easily made by documentation of a B-cell origin with CD20 immunohistochemical stains. Other lymphoid markers, intermediate filaments, myoglobin, and epithelial markers such as cytokeratin and epithelial membrane antigen, may help in the distinction of lymphoma, sarcoma, and carcinoma.

Morphologically, the main diagnostic considerations that should be included for a poorly differentiated malignant neoplasm involving the heart are metastatic carcinoma, metastatic malignant melanoma, angiosarcoma, and malignant lymphoma, all of which may be characterized by a proliferation of large atypical cells. Immunophenotypic studies should readily distinguish these neoplasms. Carcinomas exhibit immunoreactivity for cytokeratins, whereas malignant melanomas are usually immunoreactive for S-100 protein and are keratin negative. Angiosarcomas are positive for vascular markers, such as CD31 and CD34. Malignant lymphomas are defined on the basis of the reactivity for leukocyte common antigen and pan-B-cell markers such as CD20 or a pan-T-cell marker such as CD3.

For a low-grade lymphoma, the differential diagnosis includes post-transplant lymphoproliferative disorder, which is a heterogeneous infiltrate of reactive lymphocytes. Immunohistochemical studies for S-100 protein, HMB-45, and other melanoma-specific antigens help exclude metastatic melanoma.

Rarely, chloromas (granulocytic sarcomas) occur within the heart (see below). For this reason, immunohistochemical stains for granulocytic precursors, such as lysozyme, cathepsin G, and leukocyte elastase, can be performed in tumors with a histologic appearance of atypical high-grade lymphoma.

**Treatment and Prognosis.** The prognosis of patients with cardiac lymphoma is poor. In a review of 40 patients from the literature, complete remission was obtained in only 15 (50). In a more recent review, regardless of treatment, 60 percent of the patients died of their tumor 1.8 months after diagnosis (12). Survival is generally less than a month without treatment, but survival up to 5 years with treatment has been documented (12).

Treatment is similar to that of B-cell lymphomas in extracardiac sites, specifically, anthracycline-based chemotherapy and anti-CD20 (Rituximab) (83,120). Chemotherapy is used alone or combined with radiotherapy. Similarly, palliative cardiac surgery may be performed, mainly for tumor debulking. Multimodality treatment includes autologous stem cell transplantation, which has prolonged survival in select patients (64,65,121–123).

The prognosis of patients with HIV-associated cardiac non-Hodgkin lymphoma is poor, with limited survival (104). Many cases remain undetected secondary to nonspecific symptoms. Chemotherapy may produce remission in some cases (49). In AIDS patients, HAART and chemotherapy together may result in rare long-term survivors (103).

## Cardiac Lymphomas in Immunocompromised Patients

The incidence of cardiac lymphoma may be increasing due to EBV-associated lymphoproliferative disorders in AIDS patients and allograft recipients. In general, *post-transplant lymphoproliferative disorder* may develop within months or years after transplant. In AIDS patients, benign proliferations that precede malignant lymphomas have also been identified, and are termed *AIDS-associated lymphoproliferative disorder*.

The incidence of post-transplant lymphomas, at any site, is greater in patients with heart and lung transplants, approximately 6 percent, than in those with renal transplants, less than 1 percent. Cardiac lymphomas, however, comprise less than 5 percent of all lymphomas arising in patients with AIDS and organ transplants, and the presence of a tumor in the donor heart is the exception rather than the rule (85,90). In one autopsy series of 440 AIDS patients, only 1 demonstrated myocardial involvement with lymphoma (90). In a series of 90 lymphomas developing in presumed AIDS patients, only 3 involved the heart or pericardium (91). The central nervous system, bone marrow, gastrointestinal tract, and mucocutaneous sites are the most common sites of extranodal lymphomas in immunosuppressed patients. Only rare cardiac lymphomas have been described in a cardiac allograft recipient (92,93). Therefore, despite the increased prevalence of EBV-associated lymphomas, most cardiac lymphomas still occur in immunocompetent patients.

There have been approximately 40 reports of cardiac lymphoma, generally associated with extracardiac lymphoma, in patients with AIDS or allografts (4,35,49,67,73,85,92,94–103), as well as several reviews of cardiac lymphomas in immunosuppressed patients (49,85,90,93,104). Additionally, several reports have described diffuse large B-cell lymphomas associated with prosthetic valves and synthetic grafts (105–108). The precise mechanism for the development of lymphoma in these cases is unclear, but may have be related to the inflammatory reaction to the foreign body. Interestingly, some of these reported tumors were shown to be EBV positive and were not in immunocompromised patients. They may be similar to the relatively newly recognized entity, *diffuse large B-cell lymphoma with chronic inflammation* (DLBCL-CI), although the cardiac variety does not appear to share the poor prognosis with this entity (109,110).

Clinically, cardiac lymphomas in patients with AIDS usually occur in 30- to 50-year-old men and cause cardiac symptoms (85). The cardiac symptoms were nonspecific, and often masked by other conditions. The clinical findings were also nonspecific, but rapid progression of cardiac dysfunction was common after the symptoms appeared (85). Cardiac lymphoma should be suspected in lymphoma patients who present with nonspecific heart symptoms (104). Endomyocardial biopsy is a useful diagnostic tool in this patient cohort (95). In 5 of the 14 cardiac lymphomas in AIDS patients reported before 1992 (98), there was no apparent extracardiac involvement. Other extranodal sites, especially the gastrointestinal tract and lung, were involved in the remaining cases. Almost any site in the heart may be involved by cardiac lymphoma (98).

Cardiac and other extranodal lymphomas that arise in immunocompromised patients are most often high grade. *Plasmacytoid immunoblastic lymphoma, low-grade B-cell lymphomas,* and *diffuse large cell lymphomas* are the most common histologic types (33,35). Many other types of B-cell lymphoma have been described in extracardiac locations (44). Primary T-cell lymphomas are rare in immunocompromised patients and have not been found in the heart, although one report described involvement of the heart by human immunodeficiency virus (HIV)-associated peripheral T-cell lymphoma causing left ventricular rupture (111).

In two cases of cardiac lymphoma in patients with AIDS, the apparent histologic progression from a polyclonal, polymorphous infiltrate to a monoclonal, monomorphous high-grade lymphoma was demonstrated (99).

Although pericardial effusions are common with epicardial involvement by B-cell lymphomas, *primary effusion lymphoma* is a distinct type of lymphoma associated with human herpesvirus (HHV)-8 infection in immunocompromised patients (fig. 17-19). Histologically, primary effusion lymphomas have features of both large cell immunoblastic and large cell anaplastic lymphomas. Most of these cases comprise a unique subgroup of B-cell lymphomas, but T-cell or natural killer cell immunophenotypes are described (112). Formerly known as body cavity lymphoma, primary effusion lymphoma accounts for about 4 percent of all HIV-associated non-Hodgkin lymphomas and is associated with a concomitant diagnosis of Kaposi sarcoma (113). The prognosis is generally poor, although response to HAART therapy and chemotherapy has been reported. Confirmation of viral infection by HHV-8 in the neoplastic cells using in situ hybridization is considered essential for the diagnosis. The pericardium is an unusual site for primary effusion lymphoma, and the criteria for diagnosis, including CD20 phenotype and HHV-8 positivity, have not been entirely established (114–119).

Primary cardiac lymphomas in patients with prior renal or heart transplants are similar to those seen in AIDS patients (4,92–94,97,100), and are occasionally confined to the heart at autopsy (100). They are generally high-grade B-cell lymphomas that arise within a polymorphous proliferation that is identified on biopsies for the evaluation of chronic rejection. These proliferations rapidly progress to high-grade lymphomas, and may occur within months of the transplant (94).

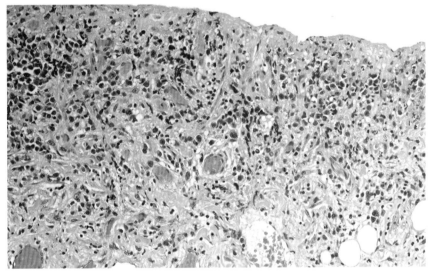

**Figure 17-19**

**PRIMARY EFFUSION LYMPHOMA: PERICARDIUM**

Top: The pericardium shows a densely cellular area on the surface, with central hemorrhage.

Bottom: At higher magnification, an infiltrate of atypical lymphoid cells is seen.

## Secondary Cardiac Involvement in Lymphoma

The incidence of secondary cardiac lymphomas in patients with malignant lymphoma ranges from 9 to 24 percent. Secondary cardiac lymphomas include Hodgkin disease (124), T-cell lymphomas (125), and the more common B-cell lymphomas. T-cell lymphomas may be more aggressive in the heart (89).

In early series (11,126), approximately 10 percent of patients with secondary cardiac involvement had symptoms that were attributable to infiltration of the heart by lymphoma, and cardiac lymphoma was suspected only rarely before autopsy. Manifestations attributable to cardiac disease include chest pain, dyspnea, large pericardial effusions, left ventricular dysfunction (127), and congestive heart failure from intracavitary masses (128). Today, secondary cardiac involvement in patients with malignant lymphoma is diagnosed antemortem in up to 40 percent of patients with cardiac involvement at autopsy (129). MRI is very sensitive, and superior to two-dimensional echocardiography, in demonstrating cardiac infiltration in patients with mediastinal lymphoma (130), and may lead to early treatment. Because patients may respond to chemotherapy or combined radiation and chemotherapy, early diagnosis of cardiac involvement is essential (129).

Lymphomas spread to the heart by three pathways: direct extension from mediastinal lymphoma, retrograde lymphatic spread in lymphatic vessels along the coronary arteries and in the epicardium, and hematogenous spread. Hematogenous spread, which is characterized by interstitial and epicardial masses that resemble abscesses, is more typical of low-grade and intermediate-grade follicular lymphomas. Both Hodgkin lymphomas and high-grade non-Hodgkin lymphomas are more likely to spread to the heart by direct extension or lymphatic routes (126).

## MISCELLANEOUS HEMATOLOGIC LESIONS OF THE HEART

### Granulocytic Sarcoma

Leukemic infiltrates are found at autopsy within the heart or pericardium in 37 percent of patients dying of acute leukemia (131,132). Symptoms directly attributable to these deposits are uncommon, however (see chapter 15) (133).

There have been several reports of *granulocytic sarcoma* within the pericardium, adherent to the pericardium, and within the myocardium or right atrium (134–139). In most of these cases, the granulocytic sarcoma occurred prior to the leukemic manifestations (137). In one patient, right ventricular failure developed as a result of the leukemic infiltrate (139).

### Erdheim-Chester Disease

Considered a histiocytosis in the juvenile xanthogranuloma group, *Erdheim-Chester disease* typically involves the eye, lung, pituitary gland, kidney, and long bones (with characteristic radiologic abnormalities). Cardiac involvement has been only recently reported, but is not considered rare (140–148). Cardiac involvement is generally determined by imaging, including CT and MRI (146). A literature review of 72 cases of cardiac Erdheim-Chester disease showed that 56 percent of patients had periaortic fibrosis; 44.4 percent, pericardial involvement; and 31 percent, myocardial involvement, with 6 right atrial masses (145). Symptomatic valve disease and severe heart failure also occur (145). The treatment is anti-inflammatory, including steroids (147).

Histologically, Erdheim-Chester xanthogranulomatous lesions contain foamy and lipid-laden macrophages, multinucleated xanthogranulomatous giant cells, monocytes, and lymphocytes in a mesh of fibrosis (fig. 17-20). There is typically infiltration of fibrous tissues and myocytes, in the case of myocardial involvement. The macrophages express CD14, CD68, factor XIIIa, and fascin, and are negative for HLA-DR, CD1a, CD163, langerin, S-100 protein, and lysozyme. Ultrastructurally, there are no Birbeck granules.

### Giant Lymph Node Hyperplasia of Mediastinum (Castleman Disease)

*Giant lymph node hyperplasia of the mediastinum* (*Castleman disease*) was originally described by Castleman et al. in 1956. Synonyms include *angiofollicular lymph node hyperplasia, angiomatous lymphoid hamartoma*, and *follicular lymphoreticuloma*. Rarely, giant lymph node hyperplasia is entirely intrapericardial and results in a pericardial mass and cardiac symptoms (149,150). The histologic features include follicular hyperplasia, intrafollicular capillary proliferation and hyalinization, and perifollicular plasmacytosis.

### Rosai-Dorfman Disease

Also known as *sinus histiocytosis with massive lymphadenopathy, Rosai-Dorfman disease* typically presents as painless cervical adenopathy in young individuals. The characteristic histologic features in the lymph nodes are dark-staining bands containing numerous small blue plasma cells and lymphocytes alternating with dilated sinuses containing pale-staining collections of macrophages that demonstrate phagocytosis of immune cells (emperipolesis) (figs. 17-21–17-23).

Extranodal involvement occurs in about 9 percent of patients, most commonly in skin, bone, and soft tissue. Cardiac involvement has been only rarely reported, with less than 10 cases in the literature as of this writing (151–154). Lesions may arise in any cardiac chamber from either epicardium, myocardium, or endocardium (151,155). Immunohistochemically, the histiocytes in Rosai-Dorfman disease express CD14, CD68, S-100 protein, lysozyme, CD163, HLA-DR, and fascin, and are negative for CD1a, factor XIIIa, and langerin.

### Langerhans Cell Histiocytosis

A child who died with cardiac and periaortic involvement with *Langerhans cell histiocytosis* has been reported (156). The immunophenotypic

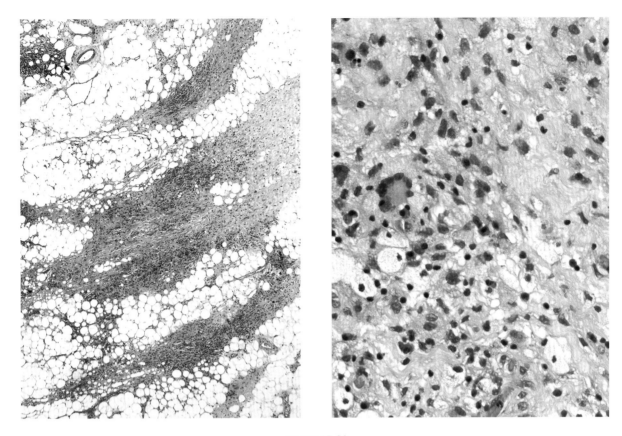

**Figure 17-20**

**ERDHEIM-CHESTER DISEASE: EPICARDIUM**

Left: The epicardial fat is infiltrated by a fibroinflammatory infiltrate.

Right: At higher magnification, a mixed inflammatory infiltrate with focal xanthoma cells and multinucleated Touton-like macrophages is seen. The diagnosis depends on the characteristic immunophenotype (factor XIIIa positive, S-100 protein negative, fascin positive).

profile of Langerhans cells, in contrast to Rosai-Dorfman disease and Erdheim-Chester disease, is positivity for HLA-DR, CD1a, S-100 protein, and langerin, and negativity for factor XIIIa, CD14, lysozyme, CD163, and fascin. Langerhans cells contain Birbeck granules as seen by electron microscopy, contain characteristic nuclear grooves, and possess dark, moderate amounts of cytoplasm.

## Crystal-Storing Histiocytosis

*Crystal-storing histiocytosis* is a rare manifestation of disorders that express monoclonal immunoglobulins, such as multiple myeloma, monoclonal gammopathy of undetermined significance, and lymphoplasmacytic lymphoma. Histologically, there is an infiltrate of macrophages with abundant cytoplasm that contain phagocytosed light chain crystals. The cells are most frequent in bone marrow, lung, lymph nodes, thymus, and spleen. The monoclonal light chains are typically of kappa isotype, with no specific heavy chain association. A single case has been reported that presented as a right atrial mass, in a patient with a poorly defined lymphoproliferative syndrome (figs. 17-24–17-26) (157).

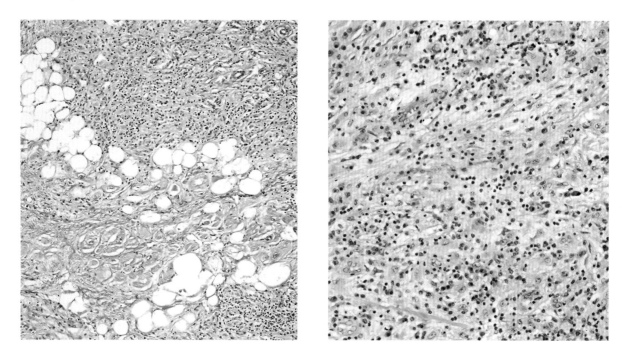

**Figure 17-21**

**ROSAI-DORFMAN DISEASE: EPICARDIUM**

Left: On low magnification, there is a fibroinflammatory infiltrate.
Right: At higher magnification, a macrophage infiltrate with focal lymphocyte emperipolesis is seen.

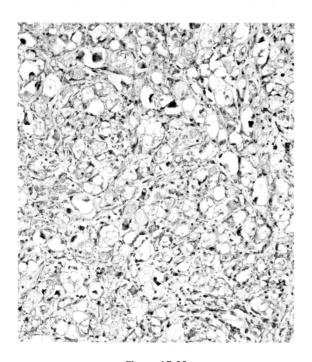

**Figure 17-22**

**ROSAI-DORFMAN DISEASE: EPICARDIUM**

Unlike Erdheim-Chester disease, the macrophages are CD163 positive.

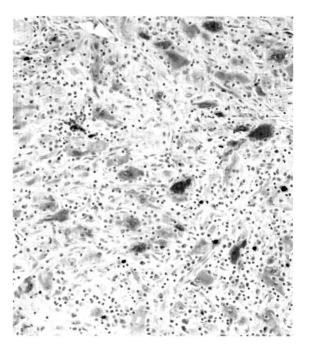

**Figure 17-23**

**ROSAI-DORFMAN DISEASE: EPICARDIUM**

The macrophages express S-100 protein.

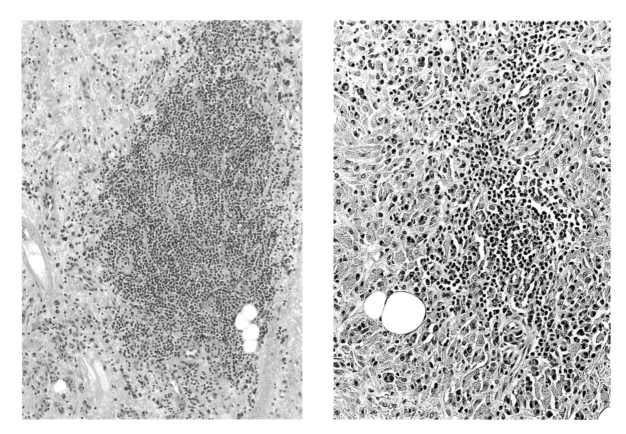

**Figure 17-24**

**CRYSTAL-STORING HISTIOCYTOSIS: RIGHT ATRIUM**

Left: There is an infiltrate of small lymphocytes, with surrounding macrophages within the atrial myocardium.
Right: At high magnification, the central lymphocytes with surrounding macrophages are seen.

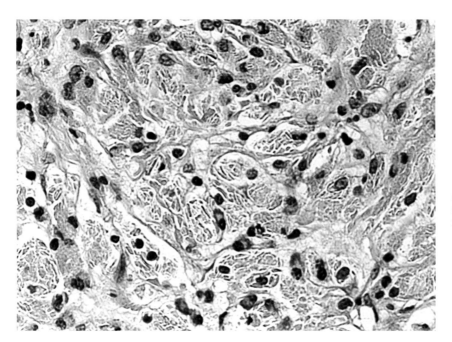

**Figure 17-25**

**CRYSTAL-STORING
HISTIOCYTOSIS:
RIGHT ATRIUM**

The macrophages contain
characteristic crystals, which
are composed of monotypic im-
munoglobulin.

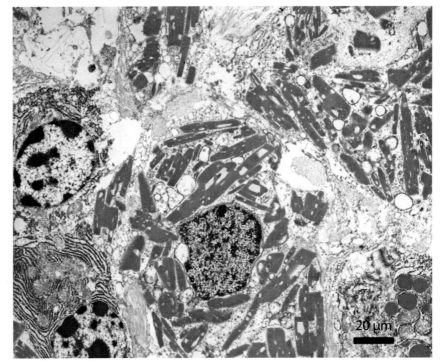

**Figure 17-26**

**CRYSTAL-STORING
HISTIOCYTOSIS:
RIGHT ATRIUM**

Electron microscopy demonstrates the characteristic crystals within the macrophage cytoplasm.

## REFERENCES

1. Curtsinger CR, Wilson MJ, Yoneda K. Primary cardiac lymphoma. Cancer 1989;64:521-525.
2. Zaharia L, Gill PS. Primary cardiac lymphoma. Am J Clin Oncol 1991;14:142-145.
3. Burke A, Virmani R. Primary cardiac sarcomas. AFIP Atlas of Tumor Pathology. Tumors of the heart and great vessels, 3rd Series, Fascicle 16. Washington, DC: American Registry of Pathology; 1996:171-180.
4. Case records of the Massachusetts General Hospital. Weekly clinicopathological exercises. Case 4-1985. A 36-year-old man with a cardiac mass three years after renal transplantation. N Engl J Med 1985;312:226-237.
5. Johnson RA, Blake TM. Lymphatics of the heart. Circulation 1966;33:137-142.
6. Shimada T, Morita T, Oya M, Kitamura H. Morphological studies of the cardiac lymphatic system. Arch Histol Cytol 1990;53 Suppl:115-126.
7. Miller AJ. The study of the lymphatics of the heart: an overview. Microcirc Endothelium Lymphatics 1985;2:349-360.
8. Bradham RR, Parker EF. The cardiac lymphatics. Ann Thorac Surg 1973;15:526-535.
9. Bradham RR, Parker EF, Greene WB. Lymphatics of the atrioventricular valves. Arch Surg 1973; 106:210-213.
10. Leblond V, Sutton L, Dorent R, et al. Lymphoproliferative disorders after organ transplantation: a report of 24 cases observed in a single center. J Clin Oncol 1995;13:961-968.
11. Roberts WC, Glancy DL, DeVita VT. Heart in malignant lymphoma (Hodgkin's disease, lymphosarcoma, reticulum cell sarcoma and mycosis fungoides). A study of 196 autopsy cases. Am J Cardiol 1968;22:85-107.
12. Gowda RM, Khan IA. Clinical perspectives of primary cardiac lymphoma. Angiology 2003;54: 599-604.
13. Agarwal V, Agarwal SK, Srivastava AK, Kapoor S. Primary cardiac tumors: surgical experience and follow-up. Indian Heart J 2003;55:632-636.
14. Bakaeen FG, Reardon MJ, Coselli JS, et al. Surgical outcome in 85 patients with primary cardiac tumors. Am J Surg 2003;186:641-647; discussion 647.

15. Endo A, Ohtahara A, Kinugawa T, et al. Characteristics of 161 patients with cardiac tumors diagnosed during 1993 and 1994 in Japan. Am J Cardiol 1997;79:1708-1711.

16. Grande AM, Ragni T, Vigano M. Primary cardiac tumors. A clinical experience of 12 years. Tex Heart Inst J 1993;20:223-230.

17. Lam KY, Dickens P, Chan AC. Tumors of the heart. A 20-year experience with a review of 12,485 consecutive autopsies. Arch Pathol Lab Med 1993;117:1027-1031.

18. Miralles A, Bracamonte L, Soncul H, et al. Cardiac tumors: clinical experience and surgical results in 74 patients. Ann Thorac Surg 1991;52:886-895.

19. Perchinsky MJ, Lichtenstein SV, Tyers GF. Primary cardiac tumors: forty years' experience with 71 patients. Cancer 1997;79:1809-1815.

20. Veinot JP, Burns BF, Commons AS, Thomas J. Cardiac neoplasms at the Canadian Reference Centre for Cancer Pathology. Can J Cardiol 1999;15:311-319.

21. Bossert T, Gummert JF, Battellini R, et al. Surgical experience with 77 primary cardiac tumors. Interact Cardiovasc Thorac Surg 2005;4:311-315.

22. Elbardissi AW, Dearani JA, Daly RC, et al. Survival after resection of primary cardiac tumors: a 48-year experience. Circulation 2008;118:S7-15.

23. Giusca S, Jurcut R, Serban M, Popescu BA, Apetrei E, Ginghina C. Cardiac tumors: the experience of a tertiary cardiology center. Rom J Intern Med 2007;45:333-339.

24. Kajihara N, Tanoue Y, Eto M, Tomita Y, Masuda M, Morita S. Surgical experience of cardiac tumors: early and late results. Surg Today 2006;36:602-607.

25. Mariano A, Pita A, Leon R, et al. Primary cardiac tumors in children: a 16-year experience. Rev Port Cardiol 2009;28:279-288.

26. Simpson L, Kumar SK, Okuno SH, et al. Malignant primary cardiac tumors: review of a single institution experience. Cancer 2008;112:2440-2446.

27. Yu K, Liu Y, Wang H, Hu S, Long C. Epidemiological and pathological characteristics of cardiac tumors: a clinical study of 242 cases. Interact Cardiovasc Thorac Surg 2007;6:636-639.

28. Whorton CM. Primary malignant tumors of the heart; report of a case. Cancer 1949;2:245-260.

29. Brucker EA Jr, Glassy FJ. Primary reticulum-cell sarcoma of the heart with review of the literature. Cancer 1955;8:920-931.

30. Burke A, Virmani R. Primary cardiac sarcomas. AFIP Atlas of Tumor Pathology. Tumors of the heart and great vessels, 3rd Series, Fascicle 16. Washington, DC: American Registry of Pathology; 1996.

31. Bestetti RB, Soares FA, Soares EG, Oliveira JS. Primary lymphoma of the right atrium with fatal neoplastic pulmonary embolism. Am Heart J 1992;124:1088-1090.

32. Castelli MJ, Mihalov ML, Posniak HV, Gattuso P. Primary cardiac lymphoma initially diagnosed by routine cytology. Case report and literature review. Acta Cytol 1989;33:355-358.

33. Chou ST, Arkles LB, Gill GD, Pinkus N, Parkin A, Hicks JD. Primary lymphoma of the heart. A case report. Cancer 1983;52:744-747.

34. Gardiner DS, Lindop GB. Coronary artery aneurysm due to primary cardiac lymphoma. Histopathology 1989;15:537-540.

35. Gill PS, Chandraratna PA, Meyer PR, Levine AM. Malignant lymphoma: cardiac involvement at initial presentation. J Clin Oncol 1987;5:216-224.

36. Kasai K, Kuwao S, Sato Y, Murayama M, Harano Y, Kameya T. Case report of primary cardiac lymphoma. The applications of PCR to the diagnosis of primary cardiac lymphoma. Acta Pathol Jpn 1992;42:667-671.

37. Moore JA, DeRan BP, Minor R, Arthur J, Fraker TD Jr. Transesophageal echocardiographic evaluation of intracardiac lymphoma. Am Heart J 1992;124:514-516.

38. Nand S, Mullen GM, Lonchyna VA, Moncada R. Primary lymphoma of the heart. Prolonged survival with early systemic therapy in a patient. Cancer 1991;68:2289-2292.

39. Pozniak AL, Thomas RD, Hobbs CB, Lever JV. Primary malignant lymphoma of the heart. Antemortem cytologic diagnosis. Acta Cytol 1986;30:662-664.

40. Proctor MS, Tracy GP, Von Koch L. Primary cardiac B-cell lymphoma. Am Heart J 1989;118:179-181.

41. Roh LS, Paparo GP. Primary malignant lymphoma of the heart in sudden unexpected death. J Forensic Sci 1982;27:718-722.

42. Somers K, Lothe F. Primary lymphosarcoma of the heart: review of the literature and report of 3 cases. Cancer 1960;13:449-457.

43. Takagi M, Kugimiya T, Fujii T, et al. Extensive surgery for primary malignant lymphoma of the heart. J Cardiovasc Surg (Torino) 1992;33:570-572.

44. Antoniades L, Eftychiou C, Petrou PM, Bagatzounis A, Minas M. Primary cardiac lymphoma: case report and brief review of the literature. Echocardiography 2009;26:214-219.

45. Ban-Hoefen M, Zeglin MA, Bisognano JD. Diffuse large B cell lymphoma presenting as a cardiac mass and odynophagia. Cardiol J 2008;15:471-474.

46. Faganello G, Belham M, Thaman R, Blundell J, Eller T, Wilde P. A case of primary cardiac lymphoma: analysis of the role of echocardiography in early diagnosis. Echocardiography 2007;24:889-892.

47. Jang JJ, Danik S, Goldman M. Primary cardiac lymphoma: diagnosis and treatment guided by transesophageal echocardiogram perfusion imaging. J Am Soc Echocardiogr 2006;19:1073.e7-9.

48. Takenaka S, Mitsudo K, Inoue K, et al. Successful treatment of primary cardiac lymphoma with atrioventricular nodal block. Int Heart J 2005;46:927-931.

49. Khan NU, Ahmed S, Wagner P, Rumley RL, Movahed A. Cardiac involvement in non-Hodgkin's lymphoma: with and without HIV infection. Int J Cardiovasc Imaging 2004;20:477-481.

50. Ikeda H, Nakamura S, Nishimaki H, et al. Primary lymphoma of the heart: case report and literature review. Pathol Int 2004;54:187-195.

51. Kang SM, Rim SJ, Chang HJ, et al. Primary cardiac lymphoma diagnosed by transvenous biopsy under transesophageal echocardiographic guidance and treated with systemic chemotherapy. Echocardiography 2003;20:101-103.

52. Hayes D Jr, Liles DK, Sorrell VL. An unusual cause of new-onset atrial flutter: primary cardiac lymphoma. South Med J 2003;96:799-802.

53. Rolla G, Bertero MT, Pastena G, et al. Primary lymphoma of the heart. A case report and review of the literature. Leuk Res 2002;26:117-120.

54. Chalabreysse L, Berger F, Loire R, Devouassoux G, Cordier JF, Thivolet-Bejui F. Primary cardiac lymphoma in immunocompetent patients: a report of three cases and review of the literature. Virchows Arch 2002;441:456-461.

55. Alter P, Grimm W, Tontsch D, Maisch B. Diagnosis of primary cardiac lymphoma by endomyocardial biopsy. Am J Med 2001;110:593-594.

56. Montalbetti L, Della Volpe A, Airaghi ML, Landoni C, Brambilla-Pisoni G, Pozzi S. Primary cardiac lymphoma. A case report and review. Minerva Cardioangiol 1999;47:175-182.

57. Cabin HS, Costello RM, Vasudevan G, Maron BJ, Roberts WC. Cardiac lymphoma mimicking hypertrophic cardiomyopathy. Am Heart J 1981;102:466-468.

58. Cairns P, Butany J, Fulop J, Rakowski H, Hassaram S. Cardiac presentation of non-Hodgkin's lymphoma. Arch Pathol Lab Med 1987;111:80-83.

59. Fiester RF. Reticulum cell sarcoma of the heart. Arch Pathol 1975;99:60-61.

60. Kissin M, Eisinger R. Reticulum cell sarcoma of the heart simulating viral pericarditis. Am Heart J 1961;62:549-552.

61. Monsuez JJ, Frija J, Hertz-Pannier L, Miclea JM, Extra JM, Boiron M. Non-Hodgkin's lymphoma with cardiac presentation: evaluation and follow-up with echocardiography and mr imaging. Eur Heart J 1991;12:464-467.

62. Rucks WW Jr, Russell HT, Motley RF. Primary reticulum cell sarcoma of the heart. Report of a case. Am Heart J 1963;66:97-103.

63. Stein M, Zyssman I, Kantor A, Spencer D, Lewis D, Bezwoda W. Malignant lymphoma with primary cardiac manifestations: a case report. Med Pediatr Oncol 1994;22:292-295.

64. Fuchida S, Yamada N, Uchida R, et al. Malignant lymphoma presenting as a cardiac tumor and superior vena caval syndrome successfully treated by haploidentical stem cell transplantation. Leuk Lymphoma 2005;46:1517-1521.

65. Anghel G, Zoli V, Petti N, Remotti D, Feccia M, Pino P, Majolino I. Primary cardiac lymphoma: report of two cases occurring in immunocompetent subjects. Leuk Lymphoma 2004;45:781-788.

66. Nonami A, Takenaka K, Kamezaki K, et al. Successful treatment of primary cardiac lymphoma by rituximab-CHOP and high-dose chemotherapy with autologous peripheral blood stem cell transplantation. Int J Hematol 2007;85:264-266.

67. Jeudy J, Kirsch J, Tavora F, et al. From the radiologic pathology archives: cardiac lymphoma: Radiologic-pathologic correlation. Radiographics 2012;32:1369-1380.

68. Chim CS, Chan AC, Kwong YL, Liang R. Primary cardiac lymphoma. Am J Hematol 1997;54:79-83.

69. Delmas-Marsalet B, Molinie V, Jary L, et al. Cardiac localization of non-Hodgkin's lymphoma: two case reports and review of the literature. Nouv Rev Fr Hematol 1995;37:223-230.

70. Bambury R, Gallagher F, Dodd JD, Fennelly D. Primary cardiac lymphoma: diagnostic tools and treatment challenges. Ir J Med Sci 2011;180:271-273.

71. O'Mahony D, Peikarz RL, Bandettini WP, Arai AE, Wilson WH, Bates SE. Cardiac involvement with lymphoma: a review of the literature. Clin Lymphoma Myeloma 2008;8:249-252.

72. Hsueh SC, Chung MT, Fang R, Hsiung MC, Young MS, Lu HF. Primary cardiac lymphoma. J Chin Med Assoc 2006;69:169-174.

73. Knowles JW, Elliott AB, Brody J. A case of complete heart block reverting to normal sinus rhythm after treatment for cardiac invasive Burkitt's lymphoma. Ann Hematol 2007;86:687-690.

74. Clifford SM, Guerra SM, Mangion JR. Massive metastatic intracardiac lymphoma presenting with complete heart block with resolution following chemotherapy. Echocardiography 2003;20:201-202.

75. Wilhite DB, Quigley RL. Occult cardiac lymphoma presenting with cardiac tamponade. Tex Heart Inst J 2003;30:62-64.

76. Binder J, Pfleger S, Schwarz S. Images in cardiovascular medicine. Right atrial primary cardiac lymphoma presenting with stroke. Circulation 2004;110:e451-452.

77. Quigley MM, Schwartzman E, Boswell PD, et al. A unique atrial primary cardiac lymphoma mimicking myxoma presenting with embolic stroke: a case report. Blood 2003;101:4708-4710.

78. Timperley J, Mitchell AR, Becher H. Primary cardiac lymphoma. Eur J Echocardiogr 2003;4:327-330.

79. Araoz PA, Eklund HE, Welch TJ, Breen JF. CT and MR imaging of primary cardiac malignancies. Radiographics 1999;19:1421-1434.

80. Dorsay TA, Ho VB, Rovira MJ, Armstrong MA, Brissette MD. Primary cardiac lymphoma: CT and MR findings. J Comput Assist Tomogr 1993; 17:978-981.

81. Khuddus MA, Schmalfuss CM, Aranda JM, Pauly DF. Magnetic resonance imaging of primary cardiac lymphoma. Clin Cardiol 2007;30:144-145.

82. Ryu SJ, Choi BW, Choe KO. CT and MR findings of primary cardiac lymphoma: report upon 2 cases and review. Yonsei Med J 2001;42:451-456.

83. Bley TA, Zeiser R, Ghanem NA, Hackanson B, Brink I, Langer M. High grade cardiac lymphoma vitality monitoring by gadolinium-enhanced magnetic resonance imaging (MRI). In Vivo 2005;19:689-693.

84. Saito T, Tamaru J, Kayao J, Kuzuu Y, Wakita H, Mikata A. Cytomorphologic diagnosis of malignant lymphoma arising in the heart: a case report. Acta Cytol 2001;45:1043-1048.

85. Holladay AO, Siegel RJ, Schwartz DA. Cardiac malignant lymphoma in acquired immune deficiency syndrome. Cancer 1992;70:2203-2207.

86. Zakynthinos E, Tassopoulos G, Haritos C, et al. Huge biatrial primary cardiac B-cell lymphoma resulting in bilateral atrioventricular valve obstruction. Leuk Lymphoma 2004;45:2339-2342.

87. Giunta R, Cravero RG, Granata G, et al. Primary cardiac T-cell lymphoma. Ann Hematol 2004;83:450-454.

88. Burke A, Jeudy J Jr, Virmani R. Cardiac tumours: an update. Heart 2008;94:117-123.

89. Chinen K, Izumo T. Cardiac involvement by malignant lymphoma: A clinicopathologic study of 25 autopsy cases based on the WHO classification. Ann Hematol 2005;84:498-505.

90. Barbaro G, Di Lorenzo G, Grisorio B, Barbarini G. Cardiac involvement in the acquired immunodeficiency syndrome: a multicenter clinical-pathological study. Gruppo Italiano per lo Studio Cardiologico dei pazienti affetti da AIDS investigators. AIDS Res Hum Retroviruses 1998;14:1071-1077.

91. Ziegler J, Beckstead JA, Volberding PA, et al. Non-Hodgkin's lymphoma in 90 homosexual men. Relation to generalized lymphadenopathy and the acquired immunodeficiency syndrome. N Engl J Med 1984;311:565-570.

92. Burtin P, Guerci A, Boman F, et al. Malignant lymphoma in the donor heart after heart transplantation. Eur Heart J 1993;14:1143-1145.

93. Nart D, Nalbantgil S, Yagdi T, et al. Primary cardiac lymphoma in a heart transplant recipient. Transplant Proc 2005;37:1362-1364.

94. Abu-Farsakh H, Cagle P, Buffone G, Bruner J, Weilbacher D, Greenberg SD. Heart allograft involvement with Epstein-Barr virus-associated posttransplant lymphoproliferative disorder. Arch Pathol Lab Med 1992;116:93-95.

95. Andress JD, Polish LB, Clark DM, Hossack KF. Transvenous biopsy diagnosis of cardiac lymphoma in an AIDS patient. Am Heart J 1989; 118:421-423.

96. Balasubramanyam A, Waxman M, Kazal HL, Lee MH. Malignant lymphoma of the heart in acquired immune deficiency syndrome. Chest 1986;90:243-246.

97. Chang H, Wu JD, Cheng KK, Tseng HH. Epstein-Barr virus-associated lymphoproliferative disorders in oral cavity after heart transplantation: report of a case. J Formos Med Assoc 1994; 93:332-336.

98. Goldfarb A, King CL, Rosenzweig BP, et al. Cardiac lymphoma in the acquired immunodeficiency syndrome. Am Heart J 1989;118:1340-1344.

99. Guarner J, Brynes RK, Chan WC, Birdsong G, Hertzler G. Primary non-Hodgkin's lymphoma of the heart in two patients with the acquired immunodeficiency syndrome. Arch Pathol Lab Med 1987;111:254-256.

100. Rodenburg CJ, Kluin P, Maes A, Paul LC. Malignant lymphoma confined to the heart, 13 years after a cadaver kidney transplant. N Engl J Med 1985;313:122.

101. Gaspar A, Salome N, Nabais S, et al. Echocardiographic assessment of a cardiac lymphoma: beyond two-dimensional imaging. Eur J Echocardiogr 2009;10:975-978.

102. Kadhim H, Ntoutoume Sima F, Corazza F, Gottignies P, Dehou MF, Deprez C. Cardiac lymphoma presenting as concentric pseudohypertrophic cardiomyopathy in a previously unrecognised HIV patient. Pathology 2009; 41:706-709.

103. Tanaka PY, Atala MM, Pereira J, Caterino-de-Araujo A. Primary effusion lymphoma with cardiac involvement in HIV positive patient-complete response and long survival with chemotherapy and HAART. J Clin Virol 2009; 44:84-85.

104. Sanna P, Bertoni F, Zucca E, et al. Cardiac involvement in HIV-related non-Hodgkin's lymphoma: a case report and short review of the literature. Ann Hematol 1998;77:75-78.

105. Miller DV, Firchau DJ, McClure RF, Kurtin PJ, Feldman AL. Epstein-Barr virus-associated diffuse large B-cell lymphoma arising on cardiac prostheses. Am J Surg Pathol 2010;34:377-384.

106. Albat B, Messner-Pellenc P, Thevenet A. Surgical treatment for primary lymphoma of the heart simulating prosthetic mitral valve thrombosis. J Thorac Cardiovasc Surg 1994;108:188-189.

107. Bagwan IN, Desai S, Wotherspoon A, Sheppard MN. Unusual presentation of primary cardiac lymphoma. Interact Cardiovasc Thorac Surg 2009;9:127-129.

108. Durrleman NM, El-Hamamsy I, Demaria RG, Carrier M, Perrault LP, Albat B. Cardiac lymphoma following mitral valve replacement. Ann Thorac Surg 2005;79:1040-1042.

109. Nakatsuka S, Yao M, Hoshida Y, Yamamoto S, Iuchi K, Aozasa K. Pyothorax-associated lymphoma: a review of 106 cases. J Clin Oncol 2002;20:4255-4260.

110. Narimatsu H, Ota Y, Kami M, et al. Clinicopathological features of pyothorax-associated lymphoma; a retrospective survey involving 98 patients. Ann Oncol 2007;18:122-128.

111. Armstrong EJ, Bhave P, Wong D, et al. Left ventricular rupture due to HIV-associated T-cell lymphoma. Tex Heart Inst J 2010;37:457-460.

112. Das DK. Serous effusions in malignant lymphomas: a review. Diagn Cytopathol 2006;34:335-347.

113. Simonelli C, Spina M, Cinelli R, et al. Clinical features and outcome of primary effusion lymphoma in HIV-infected patients: a single-institution study. J Clin Oncol 2003;21:3948-3954.

114. Bhargava P, Glass E, Brown J, Eapen E, Ames E. FDG PET in primary effusion lymphoma (PEL) of the pericardium. Clin Nucl Med 2006;31:18-19.

115. Chen YB, Rahemtullah A, Hochberg E. Primary effusion lymphoma. Oncologist 2007;12:569-576.

116. Inoue Y, Tsukasaki K, Nagai K, Soda H, Tomonaga M. Durable remission by sobuzoxane in an HIV-seronegative patient with human herpesvirus 8-negative primary effusion lymphoma. Int J Hematol 2004;79:271-275.

117. Kishimoto K, Kitamura T, Hirayama Y, Tate G, Mitsuya T. Cytologic and immunocytochemical features of EBV negative primary effusion lymphoma: report on seven Japanese cases. Diagn Cytopathol 2009;37:293-298.

118. Nakakuki T, Masuoka H, Ishikura K, et al. A case of primary cardiac lymphoma located in the pericardial effusion. Heart Vessels 2004;19:199-202.

119. Won JH, Han SH, Bae SB, et al. Successful eradication of relapsed primary effusion lymphoma with high-dose chemotherapy and autologous stem cell transplantation in a patient seronegative for human immunodeficiency virus. Int J Hematol 2006;83:328-330.

120. Nakagawa Y, Ikeda U, Hirose M, et al. Successful treatment of primary cardiac lymphoma with monoclonal CD20 antibody (rituximab). Circ J 2004;68:172-173.

121. Lo SS, Yeager AM, Peel RL, Katz WE, Ramanathan RK. Multimodality treatment in a case of primary cardiac lymphoma. Clin Lymphoma 2003;4:112-114.

122. Arimura K, Arima N, Hamada H, Kukita T, Matsushita K, Tei C. Cardiac lymphoma successfully treated with high dose chemotherapy followed by autologous haematopoietic stem cell transplantation. Haematologica 2003;88:ECR34.

123. Bestetti RB, Miguel CE. Can stem blood cell transplantation be an adjuvant treatment for primary cardiac lymphoma? Int J Hematol 2007;86:286.

124. Retter A, Ardeshna KM, O'Driscoll A. Cardiac tamponade in Hodgkin lymphoma. Br J Haematol 2007;138:2.

125. Iemura A, Yano H, Kojiro M, Nouno R, Kouno K. Massive cardiac involvement of adult T-cell leukemia/lymphoma. An autopsy case. Arch Pathol Lab Med 1991;115:1052-1054.

126. McDonnell PJ, Mann RB, Bulkley BH. Involvement of the heart by malignant lymphoma: a clinicopathologic study. Cancer 1982;49:944-951.

127. Roistacher N, Preminger M, Macapinlac H, Pierri MK. Myocardial entrapment by lymphoma: a cause of reversible segmental left ventricular dysfunction. Am Heart J 1992;124:516-521.

128. Sato H, Takahashi M. Non-Hodgkin's malignant lymphoma of the bone with intracavitary cardiac involvement. Intern Med 1993;32:502-507.

129. Petersen CD, Robinson WA, Kurnick JE. Involvement of the heart and pericardium in the malignant lymphomas. Am J Med Sci 1976;272:161-165.

130. Tesoro-Tess JD, Biasi S, Balzarini L, et al. Heart involvement in lymphomas. The value of magnetic resonance imaging and two-dimensional echocardiography at disease presentation. Cancer 1993;72:2484-2490.

131. Roberts WC, Bodey GP, Wertlake PT. The heart in acute leukemia. A study of 420 autopsy cases. Am J Cardiol 1968;21:388-412.

132. Cash T, Becton D, Mian A. Cardiac myeloid sarcoma: a case report and review of literature. J Pediatr Hematol Oncol 2011;33:e330-332.

133. Potenza L, Luppi M, Morselli M, et al. Cardiac involvement in malignancies. Case 2. Right ventricular lesion as presenting feature of acute promyelocytic leukemia. J Clin Oncol 2004; 22:2742-2744.

134. Erdol C, Ovali E, Baykan M. Granulocytic sarcoma presenting as a right atrial mass. Acta Cardiol 2003;58:155-158.

135. Foucar K, Foucar E, Willman C, Horvath A, Gerety RL. Nonleukemic granulocytic sarcoma of the heart: a report of a fatal case. Am J Hematol 1987;25:325-332.

136. Javier BV, Yount WJ, Crosby DJ, Hall TC. Cardiac metastasis in lymphoma and leukemia. Dis Chest 1967;52:481-484.

137. Krause JR. Granulocytic sarcoma preceding acute leukemia: a report of six cases. Cancer 1979;44:1017-1021.

138. Kubonishi I, Ohtsuki Y, Machida K, et al. Granulocytic sarcoma presenting as a mediastinal tumor. Report of a case and cytological and cytochemical studies of tumor cells in vivo and in vitro. Am J Clin Pathol 1984;82:730-734.

139. Tillawi IS, Variakojis D. Refractory right ventricular failure due to granulocytic sarcoma. Arch Pathol Lab Med 1990;114:983-985.

140. Ammann P, Bosch B, Buchholz S, Genoni M, Laube I, Naegeli B. Cardiac tumor due to erdheim-chester disease. Am J Med 2001;111:672-673.

141. Bassou D, El Kharras A, Taoufik AT, et al. Cardiac Erdheim-Chester. Intern Med 2009;48:83-84.

142. Botelho A, Antunes A, Almeida JC, et al. A rare histiocytosis with severe cardiac involvement: Erdheim-Chester disease. Rev Port Cardiol 2008;27:727-740.

143. Granier M, Micheau A, Serre I. A rare cause of cardiac tumour: an Erdheim-Chester disease with cardiac involvement co-existing with an intracerebral Langerhans cell histiocytosis. Eur Heart J 2008;29:1929.

144. Gupta A, Kelly B, McGuigan JE. Erdheim-Chester disease with prominent pericardial involvement: clinical, radiologic, and histologic findings. Am J Med Sci 2002;324:96-100.

145. Haroche J, Amoura Z, Dion E, et al. Cardiovascular involvement, an overlooked feature of Erdheim-Chester disease: report of 6 new cases and a literature review. Medicine (Baltimore) 2004;83:371-392.

146. Haroche J, Cluzel P, Toledano D, et al. Images in cardiovascular medicine. Cardiac involvement in Erdheim-Chester disease: magnetic resonance and computed tomographic scan imaging in a monocentric series of 37 patients. Circulation 2009;119:e597-598.

147. Kudo Y, Iguchi N, Sumiyoshi T, Murai T, Oka T. Dramatic change of Ga-67 citrate uptake before and after corticosteroid therapy in a case of cardiac histiocytosis (Erdheim-Chester disease). J Nucl Cardiol 2006;13:867-869.

148. Loeffler AG, Memoli VA. Myocardial involvement in Erdheim-Chester disease. Arch Pathol Lab Med 2004;128:682-685.

149. Virmani R, Bewtra C, McAllister HA, Schulte RD. Intrapericardial giant lymph node hyperplasia. Am J Surg Pathol 1982;6:475-481.

150. Malaisrie SC, Loebe M, Walkes JC, Reardon MJ. Coronary pseudoaneurysm: an unreported complication of Castleman's disease. Ann Thorac Surg 2006;82:318-320.

151. Maleszewski JJ, Hristov AC, Halushka MK, Miller DV. Extranodal Rosai-Dorfman disease involving the heart: report of two cases. Cardiovasc Pathol 2010;19:380-384.

152. Yontz L, Franco A, Sharma S, Lewis K, McDonough C. A case of Rosai-Dorfman disease in a pediatric patient with cardiac involvement. J Radiol Case Rep 2012;6:1-8.

153. Sarraj A, Zarra KV, Jimenez Borreguero LJ, Caballero P, Nuche JM. Isolated cardiac involvement of Rosai-Dorfman disease. Ann Thorac Surg 2012;94:2118-2120.

154. Richter JT, Strange RG Jr, Fisher SI, Miller DV, Delvecchio DM. Extranodal Rosai-Dorfman disease presenting as a cardiac mass in an adult: report of a unique case and lack of relationship to IgG4-related sclerosing lesions. Hum Pathol 2010;41:297-301.

155. Chen J, Tang H, Li B, Xiu Q. Rosai-Dorfman disease of multiple organs, including the epicardium: an unusual case with poor prognosis. Heart Lung 2011;40:168-171.

156. Chen CY, Wu MH, Huang SF, Chen SJ, Lu MY. Langerhans' cell histiocytosis presenting with a para-aortic lesion and heart failure. J Formos Med Assoc 2001;100:127-130.

157. Sailey CJ, Alexiev BA, Gammie JS, Pinell-Salles P, Stafford JL, Burke A. Crystal-storing histiocytosis as a cause of symptomatic cardiac mass. Arch Pathol Lab Med 2009;133:1861-1864.

# 18 TUMORS METASTATIC TO THE HEART

The autopsy frequency of cardiac metastases in patients with metastatic malignancies ranges from 8 percent (1) to about 30 percent (2–4). Metastatic tumors found in the heart, by decreasing order of incidence, are metastases from the lung, lymphomas, carcinomas of the breast, leukemia, carcinomas of the stomach, malignant melanoma, hepatocellular carcinoma, and carcinomas of the colon. The following tumors have an especially high rate of cardiac metastasis if the incidence of the primary tumor is considered: leukemia, melanoma, thyroid carcinoma, extracardiac sarcomas, lymphoma, renal cell carcinoma, carcinoid tumors, and carcinomas of the lung and breast (5). Cardiac metastases from the gastrointestinal and genitourinary tracts, especially the prostate gland, are rare. In one series, a high rate of metastasis from the oral cavity was reported (3).

Of surgically excised heart tumors, about one fifth are metastases. In series of surgically resected cardiac tumors, metastatic lesions comprise 3 to 27 percent of all tumor resections, and 22 to 61 percent of malignant tumors (6–8).

## MYOCARDIAL METASTASES

### Clinical Features

The clinical symptoms attributed to metastatic cardiac tumor involvement are nonspecific and infrequently diagnosed. Cardiac metastases may result in no symptoms, and be incidental findings at autopsy or imaging (32,33). When symptoms occur, the most common is dyspnea, usually related to pericardial or pleural effusion. The patient's shortness of breath may be out of proportion to the radiographic findings in cases of pericardial effusion. The differential diagnosis of pericardial effusion in a patient with known malignancy includes malignant pericardial effusion, radiation-induced pericarditis, drug-induced pericarditis, and idiopathic pericarditis (9). Patients also present with cough,

anterior thoracic pain, pleuritic chest pain, or peripheral edema.

In addition to symptoms related to effusions, patients with myocardial metastases may have manifestations related to mass effect (10): these manifest as syncope (11,12), heart failure (10,13–16), echocardiographic low voltage effects (17), conduction block (14), supraventricular tachycardia (18), and right ventricular outflow tract obstruction (13,19–24). Syncope is generally caused by prolapse of right atrial metastases into the right ventricle or by mitral or aortic valve obstruction (11,12). Involvement of the right heart and tricuspid valves may give rise to right-sided failure (25). Myocardial ischemia from coronary occlusion or embolism is unusual (26). Metastatic tumors can mimic cardiac myxoma with embolic phenomena (27).

The time interval between the diagnosis of the primary tumor and the development of cardiac metastases may be months or years (28), especially for melanomas and sarcomas. Cardiac recurrences may be multiple after excision (29). Soft tissue sarcomas may metastasize as late as 8 years after initial diagnosis (23), and melanoma has been known to metastasize after 28 years (30).

In 8 to 32 percent of patients with metastatic cardiac disease, the cause of death is related to the cardiac tumor (1,5). In these cases, cardiac tamponade, cardiac rupture, congestive heart failure, compression of the sinoatrial node or coronary arteries, and coronary artery embolism have led to death (5,31).

In patients with carcinoid syndrome caused by metastatic carcinoid tumors of the gastrointestinal tract, the clinical distinction between carcinoid valve disease and metastatic carcinoid tumor to the heart may be difficult. In a series of 11 patients with metastatic carcinoid tumor to the heart (34), the primary lesion was in the small bowel in 83 percent, and all patients had hepatic metastases. All metastases were intramyocardial; only 55 percent were detected by

**Table 18-1**

**CARDIAC SITES OF METASTASES CAUSING SYMPTOMATIC HEART DISEASE**

| | | |
|---|---|---|
| Right atrium | Direct extension | Renal cell carcinoma |
| | | Hepatocellular carcinoma |
| | | Uterine tumors (leiomyoma, stromal tumors, carcinomas) |
| | | Renal tumors other than carcinoma |
| | Hematogenous metastases | Melanoma |
| | | Sarcoma |
| | | Lymphoma |
| | | Carcinoid tumors |
| | | Carcinomas (rare) |
| Right ventricle | Direct extension | Via right atrial tumors |
| | Hematogenous metastases | Melanoma |
| | | Sarcomas |
| | | Lymphoma |
| | | Carcinoid tumors |
| | | Carcinomas (rare, usually as extension of pericardial metastases) |
| Left atrium | Direct extension | Lung carcinoma |
| | | Lymphoma |
| | | Lung metastases (osteosarcoma, other sarcomas) |
| | Hematogenous metastases | Melanoma |
| | | Lymphoma |
| | | Carcinoma (rare) |
| | | Sarcoma (rare) |
| Left ventricle | Hematogenous metastases | Melanoma |
| | | Sarcoma (rare) |
| | | Carcinoma (rare) |
| Pericardium | Direct extension | Thymoma |
| | | Esophageal carcinoma |
| | | Lung carcinoma |
| | Lymphatic spread | Lung carcinoma |
| | | Breast carcinoma |
| | | Lymphoma |
| | | Other carcinomas |

Note: Mesotheliomas are discussed in the Fourth Series Atlas, Tumors of the Serosal Membranes (34a).

echocardiography. Carcinoid valve disease was present in 8 of the 11 patients.

### Cardiac Spread of Metastases

Malignancies spread to the heart by direct extension, usually from a mediastinal tumor; hematogenously; via lymphatics, generally by retrograde extension; and by intracavitary extension from the inferior vena cava or pulmonary veins (Table 18-1).

Thymoma and esophageal carcinoma are mediastinal tumors that involve the heart by direct extension. Obstruction of the pulmonary outflow tract may result in pulmonary stenosis, which was reported in a primary atypical thymic carcinoid tumor (35).

Lymphatic spread of metastasis is associated with a high incidence of malignant pericardial effusions, rather than the myocardial metastatic tumors associated with hematogenous spread. Lymphatic spread is generally accompanied by involvement and enlargement of pulmonary hilar or mediastinal lymph nodes (36), and histologic evidence of pericardial lymphatic infiltration. Epithelial malignancies typically spread to the heart by lymphatic vessels. Most of the lymph flow in the heart is efferent, which explains the low incidence of lymphatic cardiac metastases, which occur by retrograde lymph drainage (5).

Most cardiac metastases spread hematogenously. Melanoma, sarcomas, leukemia, and renal tumors metastasize to the heart by a hematogenous route, as do adrenal tumors, liver tumors, and uterine tumors.

A subset of hematogenous metastases is composed of those tumors that grow as direct extensions into the cardiac chambers, via the venae cavae or pulmonary veins. The most common route is the right atrium via the inferior vena cava, most commonly by renal cell carcinoma. The left atrium may be invaded by primary lung tumors or metastatic tumors to the lung.

### Sites of Origin

The distribution of cardiac metastases within the heart differs between autopsy and surgical series. In a series of 407 autopsies in which metastatic tumors were present in the heart, 19 percent involved the pericardium only, 33 percent the epicardium predominantly, 42 percent the myocardium predominantly, and 6 percent the endocardium (intracavitary tumors) (5). The right side of the heart was involved in 20 to 30 percent of cases, the left side in 10 to 33 percent of cases, and bilateral or diffuse involvement occurred in approximately 30 to 35 percent of cases. Metastatic deposits were not grossly evident and seen only microscopically in 6 of 407 hearts in this study.

In contrast to autopsy metastases, which are often incidental, surgically resected metastases tend to be myocardial or intracavitary, and right-sided lesions. These surgically resected masses represent either cavoatrial extensions from abdominal tumors, such as renal cell carcinomas or hepatocellular carcinomas (37), or hematogenous metastases. In one series of clinically detected metastases, not all of which were surgically removed, 47 percent were found in the pericardium, 32 percent in the right side of the heart, 14 percent in the left side, and 7 percent in both sides (8).

Intracardiac masses that are not direct extensions from intracaval carcinomas are often unusual tumors, such as sarcomas, melanomas (24,38), endocrine carcinomas, or germ cell tumors. Epithelial malignancies also form intracardiac tumors that mimic primary lesions (28,39).

It is extremely uncommon for cardiac metastases to be isolated lesions (40,41). In only 1 of 30 cases of sarcoma metastatic to the heart, was the heart the lone site of metastasis (14).

**Right Atrial Metastases.** Right atrial metastases are either extensions from tumors filling the inferior vena cava or distant hematogenous metastases. Right atrial extension from the inferior vena cava occurs most frequently with renal cell carcinoma (42–48) and hepatocellular carcinoma (13,49–62), and less commonly with testicular teratoma (63), renal sarcoma (64), hepatoblastoma in children (65), adrenal sarcoma or carcinoma (37,66), pelvic osteosarcoma (67), retroperitoneal liposarcoma (68), endometrial carcinosarcoma (69), endometrial stromal tumors (29,70,71), pelvic osteosarcoma (72), and uterine leiomyoma (43). Rarely, cervical squamous carcinoma from abdominal lymph node metastases spreads through the inferior vena cava (73). Tumor thrombi from right-sided lung carcinomas may result from invasion into the right atrium (74). Thymomas spread into the right atrium via the superior vena cava and brachiocephalic vein (43). Rare thyroid carcinomas directly invade the right atrium (75,76).

The right atrium is also the site of distant metastasis through hematogenous spread. Such tumors include melanoma (11,77), pancreatic adenocarcinoma (25), colonic adenocarcinoma (78), adenocarcinomas of unknown origin (79), squamous carcinoma of the oral cavity (20), squamous carcinoma of the esophagus (80), endometrial carcinoma (81), alveolar rhabdomyosarcoma (82), carcinoid tumor (34), hepatocellular carcinoma (22), and uterine choriocarcinoma (83).

**Left Atrial Metastases.** The left atrium is a rare site of hematogenous metastasis, other than direct extensions of lung tumors from the pulmonary veins, but is the most common site for primary cardiac sarcomas. A case of possible metastatic synovial sarcoma to the left atrium has been reported, but was probably a primary tumor (84). A metastatic alveolar rhabdomyosarcoma has been reported infiltrating the left atrium, coronary sinus, and right atrium (82). A gastric sarcoma metastatic to the left atrium was not well documented pathologically (85).

Malignant melanoma has metastasized to the left atrium after initial successful treatment by radiation (86), as well as a metastatic hepatocellular carcinoma 3 years after initial tumor resection (55). The left atrium is involved by metastatic disease in the case of disseminated cardiac metastases in all chambers (18), or in association with left ventricular involvement, for example, with metastatic testicular seminoma (87). Rarely, left atrial tumor thrombi are free-floating as a complication of disseminated lung carcinoma (88).

Various tumors invade the left atrium by direct extension. The most common are primary lung carcinomas (of all histologic types) that extend from the hilum into the left atrium via the pulmonary veins (89–96). In addition to lobectomy or pneumonectomy, left atrial reconstruction is necessary, sometimes with stapling devices. The preoperative extent of myocardial invasion can be assessed by imaging, such as with positron emission tomography (PET) (93,95). Both right and left lower lobe lung carcinomas can extend into the left atrium (90,91,96). Metastatic tumors to the lung, such as colonic adenocarcinomas and follicular thyroid carcinomas, may also invade the left atrium from the lung parenchyma (97,98).

Sarcomas invade the left atrium as direct extensions from metastases to the lung. The most common is osteosarcoma, with 9 cases reported (38). Other such sarcomas include leiomyosarcomas (99), malignant peripheral nerve sheath tumors (100), and ossifying fibromyxoid tumor of soft parts (101).

**Right Ventricular Metastases.** Tumors that metastasize to the right ventricle may result in outflow obstruction and necessitate surgical excision with valve repair or replacement (19,102,103). Right ventricular spread may be by direct extension through the atrium, or by distant hematogenous metastasis, in which case the tumors may be quite bulky (104). The most common malignancies that metastasize without direct extension to the right ventricle are melanoma (24,105,106), renal cell carcinoma (104,107–109), and a variety of sarcomas, including liposarcoma (110), synovial sarcoma (111), osteosarcoma (38), Ewing sarcoma (112), rhabdomyosarcoma (113–115), extraskeletal chondrosarcoma (116), malignant fibrous histiocytoma/pleomorphic undifferentiated sarcoma (21,103), and liposarcoma (117). Other epithelial neoplasms that metastasize to the right ventricle include squamous carcinomas of the bladder (118), hepatocellular carcinoma (13), squamous and neuroendocrine carcinomas of the cervix (15,28,102), and squamous carcinoma arising from an ovarian teratoma (119). A case of benign metastasizing leiomyoma from the uterus has been reported in the right ventricle (120), as well as a testicular choriocarcinoma (19).

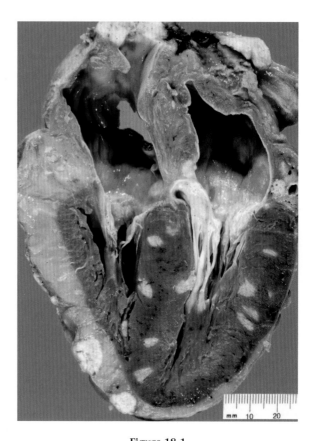

**Figure 18-1**

**METASTATIC ADENOCARCINOMA: LUNG PRIMARY**

There are multiple ventricular and epicardial metastases. The patient had disseminated carcinoma, without symptoms related to cardiac dysfunction. Epithelial malignancies, when they metastasize to the heart, are generally symptomatic when there is significant pericardial involvement.

**Left Ventricular Metastases.** The left ventricle is a rare site of metastatic tumor in surgical or clinical series. There have been reports of metastatic renal cell carcinoma (121), melanoma (122), carcinoid tumor (34), and synovial sarcoma (23) detected and treated in the left ventricle during life. Both the left and right ventricles were involved in a case of metastatic thyroid carcinoma (17), and in multichamber metastases (18,123). A metastatic carcinoid tumor metastasized to the interventricular septum (124).

### Gross Findings

Metastatic deposits may be diffuse, multinodular, or a single dominant mass (figs. 18-1–18-5). There may be diffuse studding and thickening of the pericardial surfaces with little infiltration

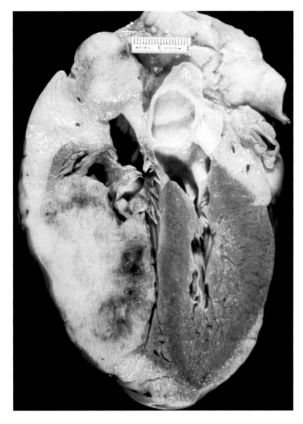

**Figure 18-2**

**METASTATIC ADENOCARCINOMA: COLONIC PRIMARY**

A single dominant mass is in the right ventricle. Dominant myocardial masses in epithelial malignancies metastatic to the heart are rare, especially in the case of adenocarcinoma.

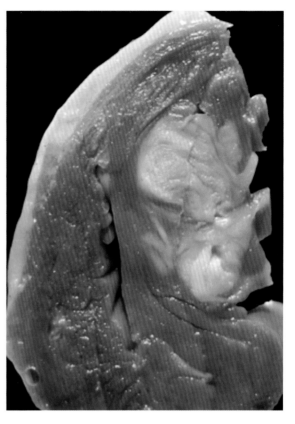

**Figure 18-3**

**METASTATIC RHABDOMYOSARCOMA: RIGHT VENTRICLE**

The patient had a head and neck rhabdomyosarcoma resected 3 years prior to death. Sarcomas are more likely to spread via the hematogenous route to the myocardium than epithelial malignancies.

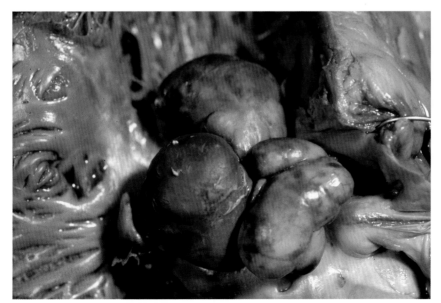

**Figure 18-4**

**METASTATIC CARCINOID TUMOR: RIGHT ATRIUM**

Neuroendocrine carcinomas may involve the heart as carcinoid syndrome, as well as metastatic deposits, which, in this autopsy case, obstructed the tricuspid valve. There were multiple liver metastases as well (not shown).

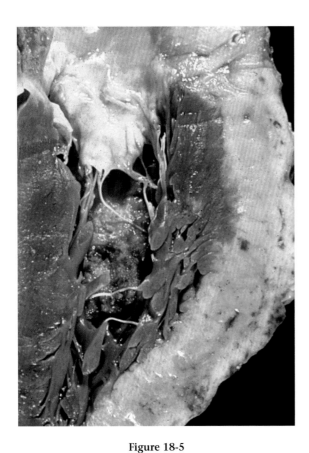

**Figure 18-5**

**METASTATIC LUNG CARCINOMA: EPICARDIUM**

In many cases of disseminated adenocarcinoma, the pericardium is diffusely involved, resulting in pericardial tamponade. In advanced cases, there is spread into superficial myocardium as well, as in this case to the right ventricle. The ventricular septum is at the left.

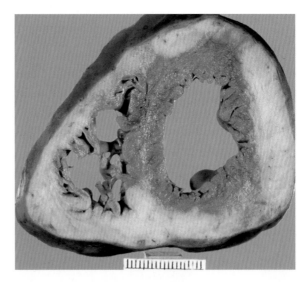

**Figure 18-6**

**MALIGNANT LYMPHOMA**

There is multifocal replacement of the myocardium involving the right ventricle and subepicardial regions of the left ventricle, predominantly in the anterior, lateral, and posteroseptal regions.

of the heart. This pattern generally occurs in carcinomatous metastases and grossly may be confused with mesothelioma, or, less commonly, benign fibrosing pericarditis. Mediastinal lymph nodes are involved in approximately 80 percent of cases of cardiac metastases (5), especially if there is pericardial involvement.

Grossly, lymphoma nodules are epicardial or myocardial, merge imperceptibly with the surrounding myocardium, and are large, homogeneous, and white to tan, with little necrosis (fig. 18-6). Leukemic infiltrates may be endocardial (fig. 18-7). Carcinomas are more variegated, gritty lesions that are usually epicardial or pericardial. Squamous cell metastases may be multiple and project into the cardiac chambers (18). The presence of melanotic pig-

ment is suggestive of metastatic melanoma. The tumor burden in the heart is the highest with melanoma, as compared to other malignancies, although there may be massive involvement in lymphoma as well (125).

Kaposi sarcoma involves the heart grossly as focal, small, firm, red-brown nodules that may coalesce; it only rarely involves the heart in the absence of systemic disease (126). Kaposi sarcoma usually involves the epicardium and pericardium and less frequently invades the myocardium and coronary arteries. Although metastatic urothelial carcinoma from the bladder is rare, it has been reported that metastatic bladder carcinoma may retain its papillary configuration within the pericardial space (127), thereby suggesting the diagnosis on gross inspection. Rarely, cardiac metastases grossly mimic endocardial-based tumors, such as myxoma (80).

Primary sarcomas are impossible to distinguish from metastatic lesions without a complete autopsy, although they are generally larger, single tumors that extend into the cardiac cavities (fig. 18-8). Sarcoidosis may result in large, firm scars, but, unlike metastatic deposits, sarcoid granulomas rarely distort the endocardial or epicardial contours of the heart.

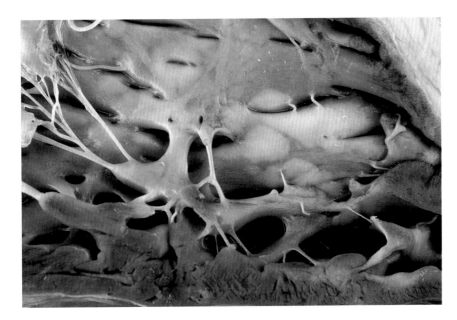

**Figure 18-7**

**ACUTE LYMPHOBLASTIC LEUKEMIA: ENDOCARDIUM**

There is diffuse endocardial thickening of the right ventricle, which histolgically proved to be a leukemic infiltrate.

**Figure 18-8**

**METASTATIC LEIOMYOSARCOMA: RIGHT VENTRICLE**

The tumor was removed and considered initially a cardiac primary, before imaging demonstrating a uterine mass that proved to be a leiomyosarcoma. The gross appearance is that of a homogeneous fleshy tumor almost suggesting lymphoma. The patient presented with outflow tract obstruction.

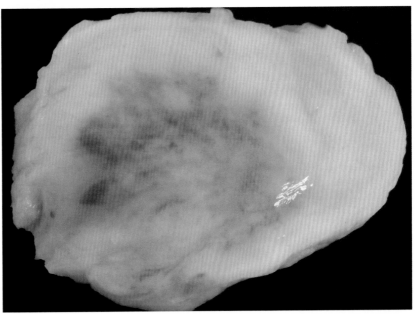

Metastatic lesions may need to be resected because of outflow tract obstruction (fig. 18-8). The primary tumor is then identified only after cardiac resection.

## Histologic Types of Metastases

**Epithelial Malignancies.** For most epithelial malignancies involving the heart, involvement is pericardial, with only superficial myocardial infiltration (see Pericardial Metastases below). The valves and endocardium are usually spared. Generally, the heart is not the only organ involved, and metastatic deposits are usually present in extracardiac sites. Although the most common epithelial malignancies to metastasize to the pericardium are carcinomas of the breast and lung, symptomatic myocardial involvement is rare for these tumors, especially for breast carcinoma. Lung cancers generally involve the myocardium by direct extension via the left atrium. In a clinical series, the most common site of origin of secondary epithelial cardiac tumors was the lung, followed by mediastinum, liver, uterus, and testis (8).

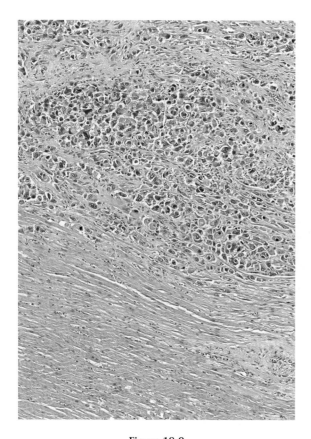

**Figure 18-9**

**METASTATIC LARGE CELL
CARCINOMA: LUNG PRIMARY**

The myocardium is infiltrated via direct spread from
the epicardium.

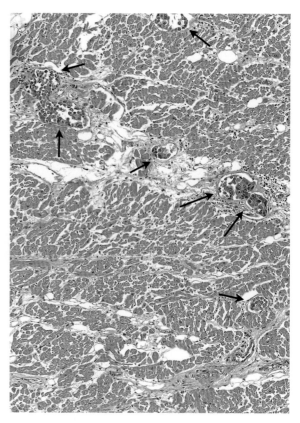

**Figure 18-10**

**METASTATIC CARCINOMA: LUNG PRIMARY**

Myocardial infiltration occurs via retrograde extension
from lymphatics (arrows).

In autopsy series, late-stage epithelial carcinomas involve the heart 8.4 percent of the
time, equally involving myocardium and
pericardium. Lung carcinoma is the most common metastasis, because of its overall high
prevalence, with a rate of 7 percent, similar to
metastases to the female genital tract. The rate
of involvement by the metastatic oral cancers in
this series was unusually high at 23 percent (3).
Although breast carcinoma is one of the most
common tumors metastatic to the pericardium,
myocardial involvement is exceptional.

**Carcinomas of the Lung.** Pericardial metastases from lung cancer are frequent; myocardial
metastases, in contrast, are rare, at least those
producing symptoms. Myocardial involvement
by lung carcinoma generally occurs via direct
invasion of the left atrium. In a minority of
patients with lung cancer, excision of the tumor

requires partial resection of the left atrium, in
addition to lobectomy or pneumonectomy.
Both right and left lower lobe tumors may infiltrate the left atrium. With appropriate surgical
resection, the long-term prognosis is reasonable, with a 5-year survival rate of 20 percent
(90). There may be concomitant invasion of the
aorta, innominate vein, or subclavian vein.

Autopsy series show hematogenous metastasis
of lung carcinoma to the ventricles (fig. 18-9),
often with a predominant subepicardial distribution. There is often involvement of lymphatics
(fig. 18-10) and subepicardial fat (fig 18-11).

The histologic subtypes vary, but metastatic
cardiac lung cancers are usually nonsmall cell
carcinomas, with a predominance of squamous
cell carcinomas, followed by adenocarcinomas,
large cell carcinomas, and sarcomatoid carcinoma (94,96). Small cell lung cancers rarely

*Tumors Metastatic to the Heart*

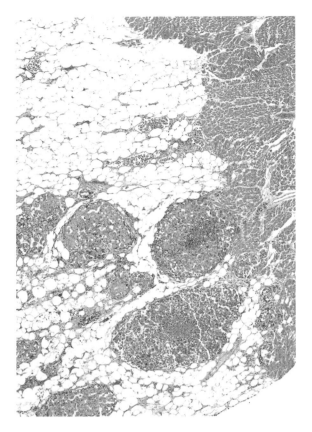

**Figure 18-11**

**POORLY DIFFERENTIATED ADENOCARCINOMA: LUNG PRIMARY WITH EPICARDIAL METASTASIS**

Pericardial metastases are common in lung and breast carcinomas, and may additionally involve the epicardial fat, by retrograde lymphatic spread into the superficial myocardium.

invade the left atrium (93). Surgical excision requires atrial reconstruction that may require stapling (92). Rarely, there are free-floating left atrial tumor thrombi without connection to the primary tumor (88), which may cause embolism and peripheral ischemia (91). Right atrial tumor thrombi have also been reported with lung carcinoma (74). Extension of primary lung tumors into the left atrium is diagnosed by imaging, including PET (93,95).

**Renal Cell Carcinomas.** Renal cell carcinomas most commonly involve the heart by direct extension through the inferior vena cava into the right atrium, with occasional extension through the tricuspid valve into the right ventricle (45,48). Atrial metastasis may occur years after the initial nephrectomy (44). Extension through the right atrium into the superior vena cava has been reported (46). Renal cell carcinoma may arise in a horseshoe kidney and spread to the right atrium, complicating surgical excision of the tumor (47). Tumor embolism into the right atrium may occur acutely during nephrectomy, and is detected by intraoperative transesophageal ultrasound (echocardiography) (128).

Renal cell carcinomas may metastasize as cavitary lesions without contiguous cardiac spread. The right ventricle is more frequently involved (42,104,107,108) than the left ventricle (121). The histology is typically that of clear cell carcinoma, although other histologic types metastasize to the heart, including the sarcomatoid variant (104).

**Hepatocellular Carcinoma.** Similar to renal cell carcinoma, hepatocellular carcinoma involves the heart usually by right-sided direct extension through the inferior vena cava (22,49–59). Surgical resection of atrial metastasis may be accomplished with or without bypass (58). Patients typically have cirrhosis, with worsening jaundice, ascites, and lower extremity edema. The diagnosis is established by serum alpha-fetoprotein determination and imaging of the liver by magnetic resonance imaging (MRI) and computed tomography (CT) (50). Tumor extension into the right atrium and ventricle may obstruct blood flow and cause sudden death by a mechanism similar to massive pulmonary embolism (56).

Right atrial metastases may be confused histologically with renal cell carcinoma because of diffuse cytoplasmic clearing (fig. 18-12). The history and appropriate immunohistochemical staining lead to the diagnosis. Hematogenous spread of hepatocellular carcinoma without direct extension is rare, but has been reported to the left atrium 3 years after surgery (55).

**Squamous Carcinomas.** Squamous carcinomas from various sites can metastasize to the myocardium and form intracavitary or intramyocardial masses (fig. 18-13). These include carcinomas of the larynx (18), maxillary sinus (33), oral cavity (20), esophagus (80), urinary bladder (118), and uterine cervix (28,39,73,102). The tumors are typically right-sided, involving the atrium, ventricle, or both.

**Other Epithelial Malignancies.** Other carcinomas that spread hematogenously to the

**Figure 18-12**

**METASTATIC HEPATOCELLULAR CARCINOMA**

There is cytoplasmic clearing, but the vascular pattern of renal cell carcinoma is not evident. The growth pattern is solid. The patient had an obstructing right atrial lesion, which was resected; only postoperatively was a primary mass detected in the liver. The diagnosis was confirmed by immunohistochemical studies, which demonstrated canalicular staining for polyclonal carcinoembryonic antigen, positivity for Hep par-1 antigen, and weak staining for alpha-fetoprotein (not shown). In general, hepatocellular carcinomas are negative for cytokeratin (CK)7 and epithelial membrane antigen (EMA), and positive for low molecular weight cytokeratins such as CK19.

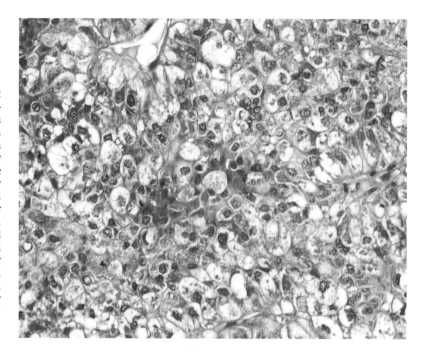

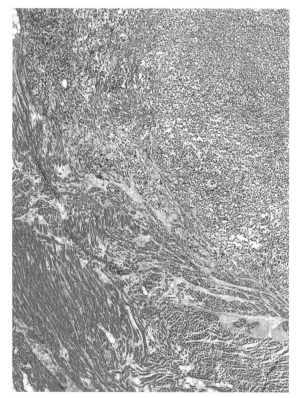

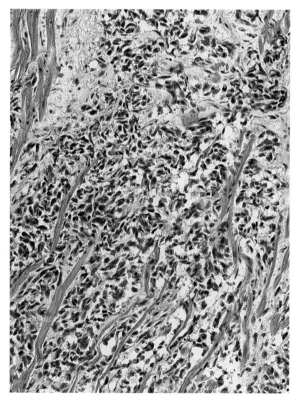

**Figure 18-13**

**METASTATIC POORLY DIFFERENTIATED SQUAMOUS CELL CARCINOMA**

Left: This patient had multiple metastases at autopsy; the primary site was a previously resected head and neck tumor. There is an infiltrating nodular lesion in the myocardium.

Right: At higher magnification, tumor cells are seen diffusely infiltrating myocytes.

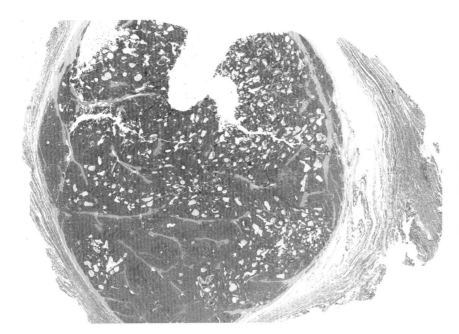

**Figure 18-14**

**METASTATIC CARCINOID TUMOR: RIGHT ATRIUM**

The tumor was an incidental finding during surgery for coronary artery disease. Carcinoid tumors, among epithelial malignancies, commonly spread to the myocardium, often as single lesions.

heart, generally to the right atrium or ventricle, include neuroendocrine cervical cancer (15), pancreatic adenocarcinoma (25), endometrial adenocarcinoma (81), thyroid carcinoma (17), and adenocarcinoma of unknown origin (79). Small bowel carcinoid tumors can coexist with carcinoid syndrome, and metastasize to the ventricles. Right-sided lesions may obstruct the right atrium (figs. 18-14, 18-15), often with tricuspid valve involvement (34,124). Thyroid carcinoma involves the right atrium by direct extension (75,76), or by extension from pulmonary metastasis (98). The histologic diagnosis is usually straightforward, but immunohistochemical staining for chromogranin shows diffuse positivity (fig. 18-16).

Mesothelioma has only rarely metastasized to the myocardium (129).

**Hematologic Malignancies.** Hematologic malignancies are especially prone to involve the heart, especially the myocardium. Approximately 35 to 40 percent of patients with leukemia have cardiac involvement at autopsy. Primary cardiac lymphomas are discussed in chapter 17. Leukemic and lymphomatous infiltrates are typically widespread, involving the epicardium (61 percent) and myocardium diffusely; the endocardium may be the sole site of involvement (fig. 18-17). The left ventricle is involved in 55 percent and right atrium in 54 percent of cases of disseminated leukemia and lymphoma.

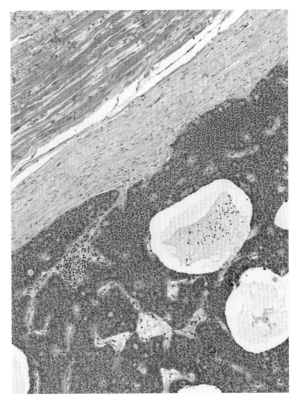

**Figure 18-15**

**METASTATIC CARCINOID TUMOR**

A higher magnification of the tumor illustrated in figures 18-4 and 18-14 shows the typical nested and pseudoglandular (cribriform) growth pattern, with regular, round nuclei having a finely stippled chromatin pattern.

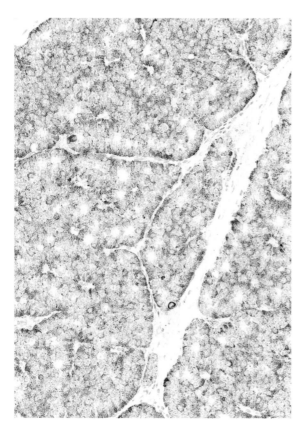

**Figure 18-16**

**METASTATIC CARCINOID TUMOR**

Low-grade endocrine carcinomas show diffuse staining for endocrine markers, including chromogranin (shown), synaptophysin, and neural cell adhesion molecule (CD56).

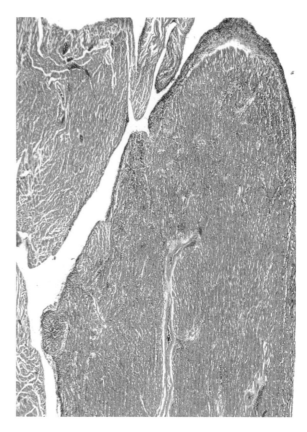

**Figure 18-17**

**ACUTE LYMPHOBLASTIC LEUKEMIA: ENDOCARDIUM**

A histologic section of the heart shown figure 18-7 shows leukemic infiltration of the endocardium.

Lymphomatous infiltrates are found in 7 to 25 percent of patients dying with lymphoma (10). Roberts et al. (130,131) reported a 16 percent incidence of cardiac involvement at autopsy in Hodgkin disease, 33 percent incidence in mycosis fungoides, and 27 percent incidence in other types of lymphoma.

**Metastatic Malignant Melanoma.** Metastatic melanoma is the malignancy most likely to spread to the heart, particularly to the right side: up to 64 percent of patients dying with melanoma have cardiac involvement at autopsy (132). The metastases seen at autopsy, however, frequently do not cause symptoms (133). Only 0.2 percent of patients with melanoma develop clinically apparent cardiac metastases, and 1.6 percent of patients with visceral metastases from melanoma develop clinically evident cardiac metastases (133). Histologically, the tumors show prominent

melanin production (figs. 18-18, 18-19) or lack melanin pigment (figs. 18-20–18-22).

In a surgical series at the Mayo Clinic (30), there were seven patients with excisions of symptomatic metastatic cardiac melanoma: four females and three males (aged 31 to 79 years). Remarkably, no patient had a history of metastatic melanoma elsewhere, and in two, no primary lesion was ever identified. In four cases, the history of primary melanoma was remote, occurring 7, 9, 13, and 28 years prior to the discovery of the cardiac mass. All patients presented with dyspnea and symptoms of outflow obstruction. Echocardiography or CT revealed an intracardiac mass (four atrial, three ventricular). Six cases involved the right side of the heart and one involved the left ventricle.

Case reports of cardiac melanoma demonstrate its propensity to occur in the right atrium

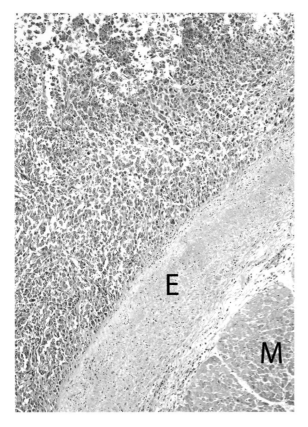

**Figure 18-18**

**METASTATIC MALIGNANT MELANOMA**

Metastatic melanoma to right ventricle grew along the thickened endocardium (E) within the ventricular lumen. Myocardial tissue (M) is present.

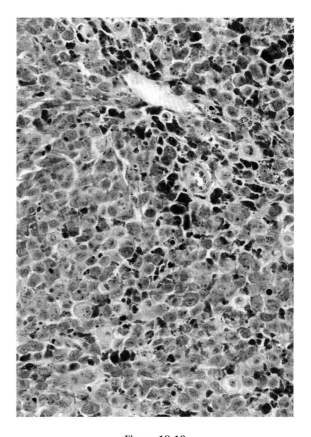

**Figure 18-19**

**METASTATIC MALIGNANT MELANOMA**

There is diffuse melanin pigmentation.

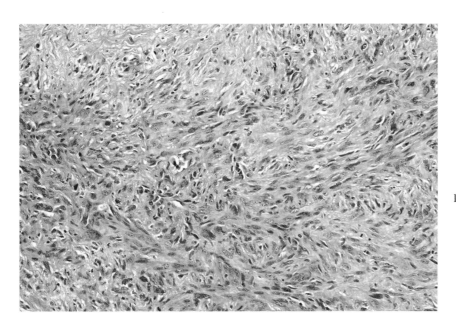

**Figure 18-20**

**METASTATIC AMELANOTIC MALIGNANT MELANOMA**

There was prominent spindling in this tumor.

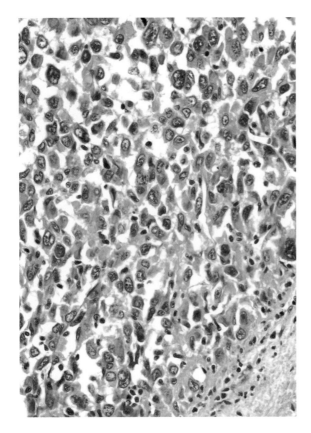

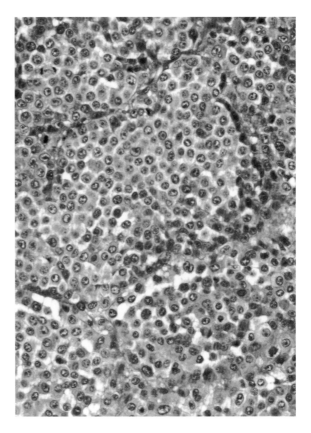

**Figure 18-21**

**METASTATIC AMELANOTIC MALIGNANT MELANOMA**

In some melanomas, the histologic features show little differentiation, and the diagnosis depends on history or immunohistochemical profiling, including positivity for S-100 protein and HMB45, and a variety of melanoma-specific markers (including melan-A). Here, undifferentiated large cells show no evidence of pigment production.

**Figure 18-22**

**METASTATIC AMELANOTIC MALIGNANT MELANOMA**

In more typical melanomas, there is an "endocrine" growth pattern, typified by nests of tumor cells with abundant eosinophilic cytoplasm and prominent nucleoli. The tumor was resected from the right atrium as an incidental finding during bypass surgery. There was a remote history of a pigmented skin lesion removed years prior, but no history of other metastases or melanoma.

(11,32,77) and to cause right ventricular outflow tract obstruction (24,105,106) and heart failure (10,16,134). Left atrial (86) and left ventricular (122) metastases are rare.

**Metastatic Osteosarcoma.** Patients with osteosarcoma metastatic to the heart are more likely female, are slightly older, and have a longer interval to the onset of secondary disease than patients with osteosarcoma metastasizing to other sites (38). The clinical characteristics involve outflow tract obstruction or symptoms of effusion, with MRI a standard of imaging diagnosis. The median age is 22 years, and there is a mean of 4 years between initial diagnosis and the development of cardiac involvement, which is a strong predictor of disease elsewhere.

Half of the patients have a primary tumor in the femur. The cardiac site in most cases is the right ventricle, followed by the right atrium and left ventricle. One third of patients have left atrial involvement as an extension of pulmonary metastasis (38). Rarely, pelvic osteosarcoma involves the right atrium by intravascular extension through the inferior vena cava (67).

Histologically, the metastatic tumors are predominantly composed of undifferentiated spindled cells (figs. 18-23, 18-24), show focal osteoid (fig. 18-24B), or demonstrate chondrosarcoma (fig. 18-24C).

**Other Metastatic Sarcomas.** The heart is affected in 8 to 25 percent of patients with metastatic soft tissue sarcomas (14). Sarcomatous

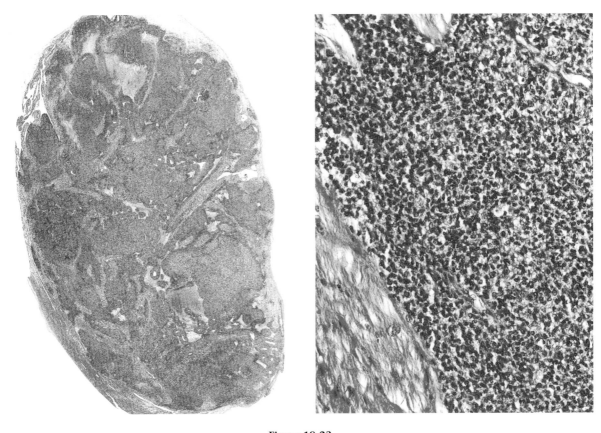

**Figure 18-23**

**METASTATIC OSTEOSARCOMA: RIGHT VENTRICLE**

Left: This well-circumscribed nodule was excised from the right ventricle. It had caused symptoms of outflow tract obstruction. The patient had an osteosarcoma of the femur treated by amputation 15 years prior.

Right: There was no evidence of osseous differentiation, and the nodule was a small cell carcinoma. Derivation from a primary bone tumor was possible only by obtaining a clinical history.

deposits are found within the myocardium (50 percent of cases), pericardium (33 percent), or both (17 percent). Valvular metastases are uncommon. Manifestations include chest pain, arrhythmias, conduction block, heart failure, or syncope related to right ventricular outflow tract obstruction. Delayed metastases, over 10 years after removal of the soft tissue lesion, has been reported (117).

The type of soft tissue sarcoma does not appear to affect the incidence of metastases to the heart (5). Histologic types of sarcoma that metastasize to the heart include uterine leiomyosarcoma (figs. 18-25, 18-26) (14,113–115), liposarcoma (68,110,117), pleomorphic sarcomas and malignant fibrous histiocytoma (14,21,103), synovial sarcoma (23,64,84,111), rhabdomyosarcoma (figs. 18-27, 18-28) (82), endometrial stromal

sarcoma (fig. 18-29) (29,70,135), and Ewing sarcoma (40,112,123).

The most common site in the heart for sarcoma metastases is the right ventricle (21,40, 103,110–112,117,135), followed by the right atrium (64,82), right atrium and ventricle (29, 68), left atrium (84), and left ventricle (23). Right atrial tumors may be extensions from renal (64) or endometrial stromal (70) sarcoma. Sarcoma metastasis to all four cardiac chambers has been reported (123). There has been a report of a benign leiomyoma metastasizing to the right ventricle (120).

**Metastatic Germ Cell Tumors.** Germ cell tumors rarely metastasize to the heart. The most common are testicular nonseminomatous germ cell tumors, including mixed germ cell tumors, embryonal carcinomas, yolk sac

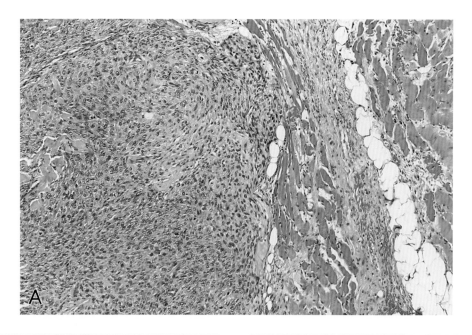

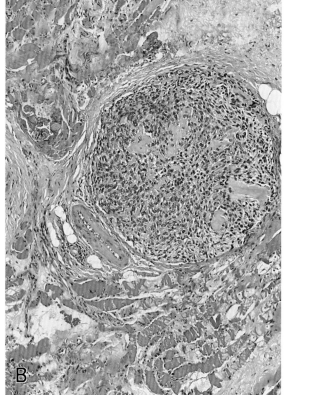

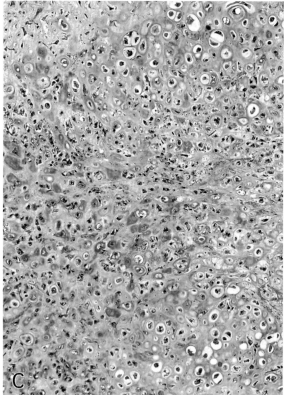

**Figure 18-24**

**METASTATIC OSTEOSARCOMA: RIGHT VENTRICLE**

A: The tumor has a pushing margin into the surrounding myocytes and a spindled appearance, with a suggestion of osteoid formation.

B: In another area there is a separate myocardial nodule. There are foci of osteoid within the tumor.

C: Other areas of the tumor showed chondrosarcoma. The primary lesion occurred in the leg 8 years prior to cardiac surgery.

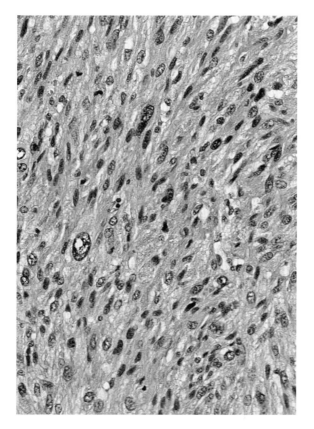

**Figure 18-25**

**METASTATIC LEIOMYOSARCOMA: RIGHT VENTRICLE**

The histologic appearance of the surgically resected specimen is typical, with fascicles of cells, abundant cytoplasm, and uniform blunt-ended nuclei. The tumor was shown grossly in figure 18-8.

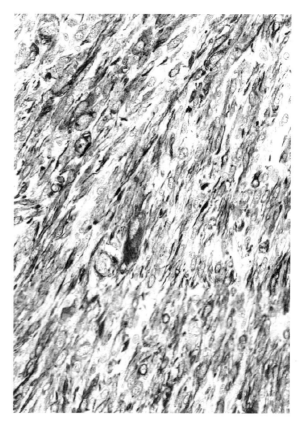

**Figure 18-26**

**METASTATIC LEIOMYOSARCOMA: RIGHT VENTRICLE**

Immunohistochemical staining with desmin confirms smooth muscle differentiation.

tumors, and teratomas, which extend into the right atrium through the inferior vena cava (12,63,136–138). The mass can extend for over 60 cm through the right heart into the superior vena cava, necessitating metastasectomy as well as orchiectomy (139). There may be concomitant lung and lymph node metastases (136). Right atrial tumors are also the result of noncontiguous tumor embolism, and occur up to 10 years after orchiectomy (140). Biatrial metastasis may be the primary manifestation of testicular seminoma (141), and right atrial metastasis may be the primary manifestation of mixed germ cell tumor in an undescended testis (139). Metastatic lesions invade the left atrium from adjacent lung metastases and may be the primary manifestation of mixed germ cell tumor of the testis (142).

A testicular choriocarcinoma has been reported metastatic to the right ventricle (19). A choriocarcinoma of the uterus metastatic to the right atrium (83) and a squamous carcinoma arising from an ovarian teratoma metastatic to the right ventricle (119) have been reported.

The histologic features of resected germ cell tumor metastases resemble the primary tumor. There may be difficulties if the metastatic deposit is a somatic malignancy, such as sarcoma, developing in a teratoma (140).

Primary germ cell tumors of the mediastinum invade the heart by direct extension (143, 144).

**Treatment**

Treatment generally includes resection of the mass, if causing symptoms, with tricuspid valve replacement for right-sided lesions (102,103,106). Venous reconstruction may be

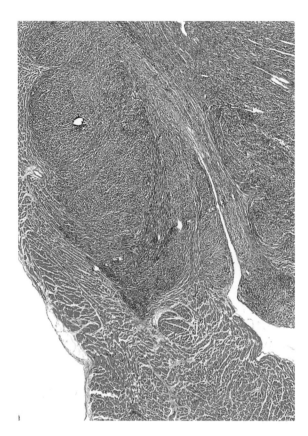 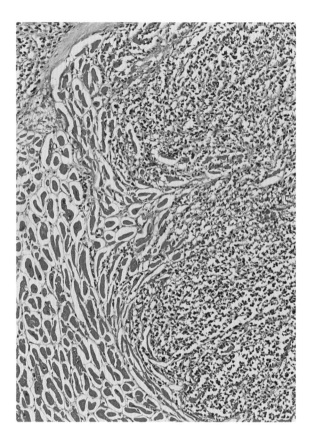

**Figure 18-27**

**METASTATIC RHABDOMYOSARCOMA: RIGHT VENTRICLE**

Left: The patient had widespread metastases from a head and neck primary. The autopsy specimen was a cellular, spindle cell neoplasm that infiltrated the myocardium by hematogenous spread. (Same tumor as seen in fig. 18-3).

Right: At higher magnification, the pushing margin of the nodules and the predominant spindled component of the tumor are seen. The primary tumor was classified as an embryonal type of rhabdomyosarcoma, the most common subtype occurring in the head and neck region.

necessary for extensive caval spread (37,43). Right atrial obstruction by metastatic tumor is a cause for emergency surgery (82). Surgery may be combined with radiation therapy, depending on tumor type (9,17,39,68,86,96,118). Sudden death has been reported during radiation therapy for intracardiac metastasis (17).

## PERICARDIAL METASTASES

### Clinical Features

At autopsy, metastatic disease to the heart often involves the pericardium as well as the subepicardial myocardium, especially with epithelial malignancies. Clinically, pericardial metastases present differently than myocardial metastases, and are sampled by pericardial biopsy with cytology. Pericardial involvement is suspected in patients with cancer if there is acute pericarditis, rapid enlargement of the heart shadow, low voltage changes on electrocardiography, serosanguinous or sanguinous effusions, or echocardiographic demonstration of echo-free spaces in pericardial effusions. Pericardial tamponade results from a variety of metastatic pericardial malignancies, including carcinomas of the lung, pancreas, kidney, breast, and ovary, as well as from lymphoma, leukemia, and rhabdomyosarcoma. Echocardiographic-guided percutaneous biopsy or pericardioscopic-guided biopsy has increased the diagnostic yield with increased sensitivity (145).

Of 60 autopsy-proven cases of pericardial metastatic disease, 26 showed significant effects on the cardiovascular system (146). Pericardial metastases were suspected in 18 of these patients before

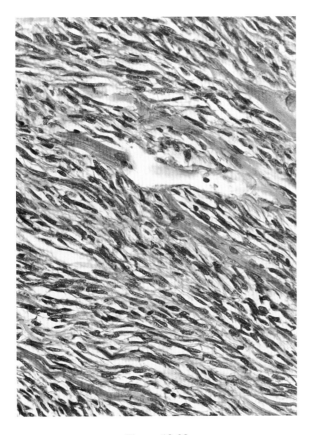

**Figure 18-28**

**METASTATIC RHABDOMYOSARCOMA:
RIGHT VENTRICLE**

Sarcomas typically have a circumscribed or pushing margin when metastatic to the heart, but in this case, the tumor diffusely infiltrates cardiomyocytes.

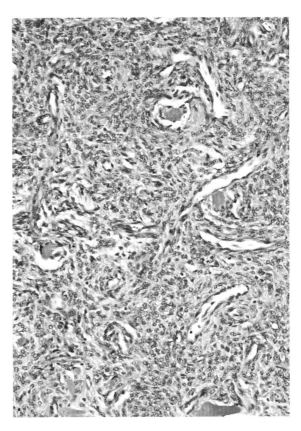

**Figure 18-29**

**METASTATIC ENDOMETRIAL
STROMAL SARCOMA: RIGHT VENTRICLE**

A variety of unusual sarcomas metastasize to the heart, necessitating surgical excision. In this case, there was no history of a previous tumor, and an unusual primary sarcoma of the heart was initially considered. Finally, a review of records revealed that the patient's hysterectomy, 15 years prior, had shown an atypical endometrial stromal proliferation. A variety of low-grade lesions from the uterus may metastasize to heart years and decades after initial resection, including benign metastasizing leiomyoma, stromomyoma, and low-grade endometrial stromal sarcoma.

death. The most common features reported were dyspnea on exertion and pleural effusion, with electrocardiographic features of ST-T changes and low voltage QRS complexes (146).

Imaging with CT, MRI, and PET has greatly improved the detection of pericardial metastatic deposits (9,147–149). The most frequent CT features of pericardial metastases include, in order of decreasing frequency, pericardial effusion, prepericardial lymph node enlargement, and pericardial thickening, enhancement, and nodules (149).

In patients with large pericardial effusions, metastatic tumor accounts for 17 to 23 percent of the cases (150,151), and is higher in cancer centers (152). In cancer patients, effusions may be idiopathic or secondary to radiation or chemotherapy. In patients with breast cancer,

small, asymptomatic effusions are likely benign, and of those that are clinically apparent, only 50 percent are malignant (153–155). Overall, 50 percent of patients with known metastatic disease and a clinically apparent pericardial effusion have malignant pericardial disease (153).

Approximately half to three fourths of patients with metastatic pericardial carcinoma have had established disease for months with recurrence. There may be prolonged intervals between the primary diagnosis of carcinoma and pericardial disease. There are reports of a 6-year remission of colonic carcinoma with death soon after pericardial spread (156), a 14-year remission before pericardial metastasis in a patient with cutaneous adenoid cystic carcinoma (157), and a 41-month remission before pericardial spread of adenocarcinoma of the fallopian tube (158).

### Sites of Origin

**Most Frequent Tumor Types.** The most common tumors diagnosed in pericardial biopsies or cytology are lung and breast carcinomas. In one third to half of the cases, a pericardial effusion was the first sign of malignancy (151). In a series of 22 patients with metastatic malignancy diagnosed on pericardial fluid cytology, most (15 of 22) patients had a previous history of cancer, most frequently lung carcinoma (8 patients), followed by carcinoma of the breast (3 patients) (159). Of the 7 patients in whom a malignant diagnosis was made initially on cytology, 4 had lung carcinoma, 1 had breast carcinoma, 1 had melanoma, and 1 had lymphoma (159). All types of lung carcinoma may present in a pericardial biopsy, including adenocarcinoma, squamous carcinoma, and small cell lung carcinoma. Squamous carcinoma is rare in effusions, including the pericardium, representing only 4 of 39 in a reported series (160). In general, most adenocarcinomas presenting as pericardial metastases originate either in the lung or an undetermined primary site (36,161). Breast carcinoma, unlike lung carcinoma, usually manifests as pericardial disease only after the primary site is known (162).

**Carcinomas of the Lung.** Metastases to the heart or pericardium represent M1 or stage IV disease in the American Thoracic Society's TNM staging system for bronchogenic carcinoma. Direct extension of tumor into the heart, pericardium, or great vessels represents T4 or stage IIIB (unresectable) disease. Lung carcinoma is the most frequent malignancy to occur in the pericardium in males, and is second to breast carcinoma in females; it is the most likely cancer to occur in the pericardium as a presenting symptom without a previous diagnosis. Concomitant malignant pleural effusions are common.

**Breast Carcinomas.** Pleural effusion occurs in 46 percent of patients with metastatic breast carcinoma. The presenting symptoms are often related to contiguous pericardial effusion, and

possible cardiac tamponade (163). Breast carcinomas are associated with the longest survival period and longest interval of latency prior to the onset of the pericardial effusion (151).

**Other Malignancies.** Gastrointestinal carcinomas rarely metastasize to the pericardium, and generally only as part of disseminated disease in patients with a previous history of cancer. Gastric adenocarcinoma, in particular, is rare in pericardial fluid or biopsies: a review found 16 cases reported between 1982 and 2005 (164). There have been other reports of gastrointestinal tumors metastasizing to the pericardium, including colorectal carcinoma (156) and gastric signet ring carcinoma after initial spread to the ovaries (165).

Ovarian carcinoma involves the pericardium in 2.4 percent of patients, and 6 percent of those with stage IV disease (166). Papillary serous carcinoma of the endometrium has also been reported in the pericardium and imparts a bad prognosis (167).

Other tumors found in pericardial biopsies include thyroid carcinoma (168), lymphoma (161), melanoma (161), angiosarcoma (161), thymoma (161), multiple myeloma (169), gynecologic carcinomas (170), urothelial carcinoma (171), thymoma (161), testicular seminoma (172), adenoid cystic carcinoma (157), sarcomas (173).

### Gross and Microscopic Findings

The pathologic diagnosis of malignancy is higher in cytologic specimens (approximately 90 percent) compared to biopsy (about 75 percent) (152). Most positive pericardial biopsies are carcinomas, and the major entities in the differential diagnosis are reactive mesothelial hyperplasia and mesothelioma, which can be difficult to distinguish. There are numerous antigens of various specificity and sensitivity to help distinguish mesothelial hyperplasia from adenocarcinoma. Markers that favor adenocarcinoma include carcinoembryonic antigen, berEP4, B72.3 antigen, epithelial membrane antigen (MUC1), MOC31, and Leu-M1 (figs. 18-30–18-32). Mesothelial antigens with high sensitivity include high molecular weight cytokeratins (CK5/6 and CK903) and calretinin (fig. 18-33) while those with intermediate sensitivity include D2-40 and WT-1; none of these markers has high specificity, however. In reactive mesothelial cells, there

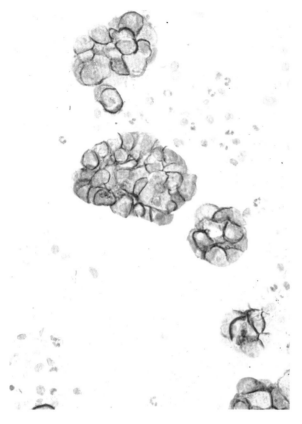

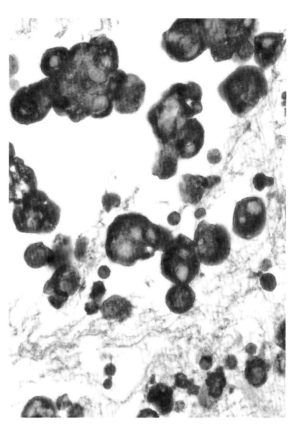

**Figure 18-30**

**METASTATIC ADENOCARCINOMA: PERICARDIAL FLUID**

Immunohistochemical stains for adenocarcinoma markers (B72.3 antigen in this example) are helpful in the distinction between carcinoma and reactive mesothelial cells.

**Figure 18-31**

**METASTATIC ADENOCARCINOMA: PERICARDIAL FLUID**

Another adenocarcinoma marker is carcinoembryonic antigen, which is rarely expressed in reactive mesothelium or mesothelioma. The polyclonal antibody also stains inflammatory cells.

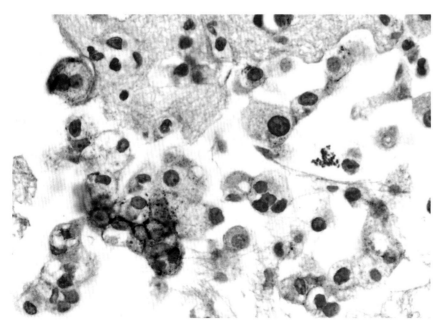

**Figure 18-32**

**METASTATIC ADENOCARCINOMA: PERICARDIAL FLUID**

Ber-EP4 stains the adenocarcinoma cells, but not the interspersed mesothelial cells.

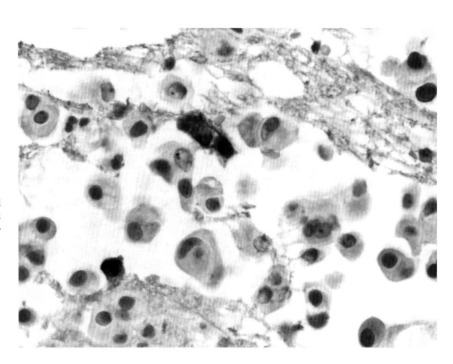

**Figure 18-33**

**METASTATIC ADENOCARCINOMA: PERICARDIAL FLUID**

The interspersed mesothelial cells stain with calretinin, which is not expressed in the adenocarcinoma.

is usually diffuse expression of vimentin, which is only weakly expressed in adenocarcinoma.

Because the most common epithelial tumors in the pericardium are pulmonary and breast, thyroid transcription factor (TTF-1), CK7 and CK20, and estrogen and progesterone receptors are useful markers in establishing a primary site. Immunostains useful in the diagnosis of undifferentiated malignancies include HMB45, S-100 protein, leukocyte common antigen (LCA), L26, and kappa and lambda light chains (159). Lymphoma markers, including LCA (CD45) and CD20, are especially useful in excluding lymphomatous involvement in the pericardium (fig. 18-34). In some cases, the primary site cannot be determined because of inconsistent immunohistochemical results, and must be based ultimately on the detection of the primary tumor clinically or at autopsy (174).

**Treatment and Prognosis**

The presence of a malignant pericardial effusion carries an ominous prognosis. In one series, 86 percent of patients with a malignant pericardial effusion died within the first year and nearly one third within the first month of diagnosis (151). The median survival period is only 5 months (164,175).

Specific tumor types that are low-grade or respond to treatment, such as lymphomas and thymomas, are associated with prolonged survival. Patients with breast carcinoma have a better prognosis than those with lung carcinoma (median survival, 23 weeks [176]) (151). Factors associated with good survival in patients with lung carcinoma metastatic to the pericardium include response to chemotherapy and the pericardium as the sole site of metastasis, a subset that responds to radiation therapy (176).

Treatment includes pericardiotomy with a pericardial-pleural or pericardial-peritoneal window (177), intracavitary chemotherapy (178,179), sclerotherapy (152,154,180), and indwelling ports for local delivery of chemotherapy (181).

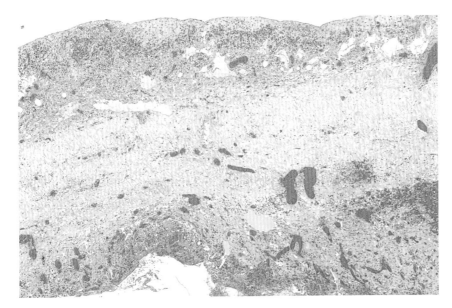

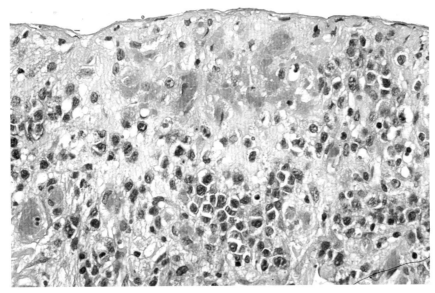

**Figure 18-34**

**MALIGNANT LYMPHOMA: PERICARDIAL RESECTION**

Top: At low magnification, hemorrhage, fibrosis, and a cellular infiltrate of the visceral surface (above) are seen.

Bottom: At higher magnification, discohesive malignant cells infiltrate the pericardium. The diagnosis of lymphoma was confirmed by immunoprofiling (not shown), with diffuse positivity for CD20. The patient had human immunodeficiency virus (HIV) of the acquired immunodeficiency syndrome (AIDS) and the diagnosis of primary effusion lymphoma was made after identification of human herpesvirus (HHV)-8 in the tumor cells.

## REFERENCES

1. MacGee W. Metastatic and invasive tumours involving the heart in a geriatric population: a necropsy study. Virchows Arch A Pathol Anat Histopathol 1991;419:183-189.
2. Abraham DP, Reddy V, Gattuso P. Neoplasms metastatic to the heart: review of 3314 consecutive autopsies. Am J Cardiovasc Pathol 1990;3: 1958-1966.
3. Manojlovic S. Metastatic carcinomas involving the heart. Review of postmortem examination. Zentralbl Allg Pathol 1990;136:657-661.
4. Sokolova IN, Shkhvatsabaia LV. [Secondary tumors of the heart (based on autopsy materials in the Oncology Research Center of the Academy of Medical Sciences of the USSR over the period of 1960-1977).] Arkh Patol 1980;42:38-41. [Russian]
5. Mukai K, Shinkai T, Tominaga K, Shimosato Y. The incidence of secondary tumors of the heart and pericardium: a 10-year study. Jpn J Clin Oncol 1988;18:195-201.

6. Miralles A, Bracamonte L, Soncul H, et al. Cardiac tumors: clinical experience and surgical results in 74 patients. Ann Thorac Surg 1991;52:886-895.

7. Murphy MC, Sweeney MS, Putnam JB Jr, et al. Surgical treatment of cardiac tumors: a 25-year experience. Ann Thorac Surg 1990;49:612-617; discussion 617-618.

8. Endo A, Ohtahara A, Kinugawa T, et al. Characteristics of 161 patients with cardiac tumors diagnosed during 1993 and 1994 in Japan. Am J Cardiol 1997;79:1708-1711.

9. Chiles C, Woodard PK, Gutierrez FR, Link KM. Metastatic involvement of the heart and pericardium: CT and MR imaging. Radiographics 2001;21:439-449.

10. Schneider B, Zienkiewicz T. Metastatic malignant melanoma presenting as congestive heart failure: diagnosis by transoesophageal echocardiography. Eur J Echocardiogr 2002;3:168-169.

11. Ozer N, Yavuz B, Atalar E. Recurrent syncope in a case of metastatic malignant melanoma—an unusual presentation of an uncommon disease. Eur J Echocardiogr 2006;7:233-234.

12. Vohra A, Saiz E, Davila E, Burkle J. Metastatic germ cell tumor to the heart presenting with syncope. Clin Cardiol 1999;22:429-433.

13. Chieng SH, Lin CH, Lu MJ, Hung CR. Intracavitary metastatic hepatocellular carcinoma of the right ventricle. Thorac Cardiovasc Surg 2005;53:123-125.

14. Hallahan DE, Vogelzang NJ, Borow KM, Bostwick DG, Simon MA. Cardiac metastases from soft-tissue sarcomas. J Clin Oncol 1986;4:1662-1669.

15. Minicucci MF, Zornoff LA, Okoshi MP, et al. Heart failure due to right ventricular metastatic neuroendocrine tumor. Int J Cardiol 2008;126: e25-26,

16. Schneider B, Zienkiewicz T, Langenstein B, Vierbuchen M, Meinertz T. Metastatic malignant melanoma initially seen as congestive heart failure: diagnosis by transesophageal echocardiography. Am Heart J 1994;128:414-416.

17. Fukuda A, Saito T, Imai M, Ishii K, Miwa K. Metastatic cardiac papillary carcinoma originating from the thyroid in both ventricles with a mobile right ventricular pedunculated tumor. Jpn Circ J 2000;64:890-892.

18. Alhakeem M, Arabi A, Arab L, Guerra RA. Unusual sites of metastatic involvement: intracardiac metastasis from laryngeal carcinoma. Eur J Echocardiogr 2008;9:323-325.

19. Gersak B, Lakic N, Gorjup V, Gulic T, Berden P, Cernic NS. Right ventricular metastatic choriocarcinoma obstructing inflow and outflow tract. Ann Thorac Surg 2002;73:1631-1633.

20. Gurvitch R, Yan BP, Aggarwal A. Metastatic squamous cell carcinoma causing right ventricular outflow tract obstruction. Heart 2007;93:697.

21. Kamlow FJ, Padaria SF, Wainwright RJ. Metastatic cardiac malignant fibrous histiocytoma presenting as right ventricular outflow tract obstruction. Clin Cardiol 1991;14:173-175.

22. Peng SY, Wu CC, Chang CP, Peng SK, Ho WM. Metastatic hepatocellular carcinoma of the right atrium causing right ventricular outflow tract obstruction during induction of anesthesia—a case report. Acta Anaesthesiol Sin 2002;40:205-208.

23. Shibata T, Suehiro S, Hattori K, Hosono M, Inoue K, Kinoshita H. Metastatic synovial sarcoma of the left ventricle. Jpn Heart J 2001;42:387-391.

24. Petropoulakis PN, Steriotis JD, Melanidis JG, Asimakopoulos PJ. Metastatic malignant melanoma as an intracavitary obstructive mass in the right heart. Eur J Cardiothorac Surg 1998;14:538-540.

25. Bowman AR, Siegel RJ, Blanche C, et al. Metastatic pancreatic adenocarcinoma to the heart diagnosed antemortem. J Am Soc Echocardiogr 2000;13:415-416.

26. Kitkungvan D, Sharma S, Pacifico L, Spodick DH. Metastatic renal cell carcinoma masquerading as ST-segment elevation myocardial infarction. J Invasive Cardiol 2009;21:256-257.

27. Arzouman DA, Danetz J, Newman JH, Spotnitz AJ, MacKenzie JW. Metastatic mucinous adenocarcinoma of the heart. J Card Surg 1997;12:49-50.

28. Inamura K, Hayashida A, Kaji Y, et al. Recurrence of cervical carcinoma manifesting as cardiac metastasis three years after curative resection. Am J Med Sci 2004;328:167-169.

29. Kronzon I, Goodkin GM, Culliford A, et al. Right atrial and right ventricular obstruction by recurrent stromomyoma. J Am Soc Echocardiogr 1994;7:528-533.

30. Wood A, Markovic SN, Best PJ, Erickson LA. Metastatic malignant melanoma manifesting as an intracardiac mass. Cardiovasc Pathol 2010; 19:153-157.

31. Virmani R, Khedekar RR, Robinowitz M, McAllister HA Jr. Tumor embolization in coronary artery causing myocardial infarction. Arch Pathol Lab Med 1983;107:243-245.

32. Morelli F, Piano A, Criconia GM, Fanelli R, Caparrotti S, Maiello E. Malignant melanoma metastatic to the right atrium: Clinical findings of an asymptomatic case. Minerva Cardioangiol. 2008;56:708-709.

33. Calvert RJ, Quinn CM. Squamous cell carcinoma of the maxillary antrum metastatic to the heart and skin. J Laryngol Otol 1994;108:896-897.

34. Pandya UH, Pellikka PA, Enriquez-Sarano M, Edwards WD, Schaff HV, Connolly HM. Metastatic carcinoid tumor to the heart: echocardiographic-pathologic study of 11 patients. J Am Coll Cardiol 2002;40:1328-1332.

34a.Churg A, Cagle PT, Roggli VL. Tumors of the serosal membranes. AFIP Atlas of Tumor Pathology, 4th Series, Fascicle 3. Silver Spring, MD: ARP Press; 2006.

35. Lynch M, Blevins LS, Martin RP. Acquired supravalvular pulmonary stenosis due to extrinsic compression by a metastatic thymic carcinoid tumor. Int J Card Imaging 1996;12:61-63.

36. Tamura A, Matsubara O, Yoshimura N, Kasuga T, Akagawa S, Aoki N. Cardiac metastasis of lung cancer. A study of metastatic pathways and clinical manifestations. Cancer 1992;70:437-442.

37. Hayashi J, Ohzeki H, Tsuchida S, et al. Surgery for cavoatrial extension of malignant tumors. Thorac Cardiovasc Surg 1995;43:161-164.

38. Platonov MA, Turner AR, Mullen JC, Noga M, Welsh RC. Tumour on the tricuspid valve: metastatic osteosarcoma and the heart. Can J Cardiol 2005;21:63-67.

39. Feys A, Herregods MC, Ector H. Cardiac metastasis from a stage IIIb cervix carcinoma. Acta Cardiol 2005;60:73-75.

40. Janssen DP, Van de Kaa CA, Noyez L, Van Haelst UJ, Lacquet LK. A solitary metastasis in the heart from Ewing's sarcoma. Eur J Cardiothorac Surg 1994;8:51-53.

41. Steinherz LJ, Rosen G, Steinherz PG, Robins J, Huvos A, Exelby PR. Isolated cardiac metastatic recurrence of epithelioid sarcoma after two and a half disease-free years. N Y State J Med 1987;87:231-233.

42. Hakim JP, Jain AC, Hill RC. Intramyocardial metastatic renal cell cancer. Echocardiography 2000;17:697-698.

43. Tsuji Y, Yamashita C, Wakiyama H, et al. Surgical treatment for transvenous tumor extension into the heart: four cases. J Vasc Surg 1998;27:740-744.

44. Ioannis V, Panagiotis S, Anastasios A, et al. Tumor extending through inferior vena cava into the right atrium. A late recurrence of renal cell carcinoma. Int J Cardiovasc Imaging 2003;19:179-182.

45. Slimani EK, Lance DG. Repeat sternotomy and hypothermic circulatory arrest for resection of renal cell carcinoma with tumour thrombus extension into the right atrium. Heart Lung Circ 2009;18:143-145.

46. Ozer N, Deniz A, Piskinpasa S, et al. Renal cell carcinoma extending from superior vena cava into right atrium. J Am Soc Echocardiogr 2007;20:538 e7-8.

47. Greene GF, Bissada NK, Madi R. Renal cell carcinoma with caval thrombus extending to the right atrium in a horseshoe kidney: a unique surgical challenge. Can Urol Assoc J 2009;3:E55-57.

48. Jiang H, Zhang ZG, Chen ZD, Shi SF, Cai SL, Wang S. Renal cell carcinoma with vena caval tumor thrombus extending into the right atrium. Chin Med J (Engl) 2006;119:1934-1936.

49. Vlasseros I, Tapanlis E, Katsaros A, Kountouras D, Gialafos I. Metastatic hepatocellular carcinoma into the right atrium and ventricle: echocardiographic diagnosis and follow-up. Echocardiography 2003;20:387-388.

50. Agelopoulou P, Kapatais A, Varounis C, et al. Hepatocellular carcinoma with invasion into the right atrium. Report of two cases and review of the literature. Hepatogastroenterology 2007; 54:2106-2108.

51. Georgen M, Regimbeau JM, Kianmanesh R, Marty J, Farges O, Belghiti J. Removal of hepatocellular carcinoma extending in the right atrium without extracorporal bypass. J Am Coll Surg 2002; 195:892-894.

52. Hayashi P, Trotter JF, Everson GT. Hepatocellular carcinoma extension into the right atrium. Liver Transpl. 2003;9:1225-1226.

53. Kumar B, Jha S. Hepatocellular carcinoma with extension into the right atrium. Am J Med 2005; 118:1436-1437.

54. Lazaros G, Samara C, Nikolakopoulou Z, Tassopoulos N. Growth of hepatocellular carcinoma into the right atrium. A case of antemortem diagnosis with magnetic resonance imaging of the heart. Acta Cardiol 2003;58:563-565.

55. Nam SW, Baek JT, Kang SB, et al. A case of the hepatocellular carcinoma during the pregnancy and metastasis to the left atrium. Korean J Hepatol 2005;11:381-385.

56. Saynak M, Ozen A, Kocak Z, Cosar-Alas R, Uzal C. Sudden death: a case report of hepatocellular carcinoma with tumor thrombus extending into the right atrium. J BUON 2007;12:556.

57. Tsai JJ, Su CW, Lin HC. Hepatocellular carcinoma with invasion into right atrium. Clin Gastroenterol Hepatol 2008;6:e39-40.

58. Uemura M, Sasaki Y, Yamada T, et al. Surgery for hepatocellular carcinoma with tumor thrombus extending into the right atrium: report of a successful resection without the use of cardiopulmonary bypass. Hepatogastroenterology 2004;51: 1259-1262.

59. Yogita S, Tashiro S, Harada M, Kitagawa T, Kato I. Hepatocellular carcinoma with extension into the right atrium: report of a successful liver resection by hepatic vascular exclusion using cardiopulmonary bypass. J Med Invest 2000;47:155-160.

60. Wu CC, Hseih S, Ho WM, Tang JS, Liu TJ, P'Eng FK. Surgical treatment for recurrent hepatocellular carcinoma with tumor thrombi in right atrium: using cardiopulmonary bypass and deep hypothermic circulatory arrest. J Surg Oncol 2000;74:227-231.

61. Ulus T, Birdane A, Dundar E, Tunerir B. Asymptomatic course of a metastatic mass completely filling the right atrium in a patient with hepatocellular carcinoma. Turk Kardiyol Dern Ars 2012;40:52-54.

62. Dedeilias P, Nenekidis I, Koukis I, et al. Acute heart failure caused by a giant hepatocellular metastatic tumor of the right atrium. J Cardiothorac Surg 2011;6:102.

63. Barton SJ, Ashdown DA, Ganta S, Wallace D. An unusual presentation of metastatic testicular tumour. J R Army Med Corps 2005;151:30-33.

64. Chen PC, Chang YH, Yen CC, Pan CC, Chiang H. Primary renal synovial sarcoma with inferior vena cava and right atrium invasion. Int J Urol 2003;10:657-660.

65. Kesik V, Yozgat Y, Sari E, Kocaoglu M, Kismet E, Koseoglu V. Hepatoblastoma metastatic to the right atrium responding to chemotherapy alone. Pediatr Hematol Oncol 2009;26:583-588.

66. Swan RZ, Hanna EM, Sindram D, Iannitti DA, Martinie JB. Adrenocortical carcinoma with intracaval extension to the right atrium: resection on cardiopulmonary bypass. Ann Surg Oncol 2012;19:1275.

67. Jani JC, Massad M, Kpodonu J, Alagiozian-Angelova V, Guzman G. High-grade pelvic osteosarcoma with intravascular extension to the right side of the heart: a case report and review of the literature. Arch Pathol Lab Med 2005;129:241-243.

68. Kono T, Amano J, Sakaguchi M, Kitahara H. Successful resection of cardiac metastatic liposarcoma extending into the SVC, right atrium, and right ventricle. J Card Surg 2005;20:364-365.

69. Kim SA, Jung JS, Ju SJ, Kim YT, Kim KR. Mullerian adenosarcoma with sarcomatous overgrowth in the pelvic cavity extending into the inferior vena cava and the right atrium. Pathol Int 2011; 61:445-448.

70. Phillips MR, Bower TC, Orszulak TA, Hartmann LC. Intracardiac extension of an intracaval sarcoma of endometrial origin. Ann Thorac Surg 1995;59:742-744.

71. Gabal S, Ashour Z, Hamada G, et al. Low-grade endometrial stromal sarcoma with intravenous extension to the heart. Medscape J Med 2009;11:23.

72. Mavrogenis AF, Angelini A, Sakellariou VI, Skarpidi E, Ruggieri P, Papagelopoulos PJ. Osteosarcoma invasion of the inferior vena cava and right atrium. J Surg Orthop Adv 2012;21:107-112.

73. Nakao Y, Yokoyama M, Yasunaga M, Hara K, Nakahashi H, Iwasaka T. Metastatic tumor extending through the inferior vena cava into the right atrium: a case report of carcinoma of the uterine cervix with para-aortic lymph node metastases. Int J Gynecol Cancer 2006;16:914-916.

74. Alexandrescu C, Civaia F, Dor V. Tumor thrombus in right atrium from lung adenocarcinoma. Ann Thorac Surg 2009;87:e11-12.

75. Dogan OF, Hanci D, Sungur A, Unal OF, Demircin M. An unusual case of thyroid Hurtle cell carcinoma with direct extension to the right brachiocephalic vein, right auricle, and right atrium: case report. Heart Surg Forum 2005;8:E114-117.

76. Taib NA, Hisham AN. Follicular thyroid carcinoma with direct tumour extension into the great cervical veins and right atrium: is transcervical thrombectomy a safe option? Asian J Surg 2007;30:216-219.

77. Chong JJ, Richards DA, Chard R, McKay T, Thomas L. Two-dimensional and three-dimensional transthoracic echocardiography in surgical planning for right atrial metastatic melanoma. Eur J Echocardiogr 2008;9:286-288.

78. Patel SA, Herfel BM, Nolan MA. Metastatic colon cancer involving the right atrium. Tex Heart Inst J 2012;39:79-83.

79. Gokce M, Korkmaz L, Oz D, Orem C, Kiris A, Ahmetoglu A. Metastatic adenocarcinoma in the right atrium and secondary Budd-Chiari syndrome (a case report). Int J Cardiol 2009;132:e1-4.

80. Nakamura Y, Nakano K, Gomi A, et al. A metastatic ball tumor in the right atrium originating from esophageal cancer: report of a case. Surg Today 2005;35:145-148.

81. Kanjwal K, Colyer W Jr. Transthoracic echocardiography-guided biopsy of a metastatic endometrial adenocarcinoma in the right atrium: a review of diagnosis and treatment of cardiac masses. Am J Ther 2010;17:e118-125.

82. Javangula KC, O'Regan DJ. Emergency surgery for left atrial metastatic alveolar rhabdomyosarcoma manifesting as a right atrial mass. Ann Thorac Surg 2008;86:1008-1011.

83. Tripathi M, D'Souza MM, Jain J, et al. Metastatic choriocarcinoma with tumor thrombus in the right atrium and pulmonary vessels: diagnosis and therapy monitoring with F-18 flurodeoxyglucose PET/CT. Clin Nucl Med 2009;34:381-385.

84. Kumar S, Chaudhry MA, Khan I, Duthie DJ, Lindsay S, Kaul P. Metastatic left atrial synovial sarcoma mimicking a myxoma. J Thorac Cardiovasc Surg 2004;128:756-758.

85. Locci G, Pili A, Pais M, Cirio E, Sanna A. Heart metastases from gastric sarcoma. A case report. Ital Heart J 2001;2:556-558.

86. Magnuson WJ, Halligan JB. Successful treatment of melanoma metastatic to the left atrium using external beam radiation therapy. Oncology (Williston Park) 2010;24:650-653.

87. Linneweber J, Magheli A, Lembcke A, Christ T, Konertz W. Intracavitary tumor spread of a metastatic testicular seminoma in the left atrium and ventricle. J Thorac Cardiovasc Surg 2011;141:583-584.

88. Ucak A, Inan K, Onan B, Temizkan V, Alp I, Yilmaz AT. Free-floating tumor thrombus in the left atrium associated with non-small cell lung cancer. J Card Surg 2009;24:686-689.

89. Lysitsas DN, Banerjee P, Shiu MF. Cardiac tamponade because of left atrium direct invasion by a large cell neuroendocrine metastatic carcinoma of the lung. Eur J Echocardiogr 2008;9:428-429.

90. Wu L, Xu Z, Zhao X, et al. Surgical treatment of lung cancer invading the left atrium or base of the pulmonary vein. World J Surg 2009;33:492-496.

91. Sadat U, Noor N, See TC, Varty K. Peripheral arterial ischemia by a primary lung tumour invading left atrium. Lung Cancer 2007;57:237-239.

92. Shimizu J, Hirano Y, Ishida Y, et al. Advanced lung cancer invading the left atrium wall treated with pneumonectomy and combined resection of the left atrium using stapling devices: report of two cases. Ann Thorac Cardiovasc Surg 2004;10:113-117.

93. Chan V, Neumann D. Small cell lung carcinoma invading the pulmonary vein and left atrium as imaged by PET/CT. Eur J Nucl Med Mol Imaging 2005;32:1493.

94. Chuah KL, Yap WM, Loh HL, Lim KH, Tan HW, Lim CH. Intravenous extension of sarcomatoid carcinoma of the lung to the left atrium. Pathology 2006;38:359-361.

95. Pitman AG, Solomon B, Padmanabhan R, McKenzie AF, Hicks RJ. Intravenous extension of lung carcinoma to the left atrium: demonstration by positron emission tomography with CT correlation. Br J Radiol 2000;73:206-208.

96. Fukuse T, Wada H, Hitomi S. Extended operation for non-small cell lung cancer invading great vessels and left atrium. Eur J Cardiothorac Surg 1997;11:664-669.

97. Zissin R, Shapiro-Feinberg M, Rachmani R, Kots E. Lung metastasis invading the left atrium—CT diagnosis. Br J Radiol 1999;72:1211-1212.

98. Shai SE, Hsieh SR, Song YM, Shen GH. Resection of follicular thyroid cancer metastasized to the left lower lobe of the lung extending into the left atrium as a huge intracardiac tumor. Thyroid 2005;15:1417-1418.

99. Collins NJ, Barlow MA, Woodford PA, Hayes PC. Intracardiac extension of metastatic pulmonary leiomyosarcoma. Heart Lung Circ 2005;14:121-122.

100. Hussain R, Neligan MC. Metastatic malignant schwannoma in the heart. Ann Thorac Surg 1993;56:374-375.

101. Sarraj A, Duarte J, Dominguez L, Pun YW. Resection of metastatic pulmonary lesion of ossifying fibromyxoid tumor extending into the left atrium and ventricle via pulmonary vein. Eur J Echocardiogr 2007;8:384-386.

102. Ferraz JG, Martins AL, de Souza JF, Matos A, Canto AP, Martins AM. Metastatic tumor of squamous cell carcinoma from uterine cervix to heart: ante-mortem diagnosis. Arq Bras Cardiol 2006;87:e104-107.

103. Harting MT, Messner GN, Gregoric ID, Frazier OH. Sarcoma metastatic to the right ventricle: surgical intervention followed by prolonged survival. Tex Heart Inst J 2004;31:93-95.

104. Atik FA, Navia JL, Krishnamurthi V, et al. Solitary massive right ventricular metastasis of renal cell carcinoma without inferior vena cava or right atrium involvement. J Card Surg 2006;21:304-306.

105. Basarici I, Demir I, Yilmaz H, Altekin RE. Obstructive metastatic malignant melanoma of the heart: Imminent pulmonary arterial occlusion caused by right ventricular metastasis with unknown origin of the primary tumor. Heart Lung 2006;35:351-354.

106. Messner G, Harting MT, Russo P, et al. Surgical management of metastatic melanoma to the ventricle. Tex Heart Inst J 2003;30:218-220.

107. Hasegawa J, Kadoba K, Maruhashi H. Metastatic renal cell carcinoma to the right ventricle complicating thrombocytopenia. J Cardiovasc Surg (Torino) 2002;43:195-197.

108. Lim KH, Brett M, Pitts-Crick J, Angelini GD, Persad R. Sarcomatoid renal cell carcinoma metastatic to right ventricle. J R Soc Med 2001;94:33-35.

109. Sato T, Takeda A, Yamada S, Numata I, Sakamoto K. Metastatic renal cell carcinoma to right ventricle without vena caval involvement. Int J Urol 2008;15:366-368.

110. Chughtai A, Cronin P, Lucas DR, Prager R, Kazerooni EA. Metastatic shoulder liposarcoma to the right ventricle: CT findings. J Thorac Imaging 2007;22:195-198.

111. Imperadore F, Catanzariti D, Recla M, Miorelli L, Vergara G. A rare metastatic tumor presenting as outflow obstruction to the right ventricle: synovial sarcoma. Ital Heart J 2002;3:337-338.

112. Pamukcu B, Bilge AK, Meric M, Atilgan D. Metastatic Ewing's sarcoma involving the right ventricle. Turk Kardiyol Dern Ars 2008;36:546-548.

113. Dencker M, Valind S, Stagmo M. Right ventricular metastasis of leiomyosarcoma. Cardiovasc Ultrasound 2009;7:20.

114. Hoy F, Boucher R, Brody A. Uterine leiomyosarcoma with cardiac metastases. Can J Surg 1988;31:418-420.

115. Keir P, Keen G. Secondary leiomyosarcoma of the right ventricle. A surgical report. Br Heart J 1978;40:328-330.

116. Banfic L, Jelic I, Jelasic D, CuZic S. Heart metastasis of extraskeletal myxoid chondrosarcoma. Croat Med J 2001;42:199-202.

117. Sugiyama K, Okubo T, Kamigaki Y, Kin H. Cardiac metastatic liposarcoma. Jpn J Thorac Cardiovasc Surg 2000;48:663-665.

118. Bonsall JM, Hughes R, Mosunjac M, Harrison D, Samady H. A rare case of squamous cell carcinoma of the bladder presenting as a metastatic right ventricular mass. Case Report Med 2010; 2010:789609.

119. Yasuda N, Ishiki R, Agetsuma H. Single large metastatic tumor growing progressively and occupying right ventricular cavity. Heart 2002; 87:328.

120. Galvin SD, Wademan B, Chu J, Bunton RW. Benign metastasizing leiomyoma: a rare metastatic lesion in the right ventricle. Ann Thorac Surg 2010;89:279-281.

121. Aburto J, Bruckner BA, Blackmon SH, Beyer EA, Reardon MJ. Renal cell carcinoma, metastatic to the left ventricle. Tex Heart Inst J 2009;36: 48-49.

122. Houmsse M, Raman SV, Leier CV, Orsinelli DA. Metastatic melanoma of the left ventricle: cardiac imaging in the diagnosis and surgical approach. Int J Cardiovasc Imaging 2004;20: 523-526; discussion 527-528.

123. Chandramohan NK, Hussain MB, Nayak N, Kattoor J, Pandey M, Krishnankutty R. Multiple cardiac metastases from Ewing's sarcoma. Can J Cardiol 2005;21:525-527.

124. Wee JO, Sepic JD, Mihaljevic T, Cohn LH. Metastatic carcinoid tumor of the heart Ann Thorac Surg 2003;76:1721-1722.

125. Iemura A, Yano H, Kojiro M, Nouno R, Kouno K. Massive cardiac involvement of adult T-cell leukemia/lymphoma. An autopsy case. Arch Pathol Lab Med 1991;115:1052-1054.

126. Steigman CK, Anderson DW, Macher AM, Sennesh JD, Virmani R. Fatal cardiac tamponade in acquired immunodeficiency syndrome with epicardial Kaposi's sarcoma. Am Heart J 1988; 116:1105-1107.

127. Gibbs JL, Rao RS, Williams GJ. Polypoid tumour of the pericardium—a previously unrecognised macroscopic appearance of metastatic bladder carcinoma. Int J Cardiol 1985;8:205-208.

128. Komanapalli CB, Tripathy U, Sokoloff M, Daneshmand S, Das A, Slater MS. Intraoperative renal cell carcinoma tumor embolization to the right atrium: incidental diagnosis by transesophageal echocardiography. Anesth Analg 2006;102:378-379.

129. Senkottaiyan N, Seacord LM, Fulling KH, Birchem JA, Fraley MA, Alpert MA. Sarcomatous pleural mesothelioma metastatic to left ventricular endocardium. Angiology 2006;57:517-521.

130. Roberts WC, Bodey GP, Wertlake PT. The heart in acute leukemia. A study of 420 autopsy cases. Am J Cardiol 1968;21:388-412.

131. Roberts WC, Glancy DL, DeVita VT Jr. Heart in malignant lymphoma (Hodgkin's disease, lymphosarcoma, reticulum cell sarcoma and mycosis fungoides). A study of 196 autopsy cases. Am J Cardiol 1968;22:85-107.

132. Glancy DL, Roberts WC. The heart in malignant melanoma. A study of 70 autopsy cases. Am J Cardiol 1968;21:555-571.

133. Savoia P, Fierro MT, Zaccagna A, Bernengo MG. Metastatic melanoma of the heart. J Surg Oncol 2000;75:203-207.

134. Schraml FV, Yudt WM, Gormley TS, Ho VB. Metastatic melanoma to the heart. Eur J Nucl Med Mol Imaging 2005;32:1349.

135. McKenna CJ, McCann HA, Sugrue DD. Endometrial stromal sarcoma of the heart. Ir Med J 1997;90:194.

136. Kinebuchi Y, Ogawa T, Kato H, Igawa Y, Nishizawa O, Miyagawa S. Testicular cancer with tumor thrombus extending to the inferior vena cava successfully removed using veno-venous bypass: a case report. Int J Urol 2007;14:458-460.

137. Paule B, Brion N, Grunenwald D, Andre-Bougaran J. Right atrial extension of an embryonal carcinoma of the testis. Cancer 1991;68:198-201.

138. Geffen DB, Kaneti J, Hendler N, Hertzanu Y. Testicular carcinoma with inferior vena cava thrombosis extending into the right atrium treated with chemotherapy and anticoagulation. Eur Urol 1992;21:82-84.

139. May M, Finkbeiner Y, Gunia S, Seehafer M, Knorig J, Hetzer R. Metastasizing testicular germ-cell tumor with infiltration of the right heart: indication for primary metastasectomy. Heart Vessels 2006;21:63-65.

140. Stefka J, Cleveland JC, Lucia MS, Singh M. Sarcomatoid intracardiac metastasis of a testicular germ cell tumor closely resembling primary cardiac sarcoma. Hum Pathol 2003;34:1074-1077.

141. Jo JC, Lee DH, Kang BW, et al. Both-sided intra-atrial intracardiac metastases as the initial presentation of testicular seminoma. Jpn J Clin Oncol 2007;37:463-468.

142. Singh A, Jenkins DP, Dahdal M, Dhar S, Ratnatunga CP. Recurrent arterial embolization from a metastatic germ cell tumor invading the left atrium. Ann Thorac Surg 2000;70:2155-2156.

143. Fang FM, Ko SF, Hwang CH, Wang CJ. Healing of superior vena cava defect in mediastinal seminoma with invasion. Ann Thorac Surg 2000;70:667-669.

144. Saraiva LR, Brindeiro Filho DB, Saraiva TB, Arruda MB, Lira V. Cardiac extension of primary mediastinal seminoma compressing the right ventricular outflow tract. Arq Bras Cardiol 2001;76:149-154.

145. Seferovic PM, Ristic AD, Maksimovic R, Tatic V, Ostojic M, Kanjuh V. Diagnostic value of pericardial biopsy: improvement with extensive sampling enabled by pericardioscopy. Circulation 2003;107:978-983.

146. Adenle AD, Edwards JE. Clinical and pathologic features of metastatic neoplasms of the pericardium. Chest 1982;81:166-169.

147. Douroukas A, Arena V, Pelosi E. Detection of metastatic involvement of the pericardium on F-18 FDG-PET/CT imaging. Clin Nucl Med 2009;34:40-41.

148. Han SH, Koh KK, Lee SJ, Seo JG, Choi SJ, Ha SY. Malignant pericardial effusion not diagnosed by pericardial fluid and biopsy: Importance of CT scan. Int J Cardiol 2007;117:e53-55.

149. Prakash P, Kalra MK, Stone JR, Shepard JA, Digumarthy SR. Imaging findings of pericardial metastasis on chest computed tomography. J Comput Assist Tomogr 2010;34:554-558.

150. Corey GR, Campbell PT, Van Trigt P, et al. Etiology of large pericardial effusions. Am J Med 1993;95:209-213.

151. Garcia-Riego A, Cuinas C, Vilanova JJ. Malignant pericardial effusion. Acta Cytol 2001;45:561-566.

152. Wilkes JD, Fidias P, Vaickus L, Perez RP. Malignancy-related pericardial effusion. 127 cases from the Roswell Park Cancer Institute. Cancer 1995;76:1377-1387.

153. Buck M, Ingle JN, Giuliani ER, Gordon JR, Therneau TM. Pericardial effusion in women with breast cancer. Cancer 1987;60:263-269.

154. Hancock EW. Neoplastic pericardial disease. Cardiol Clin 1990;8:673-682.

155. Kralstein J, Frishman W. Malignant pericardial diseases: diagnosis and treatment. Am Heart J 1987;113:785-790.

156. Lattuada S, Saggia C, Biaggi G, et al. Pericardial metastases in a long-surviving patient with sigmoid carcinoma. Tumori 2005;91:101-102.

157. Benchetritt M, Butori C, Long E, Ilie M, Ferrari E, Hofman P. Pericardial effusion as primary manifestation of metastatic cutaneous adenoid cystic carcinoma: diagnostic cytopathology from an exfoliative sample. Diagn Cytopathol 2008;36:351-354.

158. Buyukkurt S, Vardar MA, Zeren H, Guzel B, Tuncer I. Fallopian tube carcinoma metastatic to the pericardium and breast. Eur J Gynaecol Oncol 2009;30:335-337.

159. Gupta RK, Kenwright DN, Fauck R, Lallu S, Naran S. The usefulness of a panel of immunostains in the diagnosis and differentiation of metastatic malignancies in pericardial effusions. Cytopathology 2000;11:312-321.

160. Hoda RS, Cangiarella J, Koss LG. Metastatic squamous-cell carcinoma in pericardial effusion: report of four cases, two with cardiac tamponade. Diagn Cytopathol 1998;18:422-424.

161. Loire R, Hellal H. [Neoplastic pericarditis. Study by thoracotomy and biopsy in 80 cases.] Presse Med 1993;22:244-248. [French]

162. Millaire A, Wurtz A, de Groote P, Saudemont A, Chambon A, Ducloux G. Malignant pericardial effusions: usefulness of pericardioscopy. Am Heart J 1992;124:1030-1034.

163. Yeste L, Murillo J, Galbis JM, Torre W. [Thoracic metastasis of breast carcinoma. Current status.] Rev Med Univ Navarra 2003;47:17-21. [Spanish]

164. Kobayashi M, Okabayashi T, Okamoto K, Namikawa T, Araki K. Clinicopathological study of cardiac tamponade due to pericardial metastasis originating from gastric cancer. World J Gastroenterol 2005;11:6899-6904.

165. Baba Y, Ishikawa S, Ikeda K, et al. A patient with 43 synchronous early gastric carcinomas with a Krukenberg tumor and pericardial metastasis. Gastric Cancer 2007;10:135-139.

166. Dauplat J, Hacker NF, Nieberg RK, Berek JS, Rose TP, Sagae S. Distant metastases in epithelial ovarian carcinoma. Cancer 1987;60:1561-1566.

167. Ramirez PT, Ramondetta LM, Burke TW, Gershenson DM, Brewer MA. Metastatic uterine papillary serous carcinoma to the pericardium. Gynecol Oncol 2001;83:135-137.

168. Chiewvit S, Pusuwan P, Chiewvit P, Pleehachinda R, Attanatho V, Mongkharuk J. Metastatic follicular carcinoma of thyroid to pericardium. J Med Assoc Thai 1998;81:799-802.

169. Santana O, Vivas PH, Ramos A, Safirstein S, Agatston AS. Multiple myeloma involving the pericardium associated with cardiac tamponade and constrictive pericarditis. Am Heart J 1993;126:737-740.

170. Nagarsheth NP, Harrison M, Kalir T, Rahaman J. Malignant pericardial effusion with cardiac tamponade in a patient with metastatic vaginal adenocarcinoma. Int J Gynecol Cancer 2006;16:1458-1461.

171. Fabozzi SJ, Newton JR Jr, Moriarty RP, Schellhammer PF. Malignant pericardial effusion as initial solitary site of metastasis from transitional cell carcinoma of the bladder. Urology 1995;45:320-322.

172. White JE, Fincher RM, D'Cruz IA. Pericardial metastasis from testicular seminoma: appearance and disappearance by echocardiography. Am J Med Sci 1991;301:182-185.

173. Aoyama A, Isowa N, Chihara K, Ito T. Pericardial metastasis of myxoid liposarcoma causing cardiac tamponade. Jpn J Thorac Cardiovasc Surg 2005;53:193-195.

174. Hill HC. Challenges of utilizing immunostains to facilitate the diagnosis and management of metastatic adenocarcinoma. J Natl Med Assoc 2008;100:1469-1473.

175. Neragi-Miandoab S, Linden PA, Ducko CT, et al. VATS pericardiotomy for patients with known malignancy and pericardial effusion: Survival and prognosis of positive cytology and metastatic involvement of the pericardium: a case control study. Int J Surg 2008;6:110-114.

176. Quraishi MA, Costanzi JJ, Hokanson J. The natural history of lung cancer with pericardial metastases. Cancer 1983;51:740-742.

177. Olson JE, Ryan MB, Blumenstock DA. Eleven years' experience with pericardial-peritoneal window in the management of malignant and benign pericardial effusions. Ann Surg Oncol 1995;2:165-169.

178. Colleoni M, Martinelli G, Beretta F, et al. Intracavitary chemotherapy with thiotepa in malignant pericardial effusions: An active and well-tolerated regimen. J Clin Oncol 1998;16:2371-2376.

179. Tondini M, Rocco G, Bianchi C, Severi C, Corbellini D. Intracavitary cisplatin (CDDP) in the treatment of metastatic pericardial involvement from breast and lung cancer. Monaldi Arch Chest Dis 1995;50:86-88.

180. Fiocco M, Krasna MJ. The management of malignant pleural and pericardial effusions. Hematol Oncol Clin North Am 1997;11:253-265.

181. Melfi FM, Menconi GF, Chella A, Angeletti CA. The management of malignant pericardial effusions using permanently implanted devices. Eur J Cardiothorac Surg 2002;21:345-347.

# 19 TUMORS OF THE GREAT VESSELS

Malignant neoplasms of arterial origin usually arise in the inner arterial lining (intima) and exhibit primarily intraluminal growth (especially in early stages). For these reasons, the term *intimal sarcoma* is often used for these tumors. In contrast to venous sarcomas, which typically arise from the medial smooth muscle, intimal sarcomas of large arteries are usually pleomorphic and are not typically desmin-producing smooth muscle tumors (1). Tumors of veins are invariably leiomyomas or leiomyosarcomas, and are essentially indistinguishable from those of soft tissue.

The human arterial intima is composed of a small population of myofibroblastic cells, which populate the region between the internal elastic lamina and the endothelial layer. These cells contain precursors that differentiate, when they become malignant, along a variety of mesenchymal lineages. These include sarcomas with endothelial differentiation (angiosarcomas), undifferentiated pleomorphic sarcomas, and sarcomas with heterologous elements, such as malignant bone and cartilage.

## AORTIC INTIMAL SARCOMAS

**General Features.** *Aortic intimal sarcomas* are rare, with only five published series, each consisting of 4 to 12 cases (2–5). Over two dozen case reports have been published since 1996, the writing of the last Fascicle (2,6–39), at which time at least 50 had been reported (40).

**Clinical Features.** Most patients with sarcomas of the aorta are middle aged: in two series the average age was 62 to 66 years (3,4). There appears to be no sex predilection (3,4).

Because most aortic sarcomas are intraluminal, the most common symptoms are related to embolic phenomena (28). Rarely, symptoms relate to narrowing or pseudocoarctation of the occluded segment (41). Claudication and absent pulses, usually of the lower extremities, are common manifestations (30), due to either tumor embolism or obstruction of the abdominal aorta (24). Occasionally, the diagnosis is made when embolized fragments, especially in the iliac and femoral arteries, are found. Upper extremity embolization is less common, and may occur with thoracic aortic tumors (22), and occlusion of the thoracic aorta may result in upper extremity hypertension (33). Some aortic intimal sarcomas present as diffuse thrombotic disease (31). Rarely, coronary ischemia results from an aortic sarcoma growing proximally (6). Metastatic disease may cause the initial presenting symptoms (8).

About 10 percent of patients present with an abdominal aortic aneurysm. The histologic diagnosis is often unsuspected in such cases, and the diagnosis is made by the surgical pathologist (16). The tumor may initially manifest as renal artery stenosis (renovascular hypertension) (2,42), aortic rupture (32,39), systemic vasculitis (43), and bowel ischemia caused by embolic tumor (20). The tumor may be an incidental finding on imaging (44).

Several aortic sarcomas have been reported at the site of prior Dacron graft anastomoses (32). A sarcoma occurring years after endovascular repair for inflammatory abdominal aortic aneurysm has been reported (45).

**Radiologic Findings.** The aortic lumen and wall are imaged by angiography (aortograms), computed tomography (CT), CT angiography, or magnetic resonance imaging (MRI). These modalities identify intimal sarcomas as atherosclerotic-like occlusive lesions, typically in the thoracic, abdominal, or thoracoabdominal aorta, and occasionally extending to the descending thoracic aorta, visceral arteries, or infrarenal aorta (2,27). CT shows an intraluminal mass, with extravascular extension only in advanced cases (26). Transesophageal echocardiography helps delineate the intraluminal mass (23). A multimodality approach is most frequently used for disease characterization, given the rarity of these tumors (46).

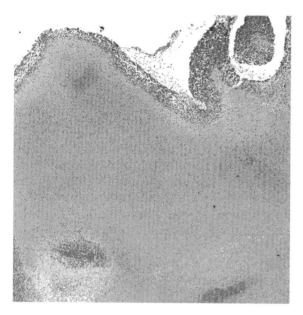

**Figure 19-1**

**AORTIC EPITHELIOID ANGIOSARCOMA**

Low magnification shows a necrotic tumor intermixed with fibrin and a cellular surface. The tumor was removed from the lumen of the aorta.

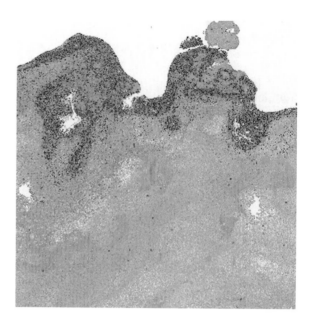

**Figure 19-2**

**AORTIC INTIMAL OSTEOSARCOMA**

The typical layering of pleomorphic tumor cells over an acellular area of fibrin mixed with necrotic tumor cells is seen. The tumor presented as a thoracic aortic aneurysm, which clinically was considered mycotic. The tumor was largely luminal.

**Gross Findings.** By definition, intimal sarcomas are either entirely intraluminal, in which case they grossly resemble thrombi, or are predominantly luminal with focal extension into the wall or adventitia (37). Occasionally, intimal sarcomas cause thinning and aneurysmal dilatation of the aortic wall. When they occur in the abdominal aorta, they may be mistaken for an atherosclerotic aneurysm. It is not unusual for the initial diagnosis to be made on embolectomy material, grossly considered by the surgeon to be a thrombus (2,3,35,40,47). Occasionally, the primary tumor is excised with a portion of the aorta, resulting in grafting or bypass (27).

Unlike sarcomas of the venae cavae, aortic sarcomas rarely arise in the wall of the great vessel. Those rare examples that have a small luminal component and are predominantly mural are histologically more likely to be leiomyosarcomas or angiosarcomas (3,40,47).

Most aortic sarcomas occur in the abdominal aorta between the celiac artery and the iliac bifurcation; approximately 30 percent occur in the descending thoracic aorta or aortic arch (6,8,36,37). In one series of 22 cases, 13 were present in the abdominal aorta, 8 in the descending

thoracic aorta, and only 1 in the ascending aorta (44). There have been several reported cases of aortic sarcomas arising at the site of a synthetic aortic graft anastomosis (3,32,48).

**Microscopic Findings.** In over half the cases, intimal aortic sarcomas are angiosarcomas, generally with an epithelioid appearance (4,12,13,20,28,33,34). The remainder are poorly differentiated sarcomas of fibroblastic or myofibroblastic differentiation. Unlike pulmonary intimal sarcomas, less than 10 percent of aortic intimal sarcomas contain areas of bone matrix production. Therefore, the most common differentiated type of aortic intimal sarcoma is *epithelioid angiosarcoma* (13,34).

The luminal surface of aortic sarcomas, regardless of the histologic subtype (undifferentiated or angiosarcoma), is often stratified into a layer of cellular neoplasm overlying a second layer of fibrin thrombus with necrotic material (figs. 19-1, 19-2). There may be an epithelioid appearance to the tumor cells, especially in cases of epithelioid angiosarcoma (figs. 19-3, 19-4). In some cases, the tumor cells are infiltrated by inflammatory cells (fig. 19-5, left). In poorly

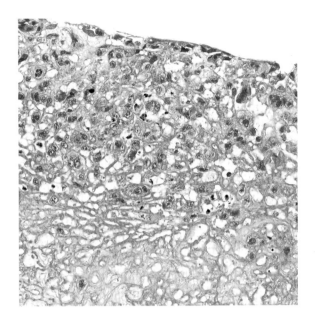

**Figure 19-3**

**AORTIC EPITHELIOID ANGIOSARCOMA**

The tumor cells form a lattice-like sheet over a layer of necrotic cells and fibrin. The distinction between angiosarcoma and pleomorphic undifferentiated sarcoma is determined by immunohistochemical staining. In this case, there was diffuse positivity for CD31 and CD34 (not shown).

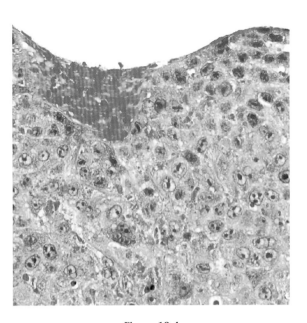

**Figure 19-4**

**AORTIC EPITHELIOID ANGIOSARCOMA**

The inflammatory infiltrate in the tumor layer is predominantly of neutrophils.

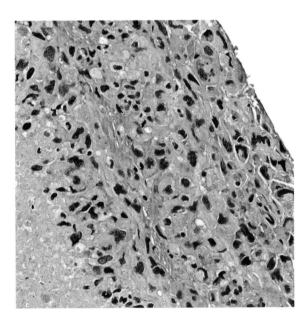

**Figure 19-5**

**PLEOMORPHIC AORTIC INTIMAL SARCOMA**

Left: The distinction between epithelioid angiosarcoma and pleomorphic undifferentiated sarcoma (malignant fibrous histiocytoma) is difficult on routine staining. In this case, epithelioid and endothelial markers were negative, with focal actin staining.

Right: At higher magnification, markedly pleomorphic cells and an atypical mitotic figure are seen.

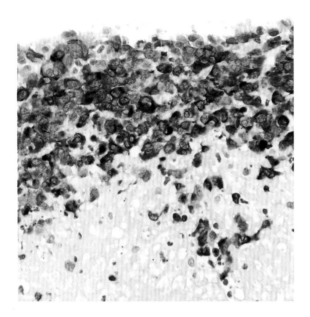

**Figure 19-6**

**AORTIC EPITHELIOID ANGIOSARCOMA: CYTOKERATIN**

Epithelioid angiosarcomas typically express epithelial markers (low- and high-molecular weight).

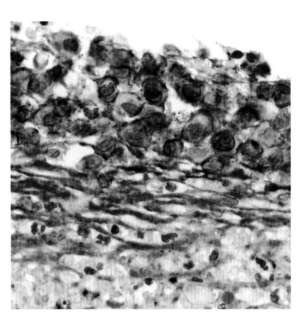

**Figure 19-8**

**AORTIC EPITHELIOID ANGIOSARCOMA: CD31**

The tumor cells of epithelioid angiosarcoma typically coexpress diverse endothelial markers, including CD31, CD34, and factor VIII-related antigen.

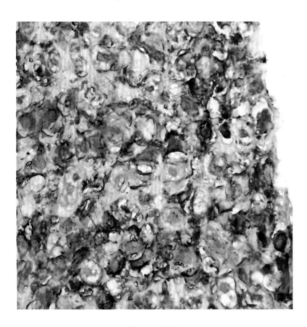

**Figure 19-7**

**AORTIC EPITHELIOID ANGIOSARCOMA: CD34**

As is typical of epithelioid angiosarcomas of other sites, aortic tumors coexpress endothelial markers.

differentiated tumors, the appearance is that of an undifferentiated sarcoma (fig. 19-5). Immunohistochemical stains demonstrate both epithelioid (fig. 19-6) and endothelial (figs. 19-7, 19-8) markers.

The invasive areas of aortic sarcomas demonstrate an undifferentiated morphology with epithelioid features. *Undifferentiated aortic sarcomas,* the second most common histologic subtype, are composed of mitotically active spindle cells with varying degrees of atypia, necrosis, and pleomorphism. The tumor cells line the luminal surface, over a mass of necrotic material and fibrin, similar to epithelioid angiosarcomas of the aorta, from which they are indistinguishable on routine stains. The tumor cells show mild to severe atypia, and a mixture of pleomorphic fibrocytic and histiocytic cells resembling malignant fibrous histiocytoma. Some intimal aortic sarcomas have, for this reason, been classified as *undifferentiated pleomorphic sarcoma (malignant fibrous histiocytoma)* (49). Immunohistochemically, they are negative for endothelial and epithelial markers, but may express smooth muscle actin (fig. 19-9).

The intimal surface of the aorta adjacent to the gross tumor may be lined by atypical cells, which is termed "dysplasia." These cells only rarely demonstrate endothelial differentiation (50).

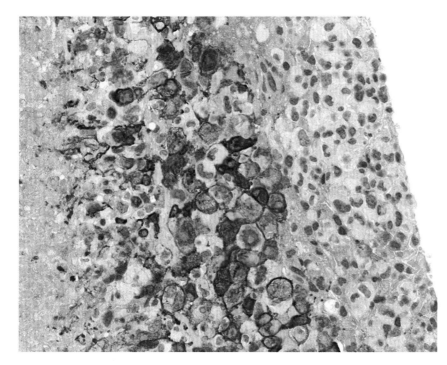

**Figure 19-9**

**AORTIC PLEOMORPHIC INTIMAL SARCOMA: SMOOTH MUSCLE ACTIN**

In contrast to aortic intimal angiosarcomas, there is no expression of endothelial or epithelial markers, but there may be actin expression, as shown here.

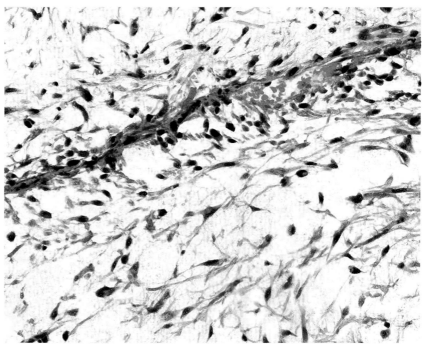

**Figure 19-10**

**AORTIC INTIMAL SARCOMA WITH PROMINENT MYXOID BACKGROUND**

Sometimes, areas of intimal sarcoma are fairly bland, with a prominent matrix, resembling myxofibrosarcoma (or fibromyxosarcomas) of soft tissue.

Aortic intimal sarcomas may have a prominent myxoid matrix (*myxofibrosarcoma*) (fig. 19-10) or show *chondrosarcomatous* and *osteosarcomatous* differentiation (figs. 19-11, 19-12) (40).

Sarcomas of the aorta that have a minor luminal component are, in contrast to intimal sarcomas, better differentiated. The few reported examples are *leiomyosarcomas*, similar to sarcomas of the venae cavae (3). Leiomyosarcomas, with characteristic fascicular growth, intracytoplasmic glycogen, and ultrastructural characteristics of smooth muscle cells are rare as luminal (intimal) aortic sarcomas. There are rare reports of aortic intimal *rhabdomyosarcoma* (15,19).

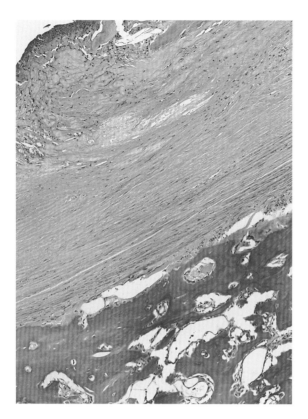
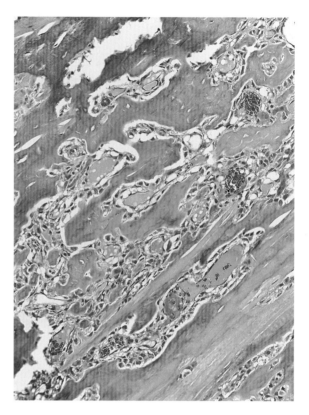

**Figure 19-11**

**AORTIC INTIMAL OSTEOSARCOMA**

Left: The aortic media is on the top and osteoid-forming sarcoma, which in this area is very bland, is on the bottom.
Right: At higher magnification, a cellular area with overtly malignant spindled cells is seen.

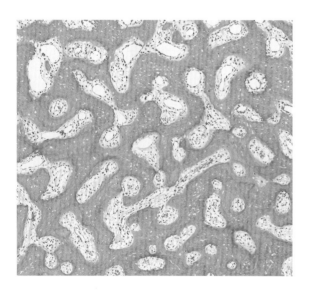
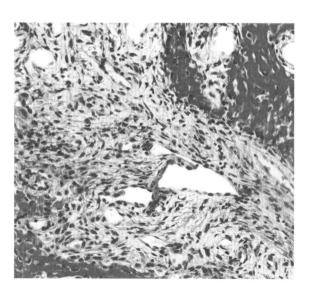

**Figure 19-12**

**AORTIC INTIMAL OSTEOSARCOMA**

Left: In this tumor, which was luminal, there are large areas of bland osteoid formation.
Right: In other areas, malignant osteoid-producing spindled cells are seen.

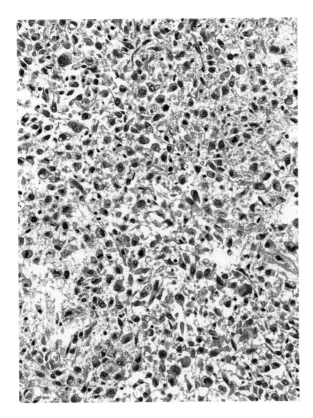

**Figure 19-13**

**AORTIC INTIMAL SARCOMA: METASTATIC TO KIDNEY**

The appearance is that of an undifferentiated pleomorphic neoplasm.

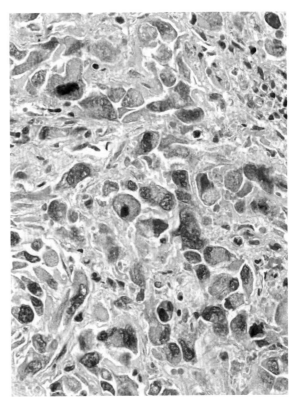

**Figure 19-14**

**AORTIC INTIMAL SARCOMA: METASTATIC TO BONE**

This tumor had metastasized to bone. The appearance is that of a pleomorphic undifferentiated malignant neoplasm.

**Spread and Metastases.** Because of their intraluminal site, aortic intimal sarcomas have the propensity for disseminated metastases. Tumor emboli in the mesenteric arteries can cause intestinal ischemia and infarction (44). Other metastatic sites include bone (10,12,42), adrenal gland, spleen (18), brain (38), heart, kidney, liver, spleen (25), lung (42), and skin (8). The histologic appearance of the metastatic deposits is usually that of an undifferentiated malignant neoplasm (figs. 19-13, 19-14).

**Treatment and Prognosis.** The treatment of aortic sarcoma consists of excision of the luminal tumor (endarterectomy), peripheral embolectomy (2), and surgical removal of the affected aortic segment with repair by synthetic graft, typically Dacron (30). Simple endarterectomy may not be sufficient if there is medial infiltration by tumor (37). In the case of thoracic aortic involvement, arch replacement with bifurcating grafts may be necessary (36,51). If the tumor is not resectable, bypass with synthetic grafts can be performed for palliation (2). Surgical treatment is often supplemented by multimodality proton beam radiation and chemotherapy (12,24).

The prognosis for patients with intimal sarcomas of the aorta is generally poor. The mean overall survival period is less than 16 months (3), with a 5-year survival rate of 8 percent (2). There are exceptional patients, especially those with mural tumors, who live years without symptoms after surgery: there are scattered reports of prolonged survival of 2 to 27 years (4,12,24,30).

## SARCOMAS OF PERIPHERAL ARTERIES

*Sarcomas of peripheral arteries* are rare, probably 5 to 20 percent of the incidence of aortic sarcomas. Sarcomas of the peripheral arteries are most common in the iliac and femoral arteries, where they result in the symptoms of arterial occlusion. One of 13 arterial sarcomas in one series was located in the iliofemoral artery, the remainder in the aorta (4). Four of 25 arterial sarcomas in a different series were located in the iliac and femoral arteries (44).

Femoral artery sarcomas occur after prosthetic bypass grafting (44,52) or present as pseudoaneurysms (53). Rare sites of intimal sarcoma include the renal and carotid arteries (13). Mesenteric occlusion can result from embolized sarcoma from an aortic intimal tumor (44). There is a report of a low-grade inflammatory myofibroblastic tumor of the carotid artery wall (9).

The few reports of peripheral artery sarcomas include undifferentiated sarcoma, epithelioid angiosarcoma, and osteosarcoma (44). In order to confirm an intimal origin, the tumor should be primarily luminal, with areas of intimal growth (figs. 19-15, 19-16).

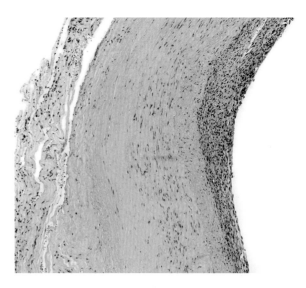

**Figure 19-15**

**PLEOMORPHIC SARCOMA: FEMORAL ARTERY**

The intima (right) is lined by pleomorphic atypical cells.

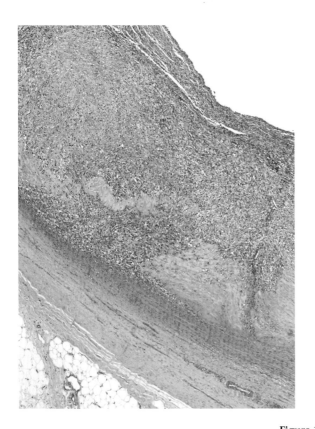

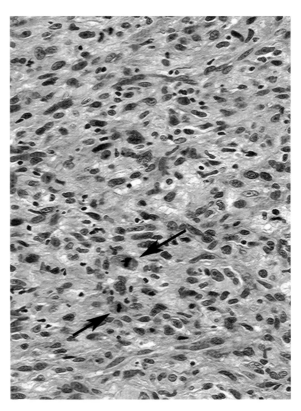

**Figure 19-16**

**PLEOMORPHIC SARCOMA: ILIAC ARTERY**

Left: There is a densely cellular tumor within the intima of the artery. The lumen is at the right, and the adventitial fat below left.

Right: Higher magnification demonstrates a cellular pleomorphic sarcoma, without evidence of specific differentiation.

## PULMONARY ARTERY INTIMAL SARCOMAS

**General Features.** *Pulmonary artery sarcomas* are rare, similar in incidence to primary parenchymal lung sarcomas. Approximately 250 have been reported (54). In the last 15 years, there have five series of more than 5 patients each (54–57), the largest with 43 patients (58). Other series of pulmonary sarcomas include parenchymal tumors, which are not of intimal origin (59,60).

**Clinical Features.** The average age of patients with pulmonary artery sarcoma is 45 to 50 years, and there is no sex predilection (3,58). Those patients with the subtype of *low-grade myofibroblastic sarcoma* are younger, with a mean age of 20 years (58).

The presenting symptoms are typically related to recurrent chronic thromboembolism (61–69), as manifested by shortness of breath (70), dyspnea, cough, and chest pain (71). Weight loss often occurs (72). The diagnosis may be missed for months, until high-resolution imaging demonstrates the characteristics of a luminal sarcoma rather than an embolism. The symptoms may initially be interpreted as pulmonary valve stenosis (55). Unilateral pulmonary artery occlusion, without a hypercoagulability syndrome or a history of thromboembolism, may suggest the diagnosis of pulmonary artery sarcoma and prompt angiographic-guided biopsy (74). Of 200 consecutive thromboendarterectomy specimens, 1 percent were pulmonary artery sarcomas (73).

Most patients are initially diagnosed as having a pulmonary embolism; only 1 in 5 are diagnosed correctly prior to biopsy (75). The diagnosis can be made prior to biopsy based on the finding of an irregular intraluminal mass by CT scans (72). With complete clinical and radiologic evaluation, most patients can be diagnosed soon after presentation (57). Early distinction from thromboembolism is essential for timely treatment (76).

Differentiating between intimal pulmonary artery sarcoma and saddle embolism may be difficult on CT (77–79). Low-attenuation defects filling the proximal or main pulmonary artery lumen, with expansion of the involved arteries and their branches, is characteristic of tumor, and extraluminal tumor extension is virtually diagnostic (46,70,80). CT can reliably separate pulmonary intimal sarcoma from thromboem-

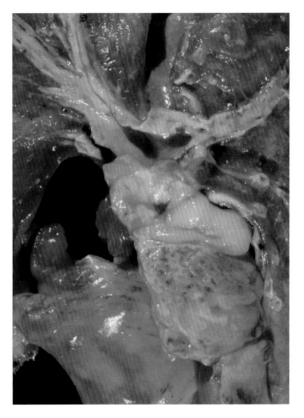

**Figure 19-17**

**PULMONARY ARTERY SARCOMA**

The gelatinous tumor fills the main pulmonary artery.

bolism, especially if there is advanced disease (81). Multiple imaging techniques, including CT and MRI, help establish the diagnosis of pulmonary artery sarcoma (82–84). CT combined with positron emission tomography (PET) shows increased uptake, in contrast to thrombus, which can coexist (85).

Long-standing pulmonary artery sarcomas may result in pulmonary hypertension (86) and increased right ventricular pressure (72), with eventual right heart failure indicative of cor pulmonale (79). The tumor may cause aneurysm formation (86) or complete or incomplete rupture, leading to pseudoaneurysm formation (85) in the case of the latter.

**Gross Findings.** Grossly, pulmonary artery sarcomas are gelatinous, soft masses that fill the arterial lumen (figs. 19-17, 18-18). There may be heterogeneous firm and calcified areas in cases of osteosarcoma. In a series of 43 cases (58), 21 occurred in the pulmonary trunk, 6 of which

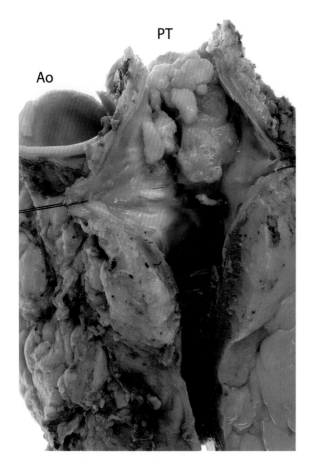

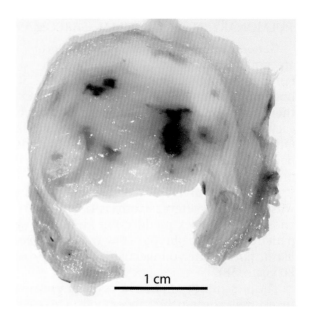

**Figure 19-18**

**PULMONARY ARTERY SARCOMA**

Left: There is a large tumor obscuring the pulmonary valve and extending toward the pulmonary trunk (PT). The aorta (AO) is uninvolved. Sarcomas of the pulmonary arterial trunk often extend retrograde to involve the valve.

Above: A cross section of the pulmonary trunk shows the tumor filling the lumen without gross extra-arterial extension.

extended into one or both major pulmonary arteries. The remaining 22 were either situated in the left (13 tumors) or right (9 tumors) pulmonary artery. Unusual locations include the pulmonary valve (60) and right ventricular outflow tract (87,88).

**Microscopic Findings.** The tissue diagnosis of pulmonary artery sarcoma is accomplished by percutaneous transvascular or open biopsy (71,89). The diagnosis is generally suspected before lobectomy or pneumonectomy, but can be an unexpected finding in thromboendarterectomy specimens.

The largest series of pulmonary artery sarcomas has shown that over half are *pleomorphic sarcomas* with a fascicular growth pattern, ranging from differentiated spindle cell myxofibrosarcoma to undifferentiated round cell sarcoma (58). In order to establish an origin in the arterial intima, imaging findings must document primarily luminal growth, at least in the initial stages of disease, and microscopically, the tumor should be primarily intraluminal (fig. 19-19). Occasion-

ally, in cases of advanced disease, the distinction between parenchymal and intimal sarcoma may be difficult, as histologic findings are nonspecific. Intimal sarcomas often show histologic heterogeneity and overlap. About 1 in 6 pulmonary artery sarcomas show heterologous elements in the form of *osteosarcoma* or *chondrosarcoma* (fig. 19-20) (56,58). Occasionally, there is extensive fibrosis with hyalinization in the central portion of the tumor, and pleomorphic tumor cells are confined to a luminal rim of neoplastic cells (*fibrosing variant*) (figs. 19-22–19-24). These tumors may be deceptively bland and mimic well-differentiated intimal sarcomas of the left atrium. Whether or not there is matrix production or a dense fibrous layer, portions of the tumor usually possess an appearance similar to that of other *pleomorphic-fascicular sarcomas* (storiform pattern or malignant fibrous histiocytoma) (figs. 19-23–19-25). Pleomorphic intimal sarcomas may have an inflammatory background (fig. 19-26), and about 1 in 10 show prominent myxoid areas (myxofibrosarcoma).

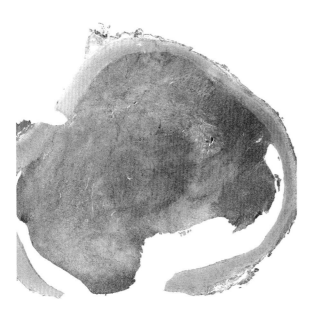
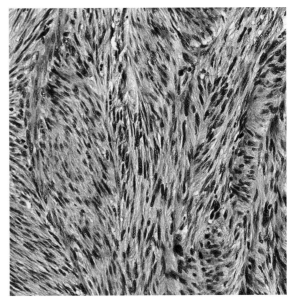

**Figure 19-19**

**PULMONARY ARTERY SARCOMA**

Left: At low magnification, the tumor fills the lumen of the artery.
Right: At higher magnification, the fascicular growth typical of leiomyosarcoma is seen.

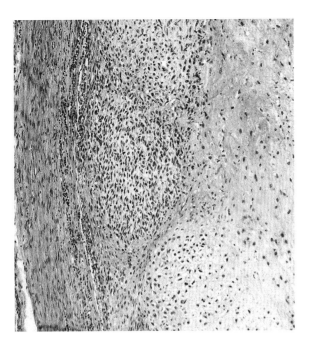
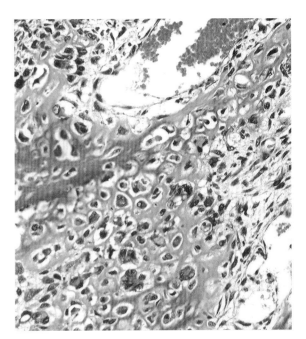

**Figure 19-20**

**PULMONARY ARTERY SARCOMA: MATRIX FORMING (CHONDROSARCOMA)**

Left: The arterial media is at the top, and the tumor is projecting into the lumen (bottom). There are nodular areas of matrix-producing sarcoma, with chondroid differentiation at the lower portion.
Right: A different area of the tumor illustrated in figure 19-18 shows areas of malignant osteoid.

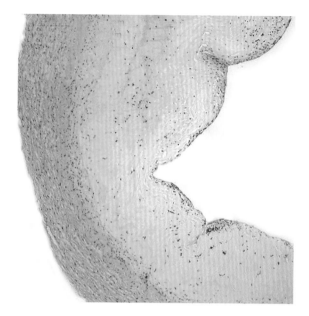

**Figure 19-21**

**PULMONARY ARTERY SARCOMA: FIBROSING VARIANT**

Bland intimal collagen is present.

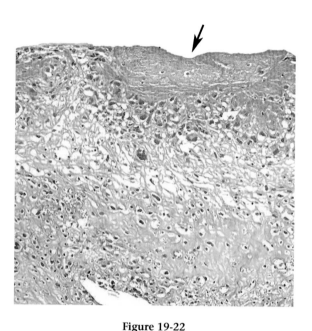

**Figure 19-22**

**PULMONARY ARTERY SARCOMA: PLEOMORPHIC TYPE**

The most common histologic type of intimal sarcoma of the pulmonary artery is the pleomorphic type, whether or not there are matrix-forming areas. This is a pleomorphic spindle cell tumor, with areas of fibrin on the luminal surface (arrow).

**Figure 19-23**

**PULMONARY ARTERY SARCOMA: PLEOMORPHIC TYPE**

At high magnification, an undifferentiated pleomorphic sarcoma with a vague storiform pattern and inflammatory background akin to inflammatory type of malignant fibrous histiocytoma is seen.

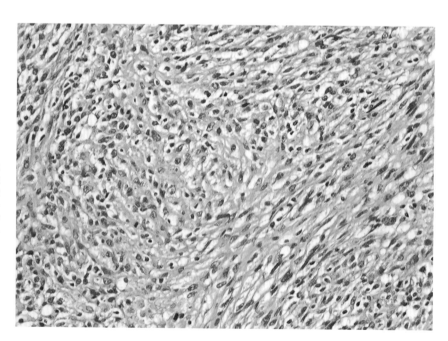

Intimal sarcomas with diffuse myogenic differentiation are uncommon, and include *leiomyosarcomas* and rarely, *rhabdomyosarcomas* (56). Leiomyosarcomas are often well differenti-ated, arise more often in the vessel wall than the lumen, and have a fairly good prognosis.

A histologic subtype of special clinical impor-tance is the *low-grade inflammatory myofibroblastic*

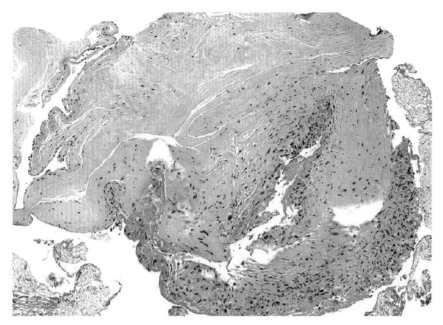

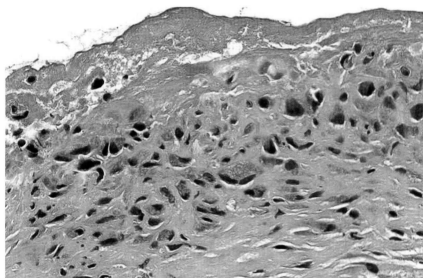

**Figure 19-24**

**PULMONARY ARTERY SARCOMA: PLEOMORPHIC TYPE**

Top: In this pulmonary endarterectomy specimen, the clinical differential diagnosis was recurrent embolism or primary sarcoma. The latter was favored, based on computerized tomography (CT) and magnetic resonance imaging (MRI).

Bottom: At higher magnification, the fibrin surface is seen overlying a sarcoma with marked cellular atypia.

*sarcoma,* which is characterized by a lack of cellularity, a variable inflammatory and myxoid background, a lack of marked pleomorphism, a myofibroblastic cellular appearance ("tissue culture" growth), and areas of fibrosis. Although an uncommon subtype, these tumors may behave in a benign fashion (fig. 19-26) (58).

Other histologic subtypes of intimal sarcoma include *fibrosarcoma* (54) and *angiosarcoma* (62). The range of histologic subtypes is more restricted than that seen in sarcomas of the lung parenchyma, which are not of intimal origin and which include synovial sarcoma, malignant peripheral nerve sheath tumor, primitive neuroectodermal tumor, and epithelioid hemangioendothelioma (59,60). In contrast to intimal sarcomas of the aorta, intimal sarcomas of the pulmonary artery are likely myxoid, more often show bone matrix, and less frequently exhibit vascular differentiation (angiosarcoma) (3,90).

Immunohistochemical results depend on histologic subtype (56). About two thirds of pleomorphic spindle cell sarcomas of the pulmonary arteries demonstrate MDM2 nuclear expression by immunohistochemistry and *MDM2* amplification by FISH (90a,91).

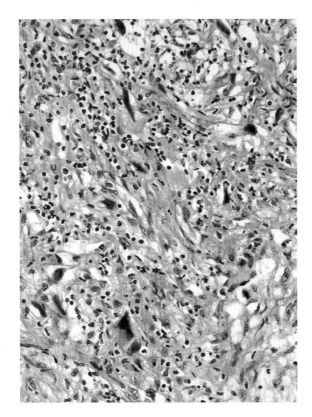

**Figure 19-25**

**PULMONARY SARCOMA: PLEOMORPHIC TYPE**

An undifferentiated pleomorphic sarcoma with a vague storiform pattern and inflammatory background akin to inflammatory type of malignant fibrous histiocytoma is seen. The diagnosis of an intimal origin rests on the location of the tumor in the lumen of the artery.

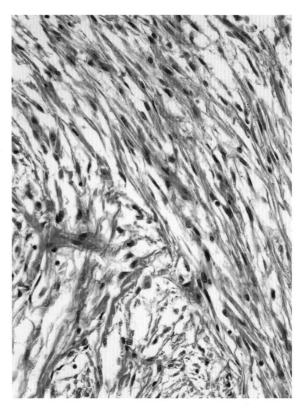

**Figure 19-26**

**PULMONARY ARTERY SARCOMA: LOW-GRADE (INFLAMMATORY MYOFIBROBLASTIC TUMOR/SARCOMA)**

In some luminal pulmonary artery sarcomas, the histologic features are fairly bland, with few mitotic figures, mild pleomorphism, and an inflammatory background. These tumors are low grade, and confer the possibility of long-term survival. Careful sampling of the lesion is important to exclude areas of high-grade sarcoma.

**Differential Diagnosis.** The diagnosis of sarcoma is typically straightforward, especially if there is significant pleomorphism or if malignant heterologous elements, such as chondrosarcoma, are present. In thromboendarterectomy specimens, the diagnosis may be subtle, with a layer of atypical cells on the surface of a fibrin thrombus the only clue of malignancy. In approximately 1 percent of pulmonary thromboembolectomies for suspected thromboembolic disease, an unexpected diagnosis of pulmonary artery sarcoma is rendered by the pathologist (73). Rarely, metastatic sarcomas to the pulmonary arteries spread from the retroperitoneum and require surgical excision (91a).

**Spread and Metastases.** About 1 in 4 patients have metastatic disease at time of surgery, most commonly to the lung parenchyma (3,58,75).

Other sites include the central nervous system (3,55,56,58,92), abdominal wall (90), kidney (3), bone (56,58), retroperitoneum (56), hilar lymph nodes (3,58,60), and skin (3).

**Treatment and Prognosis.** The prognosis for patients with pulmonary artery sarcoma with surgical treatment is considered grim, with early metastasis and death often occurring in weeks to months, especially when surgery is not possible (74,86). There are exceptions, however, with survival of several years (55,75,87,90,93). Currently, the overall survival rate is approximately 70 percent at 3 years with surgical treatment (60).

The histologic differentiation of the tumor affects the outcome. Leiomyosarcomas have a favorable outcome (56,94,95). An excellent prognosis with disease-free survival of many years has been reported for well-differentiated low-grade inflammatory myofibroblastic sarcomas arising from the pulmonary arterial intima (58), especially in younger patients (58,96).

Treatment has a significant impact on prognosis, both because of benefits from surgery and the selection of early-stage tumors amenable to surgical excision. Meta-analysis of the current body of data shows that the median survival period is 3 years for patients undergoing an attempt at curative resection compared with less than 1 year for those undergoing incomplete resection (97). The same data show a clear benefit for multimodality treatment, with a median survival of 2 years for patients undergoing multimodality treatment compared with 8 months for patients treated with single modality therapy (97).

A statistically significant survival benefit to adjuvant therapy (beyond surgical resection) has not been shown in all studies (98). Overall, there is about a 50 percent response rate to chemotherapy (71), especially when used in conjunction with radiation and surgery (multimodality treatment) (70,99,100). Regimens include combination amrubicin and carboplatin (69), ifosfamide (72,92,101), and epirubicin (102).

The surgical approach to pulmonary artery sarcoma depends on the extent of the tumor, as defined by imaging, and includes pneumonectomy (90a,93), arterial resection with Dacron grafting (102), and reconstruction of central pulmonary arteries (103,104). In some patients, right ventricular outflow tract reconstruction may be necessary if there is proximal tumor extension, in the form of bovine pericardial patching (60,105) with or without valve replacement, such as a homograft valve (60,106). Approximately 10 to 15 percent of patients present with extensive disease not amenable to surgery, and are palliated with chemotherapy and radiation.

In contrast to sarcomas of the lung parenchyma, which generally require lobectomy (60), pulmonary intimal sarcomas are often treated by endarterectomy or arterial resection with grafting and without resection of lung (57). In a series of 43 arterial sarcomas, 7 patients were not treatable and died shortly after presentation; 15 patients were initially treated with embolectomy; 9 patients were treated with lobectomy (one with prior biopsy); and 12 patients were treated with pneumonectomy (2 with prior biopsies) (58). In a series that included sarcomas of pulmonary parenchyma, surgically resected lung lobes or complete pneumonectomies showed positive resection margins in about 25 percent of cases; lymph node involvement was unusual (60).

Recurrence is manifested by the appearance of metastatic deposits or pulmonary artery stenosis, which can occur as late as 5 to 6 years after multimodality therapy (107,108). Recurrence is monitored by CT, MRI, and PET-CT (101). As is the case with the initial diagnosis, differentiation of recurrent intraluminal disease from thrombus often requires multiple imaging modalities (109). Tumor stenosis is palliated with stenting, which may prolong survival for nearly a year (110). In about 15 percent of patients with limited curative resection, recurrences necessitate subsequent pneumonectomy (60).

Other forms of treatment include combination therapy with CyberKnife excision (111) and combined heart-lung transplant (91).

## SARCOMAS OF VEINS

**General Features.** Most sarcomas of the veins are *leiomyosarcomas* of the inferior vena cava (112–115) that derive from medial smooth muscle. Rare examples of other types of sarcomas arising in the great veins have been reported (116), as well as leiomyosarcomas from pulmonary veins (117).

The incidence of caval sarcomas is difficult to ascertain with certainty, as retroperitoneal leiomyosarcomas may have originated in the inferior vena cava, although their large size precludes a definitive determination of their precise origin. In any event, those that are identified as originating clearly from the vessel wall are rare (118).

**Clinical Features.** The majority of leiomyosarcomas of the inferior vena cava arise in women, with a female to male ratio of 4.5 to 1.0. The average age at presentation is approximately 54 years (119), with a range of 15 to 83 years. The most common presenting symptoms and signs are abdominal pain, palpable abdominal mass, lower leg edema, weight loss, increased abdominal girth, and Budd-Chiari syndrome. The mean duration of symptoms is approximately 11 months prior to diagnosis. Thirty-four percent of tumors arise in the infrarenal, lower segment

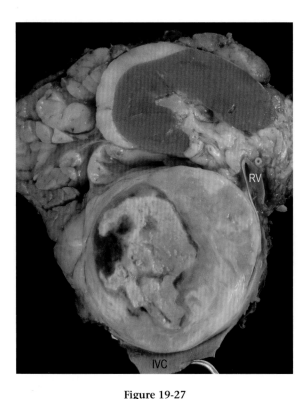

**Figure 19-27**

**PRIMARY SARCOMA: INFERIOR VENA CAVA**

The tumor was resected with the right kidney and the inferior vena cava (IVC), which was adherent to the tumor and the renal vein (RV). Histologically, the tumor was typical leiomyosarcoma.

during radiologic investigations or unrelated operations (3).

**Gross Findings.** Leiomyosarcomas of the inferior vena cava are predominantly extraluminal (fig. 19-27). Only rarely do they fill the lumen without significant spread into the vessel wall. Neoplastic thrombi occur within hepatic veins, right atrium, or iliac veins in almost 50 percent of cases. The tumors range in size from 2 to 30 cm, with a mean of 11 cm (119).

**Microscopic Findings.** Leiomyosarcomas of the inferior vena cava show similar histologic features to retroperitoneal leiomyosarcomas. About 50 percent immunohistochemically demonstrate intracytoplasmic desmin expression (119).

Unusual venous sarcomas that have been reported include *angiosarcomas* of the superior vena cava, *synovial sarcomas* of the superior vena cava, and *leiomyosarcomas* of the pulmonary, femoral, and iliac veins. Leiomyosarcomas of the pulmonary veins often show epithelioid features, with dot-like reactivity with antibodies directed against MIC-2 (117).

**Treatment and Prognosis.** Survival is longer in patients with sarcomas of the inferior vena cava than in patients with sarcomas of the aorta, with an average of about 3 years. The 5- and 10-year survival rates for patients undergoing curative surgery are 28 and 14 percent, respectively (3). Variables associated with long-term survival are radical tumor resection, the absence of a palpable abdominal mass, and patients with middle segment tumor (119). Metastases can occur to a variety of sites, including the lung, kidney, pleura, chest wall, liver, and bone (119).

Treatment consists primarily of surgery; chemotherapy has been administered without any consistent protocol, and is of questionable efficacy. Vascular resection with reconstruction of the inferior vena cava offers the best chance at prolonged survival (118).

of the vena cava; 42 percent in the middle segment, extending from the renal veins to the hepatic portion of the vena cava; and 24 percent in the superior segment between the liver and heart. Although symptoms do not correlate precisely with tumor location, Budd-Chiari syndrome is most common in leiomyosarcoma of the upper portion of the inferior vena cava (119). Rare presentations include: recurring pulmonary emboli, metastatic disease, and jaundice; fewer than five reported cases were incidental findings

## REFERENCES

1. Navarra G, Occhionorelli S, Mascoli F, Santini M, Benea G, Marzola A. Primary leiomyosarcoma of the aorta: report of a case and review of the literature. J Cardiovasc Surg (Torino) 1994;35:333-336.
2. Chiche L, Mongredien B, Brocheriou I, Kieffer E. Primary tumors of the thoracoabdominal aorta: surgical treatment of 5 patients and review of the literature. Ann Vasc Surg 2003;17:354-364.
3. Burke AP, Virmani R. Sarcomas of the great vessels. A clinicopathologic study. Cancer 1993;71: 1761-1773.
4. Sebenik M, Ricci A Jr, DiPasquale B, et al. Undifferentiated intimal sarcoma of large systemic blood vessels: report of 14 cases with immunohistochemical profile and review of the literature. Am J Surg Pathol 2005;29:1184-1193.
5. Fatima J, Duncan AA, Maleszewski JJ, et al. Primary angiosarcoma of the aorta, great vessels, and the heart. J Vasc Surg 2013;57:756-764.
6. Nanjo H, Murakami M, Ebina T, et al. Aortic intimal sarcoma with acute myocardial infarction. Pathol Int 1996;46:673-681.
7. Ruijter ET, Ten Kate FJ. Metastasising sarcoma of the aorta. Histopathology 1996;29:278-281.
8. Ingeholm P, Engel P. Metastasizing sarcoma of the aorta. A case report. APMIS 1997;105:609-611.
9. Mikami Y, Manabe T, Lie JT, Sakurai T, Endo K. Intramural sarcoma of the carotid artery with adventitial inflammation and fibrosis resembling 'inflammatory aneurysm.' Pathol Int 1997; 47:569-574.
10. Patel KR, Niazi TB, Griffiths AP, Hardy GJ, Mac Laren CA, Reid IN. Massive osteolytic bone metastases from a primary aortic sarcoma: a case report. Hum Pathol 1997;28:1306-1310.
11. Wills VL, Graham JC, Eckstein RP. Aortic intimal sarcoma: a case report. Aust N Z J Surg 1997;67: 482-485.
12. Majeski J, Crawford ES, Majeski EI, Duttenhaver JR. Primary aortic intimal sarcoma of the endothelial cell type with long-term survival. J Vasc Surg 1998;27:555-558.
13. Hottenrott G, Mentzel T, Peters A, Schroder A, Katenkamp D. Intravascular ("intimal") epithelioid angiosarcoma: clinicopathological and immunohistochemical analysis of three cases. Virchows Arch 1999;435:473-478.
14. le Rochais JP, Icard P, Coffin O, Galateau F, Khalil M, Maiza D. Intimal sarcoma of the thoracic aorta: a case report. Eur J Vasc Endovasc Surg 1999;18:181-182.
15. Miracco C, Laurini L, Santopietro R, et al. Intimal-type primary sarcoma of the aorta. Report of a case with evidence of rhabdomyosarcomatous differentiation. Virchows Arch 1999;435:62-66.
16. Neri E, Miracco C, Luzi P, Carone E, Tripodi A, Sassi C. Intimal-type primary sarcoma of the thoracic aorta presenting as a saccular false aneurysm: report of a case with evidence of rhabdomyosarcomatous differentiation. J Thorac Cardiovasc Surg 1999;118:371-372.
17. Mohsen NA, Haber M, Urrutia VC, Nunes LW. Intimal sarcoma of the aorta. AJR Am J Roentgenol 2000;175:1289-1290.
18. Nishida N, Yutani C, Ishibashi-Ueda H, Tsukamoto Y, Ikeda Y, Nakamura Y. Histopathological characterization of aortic intimal sarcoma with multiple tumor emboli. Pathol Int 2000;50:923-927.
19. Szekely E, Kulka J. Primary intimal type leiomyosarcoma with rhabdomyosarcomatous differentiation of the thoracic aorta. Virchows Arch 2000;437:208-209.
20. Santonja C, Martin-Hita AM, Dotor A, Costa-Subias J. Intimal angiosarcoma of the aorta with tumour embolisation causing mesenteric ischaemia. Report of a case diagnosed using CD31 immunohistochemistry in an intestinal resection specimen. Virchows Arch 2001;438:404-407.
21. Kim SH, Jeong JY, Kim YI, Choi YH, Chung JW, Hyung Park J. SCVIR 2002 Film Panel Case 3: aortic occlusion secondary to intimal sarcoma. J Vasc Interv Radiol 2002;13:537-541.
22. Pompilio G, Tartara P, Varesi C, Biglioli P. Intimal-type primary sarcoma of the thoracic aorta: An unusual case presenting with left arm embolization. Eur J Cardiothorac Surg 2002;21:574-576.
23. Rhee MY, Myong NH, Park YB. Primary intimal sarcoma of the aorta: role of transesophageal echocardiography. Circ J 2002;66:111-113.
24. Shuster TA, Dall'Olmo CA, Spadone D, Silver D. Abdominal aortic sarcoma: report of a case with long-term survival and review of the literature. Ann Vasc Surg 2002;16:545-549.
25. Sanchez-Munoz A, Hitt R, Artiles V, et al. Primary aortic sarcoma with widespread vascular embolic metastases. Eur J Intern Med 2003;14:258-261.
26. Crone KG, Bhalla S, Pfeifer JD. Aortic intimal sarcoma detected on helical CT. J Thorac Imaging 2004;19:120-122.
27. Hagspiel KD, Hunter YR, Ahmed HK, et al. Primary sarcoma of the distal abdominal aorta: CT angiography findings. Abdom Imaging 2004;29: 507-510.
28. Ruckert RI, Rudolph B, Rogalla P, Walter M. Primary endothelial sarcoma of the thoracic aorta. Vascular 2004;12:140-144.

29. Thalheimer A, Fein M, Geissinger E, Franke S. Intimal angiosarcoma of the aorta: report of a case and review of the literature. J Vasc Surg 2004;40:548-553.

30. Akiyama K, Nakata K, Negishi N, Henmi A. Intimal sarcoma of the thoracic aorta; clinical-course and autopsy finding. Ann Thorac Cardiovasc Surg 2005;11:135-138.

31. Tucci M, Quatraro C, Calvani N, et al. Primary intimal sarcoma of the thoracic aorta. J Exp Clin Cancer Res 2005;24:139-142.

32. Alexander JJ, Moawad J, Cai D. Primary intimal sarcoma of the aorta associated with a dacron graft and resulting in arterial rupture. Vasc Endovascular Surg 2006;40:509-515.

33. Kim JY, Chang BC, Ha JW. Images in cardiology. Intimal angiosarcoma of the descending aorta as an unusual cause of severe upper extremity hypertension. Heart 2006;92:306.

34. Dehqanzada ZA, Menezes G, Mukherjee D. Epithelioid angiosarcoma of the aorta in a 47-year-old man: a case report and literature review. J Surg Educ 2007;64:165-170.

35. Shirani S, Soleymanzadeh-Ardabili M, Arami M. Intimal sarcoma of the descending aorta. Arch Iran Med 2007;10:253-254.

36. Ishigami N, Suzuki K, Takahashi T, Neyatani H, Bashar AH, Kazui T. Intimal sarcoma of aortic arch treated with proton therapy following surgery. Asian Cardiovasc Thorac Ann 2008;16:e12-14.

37. Kato W, Usui A, Oshima H, Suzuki C, Kato K, Ueda Y. Primary aortic intimal sarcoma. Gen Thorac Cardiovasc Surg 2008;56:236-238.

38. Shimizu H, Tanibuchi A, Akaishi M, et al. Stroke due to undifferentiated aortic intimal sarcoma with disseminated metastatic lesions. Circulation 2009;120:e290-292.

39. Tanaka M, Tabata M, Shimokawa T, Takanashi S. The rupture of descending thoracic aorta due to the necrosis of aortic intimal sarcoma. Interact Cardiovasc Thorac Surg 2010;10:462-463.

40. Burke AP, Virmani R. Tumors of the heart and great vessels. AFIP Atlas of Tumor Pathology, 3rd Series, Fascicle 16. Washington, DC: American Registry of Pathology; 1996.

41. Salhab KF, Said SM, Sundt TM 3rd. Pseudocoarctation of the aorta secondary to aortic intimal sarcoma. Ann Thorac Surg 2012;94:279-281.

42. Nishikawa H, Miyakoshi S, Nishimura S, Seki A, Honda K. A case of aortic intimal sarcoma manifested with acutely occurring hypertension and aortic occlusion. Heart Vessels 1989;5:54-58.

43. Böhner H, Luther B, Braunstein S, Beer S, Sandmann W. Primary malignant tumors of the aorta: clinical presentation, treatment, and course of different entities. J Vasc Surg 2003;38:1430-1433.

44. Heath J, Tavora F, Burke AP. Intimal sarcomas of the aorta. Mod Pathol 2011;24(Suppl):75A.

45. Garg N, Lewis MA, Maleszewski JJ, Kalra M. Intimal sarcoma in an inflammatory aneurysm after endovascular aneurysm repair. J Vasc Surg 2012;55:1134-1137.

46. Bendel EC, Maleszewski JJ, Araoz PA. Imaging sarcomas of the great vessels and heart. Semin Ultrasound CT MR 2011;32:377-404.

47. Fenoglio JJ Jr, Virmani R. Primary malignant tumors of the great vessels. In: Waller B, ed. Pathology of the heart and great vessels. New York: Churchill Livingstone; 1988:429-438.

48. Weinberg DS, Maini BS. Primary sarcoma of the aorta associated with a vascular prosthesis: a case report. Cancer 1980;46:398-402.

49. Tejada E, Becker GJ, Waller BF. Malignant myxoid emboli as the presenting feature of primary sarcoma of the aorta (myxoid malignant fibrous histiocytoma): a case report and review of the literature. Clin Cardiol 1991;14:425-430.

50. Haber LM, Truong L. Immunohistochemical demonstration of the endothelial nature of aortic intimal sarcoma. Am J Surg Pathol 1988;12:798-802.

51. Sekine S, Abe T, Seki K, Shibata Y, Yamagishi I. Primary aortic sarcoma: resection by total arch replacement. J Thorac Cardiovasc Surg 1995;110:554-556.

52. Nocturne G, Sellam J, Miquel A, M'Bappe P, Berenbaum F. Is sarcoma a complication of arterial femoro-popliteal bypass? Joint Bone Spine 2010;77:358-360.

53. Ebaugh JL, Yuan M, Hu J, Chen A, Raffetto JD. Intimal sarcoma of the superficial femoral artery with osteosarcomatous differentiation. J Vasc Surg 2011;53:1394-1397.

54. Blackmon SH, Reardon MJ. Pulmonary artery sarcoma. Methodist Debakey Cardiovasc J 2010;6:38-43.

55. Hu XP, Xu JP, Liu NN. Primary pulmonary artery sarcoma: xurgical management and differential diagnosis with pulmonary embolism and pulmonary valve stenosis. J Card Surg 2009;24:613-616.

56. Huo L, Moran CA, Fuller GN, Gladish G, Suster S. Pulmonary artery sarcoma: a clinicopathologic and immunohistochemical study of 12 cases. Am J Clin Pathol 2006;125:419-424.

57. Mayer E, Kriegsmann J, Gaumann A, et al. Surgical treatment of pulmonary artery sarcoma. J Thorac Cardiovasc Surg 2001;121:77-82.

58. Tavora F, Miettinen M, Fanburg-Smith J, Franks TJ, Burke A. Pulmonary artery sarcoma: a histologic and follow-up study with emphasis on a subset of low-grade myofibroblastic sarcomas with a good long-term follow-up. Am J Surg Pathol 2008;32:1751-1761.

59. Keel SB, Bacha E, Mark EJ, Nielsen GP, Rosenberg AE. Primary pulmonary sarcoma: A clinicopathologic study of 26 cases. Mod Pathol 1999;12:1124-1131.

60. Bacha EA, Wright CD, Grillo HC, et al. Surgical treatment of primary pulmonary sarcomas. Eur J Cardiothorac Surg 1999;15:456-460.

61. Scheidl S, Taghavi S, Reiter U, et al. Intimal sarcoma of the pulmonary valve. Ann Thorac Surg 2010;89:e25-27.

62. Kim JB, Kim SH, Lim SY, et al. Primary angiosarcoma of the pulmonary trunk mimicking pulmonary thromboembolism. Echocardiography 2010;27:E23-26.

63. Abul Y, Eryuksel E, Karakurt S, et al. A malign mesenchymal tumor (sarcoma) of the pulmonary artery presenting as a form of acute thromboembolism: educational case. Clin Respir J 2010;4:e1-3.

64. Timmers L, Bove T, De Pauw M. Intimal sarcoma of the pulmonary artery: a report of two cases. Acta Cardiol 2009;64:677-679.

65. Widera E, Sulica R. Pulmonary artery sarcoma misdiagnosed as chronic thromboembolic pulmonary hypertension. Mt Sinai J Med 2005; 72:360-364.

66. Kerr KM. Pulmonary artery sarcoma masquerading as chronic thromboembolic pulmonary hypertension. Nat Clin Pract Cardiovasc Med 2005;2:108-112; quiz 113.

67. Kaplinsky EJ, Favaloro RR, Pombo G, et al. Primary pulmonary artery sarcoma resembling chronic thromboembolic pulmonary disease. Eur Respir J 2000;16:1202-1204.

68. Weijmer MC, Kummer JA, Thijs LG. Case report of a patient with an intimal sarcoma of the pulmonary trunk presenting as a pulmonary embolism. Neth J Med 1999;55:80-83.

69. Zurick AO 3rd, Lenge De Rosen V, Tan CD, Rodriguez ER, Flamm SD, Schoenhagen P. Pulmonary artery intimal sarcoma masquerading as pulmonary embolism. Circulation 2011;124:1180-1181.

70. Hirose T, Ishikawa N, Hamada K, et al. A case of intimal sarcoma of the pulmonary artery treated with chemoradiotherapy. Intern Med 2009;48:245-249.

71. Manso L, Alvarez E, Quintela M, Cortes-Funes H, Hitt R. Primary pulmonary artery sarcoma: report of three cases and review of the literature. Clin Lung Cancer 2007;8:277-281.

72. Halank M, Jakob C, Kolditz M, et al. Intimal pulmonary artery sarcoma presenting as severe dyspnea and right heart insufficiency. Onkologie 2010;33:313-316.

73. Bernard J, Yi ES. Pulmonary thromboendarterectomy: a clinicopathologic study of 200 consecutive pulmonary thromboendarterectomy cases in one institution. Hum Pathol 2007;38:871-877.

74. Levy E, Korach A, Amir G, Milgalter E. Undifferentiated sarcoma of the pulmonary artery mimicking pulmonary thromboembolic disease. Heart Lung Circ 2006;15:62-63.

75. Maruo A, Okita Y, Okada K, Yamashita T, Tobe S, Tanimura N. Surgical experience for the pulmonary artery sarcoma. Ann Thorac Surg 2006; 82:2014-2016.

76. Djordjevic I, Pejcic T, Rancic M, et al. Difficulties in establishing a timely diagnosis of pulmonary artery sarcoma misdiagnosed as chronic thrombo-embolic pulmonary disease: a case report. J Med Case Reports 2009;3:64.

77. Singla Long S, Johnson PT, Hruban RH, Fishman EK. CT features of pulmonary artery sarcoma: critical aid to a challenging diagnosis. Emerg Radiol 2010;17:153-155.

78. Lee P, Cheah FK, Huang J, Poon D, Loo CM. A suspicious clot. Thorax 2009;64:1011.

79. Huang SS, Huang CH, Yang AH, Yu WC. Images in cardiovascular medicine. Solitary pulmonary artery intima sarcoma manifesting as pulmonary embolism and subacute cor pulmonale. Circulation 2009;120:2269-2270.

80. Yi CA, Lee KS, Choe YH, Han D, Kwon OJ, Kim S. Computed tomography in pulmonary artery sarcoma: distinguishing features from pulmonary embolic disease. J Comput Assist Tomogr 2004;28:34-39.

81. Cox JE, Chiles C, Aquino SL, Savage P, Oaks T. Pulmonary artery sarcomas: a review of clinical and radiologic features. J Comput Assist Tomogr 1997;21:750-755.

82. Viana-Tejedor A, Marino-Enriquez A, Sanchez-Recalde A, Lopez-Sendon JL. Intimal sarcoma of the pulmonary artery: diagnostic value of different imaging techniques. Rev Esp Cardiol 2008;61:1363-1365.

83. Schuler PK, Weber A, Bode PK, et al. MRI of intimal sarcoma of the pulmonary arteries. Circ Cardiovasc Imaging 2009;2:e37-39.

84. Abunasser J, Colucci J, Bandyopadhyay T. Not pulmonary embolism! Conn Med 2009;73:277-280.

85. Farsad M, Pernter P, Triani A, Osele L, Wiedermann CJ. Thromboembolism in pulmonary artery sarcoma. Clin Nucl Med 2009;34:239-240.

86. Kaderli AA, Baran I, Sag S, Bicer M, Aker S. A rare reason for pulmonary hypertension: primary sarcoma of the pulmonary artery. Heart Surg Forum 2010;13:E28-30.

87. Hou Y, Shen Z, Gao W, Ye W. Pulmonary artery intimal sarcoma: case report. J Card Surg 2010; 25:29-31.

88. Ozbek C, Emrecan B, Calli AO, Gurbuz A. Intimal sarcoma of the pulmonary artery with retrograde extension into the pulmonic valve and right ventricle. Tex Heart Inst J 2007;34:119-121.

89. Winchester PA, Khilnani NM, Trost DW, Litvak B, Gold JP, Sos TA. Endovascular catheter biopsy of a pulmonary artery sarcoma. AJR Am J Roentgenol 1996;167:657-659.

90. Tsunezuka Y, Oda M, Takahashi M, Minato H, Watanabe G. Primary chondromatous osteosarcoma of the pulmonary artery. Ann Thorac Surg 2004;77:331-334.

90a. Bode-Lesniewska B, Zhao J, Speel EJ, et al. Gains of 12q13-14 and overexpression of mdm2 are frequent findings in intimal sarcomas of the pulmonary artery. Virchows Arch 2001;438:57-65.

91. Dewaele B, Floris G, Finalet-Ferreiro J, et al. Co-activated platelet-derived growth factor receptor {alpha} and epidermal growth factor receptor are potential therapeutic targets in intimal sarcoma. Cancer Res 2010;70:7304-7314.

91a. Talbot SM, Taub RN, Keohan ML, Edwards N, Galantowicz ME, Schulman LL. Combined heart and lung transplantation for unresectable primary cardiac sarcoma. J Thorac Cardiovasc Surg 2002;124:1145-1148.

92. Purandare NC, Dua SG, Rangarajan V, Shah S, Sharma AR. Pulmonary artery and femoral vein tumour thromboembolism in a patient with osteogenic sarcoma demonstrated by FDG PET/CT. Eur J Nucl Med Mol Imaging 2010;37:653.

93. Terra RM, Fernandez A, Bammann RH, Junqueira JJ, Capelozzi VL. Pulmonary artery sarcoma mimicking a pulmonary artery aneurysm. Ann Thorac Surg 2008;86:1354-1355.

94. Stella F, Davoli F, Brandolini J, Dolci G, Sellitri F, Bini A. Pulmonary artery leiomyosarcoma successfully treated by right pneumonectomy. Asian Cardiovasc Thorac Ann 2009;17:513-515.

95. Croitoru AG, Klein MJ, Galla JD, Fallon JT. Primary pulmonary artery leiomyosarcoma. Cardiovasc Pathol 2003;12:166-169.

96. Mattoo A, Fedullo PF, Kapelanski D, Ilowite JS. Pulmonary artery sarcoma: a case report of surgical cure and 5-year follow-up. Chest 2002;122:745-747.

97. Blackmon SH, Rice DC, Correa AM, et al. Management of primary pulmonary artery sarcomas. Ann Thorac Surg 2009;87:977-984.

98. Mussot S, Ghigna MR, Mercier O, et al. Retrospective institutional study of 31 patients treated for pulmonary artery sarcoma. Eur J Cardiothorac Surg 2012;43:787-793.

99. Lu S, Hong T, Wang C. Clinical treatment for pulmonary artery sarcoma. Eur J Cardiothorac Surg 2010;38:115-116; author reply 116-117.

100. Genoni M, Biraima AM, Bode B, Shan AC, Wilkler MB, Turina MI. Combined resection and adjuvant therapy improves prognosis of sarcomas of the pulmonary trunk. J Cardiovasc Surg (Torino) 2001;42:829-833.

101. Uchida A, Tabata M, Kiura K, et al. Successful treatment of pulmonary artery sarcoma by a two-drug combination chemotherapy consisting of ifosfamide and epirubicin. Jpn J Clin Oncol 2005;35:417-419.

102. Koch A, Mechtersheimer G, Tochtermann U, Karck M. Ruptured pseudoaneurysm of the pulmonary artery—rare manifestation of a primary pulmonary artery sarcoma. Interact Cardiovasc Thorac Surg 2010;10:120-121.

103. Shehatha J, Saxena P, Clarke B, Dunning J, Konstantinov IE. Surgical management of extensive pulmonary artery sarcoma. Ann Thorac Surg 2009;87:1269-1271.

104. Chhaya NC, Goodwin AT, Jenkins DP, Pepke-Zaba J, Dunning JJ. Surgical treatment of pulmonary artery sarcoma. J Thorac Cardiovasc Surg 2006;131:1410-1411.

105. Pagni S, Passik CS, Riordan C, D'Agostino RS. Sarcoma of the main pulmonary artery: an unusual etiology for recurrent pulmonary emboli. J Cardiovasc Surg (Torino) 1999;40:457-461.

106. Zerkowski HR, Hofmann HS, Gybels I, Knolle J. Primary sarcoma of pulmonary artery and valve: multimodality treatment by chemotherapy and homograft replacement. J Thorac Cardiovasc Surg 1996;112:1122-1124.

107. Tseng TW, Huang CH, Yang AH, Yu WC. Pulmonary stenosis in a patient with right pulmonary artery intima sarcoma 5 years after chemo-radiation therapy. Eur Heart J 2010;31:2432.

108. Fegbeutel C, Struber M, Becker JU, et al. Recurrent sarcoma originating from the pulmonary artery 6 years after extensive thoracic resection. J Thorac Cardiovasc Surg 2008;136:1093-1095.

109. Oberson M, Pawelczak CS, Meincke F. Paraneoplastic thrombus or relapse of a pulmonary artery sarcoma? Thorax 2010;65:941-942.

110. Meckel S, Buitrago-Tellez C, Herrmann R, Jacob AL. Stenting for pulmonary artery stenosis due to a recurrent primary leiomyosarcoma. J Endovasc Ther 2003;10:141-146.

111. Soltys SG, Kalani MY, Cheshier SH, Szabo KA, Lo A, Chang SD. Stereotactic radiosurgery for a cardiac sarcoma: a case report. Technol Cancer Res Treat. 2008;7:363-368.

112. You JS, Chung YE, Park S, Chung SP, Park JW. Diagnostically challenging tumour in a great vessel: leiomyosarcoma of inferior vena cava. Emerg Med J 2009;26:383.

113. Tranchart H, Carloni A, Balzarotti R, de Laveau-coupet J, Chapelier A, Smadja C. Leiomyosarcoma of the inferior vena cava involving the renal veins: a simple method of right renal vein reimplantation. J Vasc Surg 2008;47:209-212.

114. Ruh J, Lang H, Paul A, Dirsch O, Broelsch CE. Surgical aspects in the therapy of primary sarcoma of the vena cava. J Am Coll Surg 2006;202:559-562.

115. Kieffer E, Alaoui M, Piette JC, Cacoub P, Chiche L. Leiomyosarcoma of the inferior vena cava: experience in 22 cases. Ann Surg 2006;244:289-295.

116. Costilla VC, Adams JC, Mookadam F. Biphasic synovial sarcoma arising from superior vena cava. Eur Heart J Cardiovasc Imaging 2012; 13:713.

117. Oliai BR, Tazelaar HD, Lloyd RV, Doria MI, Trastek VF. Leiomyosarcoma of the pulmonary veins. Am J Surg Pathol 1999;23:1082-1088.

118. Fiore M, Colombo C, Locati P, et al. Surgical technique, morbidity, and outcome of primary retroperitoneal sarcoma involving inferior vena cava. Ann Surg Oncol 2012;19:511-518.

119. Thapar VB, Satoskar RR, Kanjan GM, Chaudhary AS. Leiomyosarcoma of the inferior vena cava: a case report and review of literature. Int Surg 2005;90:262-265.

# Index*

*In a series of numbers, those in boldface indicate the main discussion of the entity.